AF556783

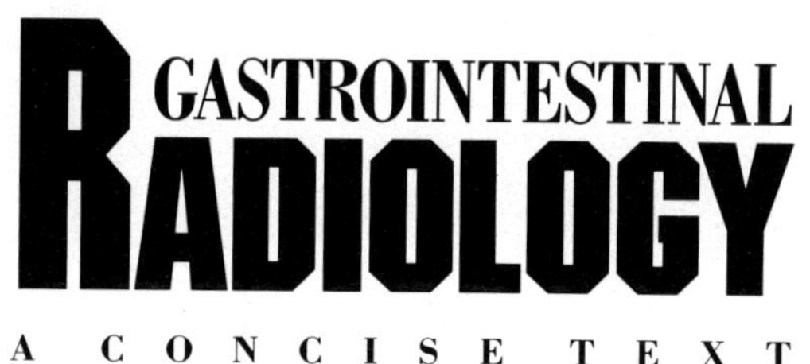

A CONCISE TEXT

NOTICE

Medicine is an ever-changing science. As new research and clinical experience broaden our knowledge, changes in treatment and drug therapy are required. The editors and the publisher of this work have checked with sources believed to be reliable in their efforts to provide information that is complete and generally in accord with the standards accepted at the time of publication. However, in view of the possibility of human error or changes in medical sciences, neither the editors nor the publisher nor any other party who has been involved in the preparation or publication of this work warrants that the information contained herein is in every respect accurate or complete. Readers are encouraged to confirm the information contained herein with other sources. For example and in particular, readers are advised to check the product information sheet included in the package of each drug they plan to administer to be certain that the information contained in this book is accurate and that changes have not been made in the recommended dose or in the contraindications for administration. This recommendation is of particular importance in connection with new or infrequently used drugs.

GASTROINTESTINAL RADIOLOGY

A CONCISE TEXT

Branko M. Plavsic, M.D., Ph.D.
Professor of Radiology and
Director of Abdominal Imaging and Research
Tulane University School of Medicine
New Orleans, Louisana
Formerly
Professor of Radiology and
Chief of Gastrointestinal Radiology
University of Zagreb, Yugoslavia

Arvin E. Robinson, M.D.
Professor of Radiology
Chair, Department of Radiology
Tulane University
New Orleans, Louisiana

R. Brooke Jeffrey, Jr., M.D.
Professor of Radiology
Chief, Abdominal Imaging Section
Department of Diagnostic Radiology and Nuclear Medicine
Stanford University
Stanford, California

McGraw-Hill
Health Professions Division
New York St. Louis San Francisco Auckland Bogotá Caracas
Lisbon London Madrid Mexico Milan Montreal New Dehli
Paris San Juan Singapore Sydney Tokyo Toronto

Gastrointestinal Radiology: A Concise Text

Copyright ©1992 by McGraw Hill, Inc. All rights reserved. Printed in the United States of America. Except as permitted under the United States Copyright Act of 1976, no part of this publication may be reproduced or distributed in any form or by any means or stored in a data base or retrieval system, without the prior written permission of the publisher.

1 2 3 4 5 6 7 8 9 0 MMN MMN 9 8 7 6 5 4 3 2 1 0

ISBN 0-07-105369-7

The Maple-Vail Book Manufacturing Group was the printer and binder.

Library of Congress Cataloging-in-Publication Data

Plavsic, Branko M

Gastrointestinal radiology : a concise text / Branko M. Plavsic, Arvin E. Robinson, R. Brooke Jeffrey, Jr.

p. cm.

Translated from Croatian.

Includes bibliographical references.

Includes index.

ISBN 0-07-105369-7

1. Gastrointestinal system--Radiography. I. Robinson, Arvin E. II. Jeffrey, R. Brooke. III. Title.

[DNLM: 1. Gastrointestinal System--radiography. WI 149 P721g]

RC804.R6P57 1991

616.3′.30757--dc20

DNLM/DLC

for Library of Congress 90-7756

CIP

British Library Cataloguing in Publication Data

Plavsic, Branko M.

Gastrointestinal radiology.

1. Man. Digestive system. Diagnosis. Radiography

I. Title. II. Robinson, Arvin E. III. Jeffrey, R Brooke.

616.30757

ISBN 0-07-105369-7

Also published in Yugoslavia as

Alimentary Tract Radiology,

Školska Knjiga, Zagreb, Yugoslavia.

To Valerie, Beverly, and Stefanie

Contents

Foreword

Alimentary radiology has undergone great changes with the introduction of cross-sectional computer-assisted techniques, which have been complementing the barium single- and double-contrast studies. The barium studies themselves, whether single or double contrast, have made great advances, partially stimulated by the competition with endoscopy, which has imposed rigorous controls over the accuracy of radiologic studies.

This book combines the European approach of exquisite illustrations and clear, well-organized text with the American strength of multimodal approaches. The book excels in superb illustrations, informative text, excellent organization, and broad scope.

The method of first presenting a concise text of anatomy and a thorough discussion of the physiology of alimentary canal motility gives a beautiful background to pathology. The technical aspects are dealt with very thoroughly, with detailed descriptions of the various techniques, and this is followed by a meticulous and eloquent presentation of radiologic abnormalities throughout the alimentary tube. This book, with its multiple illustrations, is a pleasure to read and will, hopefully, see many editions.

ALEXANDER R. MARGULIS, M.D.
PROFESSOR OF RADIOLOGY
UNIVERSITY OF CALIFORNIA, SAN FRANCISCO

Preface

This book is presented as an instructional guide and informational resource primarily for physicians interested in the examination and evaluation of alimentary tract radiology; this includes radiology residents in training, radiologists, pediatricians, surgeons and medical students.

While all aspects of the gastrointestinal tract have been mentioned for completeness's sake, primary consideration has been given to the hollow viscous organs constituting the alimentary tube. Classic radiologic techniques still dominate alimentary canal examinations and are therefore described in detail. However, discussions on ultrasonography, computed tomography, magnetic resonance imaging, angiography, and interventional radiology are also included.

This edition contains some text and illustrations previously published by Skolska Knjiga of Zagreb, Yugoslavia. Excerpts from two editions of that publication were translated from Croatian by the first author and Valerie Drnovsek, M.D. The authors are grateful to Skolska Knjiga for permission to use that material.

Several explanations of the material presented in the text are in order. Careful attention was made to be nonspecific in referring to either patient or examiner by gender. However, there were instances where this was not feasible. Consequently, reference in the male gender was utilized without the intention of being gender specific, or of being demeaning to female patients or examiners.

Every effort has been made to ensure that drug selection and dosage are in accordance with current recommendations and practices. However, it is most important that the reader refer to the package insert for every drug under consideration. Great care is required as to dosage, added warnings, and precautions. This is particularly important when the recommended agent is a new or infrequently ordered drug, or where the drug might be foreign to the reader's clinical practice. While every attempt was made to refer to all drugs in a generic nature, common brand names were occasionally utilized for the sake of clarity. There was no purposeful intent to denigrate the development efforts of drug manufacturers who have not been mentioned here. Contrast media have been treated in a similar manner. While the authors have recommended various procedures and protocols, these need to be considered in light of the technologies available and the standards of care within the reader's community.

We are not inclined a priori to support any particular radiologic-gastroenterologic school—such as those which promote exclusively double- or single-contrast examinations; to do so would mean unavoidably accepting its prejudices. Instead, we prefer a more eclectic approach to problems, applying the best from each method.

Literature cited in this book is reduced to a necessary minimum, and is intended as a guide to additional reading. It is cited according to the Vancouver declaration, uniform requirements for manuscripts submitted to medical journals.

As is often the case in the radiologic literature, a large number of illustrations are required. In addition to case material provided from the private collections of the authors, illustrations from other sources are included. We are particularly grateful to Drs. Charles M. Nice Jr., Datla G.K. Varma, and William L. Wells for case material from Tulane University Medical Center and Charity Hospital of Louisiana at New Orleans. Photography was provided by Stjepan Ivekovic and J. Richard Hutton, with graphic reproductions by John Geshner, and stenography by Terry McGuckin. We wish to acknowledge these contributions with gratitude.

Introduction

The most carefully performed radiologic examinations sometimes fail to determine the pathologic nature of a lesion. Frequently, pathologic lesions observed directly during endoscopy, surgery, or autopsy have no specific surface characteristics. Alimentary canal organs can be altered similarly or identically by different diseases. Pathologic changes are often successfully discovered using radiologic methods, but one cannot expect more than real capabilities allow. Thus, radiologic methods cannot always predict or determine microscopic properties of such lesions. The radiologist, therefore, must closely communicate with other clinicians in order to compare results of radiologic examinations with other clinical and diagnostic information.

In forming an opinion about a pathologic lesion, its morphologic properties, as well as the location of the lesion, prevalence of the predicted disease, and frequency and significance of individual radiologic signs have to be considered. Inevitably some interpretive difficulties arise in selected pathologic processes involving the gastrointestinal tract. This is a consequence of our incomplete current understanding of various abnormalities.

Chapter 1

Normal Anatomy of the Alimentary Canal

GENERAL COMPOSITION OF ALIMENTARY CANAL ORGANS

Along its entire length the alimentary tube consists of four layers. These are, from the lumen – the mucosa, submucosa, muscularis, and serosal coat or adventitia (Diagram 1.1). Characteristics such as thickness, vascularity, and nerve supply depend on functional needs of particular segments.

The *mucosa* is a wet membrane covered with epithelium; it sits on the basement membrane and attaches to the lamina propria. Smooth muscle bundles may pervade the outer portions of the lamina propria. The *submucosa* is well vascularized and contains preganglionic fibers of the parasympathetic, and postganglionic fibers of the sympathetic, nervous system. Parasympathetic ganglia and fibers create the submucosal Meissner's plexus. Secretory glands are situated in both the mucosa and submucosa.

The *muscular layer* contains smooth muscle except in the proximal two-thirds of the esophagus. The inner layer is circular and the outer longitudinal. Between the layers are ganglia of the Auerbach's parasympathetic myenteric plexus and postganglionic sympathetic fibers. The *outer surface* of the alimentary canal is

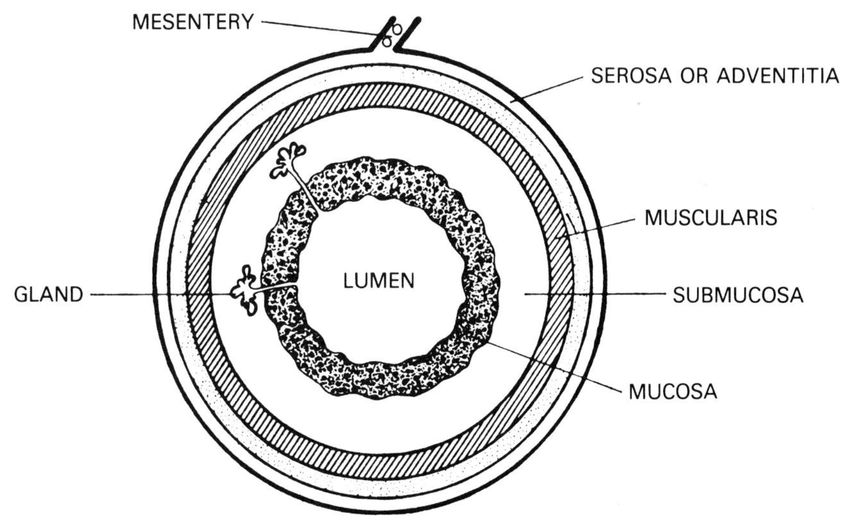

DIAGRAM 1.1. Transverse section of an alimentary canal organ.

covered with a serosal membrane such as the peritoneum. Adventitia covers the esophagus.

The stomach and intestine are bound to the posterior abdominal wall by reflections of the peritoneum. The blood vessels and nerves reach the stomach and intestine by traversing the mesogastinum, mesenterium, and mesocolon.

PHARYNX

The pharynx is an oval fibromuscular structure attached to the base of the skull. At the level of the lower edge of the cricoid cartilage, the pharynx is continuous with the esophagus. The pharynx is divided into epipharynx (nasopharynx), mesopharynx (oropharynx) and hypopharynx (laryngopharynx). It is widest at the epipharynx and narrowest at the point where it joins the esophagus. The nasopharynx is functionally part of the respiratory system. The oropharynx is continuous cranially with the nasopharynx and caudally extends to the level of the hyoid bone. It communicates with the oral cavity at its cranial part through the faucial isthmus. Caudal to the level of the faucial isthmus, the anterior wall of the oropharynx is formed by the root of the tongue and the epiglottic valleculae (Diagram 1.2, Figs. 1.1, 1.2, and 1.3). The palatine tonsils are on each side of the lateral wall of the oropharynx. The posterior wall is adjacent to the second and third cervical vertebrae.

The hypopharynx lies lateral and dorsal to the larynx. It extends from the mesopharynx cranially to the esophagus caudally, at the level of the caudal border of the cricoid cartilage. The ventral wall is adjacent to the larynx (Fig. 1.2). The pyriform recess is an elongated space of the hypopharynx lying on each side of the laryngeal aperture. An aryepiglottic fold, an arytenoid cartilage, and the cricoid cartilage constitute the medial wall of each pyriform recess. Laterally are the thyrohyoid membrane and the thyroid cartilage. The recess extends from the hyoid bone to the caudal limits of the cricoid cartilage (Diagram 1.2). The pyriform recess is a site where foreign bodies may lodge and where abscesses can develop.

Pharyngeal muscles are chiefly constrictors in function, though there are also longitudinal muscles. The superior, middle, and inferior pharyngeal constrictors constitute most of the pharyngeal musculature. These muscles are mutually overlapping, being arranged as a lattice, one within the other.

On the lateral radiograph of the hypopharynx,

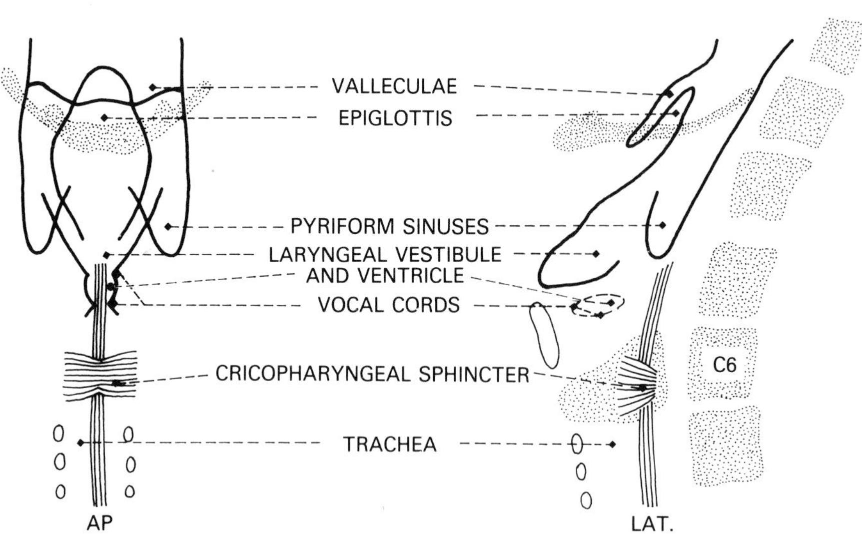

DIAGRAM 1.2. Characteristics of the hypopharynx relevant to radiologic examination. (Used by permission, Donner MW, Silbiger ML. Cinefluorographic analysis of pharyngeal swallowing in neuromuscular disorders. Am J Med Sci. 1966; 251:134.)

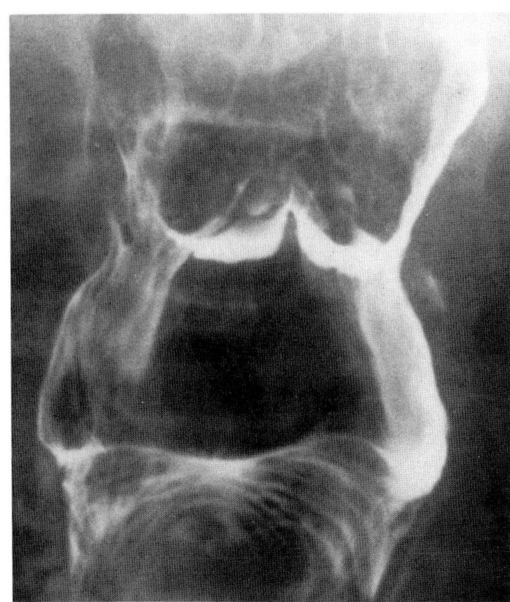

Figure 1.1. Hypopharynx in P-A projection. Double-contrast barium study. (See Diagram 1.2.)

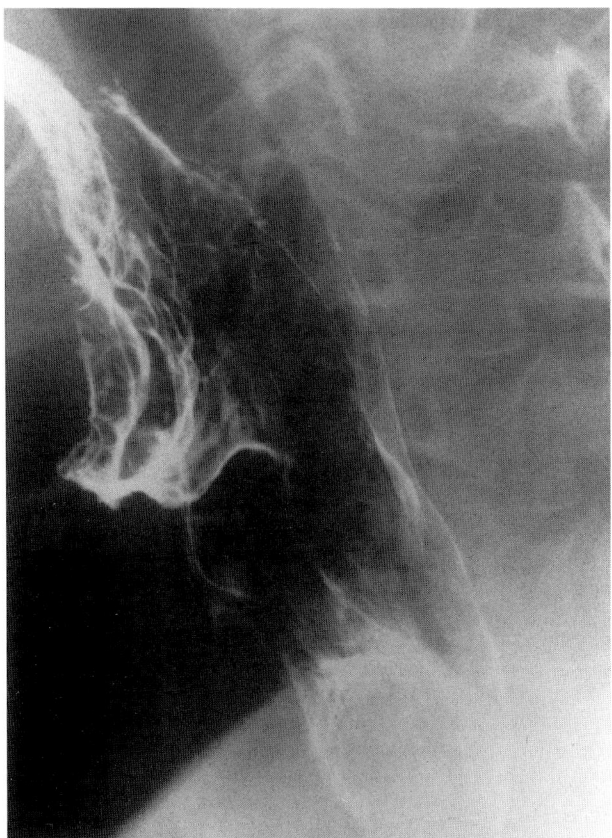

Figure 1.2. Hypopharynx in oblique projection. Double-contrast barium study. (See Diagram 1.2.)

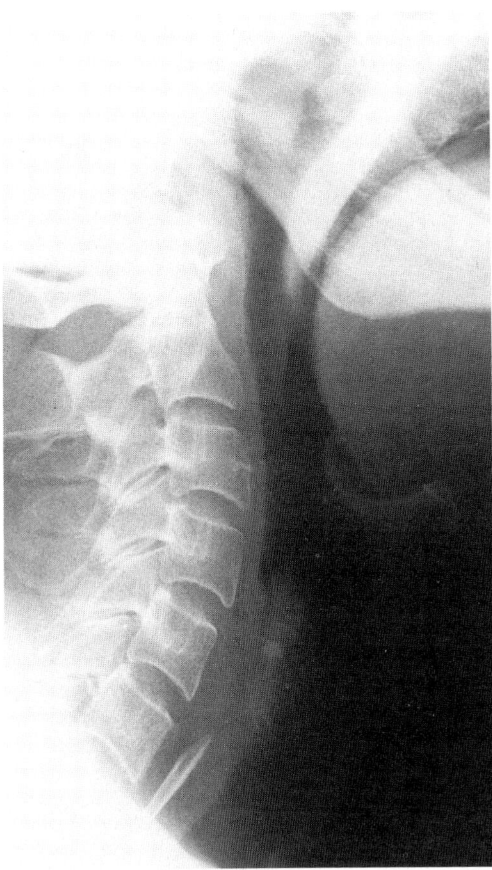

Figure 1.3. Hypopharynx and airways filled by air. Chicken bone lodged in the posterior pharyngeal wall. Non-contrast profile view.

epiglottic valleculae and pyriform recesses are visible because they are filled with air (Fig. 1.3). Detailed radiologic presentation requires the use of barium (Figs. 1.1 and 1.2).

ESOPHAGUS

The esophagus is the first segment of the digestive tube. It transports contents from the pharynx to the stomach without changing their properties. When relaxed, this muscular tube is 25–30 cm long and 2–3 cm wide. It consists of cervical, thoracic, and abdominal segments, and extends from the level of the C6 vertebra downward, mainly through the posterior mediastinum directly in front of the vertebral column. The cervical portion of the esophagus is in the midline. At the level of C7, it turns slightly to the left. About the level of T5 the esophagus is again in the midline. It turns anteriorly and left at the level of T7 (Fig. 1.4). On the lateral view, the esophagus follows the curvature of the vertebral column.

The esophagus passes through the esophageal hiatus of the diaphragm at the level of T10. This opening in the posterior part of the diaphragm is said to regulate esophageal emptying. In addition, the right crus of the diaphragm contributes a sphincteric function. The abdominal portion of the esophagus, approxi-

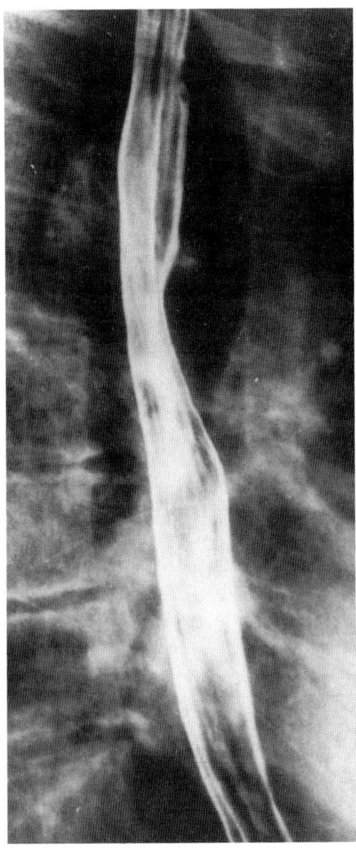

Figure 1.4. Mucosal relief of the esophagus. Barium esophagogram.

mately 2 cm in length, is directed to the left and anteriorly.

Muscles of the distal third of the inferior constrictor of the pharynx are interwoven with longitudinal muscles of the esophagus. The resultant increased intraluminal pressure maintains closure of the junction with the esophagus. This region with increased pressure is called the superior esophageal sphincter. Cineradiographically and at autopsy, the superior esophageal sphincter is verified to be part of the inferior constrictor of the pharynx. There are three anatomic narrowings of the esophagus: one at the origin, another at the level of the aortic arch, and a third where it passes through the diaphragm.

The cervical portion of the esophagus is in contact with the trachea and the left mainstem bronchus, and is separated from them only by connective tissue. The aortic arch lies close to the esophagus at the level of T3 or T4 with the descending aorta to the left. Before passing through the diaphragm, it crosses the esophagus from behind. There are several normal impressions on the esophagus produced by the aorta, the left mainstem bronchus, and, in some healthy people with an extremely asthenic constitution, by the left atrium, although only in maximal expiration (Fig. 1.5). However, inferior indentation is commonly caused by the left inferior pulmonary veins. The lumen of the esophagus in the cervical and abdominal parts is normally closed, except when a bolus is passing through. The thoracic portion may contain a small amount of air. The esophagus is the segment of the digestive tube with the least elasticity, but it has strong muscles that enable propulsion of contents without symptoms of dysphagia, even when the lumen is narrowed to half the normal size.

The distal, lower esophageal segment has a number of distinctive properties. Its anatomy and physiology are described separately.

The esophagus is lined with thick mucosa creating longitudinal folds that accommodate distension. This can be demonstrated during radiographic examination with barium suspension. Five to six folds that protrude into the esophageal lumen are in constant position. These folds are prominent during contraction of the muscularis and lamina muscularis mucosae (Fig. 1.4). When the esophagus is relaxed, the mucosal surface is smooth (Fig. 1.6). Esophageal glands are scattered throughout the tela submucosa. The inner muscle fibers of the esophagus are closely related to the inferior constrictor of the pharynx and to the oblique muscles of the stomach. While this layer has often been described as being circular, it is mostly elliptical. However, in the lower esophageal segment (gastroesophageal vestibule) fibers are not elliptical but circular. The outer longitudinal fibers are in continuity with corresponding muscles of the stomach.

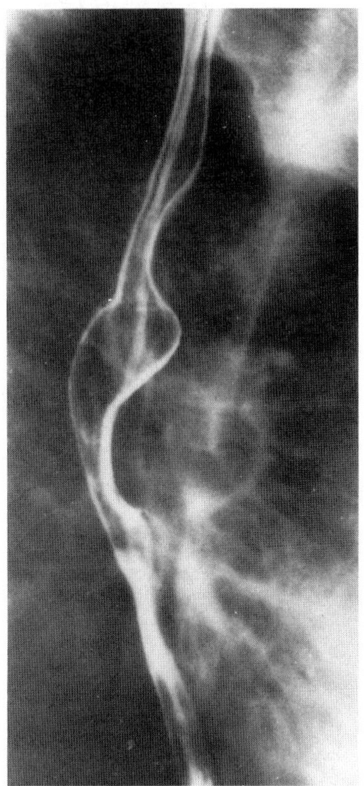

Figure 1.5. Impressions on the anterior aspect of the esophagus by the aortic arch, left main stem bronchus, and left inferior pulmonary veins.

There is striated muscle in the upper third of the esophagus, and smooth muscle in the lower third. The middle third contains both types of muscles. All esophageal muscles have

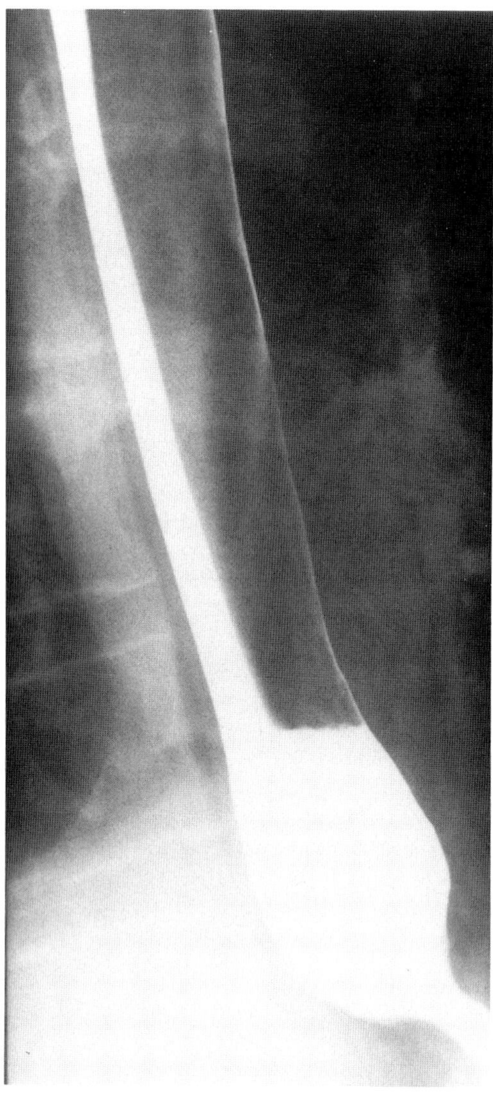

Figure 1.6. Relaxed esophagus. The inner surface is perfectly smooth. Double-contrast esophagogram.

functional properties of smooth muscle fibers. Peristalsis propagates along them following a phase of relaxation, which precedes contraction. The adventitia is a loose envelope of connective tissue around the esophagus, which permits a relative degree of mobility when compared to adjacent structures and is important in healing after injury or surgery.

Lower Esophageal Segment – Anatomy and Physiology

The most controversial part of the alimentary canal is the lower esophageal segment (LES). Its ill-defined function has led to the creation of many terms for the same structure. Some of these terms, which are not recommended for further use, are listed for correlation with the terminology of earlier literature. The most erudite hypotheses on the function of the LES have succeeded in revealing only some of the phenomena that occur in this part of the alimentary canal. Studies on the LES have also shown how complementary data may be obtained by radiologic and manometric methods.

The LES functions in the acceptance and transportation of an ingested bolus to the stomach and in the prevention of regurgitation from the distal segments of the alimentary canal.

The upper part of the esophagus is tubular down to approximately 3 cm above the esophageal hiatus – the tubular esophagus. The next segment, between the tubular esophagus and the cardia of the stomach, is called the vestibule or LES (Diagram 1.3, Figs. 1.7 and 1.8).

Opinions of radiologists, endoscopists, surgeons, and anatomists differ as to the location of the cardia. The transition of epithelium from the esophagus to the stomach is called the Z-line (*ora serrata*). Since the Z-line position is not constant, it is not a good radiographic indicator for location of the cardia. A more reliable method for locating the cardia by radiologic means is identification of the transverse fold of mucosa produced by contracted oblique muscles of the stomach (Fig. 1.8).

Increased intraluminal pressure in the resting LES can be documented manometrically, and hormonal action by gastrin will increase its tone. The LES is extremely distensible. The border between the tubular esophagus and esophageal vestibule (LES) is called the tubulovestibular junction. The portion of the LES, described as the phrenic ampulla, is actually the supradiaphragmatic segment of the esophageal vestibule. Pressure differences between the abdominal and thoracic cavity will cause the phrenic ampulla to respond independent of the infradiaphragmatic portion of the esophagus. The latter is the abdominal segment of the

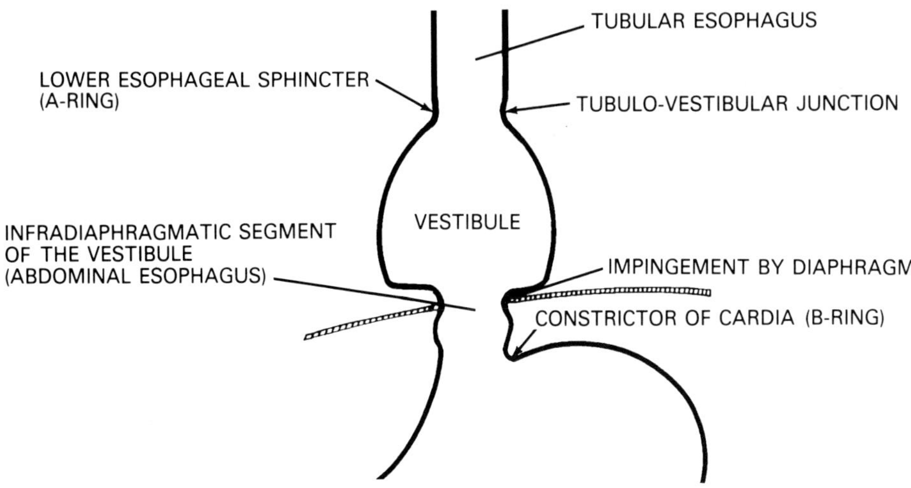

Diagram 1.3. Structures of the lower esophageal segment, the vestibule.

esophagus, earlier known as the cardiac antrum and submerged segment (Diagram 1.3). This segment varies between 1.5 and 3.5 cm in length, according to the phase of respiration. During swallowing, the whole esophagus moves upwards and the abdominal portion seemingly disappears. Thus, it is not possible to evaluate the true competence of the esophageal hiatus without knowing the phase of swallowing.

There are four main opinions on the existence of a sphincter in the LES:

1. An anatomic sphincter does not exist;
2. A ring-shaped sphincter exists at the transition of the tubular esophagus to the esophageal vestibule—a lower esophageal sphincter;
3. The whole vestibular segment has the properties of a sphincter;
4. There is a semicircular sphincter of the cardia at the esophagogastric transition.

The latter sphincter is said to be made by oblique muscular fibers of the stomach (Diagram 1.4). Recent studies show that the role of the LES in prevention of gastroesophageal reflux may have been previously overestimated. Indeed, diaphragmatic crura appear to be important in preventing reflux of contents from the stomach.

Several rings may be seen in the esophageal vestibule during an upper gastrointestinal series (Diagram 1.3). The A-ring is synonymous with the tubulovestibular junction, that is, the lower esophageal sphincter at the transition of the tubular esophagus to the esophageal vestibule. It is often seen during the course of the radiologic examination but is not precisely verified by manometry. Fluoroscopically, one may perceive that the A-ring is contracted only during swallowing. Thus, it prevents reflux of contents into the tubular segment of the esophagus during emptying of the vestibule into the stomach. Contraction of this sphincter at times other than during swallowing should be considered abnormal.

The B-ring corresponds to the sphincter of the cardia. In one-third of patients examined, the B-ring is accompanied by a transverse fold of mucosa. For that reason, it is often called the mucosal ring (Figs 1.7 and 1.8). The mucosal ring usually lies a few millimeters distal to the Z-line, and it is radiologically detectable only in cases of gastric hernia, through the esophageal hiatus.

At the site where the esophagus passes through the esophageal hiatus, muscle fibers of the diaphragm impress upon the esophageal vestibule (Diagram 1.3). During inspiration, the infradiaphragmatic portion of the esophageal vestibule (phrenic ampulla) distends, while the distal vestibular segment collapses. This is caused by differences in pressure between the thoracic and abdominal cavities, as well as by

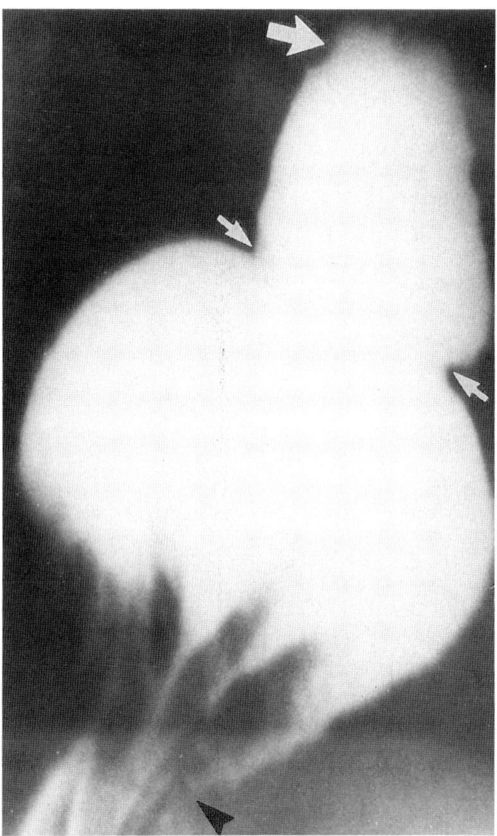

FIGURE 1.7. Hiatus hernia of the stomach. Tubulovestibular junction A-ring (upper arrow), mucosal B-ring (two white arrows), indentation of the esophageal hiatus upon the stomach (arrowhead). The gastroesophageal vestibule lies between rings A and B. (See Diagram 1.3.)

compression by diaphragmatic crura and adjacent organs.

In contrast to the aforementioned ring-shaped structures, the ring of Schatzki has a membranous appearance at the site of the B-ring; it is caused by reflux esophagitis and seen with gastric hiatus hernia.

The acute angle between the LES and the fundus of the stomach, the angle of Hiss, was previously considered to enhance closure of the cardia. However, this angle may vary between 70 and 110 degrees without affecting closure of the cardia. Thus, it may not be an important factor in the prevention of reflux. A valve mechanism was also suspected to be involved in closing the cardia. In the last three decades only one study describes such a structure, while all others deny it.

The phrenicoesophageal membrane encircles the esophageal vestibule. It consists of two membranes: the upper is continuous with the fascia which covers the thoracic face of the diaphragm, and the lower is connected to the fascia on the abdominal face of the diaphragm. Both are closely attached to each other at the edge of the esophageal hiatus, as well as to the adventitia of the esophagus. In the first four decades of life, the phrenicoesophageal membrane is of very high elasticity and enables the proximal part of the stomach to enter the thoracic cavity temporarily, in the last phase of swallowing. With aging, elasticity of the membrane diminishes, and mobility of the stomach increases, as well as the risk of hiatal herniation. When the fibers are less elastic, the membrane is not efficient in replacing the stomach back from the thoracic cavity to the abdomen.

A peristaltic wave initiated by swallowing propagates along the tubular part of the esophagus but not within the esophageal vestibule (Fig. 1.9). There is evidence that the tubular esophagus and the LES react to cholinergic and adrenergic stimulation in opposite ways. In fact, the esophageal vestibule relaxes during swallowing in the same way as the upper esophageal sphincter. Increasing pressure in the proximal portions of the esophagus creates a pressure gradient from the esophagus to the stomach. The primary peristaltic wave loses its speed and intensity as it approaches the relaxed vestibule. After closure of the tubulovestibular junction, a negative wave in the vestibule is followed by a positive, rather faint wave which is an extension of the peristalsis in the tubular esophagus. The latter may be followed by prolonged contraction of the vestibule, which is regarded as additional prevention of gastroesophageal reflux.

STOMACH

The stomach is the widest and most distensible of all alimentary canal organs. It extends from the end of the esophagus to the duodenum. The size and shape of the stomach are inconstant. The cupular portion of the stomach

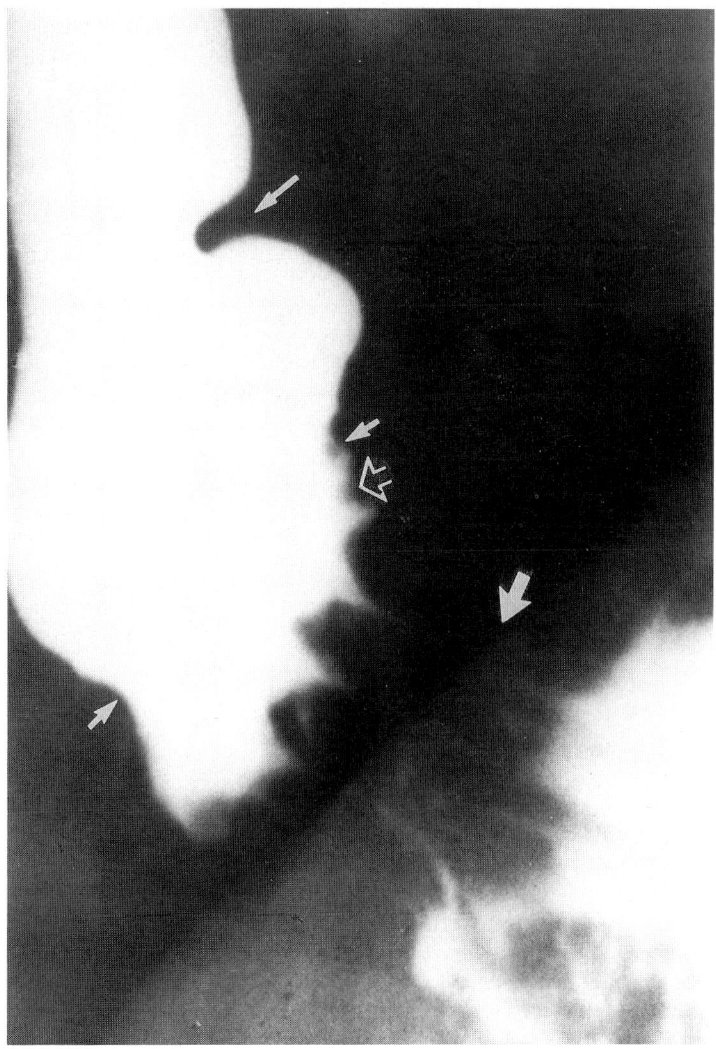

FIGURE 1.8. Hiatus hernia of the stomach. A-ring (upper arrow), B-ring, mucosal ring (two small arrows), indentation by gastric sling fibers (open arrow), and indentation of the stomach by esophageal hiatus (large closed arrow).

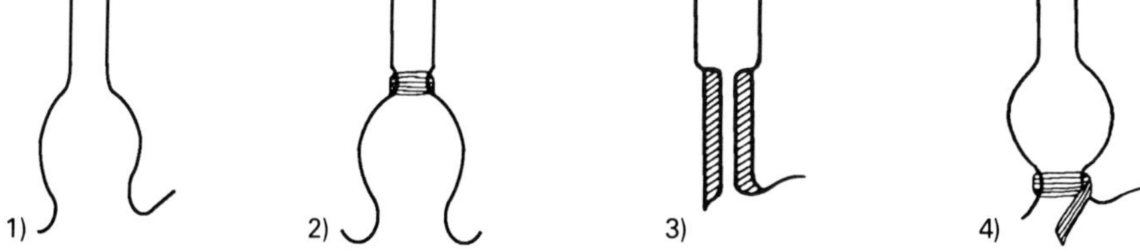

DIAGRAM 1.4. Proposed mechanisms of sphincteric function of the lower esophageal segment. (Used by permission, Friedland GW. Historical review of changing concepts of lower esophageal anatomy: 430 B.C.–1977. AJR. 1978; 131:373, © American Journal of Roentgenology.)

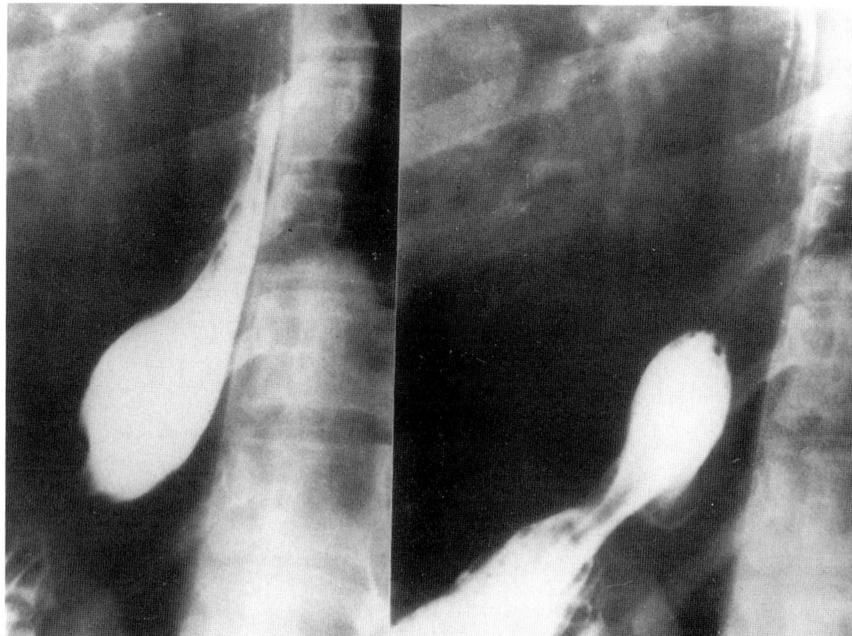

Figure 1.9. Emptying of the lower esophageal segment, the vestibule, with primary peristalsis.

situated above the cardia, the place where the esophagus becomes the stomach, lies beneath the diaphragm and is called the fundus. The pyloric portion of the stomach is distal to the angular notch and consists of the pyloric antrum and the pyloric canal (Figs. 1.10 and 1.11). The body of the stomach is limited superiorly by the cardia and fundus, and inferiorly by the pylorus (Diagram 1.5).

Mucosal folds running mainly in a longitudinal direction are called gastric rugae. They are of constant appearance except in the antrum where the pattern is more varied. Gastric folds are normally 4–5 mm thick.

The lesser curvature of the stomach is continuous with the esophageal contour. It is directed to the right, with an average length of 10 cm in adults. During X-ray examination of healthy patients, the lesser curvature is smooth. A passage along the lesser curvature produced by longitudinal mucosal folds is called the gastric canal.

Along the left margin, the posterior and anterior walls of the stomach unite to form the greater curvature. Irregularities or asymmetry

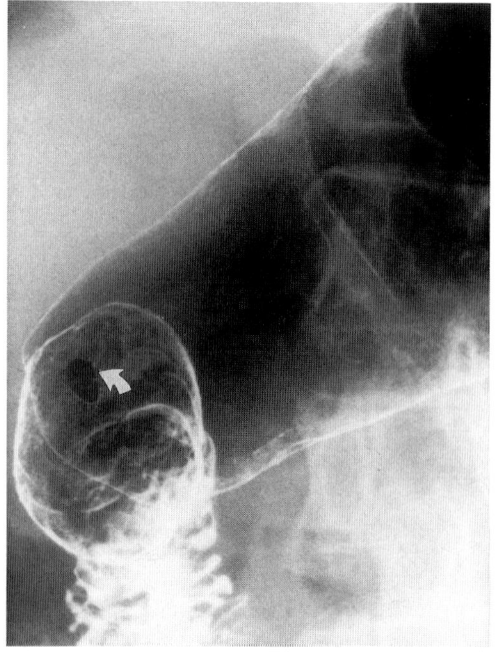

Figure 1.10. Double-contrast study of the stomach demonstrating the pylorus (arrow).

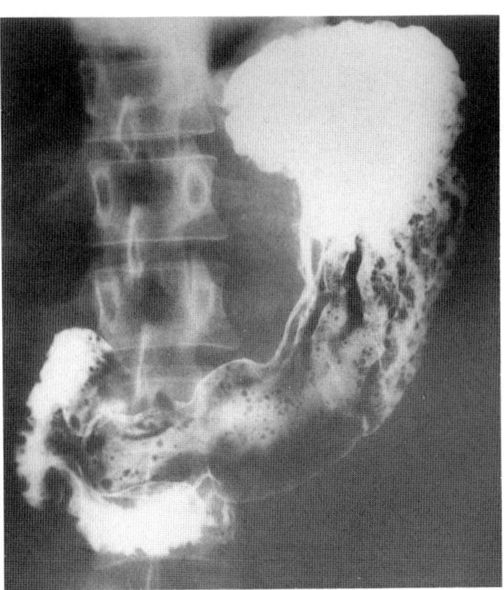

FIGURE 1.11. Roentgenogram of the stomach in the supine position. Barium accumulates in the proximal portion and gas in the distal portion of the stomach.

gus. These muscular layers of the stomach are covered with a serosa of visceral peritoneum.

The shape of the stomach depends on the constitution of the patient, gastric muscular tone, and the volume of contents. The capacity of the stomach is approximately 1 L. The relation of the stomach to adjacent organs is presented on Diagram 8.1. The stomach is fixed by the following ligaments: hepatogastric, gastrosplenic, gastrophrenic, and gastrocolic. The greater omentum is a double peritoneal apron suspended from the greater curvature of the stomach and the transverse colon.

The fundus is directed posteriorly, while distal segments of the stomach are directed anteriorly. During radiographic examination with the patient in a supine position, the fundus is filled with contrast medium and the antrum contains gas.

The cardia is the most difficult to visualize by radiological means because its appearance changes during respiration and swallowing. In different subjects, it may present any one of the following aspects: protrusion with surrounding radial mucosal folds – stellate type, radial mucosal folds alone, or no visible struc-

of the greater curvature folds need not be pathologic.

The areae gastricae are mucosal elevations 1–6 mm in diameter, bordered by shallow grooves (Fig. 1.12). The surfaces of areae gastricae are perforated by numerous gastric pits which are openings for gastric glands. There are approximately 3.5 million pits, every one receiving three to five gastric glands. There are three types of gastric glands. The type that secretes mucus is scattered throughout the whole stomach. Glands in the fundus secrete pepsin, intrinsic factor, and HCl. Pyloric glands which also secrete mucus are the least numerous.

The identification of areae gastricae on roentgenographs depends on the contraction and tone of the lamina muscularis mucosae.

In addition to the outer longitudinal and adjacent inner circular muscular layers, there is a third, innermost incomplete muscular layer of oblique fibers. These encircle the fundus and cardia and approach the greater curvature running parallel to the lesser curvature. The longitudinal and circular muscles are continuous with the corresponding layers of the esopha-

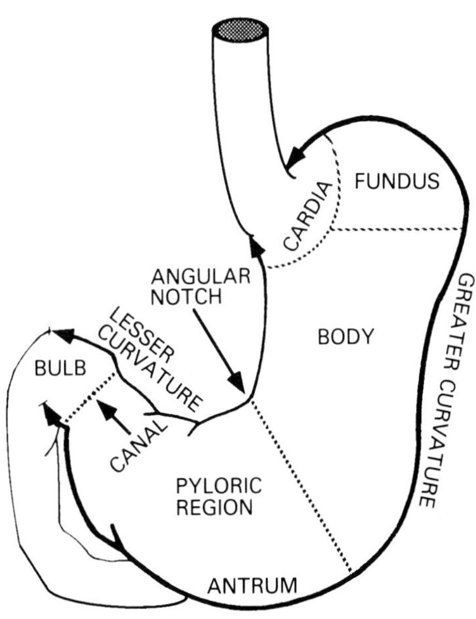

DIAGRAM 1.5. Anatomical characteristics of the stomach for the radiologic examination.

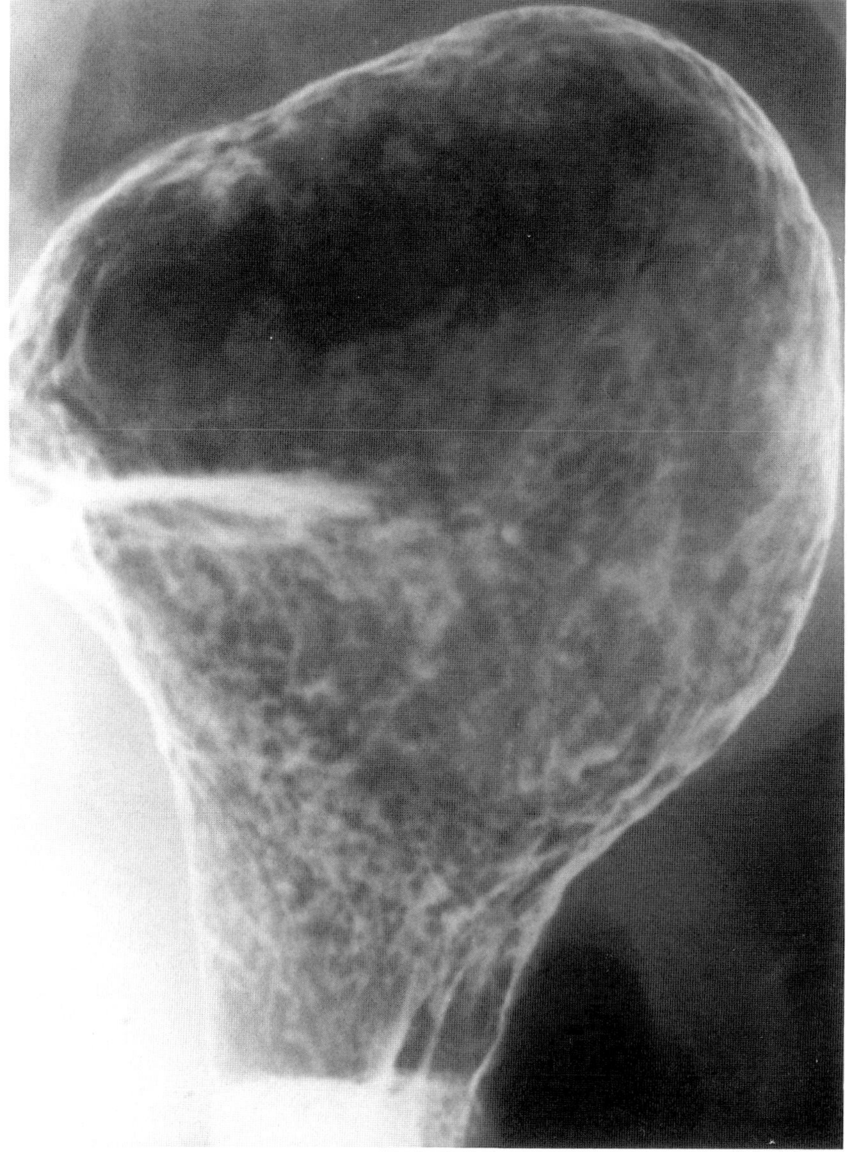

Figure 1.12. (A) Areae gastricae in proximal portion of the stomach.

ture except for a sharp line (Fig. 1.13). A double-contrast examination best visualizes the cardia.

SMALL BOWEL

The small bowel consists of the duodenum and the mesenteric small bowel. It is located in the central and inferior parts of the abdominal cavity. In healthy people, the mesenteric small bowel is partly or completely collapsed.

Duodenum

The duodenum is the shortest and widest segment of the small intestine extending from the pylorus to the duodenojejunal junction. The duodenal loop measures 25 cm in length

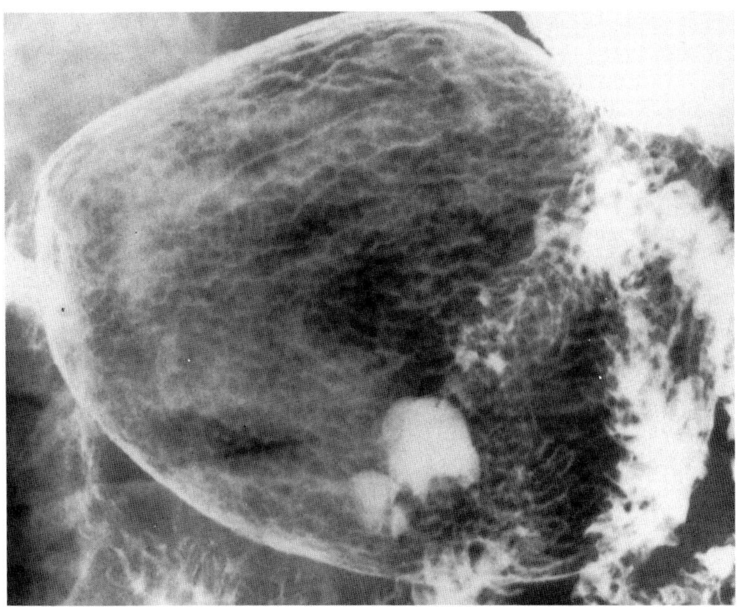

FIGURE 1.12. (B) Areae gastricae in distal portion of the stomach.

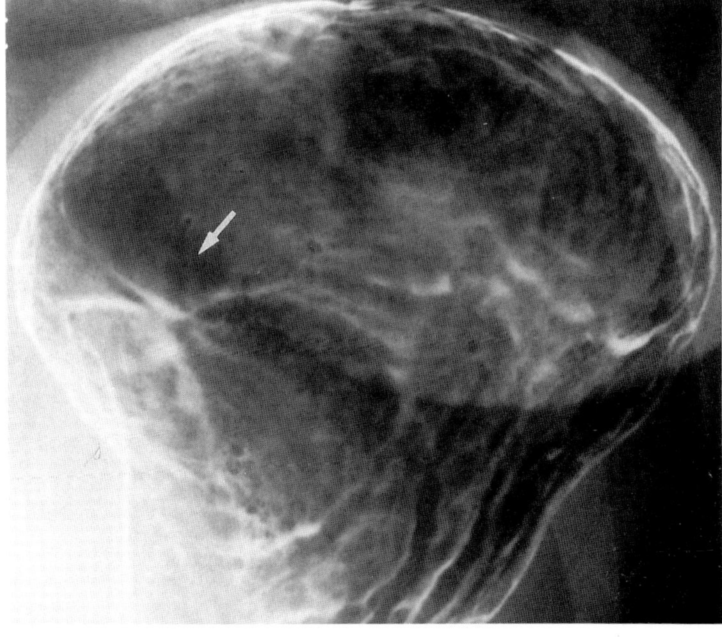

A

FIGURE 1.13. The cardia of the stomach. (A) The stellate type (arrow). (*Figure continued on overleaf.*)

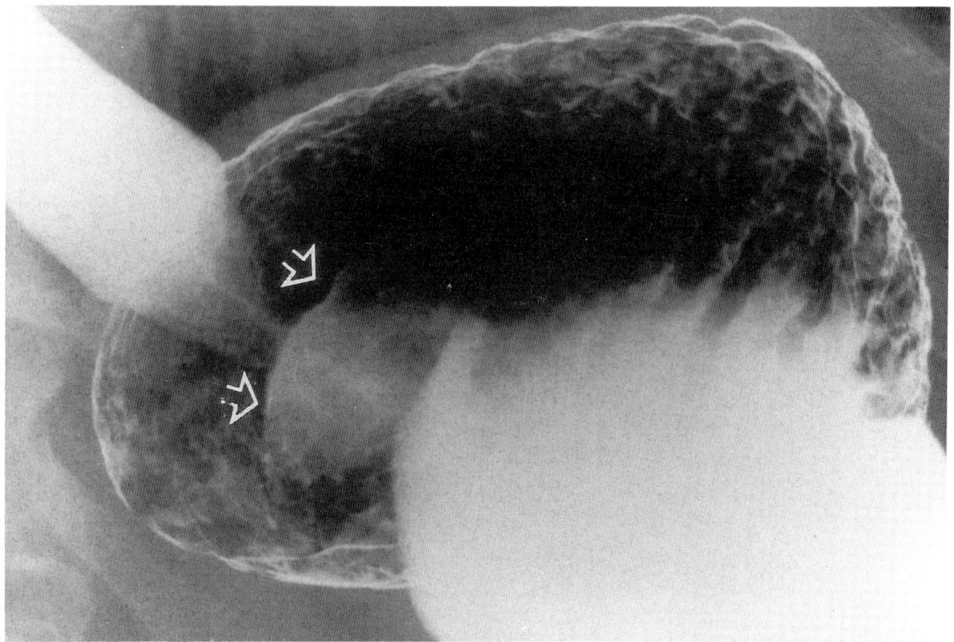

B

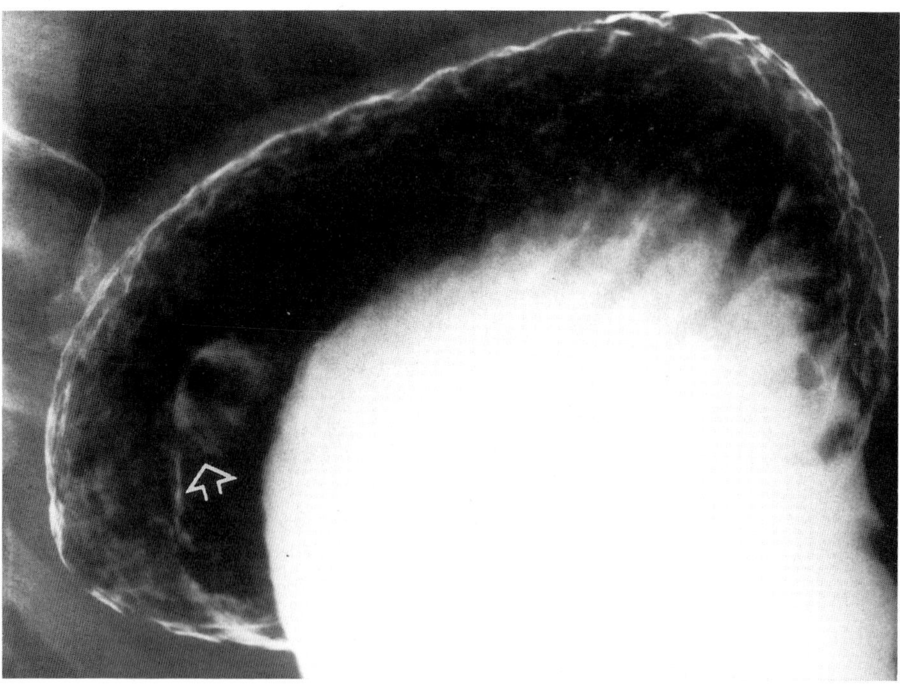

C

FIGURE 1.13. continued. (B) Apparent linear type (arrows) readily changes to (C) protruding type (arrow).

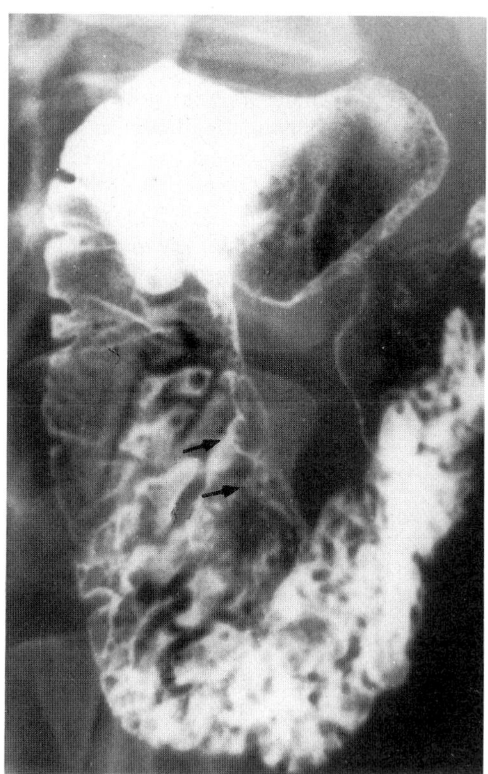

Figure 1.14. Double-contrast study of the duodenum. Impression on the bulb by the gallbladder. The major papilla (upper arrow) and the longitudinal fold (lower arrow) extend distally.

and 4 cm in width (Fig. 1.14) and is composed of four segments: first (superior), second (descending), third (horizontal), and fourth (ascending). The latter two comprise the inferior portion. The superior and inferior duodenal flexures are between the first and second, and second and third portions, respectively. The duodenum is fixed retroperitoneally to the posterior abdominal wall from the superior duodenal flexure to the duodenojejunal junction. However, the duodenum is not covered with peritoneum at the crossing of the superior mesenteric artery.

A widened area of the superior portion of the duodenum adjacent to the pylorus is called the duodenal bulb. This dilation is caused by a lower degree of tone of the muscular coat. The duodenal bulb deepens into medial and lateral recesses, which must not be mistaken for ulcer craters.

A major part of the first portion of the duodenum has longitudinal mucosal folds (Fig. 1.15). Circular Kerckring's folds, mucosal duplications, appear distal to the duodenal bulb and anastomose with one another (Fig. 1.16).

The submucosa of the superior and descending duodenum contains numerous Brunner's glands that secrete mucus which protects the duodenal mucosa from gastric acid. There is a mucosal ridge in the dorsal wall of the descending duodenum that is created by the main pancreatic and common bile ducts. The major duodenal papilla, an elevation at the proximal end of the longitudinal fold, contains an opening for the main pancreatic and common bile ducts. This papilla may be visualized in 50% of patients (Fig. 1.14). About 2 cm cranially and

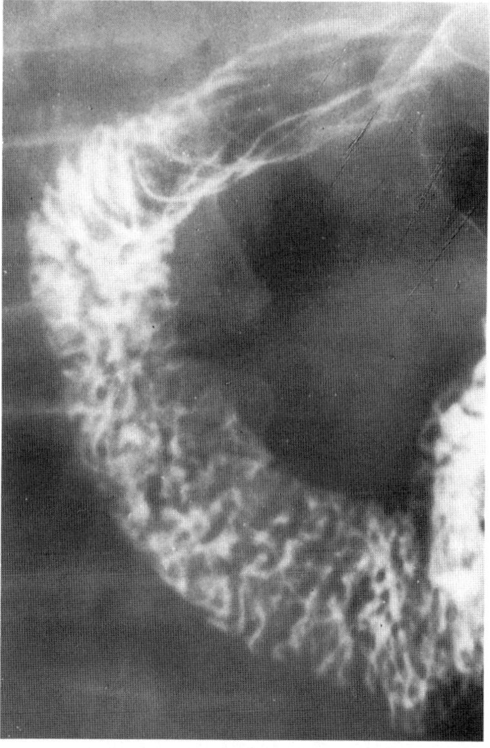

Figure 1.15. Longitudinal folds characteristic of the mucosal relief pattern of the bulb, and circular folds characteristic of the more distal segments of the duodenum.

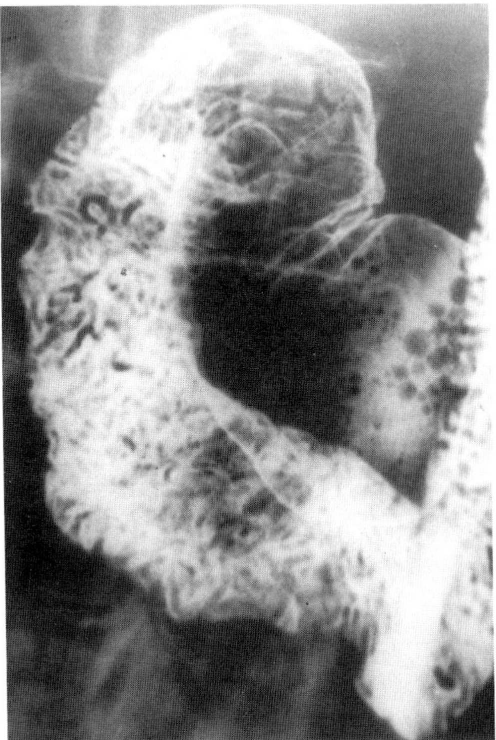

FIGURE 1.16. Anastomosis of circular folds in incompletely distended duodenum.

slightly anterior to the major duodenal papilla, lies a minor papilla containing an opening for the accessory pancreatic duct (see chapter 4, Fig. 4.57).

The liver and gallbladder lie in front of the proximal portion of the duodenum while the pancreas and inferior vena cava are behind. The second, descending portion of the duodenum is posteriorly in contact with the right kidney and the inferior vena cava. The horizontal portion abuts the head of the pancreas and superior mesenteric artery. Loops of jejunum may lie in front of the ascending portion while the uncinate process of the pancreas is behind. In 50% of patients, there is a superior duodenal recess and in a somewhat larger proportion, an inferior duodenal recess. The superior and inferior duodenal recesses are potential peritoneal spaces behind the superior and inferior duodenal folds. These may be sites of internal herniation.

MESENTERIC SMALL BOWEL

The mesenteric small bowel consists of jejunum and ileum and is approximately 5 m long. There is no sharp transition between the two segments with the proximal two-thirds representing the jejunum. The small bowel is attached to the posterior abdominal wall via a long mesentery. The root of the mesentery extends from the duodenojejunal junction to the ileocecal valve, and is 15 cm long. It crosses the third portion of the duodenum. The jejunum occupies the middle, and the ileum the inferior, part of the peritoneal cavity (Fig. 1.17). The lumen of the small bowel narrows distally, and the intestinal wall becomes thinner. The jejunum is 2.5–3.0 cm wide, and the width of the terminal ileum is 1.5–2.0 cm. Circular folds become shorter and transform into longitudinal folds at the terminal ileum. The circular folds are normally 1–2 mm thick. In a distal direction, the motility of the small bowel decreases and the quantity of lymphoid tissue increases. Single lymphoid follicles populate the lamina propria of the jejunum. In addition to single follicles, the ileum contains aggregated lymphoid follicles called Peyer's patches. These patches are 1–8 cm long and 1–2.5 cm wide. Their number varies between 20 and 30 and they are directed longitudinally, facing the mesentery. Conical elevations of mucosa called intestinal villi are hardly visible with the naked eye and are not a subject for barium studies.

LARGE BOWEL

The large intestine is divided into the following portions: cecum with appendix, colon, rectum, and anal canal. It extends distally from the ileum and lies along the periphery of the abdominal cavity. The average length is 150 cm and the approximate thickness of the wall is 1.5–3 mm. The wall is thinner in the proximal portions of the large intestine. Except for the appendix, rectum, and anal canal, all portions of the large intestine are characterized by sacculations (haustra) and longitudinal bands (teniae).

Haustra are separated by semilunar folds, which do not encircle the intestinal lumen completely but occupy only a portion of the circumference (Fig. 1.18). Longitudinal muscles of the

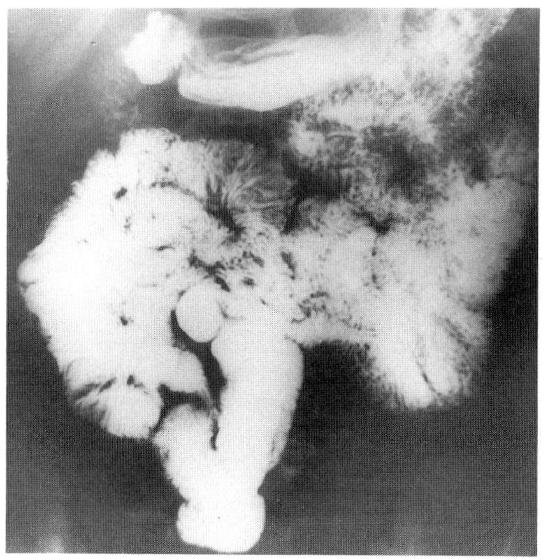

A

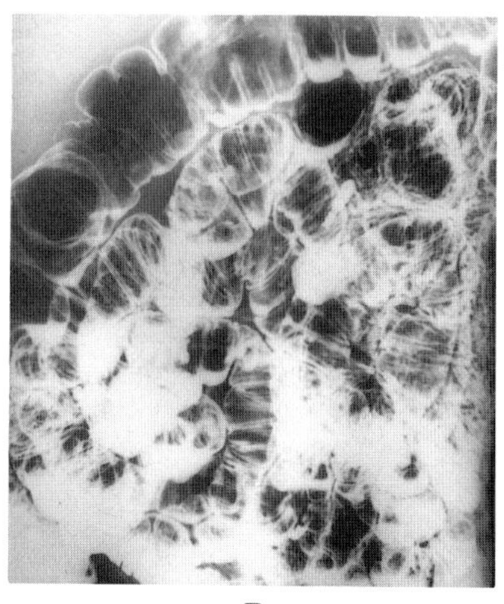

B

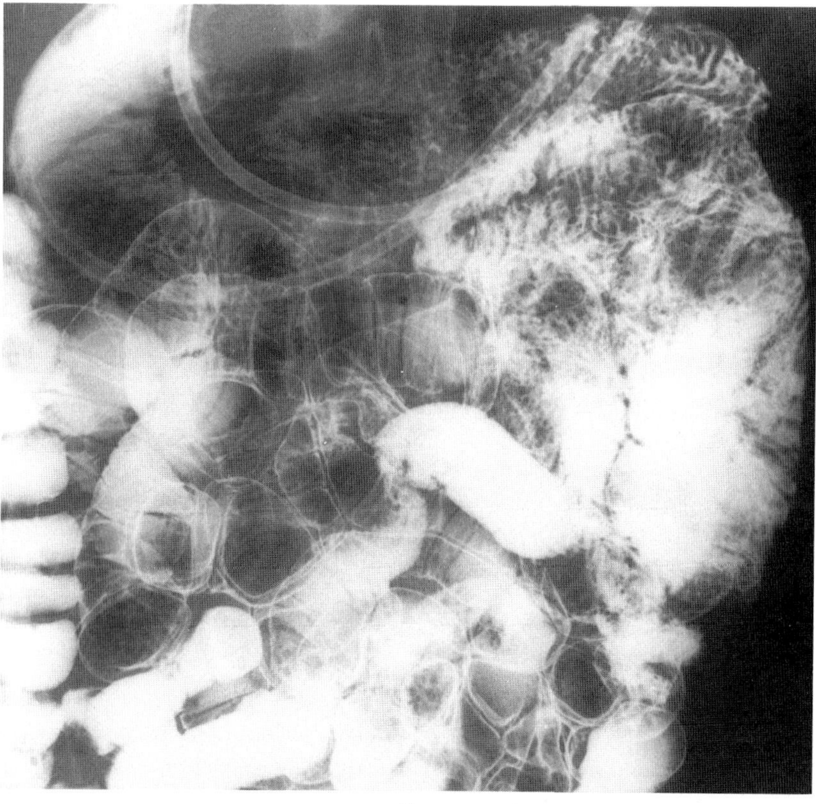

C

FIGURE 1.17. Small bowel anatomy. (A) Follow-through study. (B) and (C) Air contrast enteroclysis with proper distension of the gut. Barium has also opacified the colon.

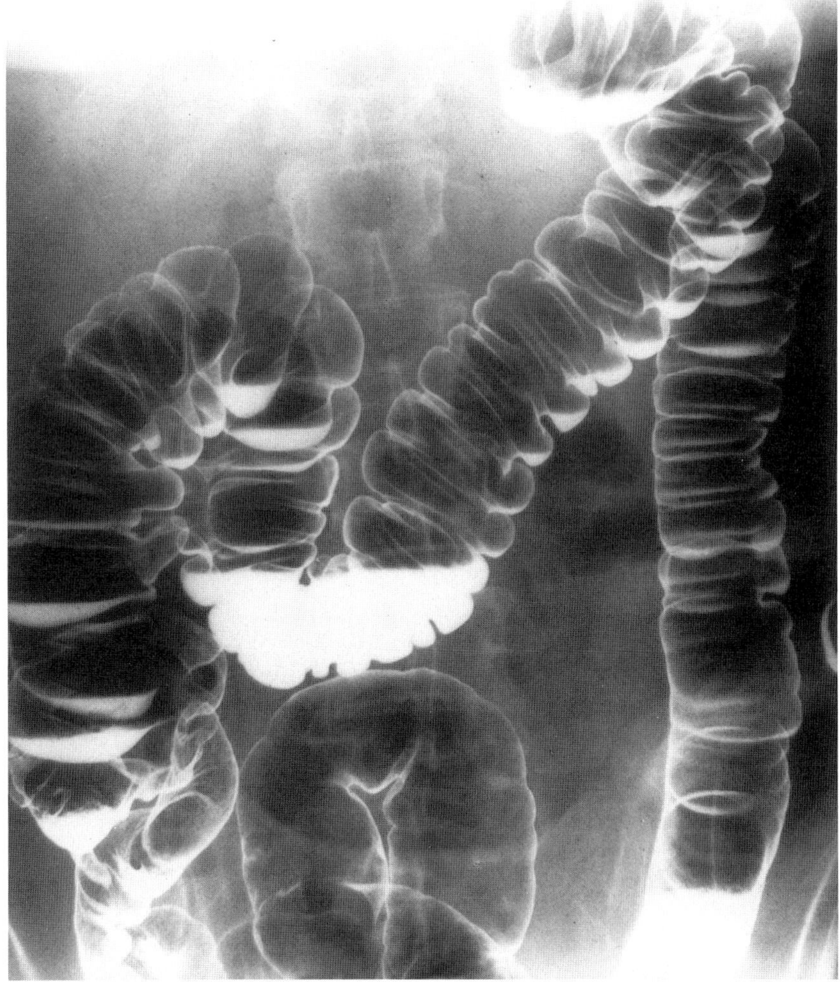

FIGURE 1.18. Air contrast barium study demonstrating cecum and colon.

colon and cecum form three teniae: omental, free, and mesocolic. Their usual width is 10 mm.

Haustra are always present down to the left colic flexure in healthy people. Hence, they are constant in the proximal segments of the large bowel and their absence is a pathologic sign. Haustra appear only during the course of contractions of teniae in the distal portions of the colon.

The cecum lies beyond the ileocecal valve which is located at the opening of the ileum into the large intestine. It is of saccular shape, measuring up to 7 cm in diameter. The ileocecal valve consists of circular muscles of ileum covered with cecal mucosa. It lies on the dorsomedial wall of the large intestine at the level of the first complete semilunar fold. The end of the ileum passes obliquely through the wall of the large intestine. Thus, this opening has valvular properties when the cecum is filled with chyme.

Two lips of the ileocecal valve unite, on both sides, to form the frenulum of the ileocecal valve. The valve's average diameter is 1.8 cm. It is elevated about 1 cm from the inner surface of the large intestine. The ileal opening may be oval, circular (Figs. 1.19, 1.20, and in chapter 12, 12.67), or may resemble a longitudinal fis-

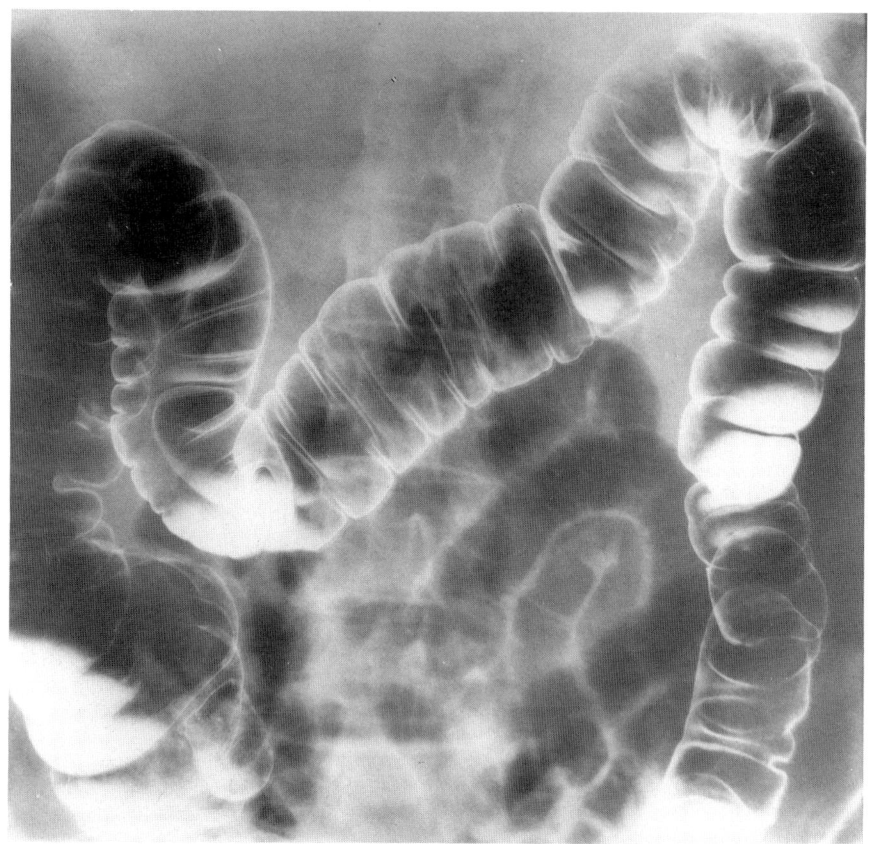

Figure 1.19. Oval shaped ileocecal valve. Double-contrast barium enema examination.

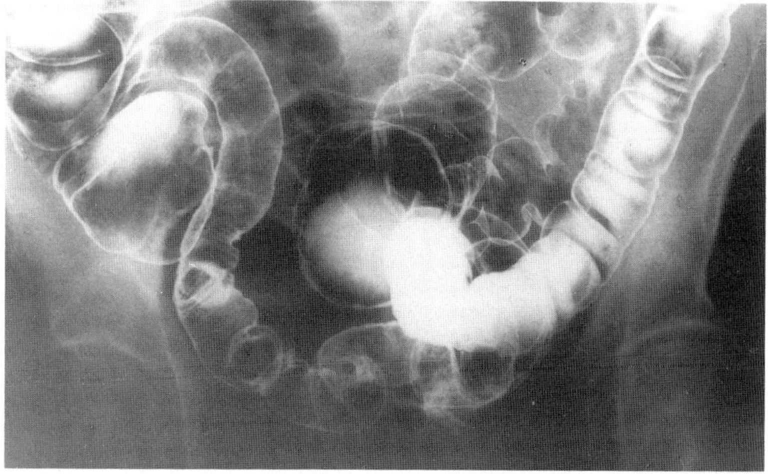

Figure 1.20. Terminal ileum demonstrated by retrograde hypotonic ileography.

sure. There are two peritoneal folds near the ileocecal opening, which border the superior and inferior ileocecal recesses. These are locations for potential herniation.

An appendage of the cecum, the vermiform appendix, originates from its dorsomedial wall.

The colon extends from the cecum to the rectum, along the periphery of the abdominal cavity. The ascending colon is about 20 cm long and two-thirds of the cecal width wide. It ascends retroperitoneally up to the hepatic flexure. The hepatic flexure may be in contact with the gallbladder anteriorly, with the right kidney, the second segment of the duodenum, and head of the pancreas posteriorly. These relationships are important in the spread of inflammation or neoplasms.

The transverse colon is intraperitoneal, extending between hepatic and splenic colic flexures. It is usually 40–50 cm long, but may vary considerably in length. It is attached to the posterior abdominal wall by the transverse mesocolon which allows extensive mobility. Superiorly, the transverse colon is adjacent to the stomach, liver, gallbladder, and spleen. Since the transverse colon lies anteriorly in the abdominal cavity, it shows the most distension when the colon is filled with gas, and the patient is supine.

The descending colon is 20–30 cm long in adults. Like the ascending colon, it is retroperitoneally located. The left paracolic gutter is narrower than the right. The ascending colon is adjacent to small intestinal loops anteriorly, and the left kidney and posterior abdominal wall posteriorly. The entrance into Douglas's cavity, the true pelvis, marks the transition between the descending and the sigmoid colon.

The sigmoid colon (Fig. 1.21) is also attached to the posterior abdominal wall via a long mesocolon which permits considerable mobility. The approximate length of the sigmoid colon is 40 cm. It extends from the entrance into Douglas's cavity to the level of the S3 vertebral segment creating one or more loops within Douglas's cavity. Distally, the transition between the sigmoid colon and the rectum is the narrowest point of the large intestine.

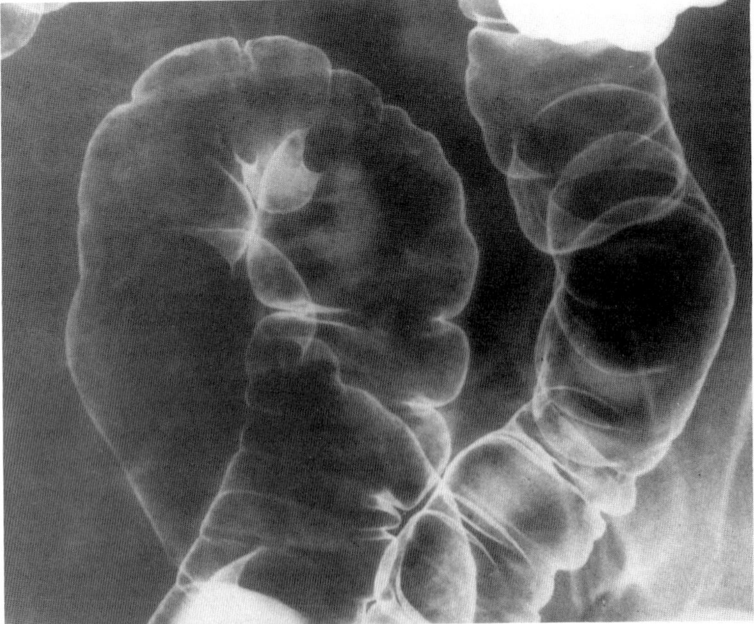

Figure 1.21. Anatomy of the sigmoid colon. Double-contrast barium enema study.

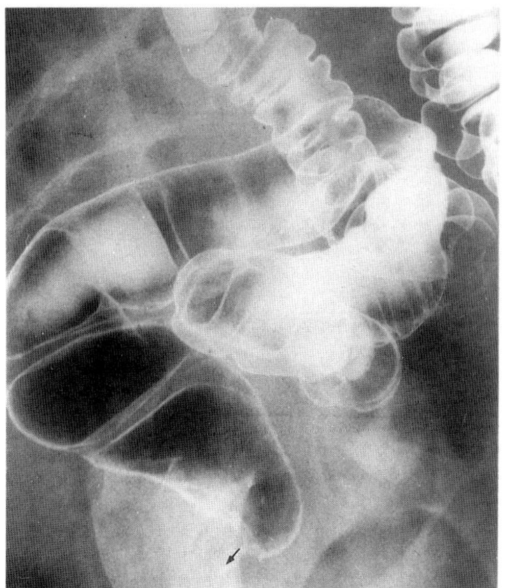

FIGURE 1.22. Double-contrast barium enema demonstrating the rectum directed anteriorly. Posterior position of the anal canal, filled with a small quantity of barium (arrow).

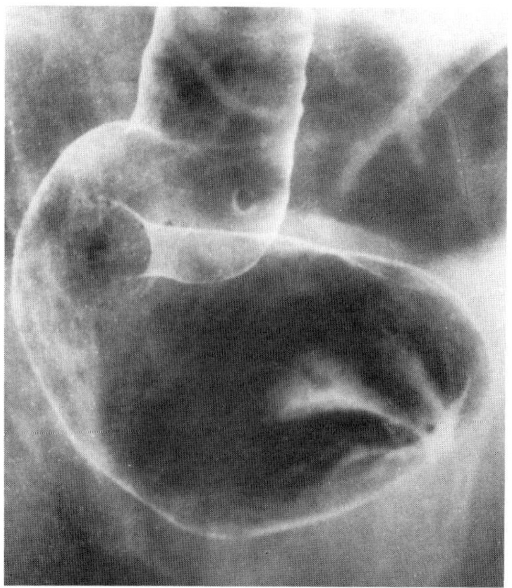

FIGURE 1.23. Double-contrast study of the rectum. Anal columns occupy the distal segment. Small sessile polyp in the proximal segment.

The rectum (Figs. 1.22 and 1.23) follows the curvature of the sacrum and coccyx with slight lateral deviations. It is 11–15 cm long. The distal portion of the rectum is widened into a distensible ampulla which lies subperitoneally. Only the upper third of the rectum is intraperitoneal. Three transverse folds which protrude into the rectal lumen are called rectal valves. The middle fold (Houston's valve) is the most prominent and may interfere with the passage of a catheter for a barium enema examination. The pouch of Douglas or rectouterine space is a peritoneal reflection separating the uterus from the rectum in females. In males, the rectum lies behind the urinary bladder, seminal vesicles, ampullas of the deferent ducts, and prostate. Anteriorly, the rectum is also adjacent to the sigmoid colon and the ileum.

The anal canal is the terminal segment of the digestive tube. It extends from the apex of the coccyx to the anus and measures 3 cm in length. In contrast to the rectum, the anal canal is directed backward. The mucosa of the upper part of the anal canal creates 8–10 longitudinal folds, called anal columns (*columnae Morgagni*). The distal ends of the anal columns are connected by transverse folds, creating anal valves.

Mucoid glands (Lieberkühn's crypts) are scattered throughout the mucosa of the large intestine. This type of gland is also present in the small intestine. Gland openings may be filled with contrast medium during the course of a normal barium enema and may be confused with discrete "rose-thorn" ulcerations seen in ulcerative colitis.

Bibliography

Adler RH, Firme CN, Lanigan JM. A valve mechanism to prevent gastroesophageal reflux and esophagitis. Surgery. 1958;44:63.

Baastrup CJ. Roentgenologic studies of inner surface of the stomach and the movements of gastric contents. Acta Radiol. 1924;3:180.

Barrett NR. Benign stricture of the lower esophagus. Proc Roy Soc Med. 1960;53:402.

Creamer B, Harrison GK, Pierce JW. Further observations of the gastroesophageal junction. Thorax. 1959;14:132.

Dornhorst AC, Harrison K, Pierce JW. Observations on the normal esophagus and cardia. Lancet. 1954;1:695.

Edwards DAW. Concepts of esophageal disorders (Editorial). J Roy Soc Med. 1980;402.

Ekberg O, Lindstrom C. The upper esophageal sphincter area. Acta Radio Diagn. 1987;28:173.

Forssell G. Studies of the mechanism of movement of the mucous membrane of the digestive tract. AJR. 1923;10:87.

Friedland GW. Historical review of changing concepts of lower esophageal anatomy: 430 B.C.–1977. AJR. 1978;131:373.

Fyke FE Jr, Code CF, Schlegel JF. The gastroesophageal sphincter in healthy human beings. Gastroenterologia (Basel). 1956;86:135.

Garry RC. Innervation of the abdominal viscera. Br Med Bull. 1958;14:212.

Haddad JK. Relation of gastroesophageal reflux to yield sphincter pressures. Gastroenterology. 1970; 58:175.

Herlinger H, Grossman R, Laufer I, Kressel HY, Ochs RH. The gastric cardia in double contrast study: its dynamic image. AJR. 1980;135:21.

Ito S. The enteric surface coat on cat intestinal microvilli. J Cell Biol. 1965;27:475.

Karan E, Rubenstein WA, Markisz JA, Whalen P, Zirinski K. Anatomy. In: Margulis AR, Burhenne HJ (eds). Alimentary Tract Radiology, vol 1. St. Louis: CV Mosby; 1989:231.

Ott DJ, Gelfand DW, Wu WC, Castell DO. Esophagogastric region and its rings. AJR. 1984;142:281.

Pope CE. Is LES enough? (Editorial) Gastroenterology. 1976;71:328.

Sanchez GC, Kramer P, Ingelfinger FJ: Motor mechanisms of the esophagus, particularly of its distal portion. Gastroenterology. 1953;25:321.

Schatzki R. The lower esophageal ring; long-term follow up of symptomatic and asymptomatic rings. AJR. 1963;90:810.

Sloan R. The mucosal pattern of the mesenteric small intestine; an anatomic study. AJR. 1957;77:651.

Solans GR. Sliding hernias through the esophageal hiatus. Br Med J. 1953;1:1029.

Chapter **2**

Gastrointestinal Physiology

MOTILITY OF THE ALIMENTARY CANAL

Alimentary canal movements may be observed by barium studies or measured by intraluminal pressure readings. Peristalsis and rhythmic contractions are the most important features identified. They result from successive contractions and relaxations of digestive tube muscles innervated by external nerves and intramural plexuses. The vagus nerve is a source of preganglionic parasympathetic nerve fibers and postganglionic sympathetic nerve fibers, originating from cervical sympathetic ganglia. This pattern of external innervation extends from the pharynx to the left colic flexure. More distal segments of the large intestine receive innervation from pelvic nerves. The functioning of the intramural intestinal plexus can be independent of external nerves. Actually, the interrelationship between local and external innervation has not been completely elucidated. The intramural nervous system is divided into subserosal, myenteric, submucosal, and mucosal plexus. Cholinergic, parasympathetic receptors, reacting with acetylcholine, are either muscarinic or nicotinic. Adrenergic α and β_2 receptors react with epinephrine or norepinephrine, or both. Stimulation of either nicotinic or muscarinic receptors provokes muscular contractions. In contrast, contractions are inhibited when β_2 adrenergic receptors are stimulated. Stimulation of α adrenergic receptors has opposite effects, either contraction or relaxation, depending on the particular section of the digestive tube involved.

Peristalsis

Peristalsis is defined as an orderly sequence of contraction and relaxation cycles of alimentary canal smooth muscle, resulting in distal transportation of intraluminal contents. The peristaltic reflex of Starling includes contraction proximal to the site of stimulation and relaxation beyond. It has not yet been elucidated why peristaltic waves spread exclusively in one direction. When a resected segment of small intestine is reanastomosed after changing direction, it does not propagate peristaltic waves. Esophageal peristalsis is dependent on preganglionic fibers of the vagal nerve. External impulses are not required to maintain peristalsis in the stomach and bowel, although they may modify it.

Local plexuses are essential in coordinating peristaltic smooth muscle activity. Namely, contraction that occurs as a response to distension of the wall is mediated by local reflexes. Cells in the submucosal plexus are sensitive to bowel distension, and stimulate motoric efferent cells of the myenteric plexus. Acetylcholine and norepinephrine are chemical transmitters of these impulses. The former increases the excitability of smooth muscles and depolarizes cellular membranes. This results in increased tone and in a higher number of rhythmic con-

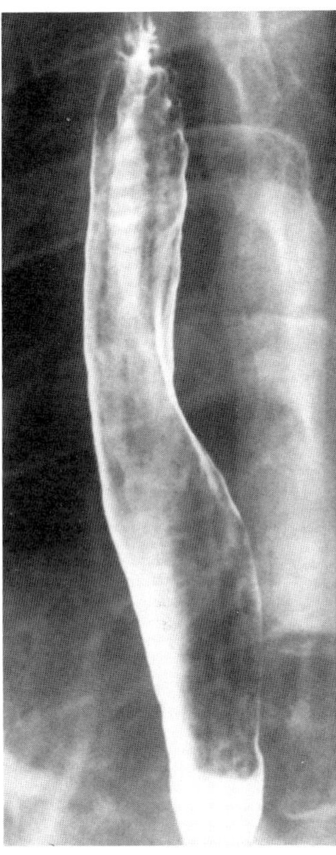

Figure 2.1. "Feline" appearance of the proximal esophagus resulting from contractions of the lamina muscularis mucosae.

tractions. However, the action of acetylcholine on areas such as the lower esophageal segment is the opposite. The effects of catecholamines and acetylcholine on smooth muscles of the gastrointestinal tract are opposed. Postganglionic parasympathetic neurons are excitatory, whereas postganglionic sympathetic neurons are inhibitory. Norepinephrine causes contraction of alimentary canal sphincters.

Autoplasticity of the Alimentary Canal Mucosa

Contraction and relaxation of lamina muscularis mucosae of the alimentary canal is termed *autoplasticity*. Such movement probably contributes to the stirring of contents. Autoplasticity may be observed during radiologic examination in almost any alimentary canal section distal to the pharynx (Fig. 2.1). Contraction of the lamina muscularis mucosae, except for the principal muscles of the esophagus, participates in the formation of longitudinal esophageal folds. The autoplasticity of gastric mucosa (Fig. 2.2) changes the caliber of gastric folds and makes areae gastricae more distinct. In normal circumstances, the elevation of gastric folds depends primarily on the hydration of the submucosa. However, the prominent movements of circular folds seen during contrast examination of the small intestine are the result of autoplasticity

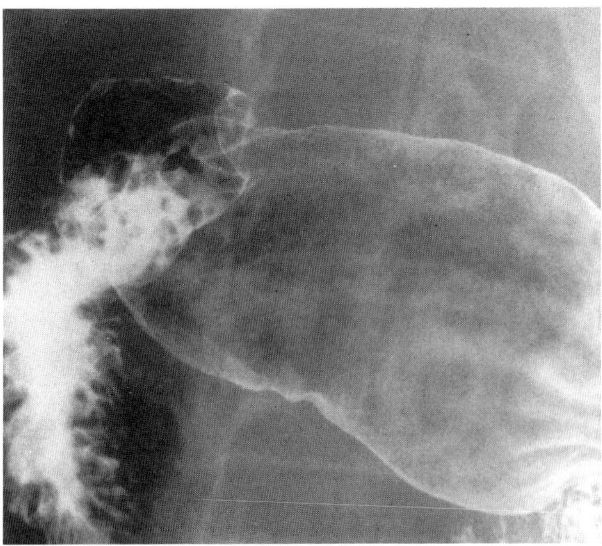

Figure 2.2. Transverse mucosal lines in the antrum, probably resulting from contraction of the lamina muscularis mucosae.

of the mucosa. Autoplasticity of the large intestinal mucosa is discussed in chapter 12 (Fig. 2.3).

REFLEXES AND ALIMENTARY CANAL MOTILITY

Both excitatory and inhibitory local reflexes affect motility of the digestive tube. These reflexes are stimulated by distension of the wall or by chemical stimulation. The pyloric reflex is stimulated by the presence of food in the duodenum and it results in the contraction of pyloric sphincter muscle. The enterogastric reflex suppresses gastric motility when the small bowel is distended. Gastroileal and gastrocolic reflexes are activated by gastric dilatation. These stimulate ileal and colonic motility, respectively. The duodenocolic reflex begins by distension of the duodenal wall and results in massive movements within the large intestine.

THE ACT OF SWALLOWING

Swallowing has two aims: to propel food from the mouth to the stomach and to protect the respiratory tract from aspiration. It is comprised of three phases. In the oral phase, contents are transported to the pharynx; they enter the esophagus in the pharyngeal phase, and finally reach the stomach in the esophageal phase. The first, oral phase, is voluntary. After the bolus enters the esophagus, swallowing continues involuntarily. The afferent limb of the reflex arch has mechanoreceptors in the mucosa of the soft palate, tonsils and tonsilar fossae, the root of the tongue, and posterior wall of the pharynx.

Swallowing is governed by a central neuronal cluster of the rhomboid fossa. Efferent fibers are part of the glossopharyngeal and hypoglossal nerves. They innervate muscles that are important for the oral and pharyngeal phases of swallowing, while the vagus nerve innervates striated muscles of the esophagus. Smooth muscles of the esophagus are influenced by a local plexus similar to the myenteric plexus of the distal segments of the alimentary canal.

The oral phase features contractions of muscles of the tongue, soft palate, and pharynx (Diagram 2.1). There are differences when swallowing a solid or liquid bolus. A chewed bolus

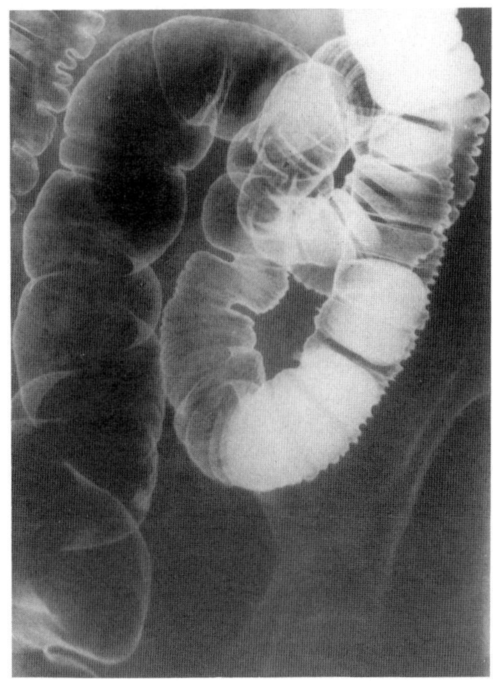

FIGURE 2.3. Irregularities of the sigmoid colon contours, resulting from contractions of the lamina muscularis mucosae. Two diverticula are on the medial contour of the proximal sigmoid colon.

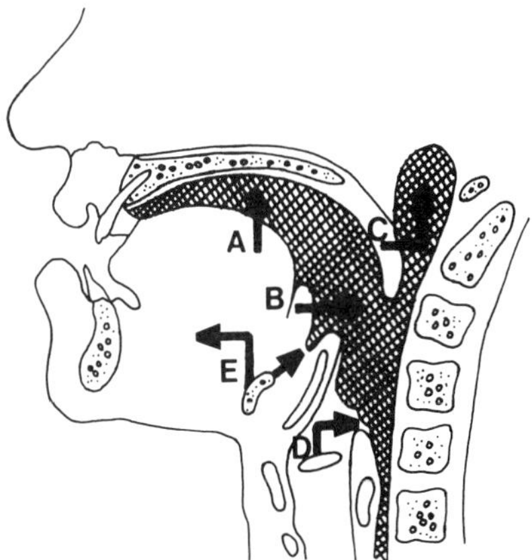

DIAGRAM 2.1. Oral and pharyngeal phase of swallowing. Letters indicate the sequence and arrows the direction of movements. (Used by permission and modified from Donner MW, Silbiger ML. Cinefluorographic analysis of pharyngeal swallowing in neuromuscular disorders. Am J Med Sci. 1966;251:134.)

is forced into the middle of the oral cavity. The top of the tongue first moves toward the hard palate, followed by the dorsum. The soft palate moves upward and closes the epipharynx. The bolus is then pushed backward with the root of the tongue, while both the larynx and esophagus elevate. A solid bolus then passes mostly alongside the epiglottis and through the pyriform recess on the same side. In contrast, fluid contents leak on both sides of the epiglottis and through both pyriform recesses (Figs. 2.4 and 2.5).

In radiographic analysis of the act of swallowing, contrast boluses of different viscosity may produce variations in motility. Progression of a very liquid bolus is considered in the following sequence. The pharynx is emptied by sequential contractions of its constrictors, completing the second phase of swallowing. Aspiration is prevented by shifting the larynx up and ahead. The root of the tongue pushes the epiglottis, closing the laryngeal opening. The speed of the bolus remains rapid until it enters the esophagus. For this reason, the whole radiologic examination should be recorded on vid-

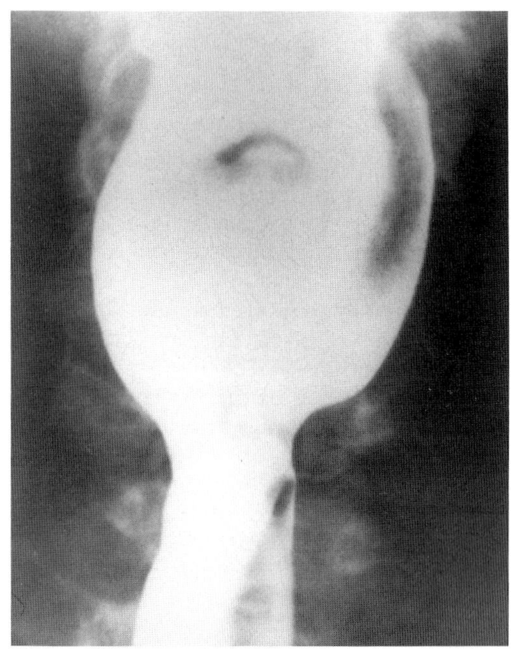

Figure 2.4. Hypopharynx filled with barium suspension.

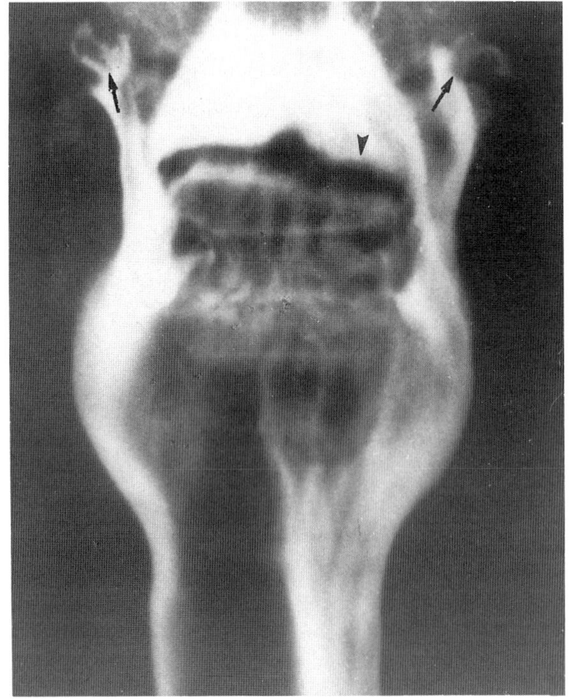

Figure 2.5. Transient lateral hypopharyngeal diverticula (arrows), lateral tilting of the epiglottis (arrowhead), and dilation of the hypopharynx are signs of altered pharyngeal phase of swallowing. A central negative defect of the contrast column is caused by the larynx.

eotape for functional analysis. In the area of the inferior pharyngeal constrictor, near the pharyngoesophageal junction, there is a section 3 cm in length with high intraluminal pressure at rest. This area is called the upper esophageal sphincter. Corresponding circular muscles are in permanent tonic contraction. Negative pressure in the esophagus is separated from positive pressure in the pharynx by this sphincteric mechanism. Immediately after swallowing commences, intraluminal pressure of the upper esophageal sphincter increases for several tenths of a second. This is followed by a drop in pressure below basal values, coinciding with the opening of the pharyngoesophageal junction. At almost the same time, the peristaltic wave caused by contraction of the superior and middle pharyngeal constrictors propels contents into the esophagus.

During an examination of esophageal peristalsis, the patient should slowly swallow one large bolus of barium. Any successive bolus would disturb peristalsis of the preceding one. Consequently, the tail of the contrast bolus should be fluoroscopically monitored.

Primary esophageal peristalsis (Fig. 2.6) is a continuation of the pharyngeal peristalsis initiated by swallowing. It may be demonstrated in 90% of healthy young examinees. The primary peristaltic wave of the esophagus begins with an inhibitory impulse originating from the superior esophageal sphincter. It is immediately followed by a peristaltic contraction 4–8 cm long which reaches the lower esophageal sphincter in six seconds. The amplitude of the esophageal peristalsis is maximal in the distal third of the esophagus. Contraction is followed by another wave of relaxation. Motor branches are supplied by the vagal nerve. Nuclei of the vagus nerve receive afferent impulses from the mucosa and submucosa as well as muscles of both the pharynx and esophagus.

Gravity plays an important role in bolus transportation. In the upright position, a contrast bolus slides down the cervical and thoracic esophagus in less than a second.

Secondary esophageal peristalsis commences by distension or local irritation of the esophageal wall. A secondary peristaltic wave spreads in a distal direction in the same way as a primary propulsive peristaltic wave. A monophasic wave of positive pressure is recorded manometrically. The secondary peristaltic wave has a smaller amplitude than the primary. If primary peristalsis does not succeed in propelling the bolus, secondary peristalsis will drive the bolus into the stomach. Secondary peristalsis empties the esophagus of food particles and regurgitated contents of the stomach, and is a normal phenomenon. It may be observed in any section of the esophagus, though it is seen more often in the distal two-thirds (Fig. 2.7).

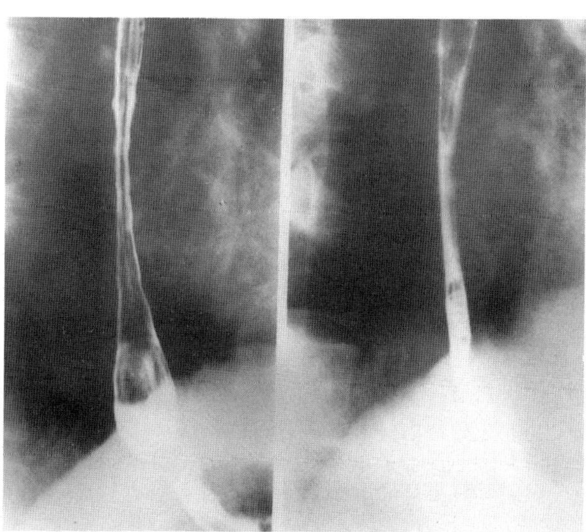

FIGURE 2.6. Primary esophageal peristalsis.

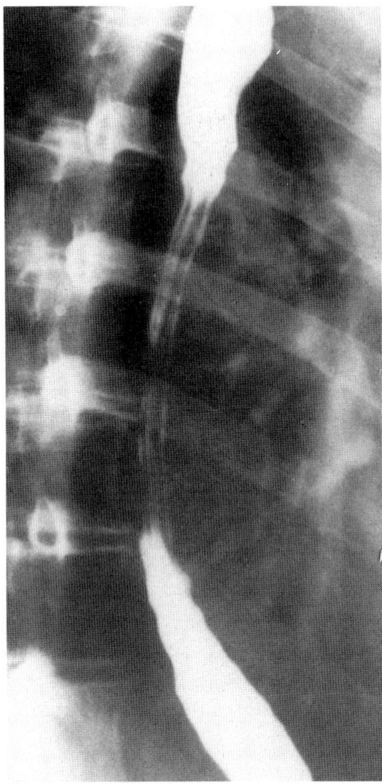

Figure 2.7. Secondary esophageal peristalsis.

Tertiary contractions of the esophagus are neither peristaltic nor coordinated. They vary in amplitude from fasciculations to pseudodiverticular contractions (Fig. 2.8). Tertiary contractions may be confined to only one section of the esophagus. They can, but need not, reflect pathological changes. Occasionally, they are clinically inapparent. If they are of high amplitude, the clinical symptoms may mimic a heart attack. Tertiary contractions may result from a break in the reflex arches above, or at the level of, myenteric ganglia, or from the absence of a motoric response to swallowing. The final phase in the act of swallowing is discussed in the paragraph on LES in chapter 1.

MOTILITY OF THE STOMACH

Fluoroscopy is a primary technique for examination of gastric peristalsis. When followed by spot films, it yields sufficient information in most cases. For a thorough analysis, gastric movements should also be recorded on videotape.

Both frequency and intensity of gastric peristaltic waves are rather variable in normal subjects. Contractions of the muscularis mucosae change the pattern of gastric folds. Tone represents permanent contraction of the gastric muscles, and along with the volume of contents and posture, it influences the shape of the stomach. Tone is inversely proportional to the average capacity of the stomach; hence, as a result of gastric compliance, intragastric pressure does not increase during filling.

The tension of the gastric wall remains constant, although the volume may change throughout a broad range. Tone is regulated by the autonomic nervous system. Mechanoreceptors in gastric mucosa register the degree of distension and, via a reflex arch, modify the tone. Corticovisceral pathways are also supposed to influence gastric tone, which is proportional to the intensity and frequency of peristaltic

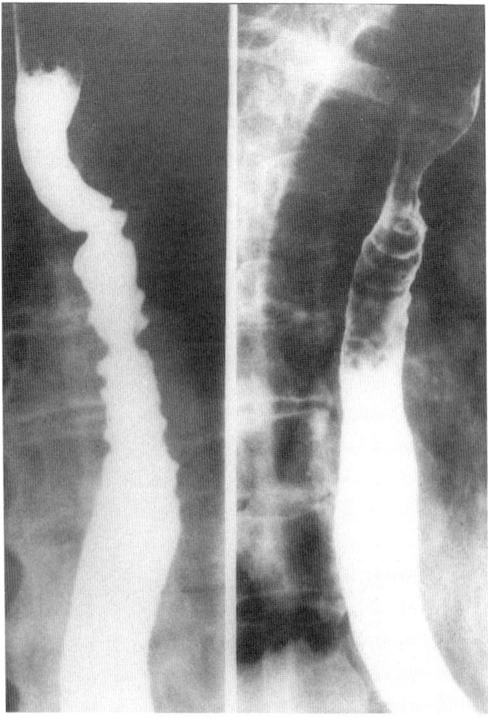

Figure 2.8. Tertiary esophageal contractions.

waves, that is, high tone stimulates peristalsis. In a standing patient, peristalsis originates on the lesser curvature of the stomach near the angular notch. In the prone position, peristalsis originates just distal to the cardia. Almost simultaneous with a peristaltic wave on the lesser curvature, a symmetric and somewhat deeper contraction indents the greater curvature. The amplitude of both waves increases toward the pylorus.

Peristalsis commences following the increase of tone. Type I waves of low amplitude mix gastric contents. These transient tonic contractions last for approximately 1 minute. Their frequency is higher in the fundus than in the antrum. Deep propulsive waves are referred to as type II, and occur about three times a minute. Three peristaltic waves are usually seen at the same time. Reaching the antrum, a peristaltic wave becomes a stationary nonperistaltic contraction of the antrum (Fig. 2.9). This is followed by a contraction of particularly arranged, crossed antral muscles—the torus. Complete antral contraction propels the bolus into the duodenum; if the contraction is incomplete, the bolus will remain in the stomach. Both the duration and strength of nonperistaltic antral contractions are proportional to the amplitude of the peristaltic wave that initiates the contraction. The contents enter the duodenum through the opened pylorus. The action of pharmacologically active substances on gastric motility is discussed in chapter 4.

Tonic rhythmic movements of the proximal

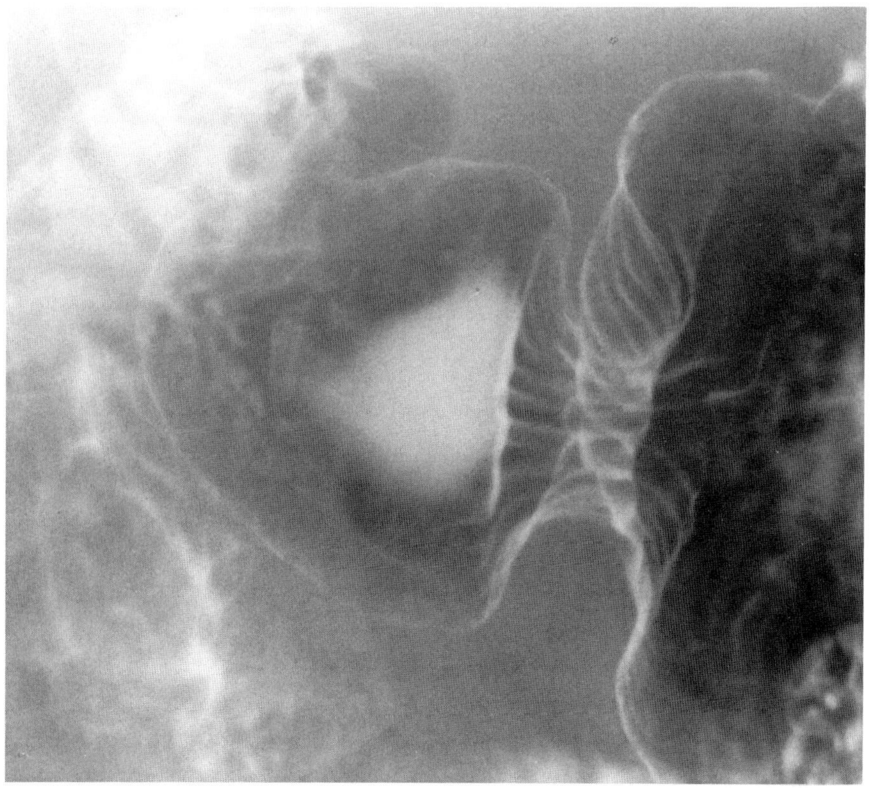

Figure 2.9. Gastric peristaltic wave transforms into stationary antral contraction.

duodenum are inhibited during the antral contraction. They reappear after contraction of the pyloric sphincter. Contractions of the duodenal bulb and the pyloric sphincter are both synchronous.

Liquid contents are evacuated from the stomach down two parallel grooves near the lesser curvature. Emptying of the stomach depends on the volume, consistency, osmolarity, and pH of the contents. It is regulated by a strong pyloric sphincter. Gastrin increases the tone of gastric muscles. Both pyloric and enterogastric reflexes and enterogastrone delay emptying of the stomach. Contact of duodenal mucosa with fatty acids is a trigger for the secretion of enterogastrone. It inhibits both secretion and motility of the stomach.

Extremely deep peristaltic waves occur in compensated stages of pyloric and duodenal obstructions. This hyperperistalsis is probably due to the absence of inhibitory enterogastric reflexes. Localized hypertonia is sometimes observed on the gastric wall opposite a peptic ulcer (Fig. 2.10). Gastric atonia accompanies vascular shock, diabetic acidosis, and surgical operations. Gastric peristalsis is absent in portions of the stomach affected by neoplastic infiltration or extensive scarring.

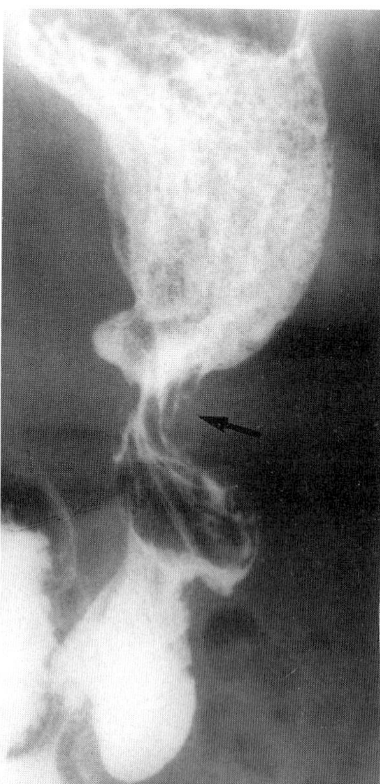

Figure 2.10. Spasm of the gastric wall (arrow) opposite a peptic ulcer.

MOTILITY OF THE SMALL BOWEL

Peristalsis of the Duodenum

The duodenal bulb is not anatomically differentiated but is the result of low tone in the proximal duodenum. Peristalsis of the duodenum is an extension of gastric peristalsis. Peristaltic contraction commences in the bulb and spreads distally (Fig. 2.11). Duodenal contents are propelled by peristalsis into the mesenteric small intestine.

There are two types of movement in the mesenteric small intestine: rhythmic segmental contraction and peristalsis.

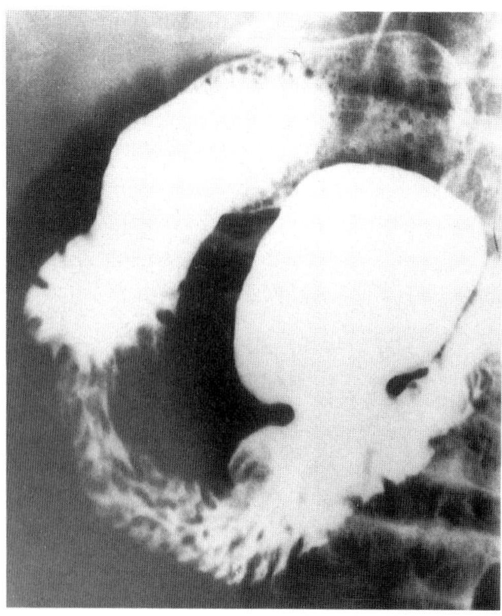

Figure 2.11. Peristaltic wave of the duodenum. Large duodenal diverticulum.

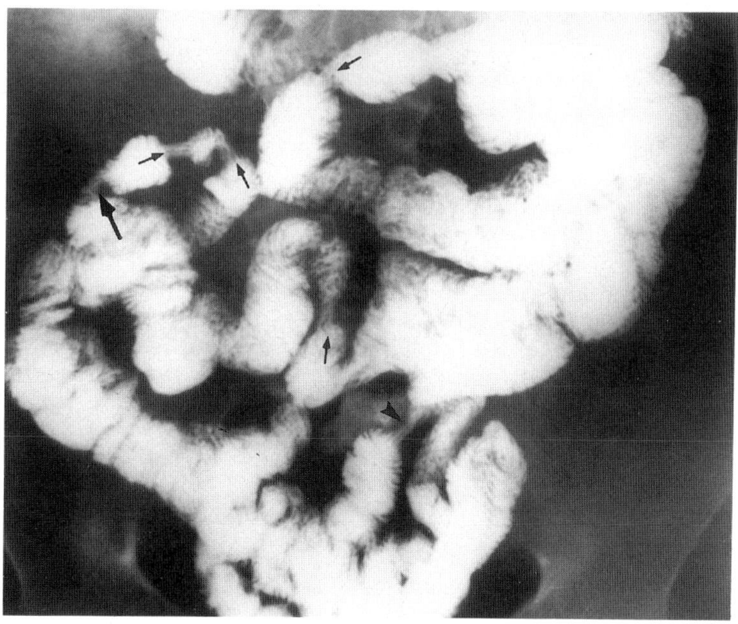

Figure 2.12. Rhythmic segmental contractions of the small bowel (arrows and arrowhead).

Rhythmic Segmental Contractions of the Small Bowel

These movements occur with constant frequency in short equidistant segments of the small bowel. Circular contractions divide the small bowel into sections only a few centimeters long. Relaxation follows the contraction of an intestinal segment while an adjacent dilated section undergoes contraction (Fig. 2.12).

Rhythmic segmental contractions may be eccentrically confined to a portion of the intestinal curvature. These eccentric contractions mix intestinal contents, while concentric contractions, which completely encircle the lumen, evacuate the corresponding segment. Segmental contractions occur with a frequency of 11 per minute and 8 per minute in the duodenum and ileum, respectively. These contractions are not depleted by denervation, suggesting that they are governed by the myenteric plexus. Nevertheless, they may be modified by the autonomic nervous system. Cholinergic stimulation activates, whereas adrenergic stimulation suppresses, segmental contractions.

Peristalsis of the Small Bowel

A series of contraction phenomena with propagation in a distal direction is referred to as peristalsis. The contraction wave slips along the bowel as it vanishes proximally. The distance covered by a peristaltic wave usually amounts to a few centimeters, but may sometimes be up to a few meters. Peristaltic waves occur in the small intestine at irregular intervals. Individual waves usually last more than a second. The degree of temporospatial integration of peristalsis in the small intestine is not as high as in the esophagus or gastric antrum.

Motility of the Ileocecal Valve. At the termination of each peristaltic wave in the terminal ileum, the circular muscle sphincter of the ileocecal valve is relaxed, permitting a few milliliters of small bowel contents to enter the cecum. A short relaxation is then replaced by a contraction. The valve regulates filling of the cecum and probably prevents regurgitation into the terminal ileum. Gastroileal reflex, initiated by distension of the gastric wall by food or liquid, stimulates peristalsis of the terminal ileum.

MOTILITY OF THE LARGE BOWEL

Movement of the large intestine is seen only exceptionally during routine contrast examination. Movements may be observed in patients with irritable colon (Fig. 2.13). Gastrocolic reflex, initiated by gastric distension, provokes lively colonic peristalsis. Motility of the cecum is minimal. In contrast, two types of movements occur in the colon. The first type mixes contents but does not transport them distally. These are *stationary rhythmic contractions and relaxations*. They are analogous to segmental contractions of the small intestine, but not as intensive. Stationary rhythmic contractions may vary in duration, but appear at regular intervals of 30 seconds and occupy a long segment, usually a few haustral compartments. *Propulsive contractions* of the large intestine

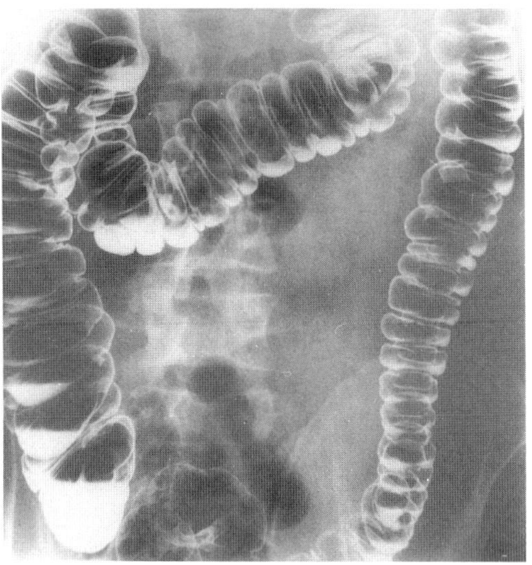

Figure 2.13. Pronounced haustral markings of the colon due to main muscular coat contractions.

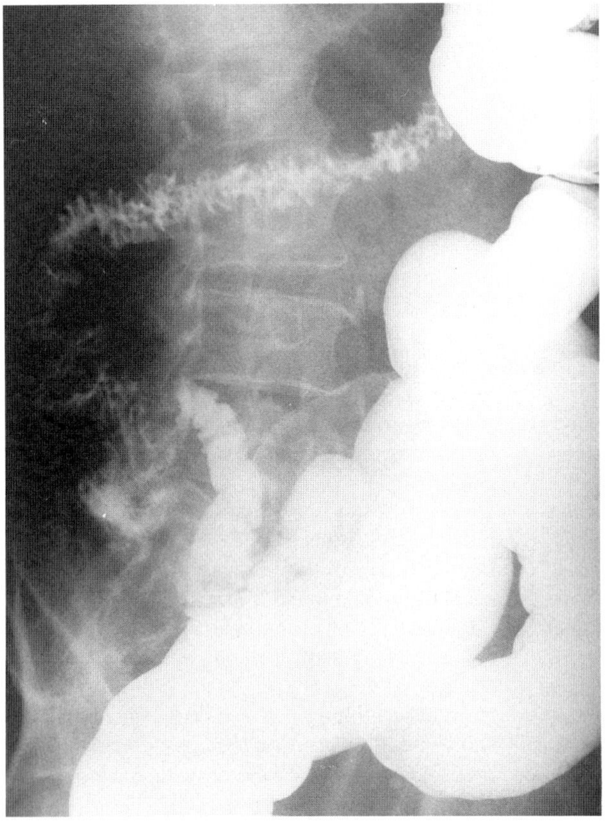

Figure 2.14. Massive movement of the colon in the barium filling phase.

also include massive movements. As in other alimentary canal organs, this motility is initiated by distension due to accumulation of contents. Peristalsis of the large intestine occurs mostly during defecation. Massive movements involving long sections appear after a meal and transport large amounts of feces (Fig. 2.14). They occur only a few times per day.

Stationary rhythmic contractions and cycles of reverse peristalsis dominate the right hemicolon. Hence, the contents of the cecum and ascending colon stagnate for more than 8 hours. In these sections water is absorbed from the 800–900 mL of liquid chyme that daily enter the cecum through the ileocecal valve.

Defecation is influenced by a series of control mechanisms. Continence is maintained by the external anal sphincter and levator ani muscle. Contraction of the latter decreases the angle between the rectum and anal canal. Distension of the rectum provokes parasympathetic stimulation from the sacral plexus and stimulation of the myenteric plexus. Thereafter, the internal anal sphincter is involuntarily relaxed, and this is followed by voluntary relaxation of the external anal sphincter. The angle between the rectum and the anal canal, measuring 100 degrees at rest, is thus practically flattened, allowing for the passage of contents.

Bibliography

Ardaran GM, Kelleher WH, Kemp FH. Closure and opening of the larynx during swallowing. Br J Radiol. 1956;29:205.

Christensen J. The controls of the gastrointestinal movements: some old and new views. N Engl J Med. 1971;285:85.

Donner MW, Silberger ML. Cinefluorographic analysis of pharyngeal swallowing in neuromuscular disorders. Am J Med Sci. 1966;261:600.

Donner MW. Normal and abnormal motility of the stomach. Radiol Clin North Am. 1976;14:441.

Durdle NG, Kingma YJ, Bowes KL, Chanbers MM. Origin of slow waves in the canine colon. Gastroenterology. 1983;84:375.

Forsell G. Studies of the mechanism of movement of the mucous membrane of the digestive tract. AJR. 1923;10:87.

Garry RC. The movements of the large intestine. Physiol Rev. 1934;13:103.

Hell KE, El-Sharkawy TY, Diamant NE. Vagal control of migrating motor complex in the dog. Am J Gastrointest Liver Physiol. 1982;6:6276.

Hinder RA. Individual and combined roles of the pylorus and the antrum in the canine gastric emptying of the liquid and a digestible solid. Gastroenterology. 1983;84:281.

Isberg A, Nilsson ME, Schiratzki H. Movement of the upper esophageal sphincter and a manometric device during deglutition. A cineradiographic investigation. Acta Radiol Diagn. 1985;26:381.

Johnstone AS. A radiological study of deglutition. J Anat (Lond). 1942;77:100.

Keet AD Jr. The prepyloric contractions in the normal stomach. Acta Radiol. 1957;48:413.

Margulis AR, Koehler RE. Radiologic diagnosis of disordered esophageal motility. Radiol Clin North Am. 1976;14:429.

Miller AJ. Deglutition. Physiol Rev. 1982;62:129.

Ramsey GH, Watson JS, Gramiak R, Weinber SA. Cinefluorographic analysis of the mechanism of swallowing. Radiology. 1955;64:498.

Rushmer RF, Hendrom JA. The act of deglutition. A cinefluoroscopic study. J Appl Physiol. 1951; 3:622.

Schulze Delrien K, Shirazi SS. Neuromuscular differentiation of the human pylorus. Gastroenterology. 1983;84:287.

Soergel KH, Zboralske FF, Amberg JR. Presbyesophagus. Esophageal manometry in nonagenarians. J Clin Invest. 1964;43:1472.

Spjut HJ. Stomach and duodenum. Pathology. In: Margulis AR, Burhenne HJ (eds). Alimentary Tract Radiology, vol 1. St. Louis: CV Mosby; 1989:513.

Talbot IC. Colon. Pathology. In: Margulis AR, Burhenne HJ (eds). Alimentary Tract Radiology, vol 1. St. Louis: CV Mosby; 1989:869.

Truelove SC. Movements of the large intestine. Physiol Rev. 1966;46:512.

Wu WC, Kisslinger SD, Gaginella TS. Functional evidence for the presence of cholinergic nerve endings in the colonic mucosa of the rat. J Pharmacol Exp Ther. 1982;221:664.

Chapter 3

Radiologic Aspects of Gastrointestinal Pathology

NORMAL AND PATHOLOGIC CHARACTERISTICS

Radiologic examination should detect most gross pathologic lesions of the alimentary canal. Fundamental characteristics of a normal alimentary canal concern position, dimension and wall integrity, mucosal relief of a typical configuration, and regular dimensions. Organs are mobile and pliable. Wall motility, such as peristalsis and segmental contractions, may be seen. The presence of gas, liquid, or solid contents may reflect normal or pathologic conditions. The alimentary canal can react to various injuries with similar radiologic appearance. Normal tissues are destroyed and excess tissues are formed. However, properties such as wall compliance can be modified without alteration in the inner or outer surfaces of the organs. Masses protruding into the lumen cause negative defects of a radiographic contrast column, contrary to positive defects caused by depressed lesions such as diverticula or ulcers (Diagram 3.1 and Figs. 3.1 and 3.2).

Pathologic processes may be divided into categories based on the length of the canal affected. A *diffuse* process involves the entire alimentary canal or some of its organs. A *segmental* process affects a major portion of an alimentary canal organ with normal proximal and distal segments. A *regional* process extends through a complete portion of an organ such as the gastric antrum or the cecum. The segments involved are shorter than with segmental distribution. A *focal* process affects an even shorter portion of the alimentary canal. Focal lesions can be solitary or multiple. When fused, focal lesions may involve longer segments of the alimentary canal.

In a *discontinuous* process, in contrast to a *continuous* one, segments of normal wall alternate with pathology, as in Crohn's disease. Regarding *depth*, a lesion can be confined to a particular layer such as the mucosa or affect deeper layers of the wall. Transmural lesions affect the entire wall thickness. Any layer of the wall may be the origin of, or be affected by, a pathologic process.

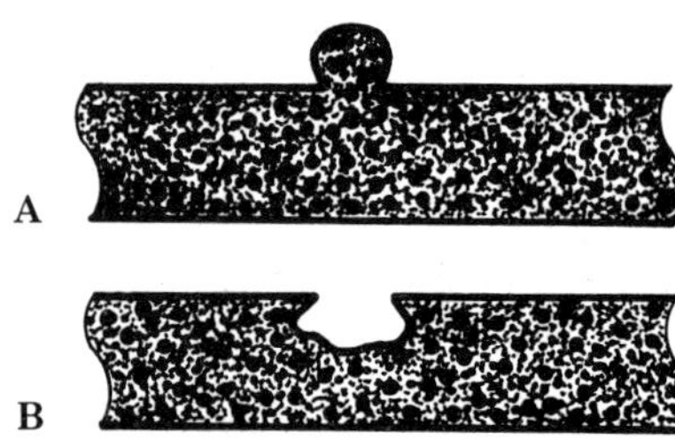

DIAGRAM 3.1. Defects of the contrast column in the alimentary canal. (A) Positive defect. (B) Negative defect.

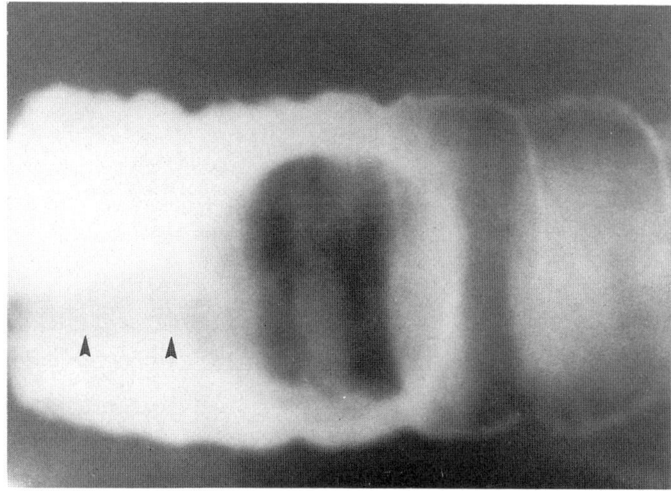

FIGURE 3.1. Colon polyp on a stalk (arrowheads), a negative defect in the contrast column.

Edema of the alimentary canal wall results in a homogenous swelling of mucosal relief elements. *Inflammatory* mucosal folds are thickened along with an appearance of ulceration, hyperplastic formation, and changes in lumen diameter. In advanced stages the mucosal surface may be smooth, as a result of atrophy, and devoid of anatomic features. *Ulcers* may be peptic, inflammatory, ischemic, malignant, or idiopathic.

Neoplasms can extend in various directions but most commonly narrow the lumen. They may be benign or malignant, primary or secondary. Distinction between primary and secondary neoplasms may be difficult. *Impressions* by adjacent organs displace the gastric mucosal pattern without causing destruction (Fig. 3.3). It may be impossible to distinguish an intramural process from a submucosal lesion solely by the use of barium studies without correlative computed tomography (CT). Large impressions and submucosal lesions can even efface the mucosal surface. Involvement of an inflammatory or neoplastic lesion originating in an adjacent anatomic structure may alter the pliability of the alimentary canal wall. Stenoses of the alimentary canal can result from either inflammations or neoplasms (Fig. 3.4). Widening of the alimentary canal may result from altered innervation, muscular lesions such as sclero-

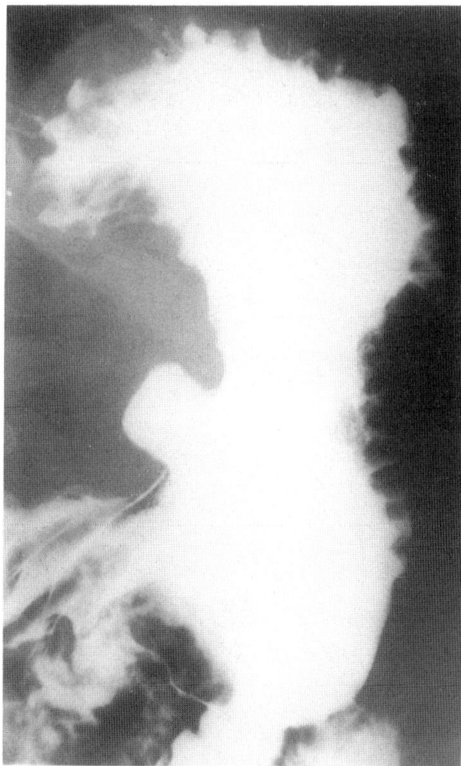

FIGURE 3.2. Peptic ulcer of the lesser gastric curvature penetrating into the lesser sac. Positive defect in the contrast column.

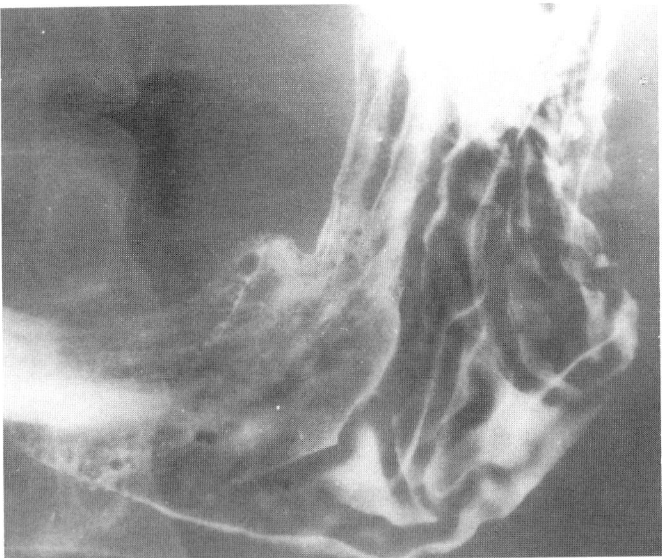

Figure 3.3. Retrogastric mass. Pseudocyst of the body of the pancreas. Gastric rugae are displaced in an arcuate manner by extrinsic compression from the mass. Identical finding may result from large submucosal masses in the gastric wall.

derma (Fig. 3.5), or growth of certain neoplasms, but it is most frequently found proximal to a stenosis.

In the radiographic analysis of a pathological process of the alimentary canal, the morphology and number of lesions, as well as the location, must be taken into consideration. Prevalence of the suspected disease, the frequency of particular symptoms, and the accurate evaluation of those symptoms should guide the diagnostic process. Pathological changes may be congenital or acquired.

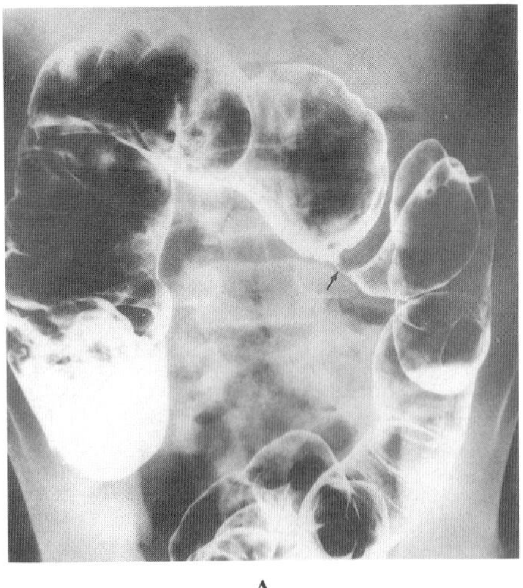

A

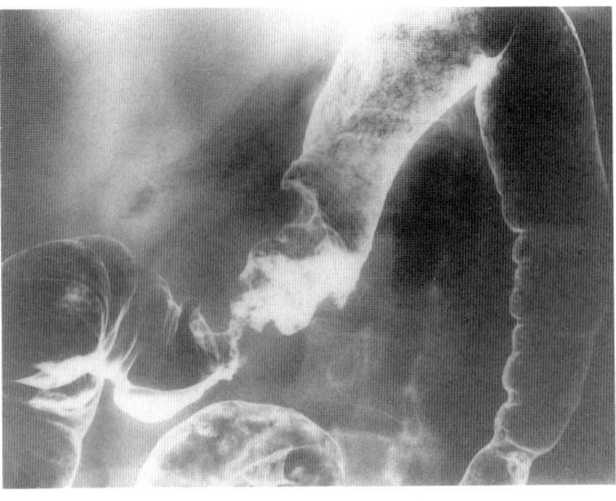

B

Figure 3.4. (A) Benign-appearing stenosis of the transverse colon (arrow) in Crohn's disease. (B) Typical malignant stenosis in the transverse colon of carcinoma.

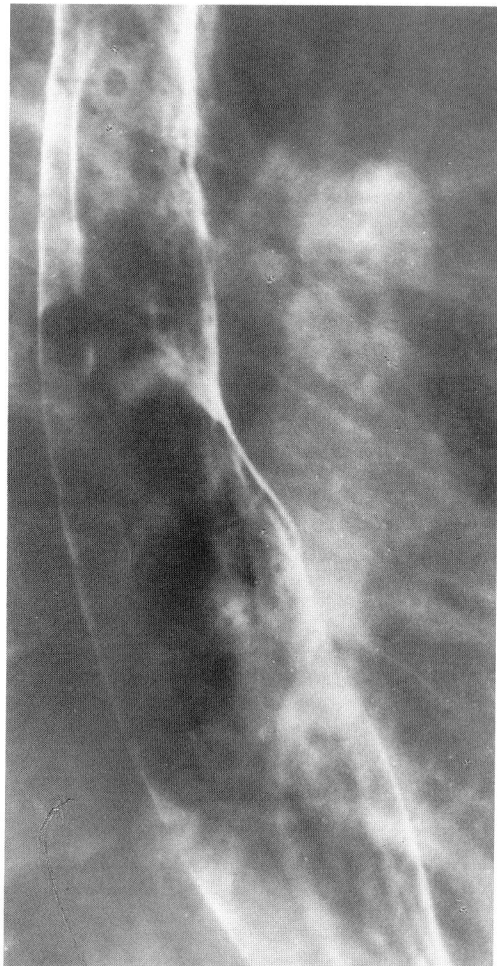

FIGURE 3.5. Dilatation of the esophageal lumen in scleroderma.

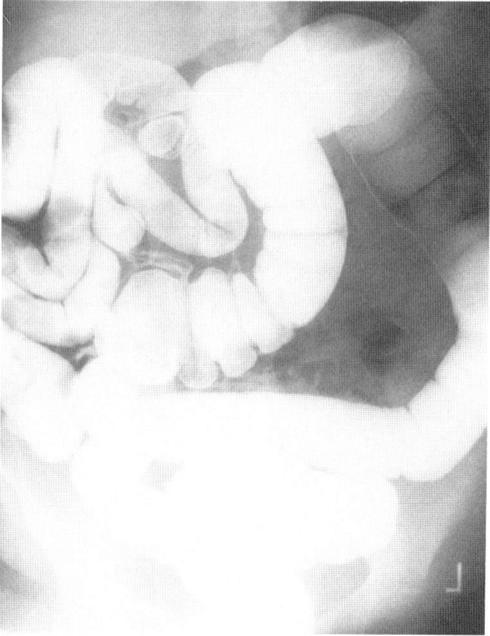

FIGURE 3.6. Common ileocolic mesentery (nonrotation of the intestine).

CONGENITAL ANOMALIES

Agenesis is partial or complete absence of an organ, and is not common. Congenital changes in the *position* of alimentary canal organs exist in *inverse situs of organs*. Furthermore, some abdominal sections of the digestive tube even may lie in the thoracic cavity. *Malrotation* is also characterized by unusual arrangements of the gastrointestinal tract (Figs. 3.6 and 3.7). Due to insufficient fixation for the posterior abdominal wall and long mesentery, sections of the alimentary canal may remain excessively

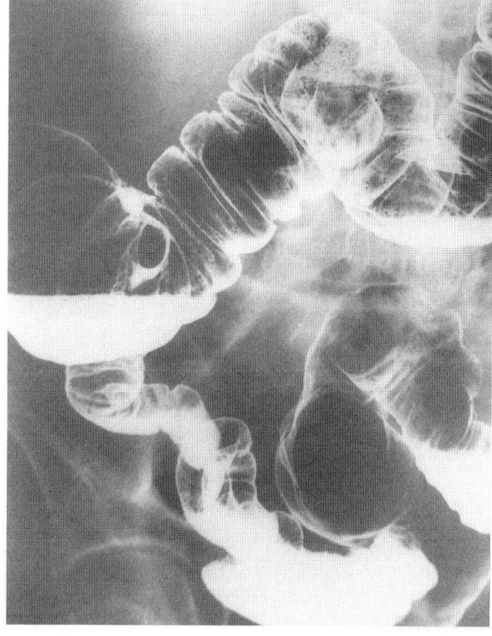

FIGURE 3.7. Congenital fixation anomaly. The tip of the cecum is cranially directed.

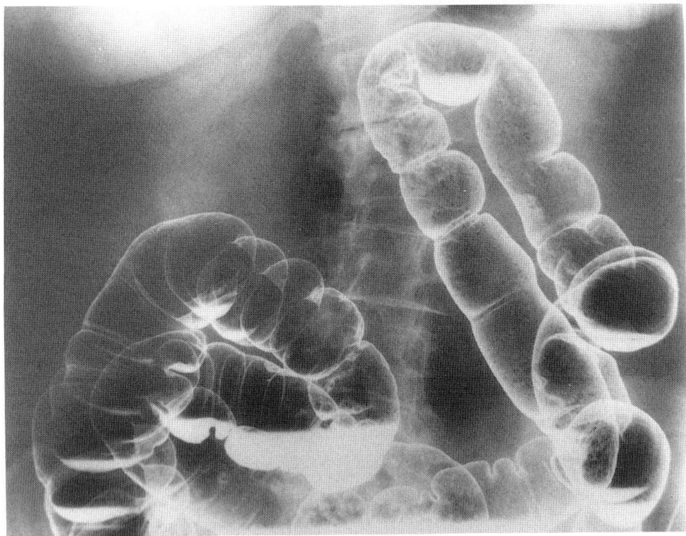

Figure 3.8. Very elongated colon.

mobile. In the condition termed "common ileocolic mesentery," both mesentery and mesocolon are mobile and in continuity with each other. Individual sections of the digestive tube may vary in *length*; the esophagus may be short and the colon elongated (Fig. 3.8). Any section of the gastrointestinal tract may have an *obturated or inadequate lumen*. Absence of lumen is termed *atresia*, and there is a solid band instead of a tube. Esophageal atresia (Fig. 3.9) is usually associated with esophagotracheal fistula. Atresias may be located in the small intestine, particularly duodenum and ileum. The colon is the least likely to be atretic. Unperforated anus is also a form of atresia. Narrowing of the lumen is termed *stenosis*. *Diverticula* may appear as developmental anomalies (Fig. 3.10). These are saccular bulges of the alimentary canal. The wall of a congenital diverticulum, as opposed to the majority of acquired diverticula, which are mucosal and submucosal prolapses, is composed of the same layers as the adjacent alimentary canal wall. Meckel's diverticulum is a remnant of an omphaloenteric duct. It originates within 1 meter of the ileocecal valve. In 25% of cases Meckel's diverticula contain islets of gastric mucosa. *Aganglionic megacolon* is characterized by absence of both myenteric and submucous plexuses in a segment of the large intestine. In 5% of patients the entire large intestine is aganglionic. The aganglionic intestinal segment is aperistaltic, creating a functional obstruction. Proximal sections are distended, with hypertrophic walls (Fig. 3.11). *Choristomas* are rare anomalies, representing heterotopic pancreatic tissue in the stomach or duodenum. *Duplications* of the alimentary ca-

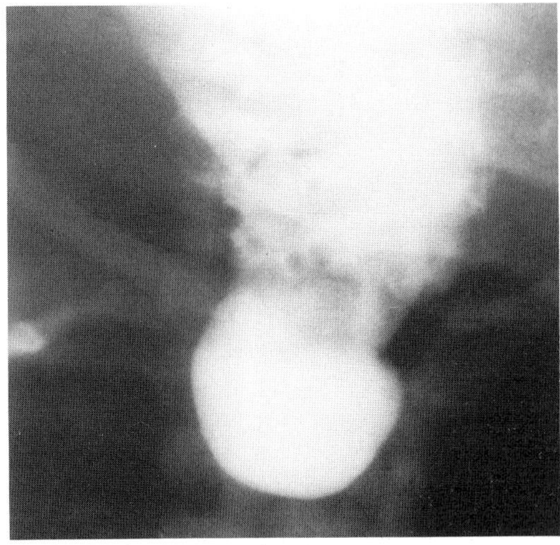

Figure 3.9. Esophageal atresia. Water soluble isotonic, nonionic contrast medium was administered under fluoroscopy and removed after examination. The figure is used only for the purpose of illustration.

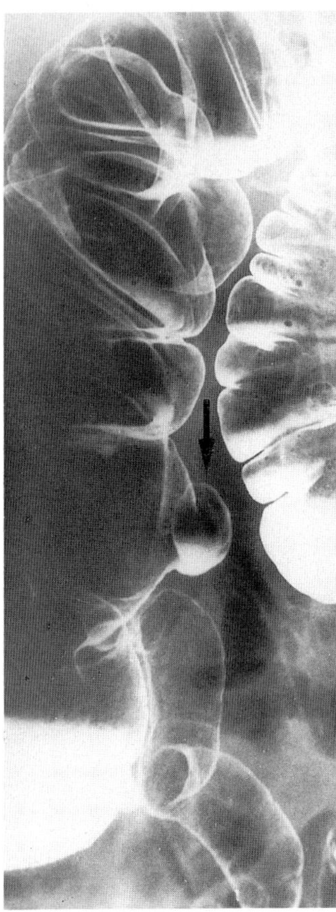

Figure 3.10. Solitary large diverticulum of the ascending colon (arrow) in a young person. Probably congenital diverticulum.

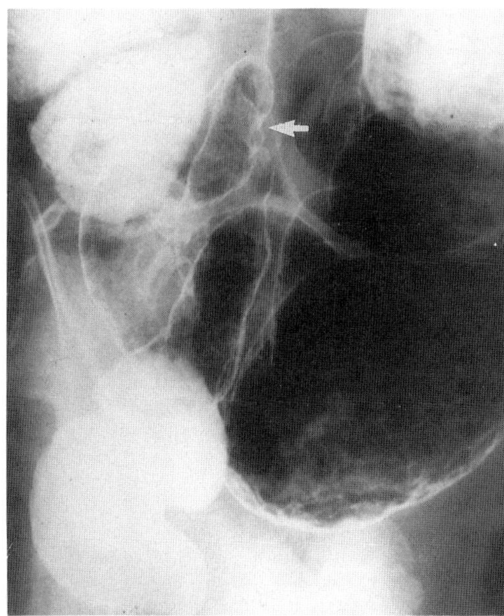

Figure 3.11. Congenital megacolon. Hirschprung's disease. Aganglionic segment in the sigmoid colon (arrow) resulting in proximal dilatation.

nal are uncommon. They may occur in any section of the digestive tube, particularly in the ileum. Duplications may share a portion of the wall or mesentery. They may, but need not, communicate with each other. If a communication exists, a duplicated section can be filled with barium during the examination (Figs. 7.19 and 9.6). Noncommunicating duplications appear on barium studies as negative defects caused by extrinsic impressions. Duplications of the digestive tube may be demonstrated by CT. In the esophagus and in the small intestine the duplications are tubular or spherical. *Cysts* are similar to duplications, but are spherical in shape and do not communicate with the lumen of the gastrointestinal tract. Pseudocysts are acquired. Unlike cysts, their internal surface is not covered with epithelium.

ACQUIRED PATHOLOGIC CONDITIONS

Hernias refer to the abnormal position of alimentary canal organs caused by protrusions of an organ or portion thereof, through normal openings in the abdominal cavity or through defects in fascia planes. Hernias may be internal or external (Fig. 3.12). The former include herniations of sections of the alimentary canal into the lesser sac or duodenojejunal, pericecal, or intersigmoid recesses. The alimentary canal lumen may be abnormally narrowed or widened. *Stenoses* are congenital or acquired, and may be either benign or malignant. However, benign stenoses, whether acquired or congenital, may lead to life-threatening obstruction. Postinflammatory stenoses are termed strictures (Fig. 3.13). Foreign bodies may lead to gastrointestinal obstruction. The alimentary canal lumen can also be narrowed by adhe-

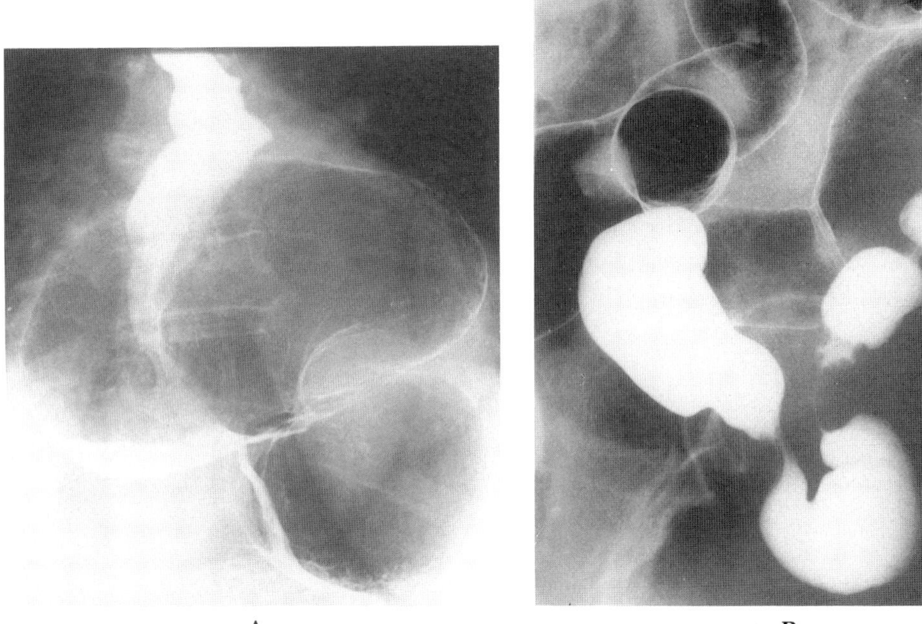

A B

Figure 3.12. (A) Paraesophageal hernia of the stomach. (B) Inguinal hernia of the sigmoid colon.

sions, torsion, strangulation, and invagination (Fig. 3.14). Malignant tumors are common causes of stenosis. *Dilatation* develops proximal to stenoses, with concomitant hypertrophy of the muscular layer. Neoplasms spreading along the intestinal wall and destroying intramural ganglia also cause dilatation. This mode of growth is more characteristic of lymphomas (Fig. 3.15A) than of carcinomas. On rare occasions, when a carcinoma grows toward the serosa, resultant dilatation corresponds to the location of the tumor. Any dilatation distal to the tumor is attributed to destruction of the intramural neuronal network (Fig. 3.15B).

Obstructions are caused by stenoses, aganglionic segments, achalasia (Fig. 3.16), and foreign bodies. The etiopathogenesis of obstructions is discussed in chapter 5. *Acquired diverticula* are false diverticula, prolapses of mucosa and submucosa only through the muscle layers (Figs. 3.17 and 3.18). They occur preferentially where blood vessels enter the intestine. These sites are weak points because they are filled with loose connective tissue. Unlike false diverticula, the walls of true diverticula are composed of the same layers as the normal intestinal wall. Pulsion diverticula, most commonly located in the sigmoid and descending colon, are false, whereas traction diverticula are true diverticula. The term "pseudodiverticula" is sometimes used to denote abnormal bulges of the wall that appear near nonelastic, fibrotic, or scarred segments of the alimentary canal, such as postulcerative deformity of the duodenal bulb or deformity adjacent to stenoses in Crohn's disease.

Cysts filled with gas located in intestinal submucosa or subserosa are called *pneumatosis intestinalis cystica* (Figs. 10.6 and 12.32). Etiologic factors include obstructions, inflammation, cough, and endoscopic maneuvers.

Vascular disorders may affect any section of the digestive tube. Significant bleeding can be caused by peptic ulcers, erosions, varices (Fig. 3.19), malformations, or tumors. The esophagus and the stomach are sites of predilection for submucosal varices. Infarctions of

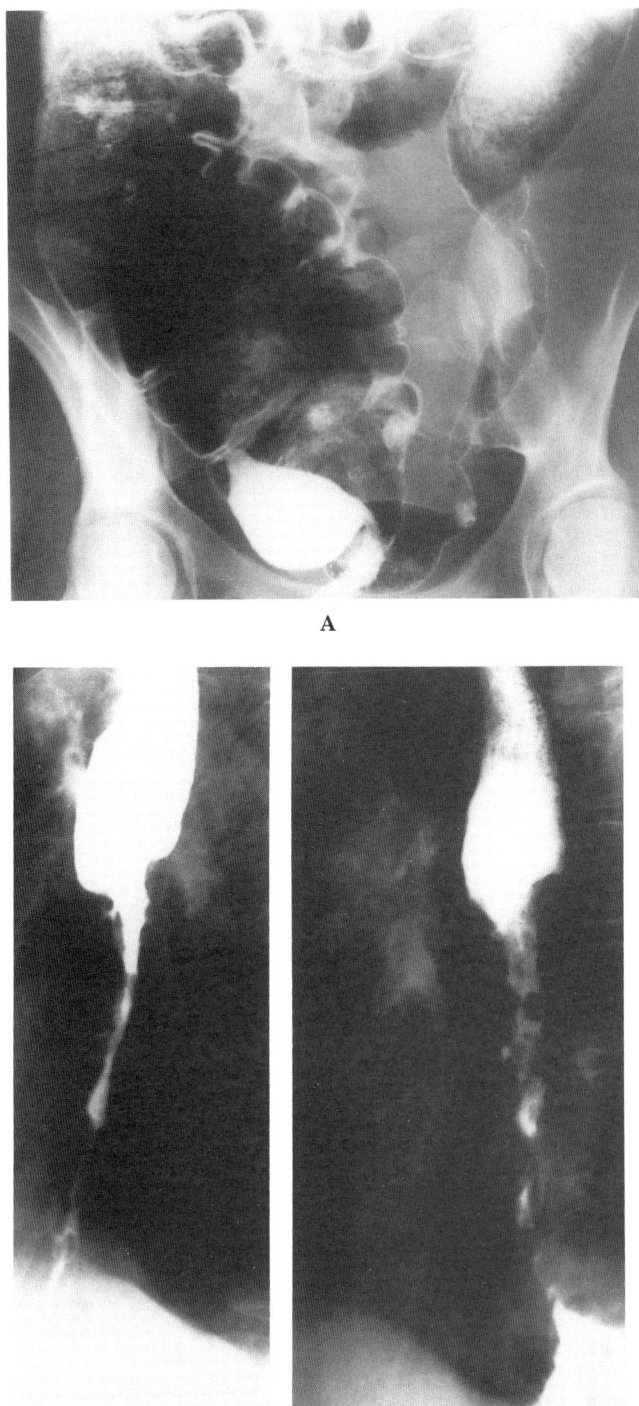

Figure 3.13. (A) Long, benign-appearing stricture of the descending and sigmoid colon with proximal dilatation in Crohn's disease. (B) Long malignant stenosis of esophageal carcinoma.

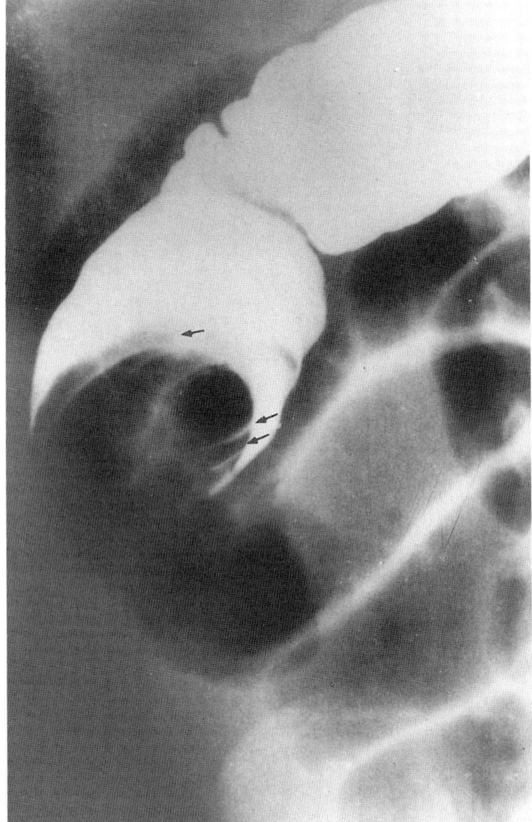

A

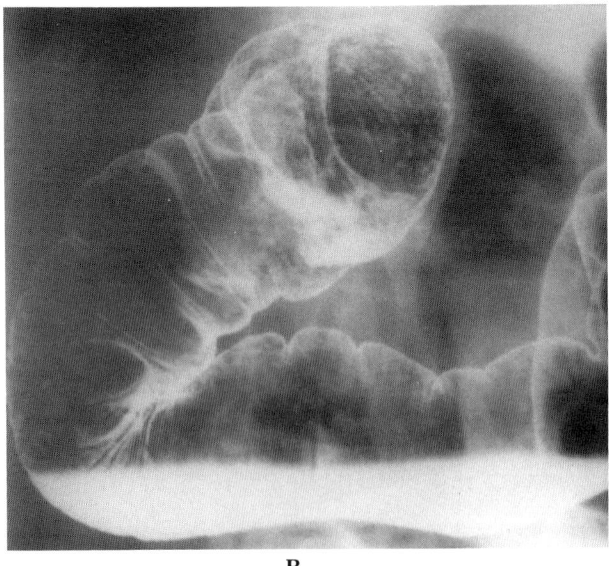

B

FIGURE 3.14. (A) Colocolic intussusception resulting in obstruction of the small bowel in a child (arrows). (B) Intussusception of the transverse colon resulting from carcinoma. Coiled spring appearance of barium entering between the intussusceptum and the intussuscipiens.

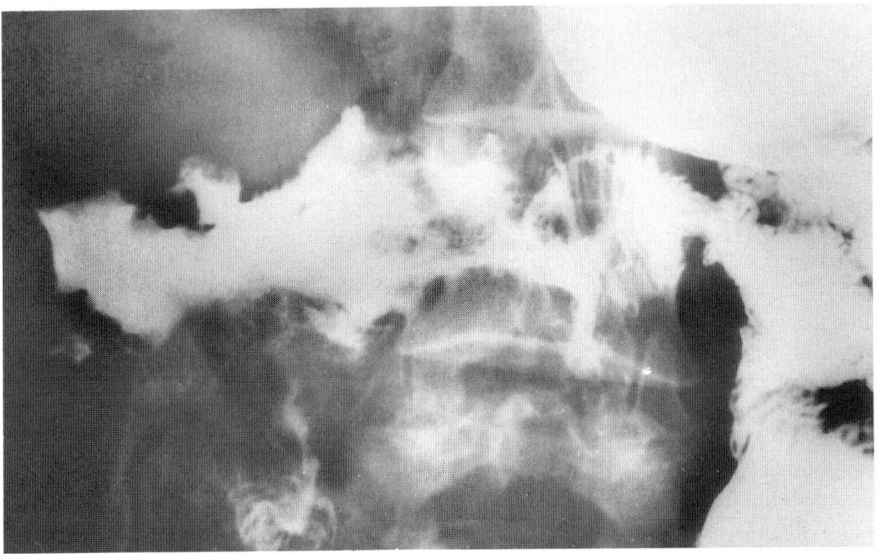

A

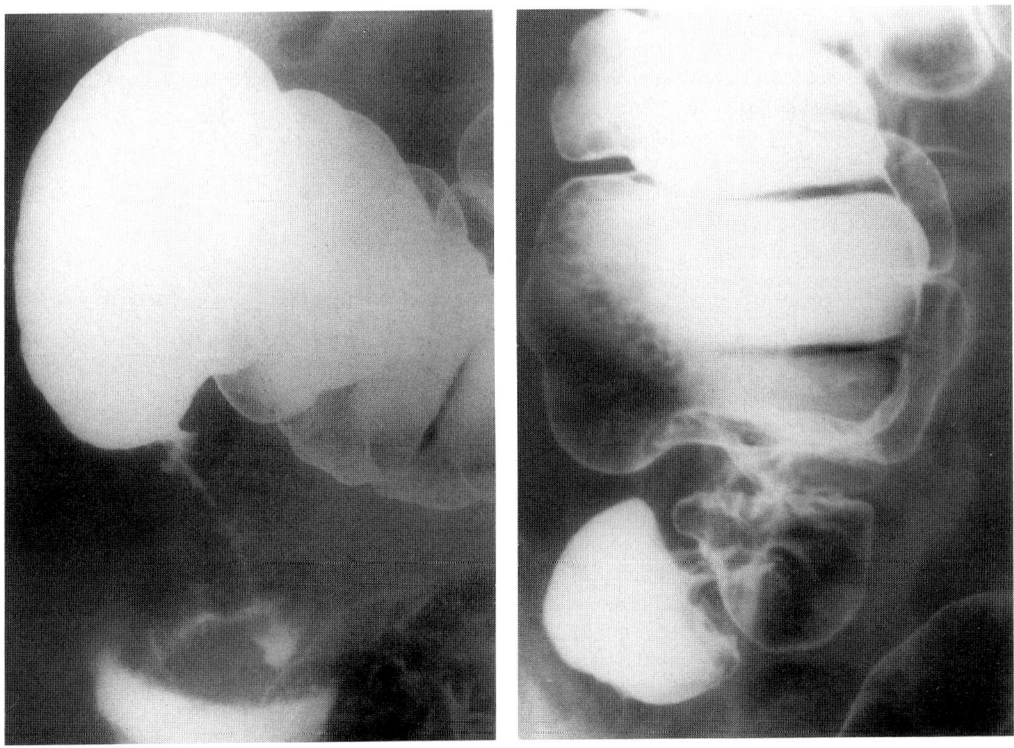

B

FIGURE 3.15. (A) Irregular dilatation of the small bowel caused by lymphoma. (B) Poststenotic dilatation, resulting from neuronal network destruction by carcinoma.

the alimentary canal are mostly hemorrhagic. Ischemic infarction results from obstruction of a branch of the mesenteric artery distal to anastomosing arcades. The amount of damage to the wall depends on the degree of arterial narrowing and anastomoses, and on rapidity of onset. In complete obstruction with insufficient collateral circulation, gangrene may develop leading to bowel perforation.

Angiodysplasias are acquired dilatations of veins, venules, and capillaries in the mucosa and submucosa of the digestive tract. Most of them are found in the large intestine, particularly in the right hemicolon. Degenerative processes and aging are possibly etiologic factors. Bleeding may be minimal, but massive hemorrhage is a potential risk. Angiography demonstrates angiodysplasias as accumulations of radiographic contrast medium in dilated vascular spaces (Fig. 4.89).

Any region of the gastrointestinal tract can be affected by *inflammation* and is subject to both specific and nonspecific changes. The clinical course may be either acute or chronic, with a spectrum of intermediate stages (Fig. 3.20). Inflammations can be catarrhal, pseudomembranous, or purulent, or can result in infected necrosis. Chronic inflammations of the stomach and the intestine are discussed separately in pertinent sections, because of their complicated pathophysiologic mechanisms.

Peptic ulcers occur exclusively on mucosa that is in contact with acidic gastric juice. Regardless of the site, the macroscopic and microscopic features of peptic ulcers are constant. In contrast to erosions that are no deeper than the lamina muscularis mucosae (Figs. 3.21 and 3.22), an active peptic ulcer extends to the main muscular coat or even deeper (Fig. 3.23A). A chronic ulcer characteristic of peptic disease often demonstrates an irregular crater and an inflammatory reaction near the edges. Healing leaves circular, linear, or stellate scars (Fig. 3.23B). Folds of the surrounding mucosa converge toward the scar. Deep and large scars may cause stenoses, particularly when located near areas of physiologic narrowings.

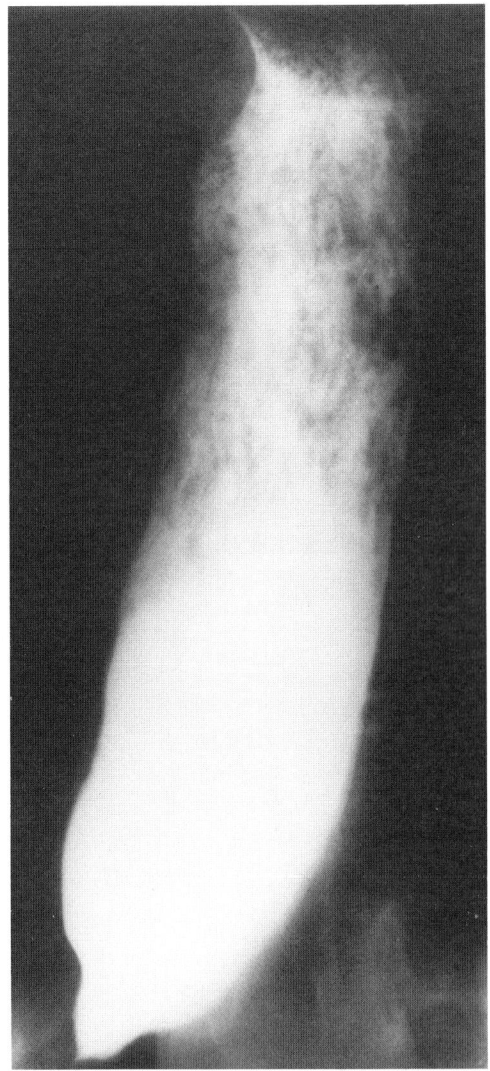

FIGURE 3.16. (A) Achalasia of the esophagus. Barium examination.

NEOPLASMS

Alimentary canal neoplasms are either epithelial or mesenchymal in origin. The neoplasms may be benign or malignant, and the degree of malignancy is subject to variation. For example, alimentary canal adenocarcinomas are very malignant and carcinoids have low malignant potential. Adenomas, fibromas, lipomas, leiomyomas, neurofibromas, and angiomas are benign tumors.

Gross pathologic features of neoplasms depend on:

1. The layer from which the tumor originates (mucosa, submucosa, muscular, serosa);

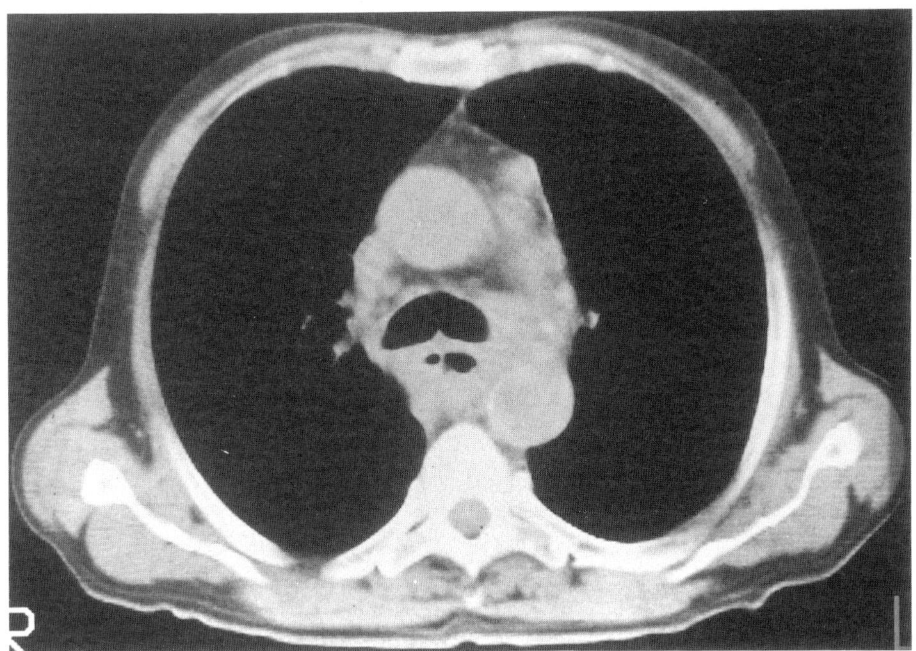

Figure 3.16. (B) Carcinoma in achalasia of the esophagus. CT examination.

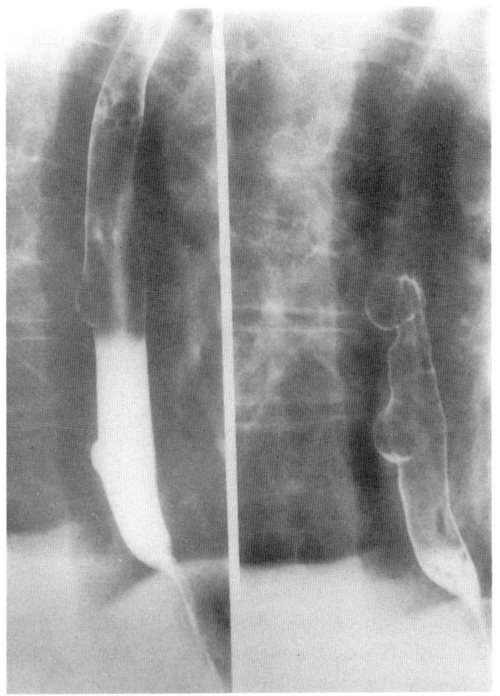

Figure 3.17. Pulsion diverticula of the esophagus.

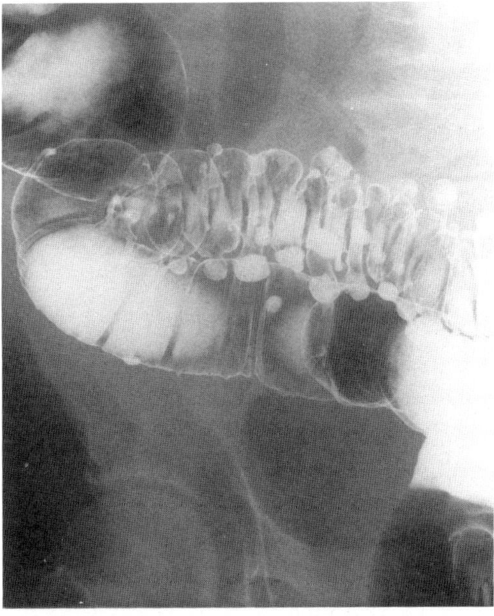

Figure 3.18. Diverticulosis of the sigmoid colon.

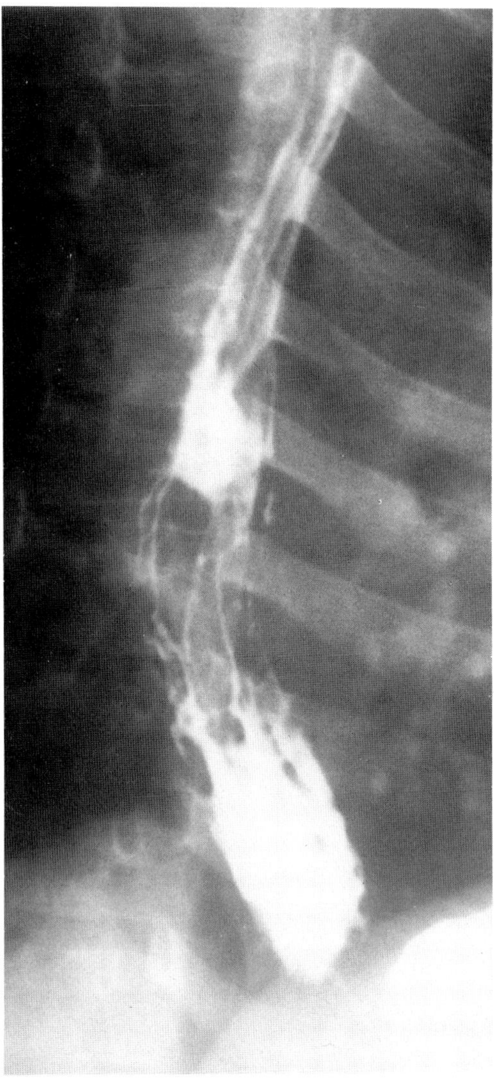

Figure 3.19. Esophageal varices.

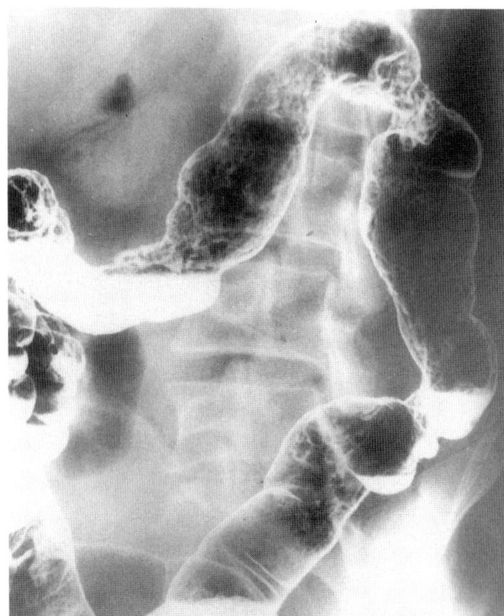

Figure 3.20. Crohn's disease affecting the colon. Involved segments alternate with skip areas.

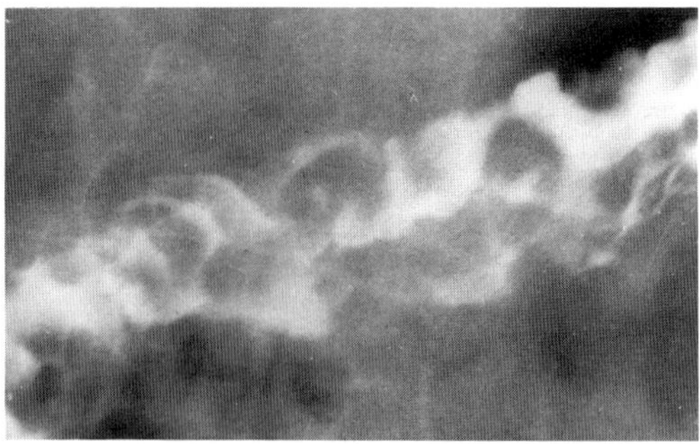

Figure 3.21. Multiple complete erosions of the gastric antrum. Controlled compression study.

2. The consistency of the tumor (for example, hemangiomas are soft and compressible whereas leiomyomas are hard);
3. The degree of invasiveness;
4. The dimensions.

Small mucosal tumors can be detected radiologically while subserosal tumors are often detected late after they assume large dimensions. The mode of growth may be assessed by analysis of the contrast column defect, the mobility of the organ or its affected part, the pliability of the wall, and the accumulation of barium in an ulcer, if one exists.

Polyps are neoplastic or inflammatory lesions that project from the mucosa into the lu-

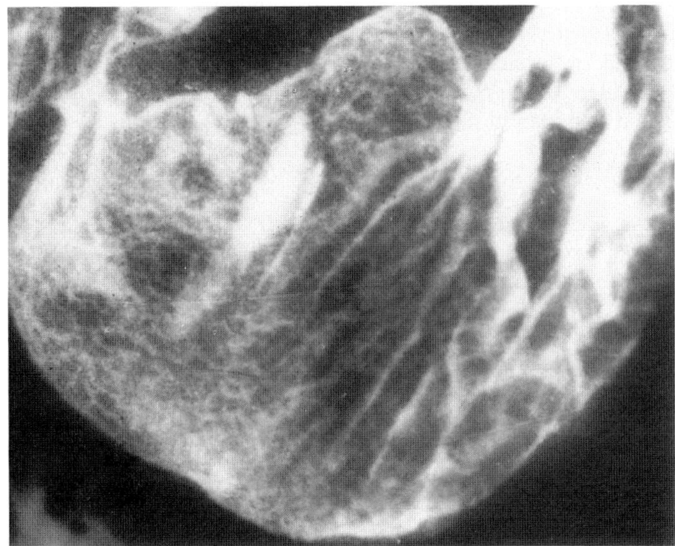

Figure 3.22. Double-contrast barium study of gastric erosions.

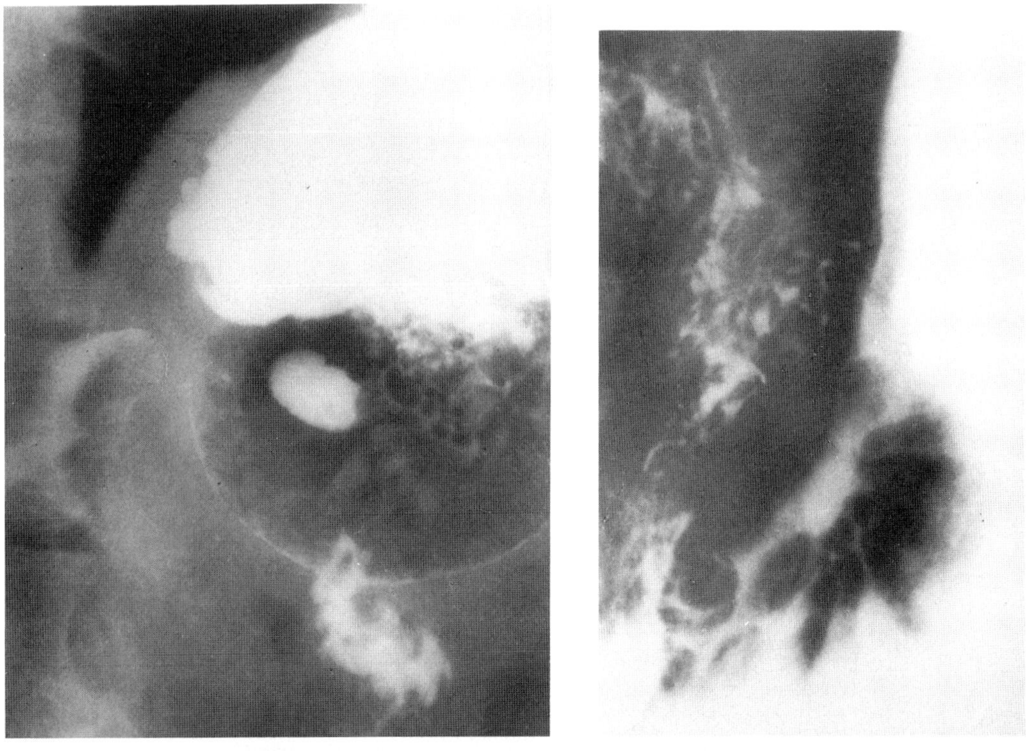

A B

Figure 3.23. (A) Acute gastric peptic ulcer. (B) Prominent scarring wtih chronic peptic ulcer.

men. Originally, the term polyp pertained solely to pedunculated growths (Fig. 3.24), but has now been extended to sessile tumors as well (Diagram 3.2). "Polyp" is a gross pathologic-clinical concept which includes:

1. Regenerative, hyperplastic, and inflammatory formations
2. Neoplastic growths such as adenomas and carcinomas (Figs. 3.25 to 3.30)
3. Hamartomas and choristomas

A series of syndromes are characterized by alimentary canal polyps. Hyperplastic and adenomatous polyps, or even malignant polypoid tumors, often cannot be distinguished from one another by means of radiologic examination.

A neoplasm may be characterized by either intraluminal, intramural, or subserosal growth (Diagram 3.3). Some neoplasms have a combined mode of growth. In typical cases, the layer from which tumors originate can be identified radiologically. Tumors arising on the mucosal surface distort or destroy visualization of the mucosal surface. Submucosal, muscular, and serosal neoplasms elevate normal mucosa and flatten folds. When they become large enough, serosal tumors displace all layers of the wall toward the lumen. However, the same radiologic appearance may be caused by neoplasms of adjacent organs. Neoplasms arising in the submucosa cannot reliably be distinguished ra-

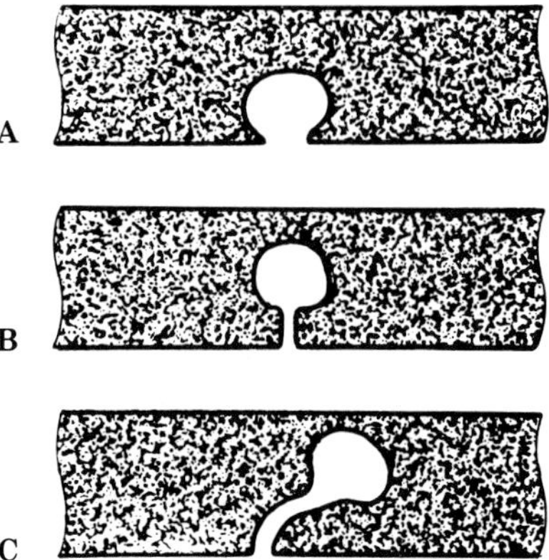

Diagram 3.2. Polyps. (A) Sessile. (B) On a short stalk. (C) On a long stalk.

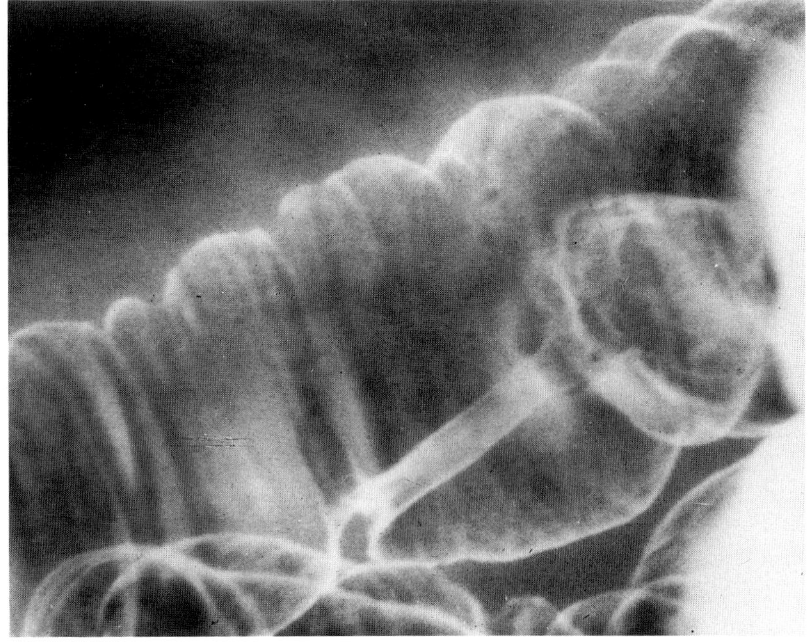

Figure 3.24. Large pedunculated adenomatous polyp of the colon.

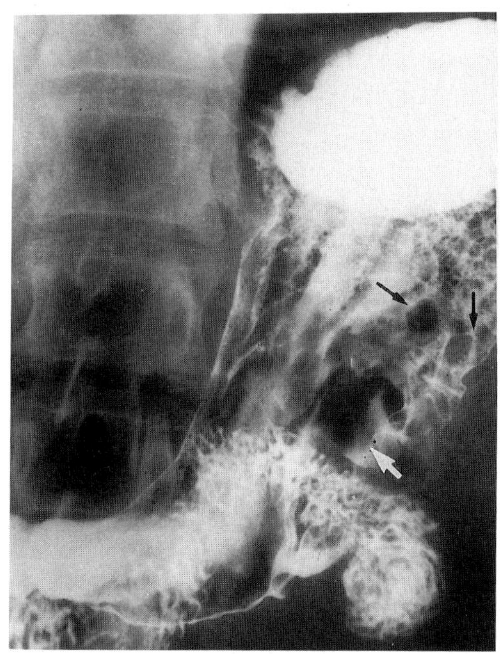

FIGURE 3.25. Sessile and pedunculated adenomatous polyps of the stomach (arrows).

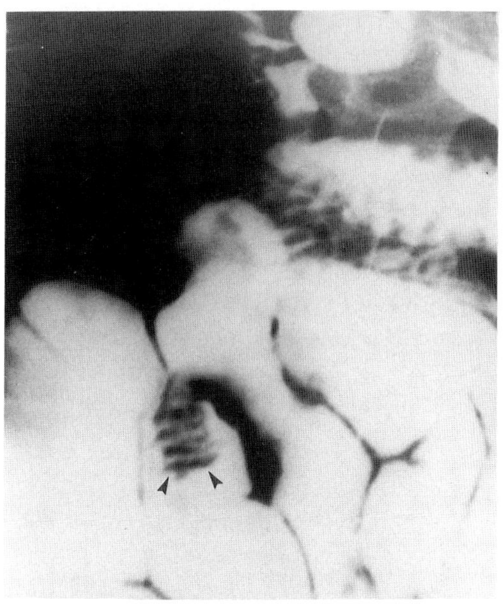

FIGURE 3.27. Adenomatous polyp of the mesenteric small bowel, demonstrated by controlled compression (arrowheads).

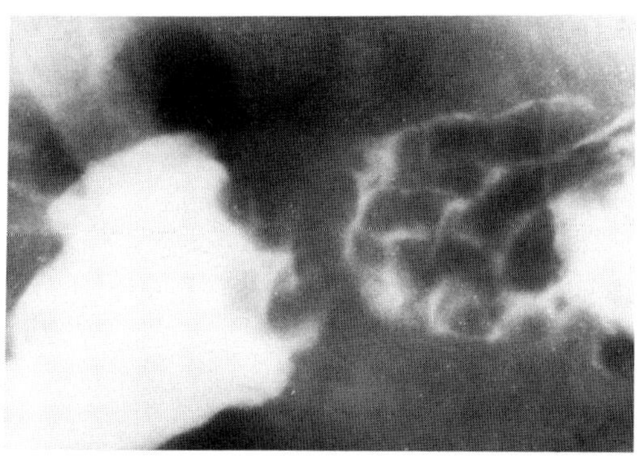

FIGURE 3.26. Hyperplastic polyps of the gastric antrum. Distal polyps prolapse into the duodenal bulb.

diologically from lesions originating in deeper layers of the alimentary canal wall, or even from extrinsic tumors that impinge on or invade the alimentary canal from adjacent organs. Even ulcerated neoplasms of gastric mucosa, as exemplified by Carman's sign (Fig. 3.31), can

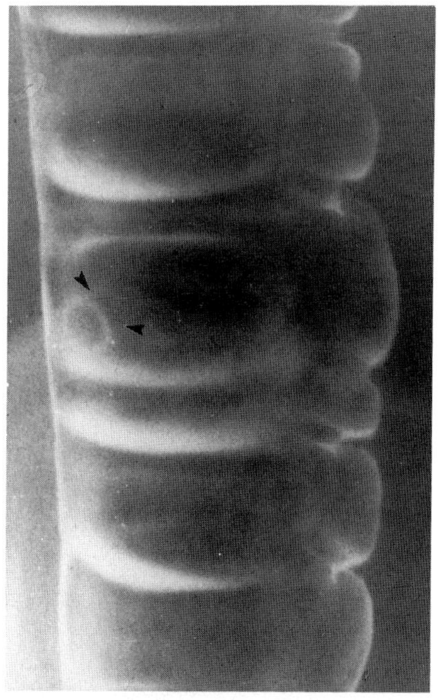

FIGURE 3.28. Sessile adenomatous polyp of the descending colon (arrowheads).

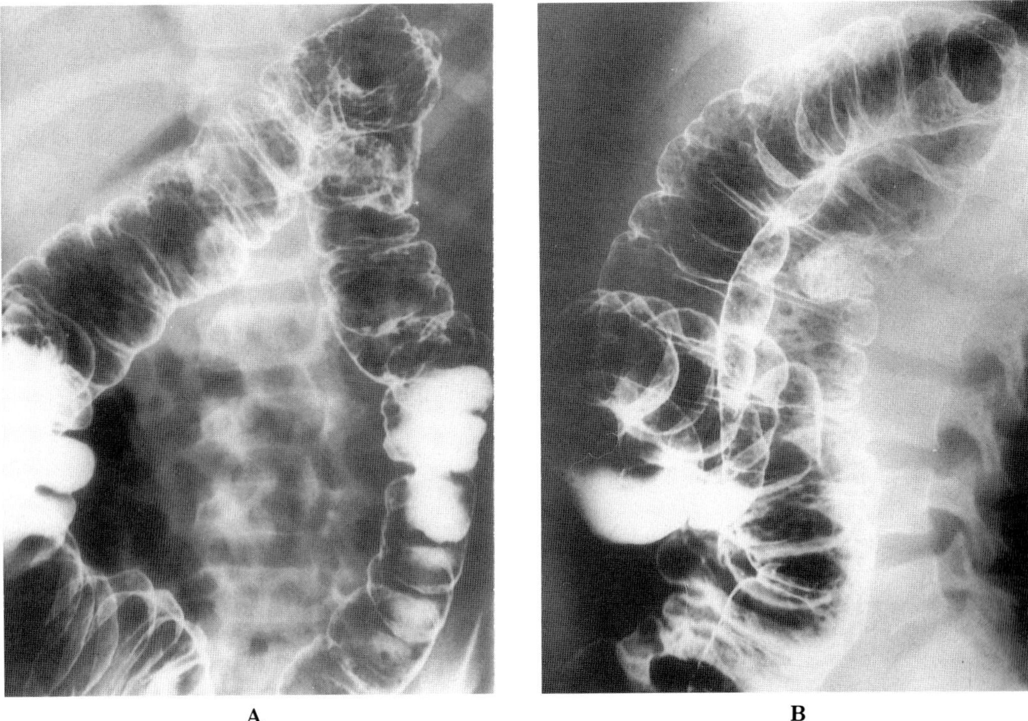

FIGURE 3.29. Familial polyposis. Double-contrast barium enema study. (A) Supine projection. (B) Profile projection demonstrating adenocarcinoma of the proximal descending colon.

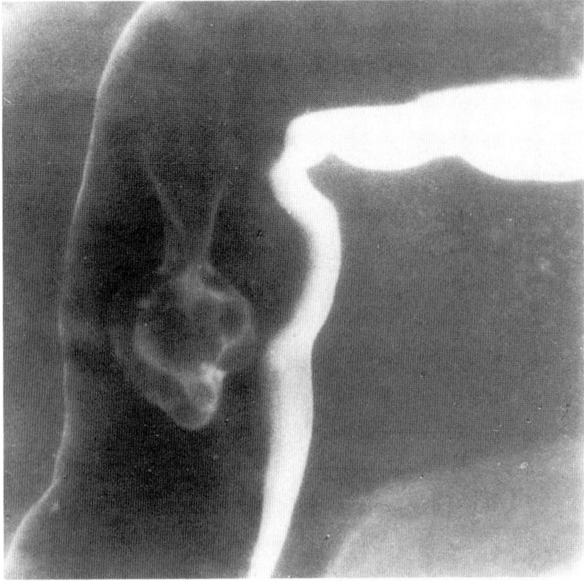

FIGURE 3.30. Lobulated adenomatous polyp of the colon on a stalk.

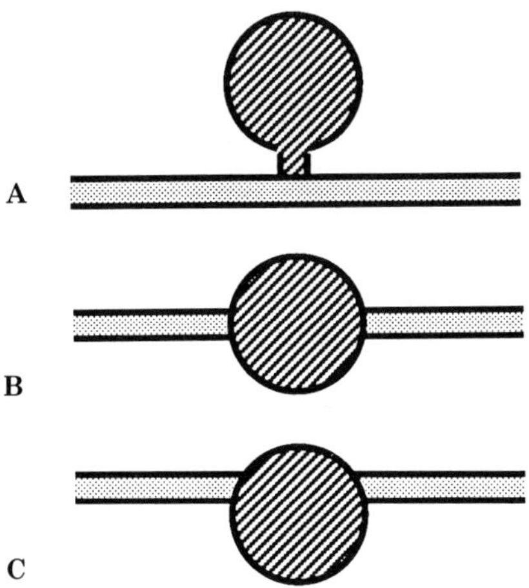

Diagram 3.3. Position of a tumor in the alimentary canal wall. (A) Intrinsic lesion on a stalk demonstrates an acute angle with the wall. (B) Intramural lesion exhibits a 90 degree or obtuse angle. However, this can also result from an extramural lesion. (C) Extramural lesion tends to create an angle much larger than 90 degrees. (Used by permission and modified from Kidd R, Freeny PC. Radiographic manifestations of extrinsic processes involving the bowel. Gastrointest Radiol. 1982;7:21-28.)

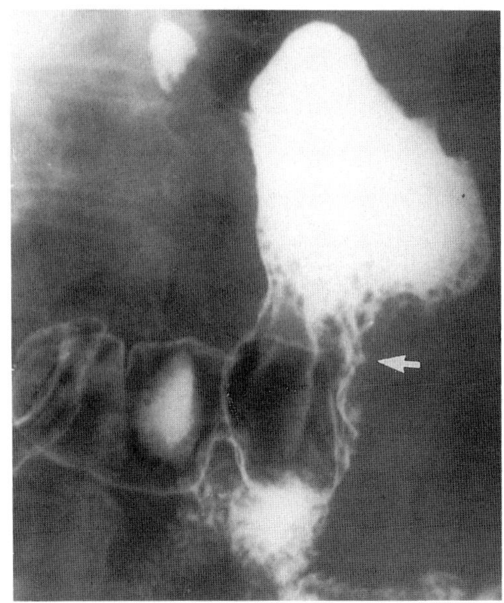

Figure 3.31. Ulcerated gastric carcinoma (arrow).

mimic exogastric neoplasms which pull the gastric wall outward, creating an "attraction cone" (Diagram 3.4 and Fig. 3.32). Furthermore, large ulcerated exogastric neoplasms (Fig. 3.33) can resemble ulcerated gastric neoplasms.

Benign neoplasms of the alimentary canal originating from the mucosa protrude into the lumen producing negative defects on single-contrast examination. On double-contrast studies these tumors appear as protruding masses covered with a thin layer of barium on the nondependent wall, and negative defects in the barium accumulations on the dependent wall. They are not coated with characteristic mucosal relief. Submucosal benign tumors impress upon the contrast column creating a negative defect. The double-contrast technique allows optimal demonstration of the derangement and separation of normal mucosal relief elements.

Malignant neoplasms of the alimentary canal assume one of several macroscopic forms (Diagram 3.5). The most common are *irregular polypoid growths* (Fig. 3.34).

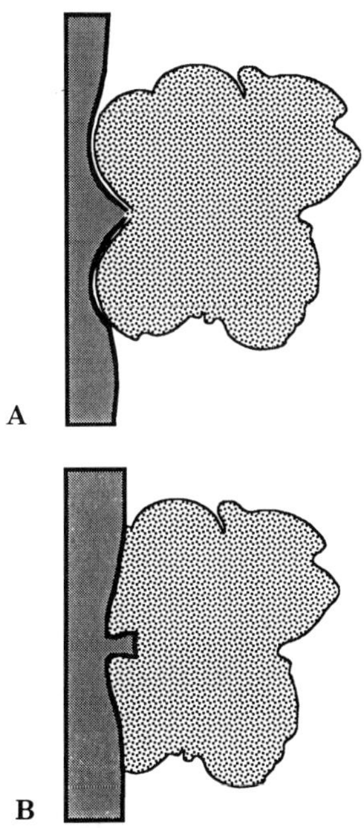

Diagram 3.4. Exogastrically growing tumor. (A) Resembles endogastric ulcerated neoplasm. (B) Ulcerated serosal tumor may mimic an ulcer in the gastric wall.

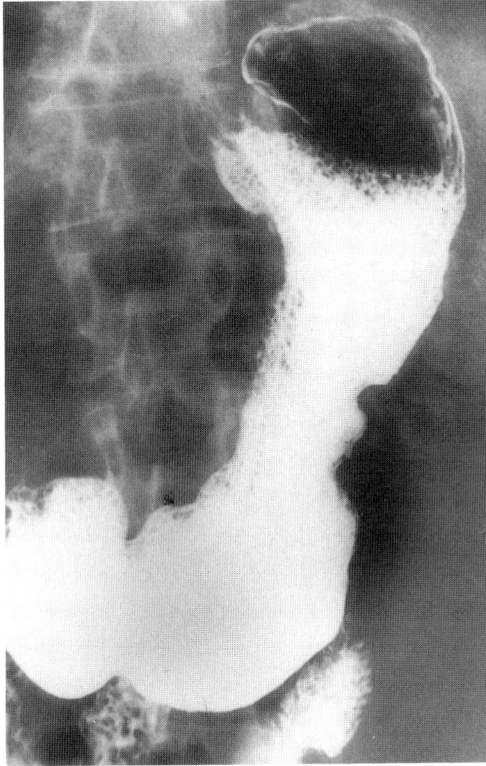

Figure 3.32. Neoplasm of an outer layer of the gastric wall. Predominant exogastric growth forms an "attraction cone." (See Diagram 3.4.)

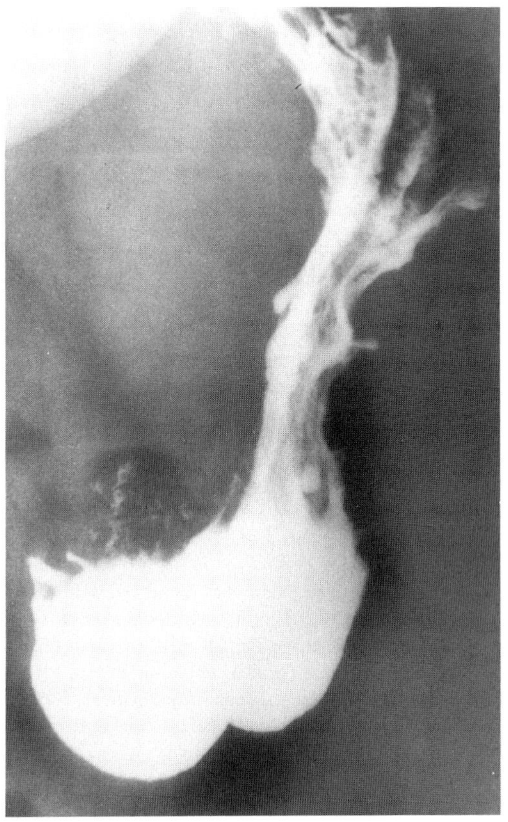

Figure 3.33. Large exogastrically growing gastric neoplasm with an ulcer at the base. (See Diagram 3.4.)

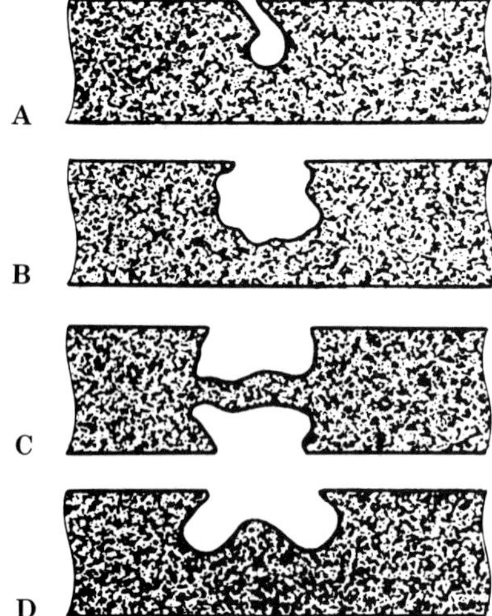

Diagram 3.5. Alimentary canal carcinomas. (A) Polypoid. (B) Large polypoid mass with irregular surface. (C) Annular. (D) Ulcerated.

Stenoses caused by malignant neoplasms differ from inflammatory, granulomatous, and corrosive strictures (Table 3.1, Fig. 3.13, and Figs. 3.35 to 3.38). The stenotic area tends to be relatively shorter, mucosal relief is destroyed, and the tumor mass can protrude into the lumen. The transition to normal wall is abrupt and tumor masses can create overhanging margins, producing a "shouldering" effect (Diagram 3.6). The wall of the digestive tube in the area affected by tumor is rigid. However, decreased elasticity of the wall may also be observed in inflamed or scarred organs. Some malignant tumors are purely circumferential (Figs. 3.42 and 3.43).

A *volcano-like* appearance of ulcerated gastrointestinal neoplasms is quite common. Within a negative defect in the contrast column, corresponding to the tumor, there is a positive de-

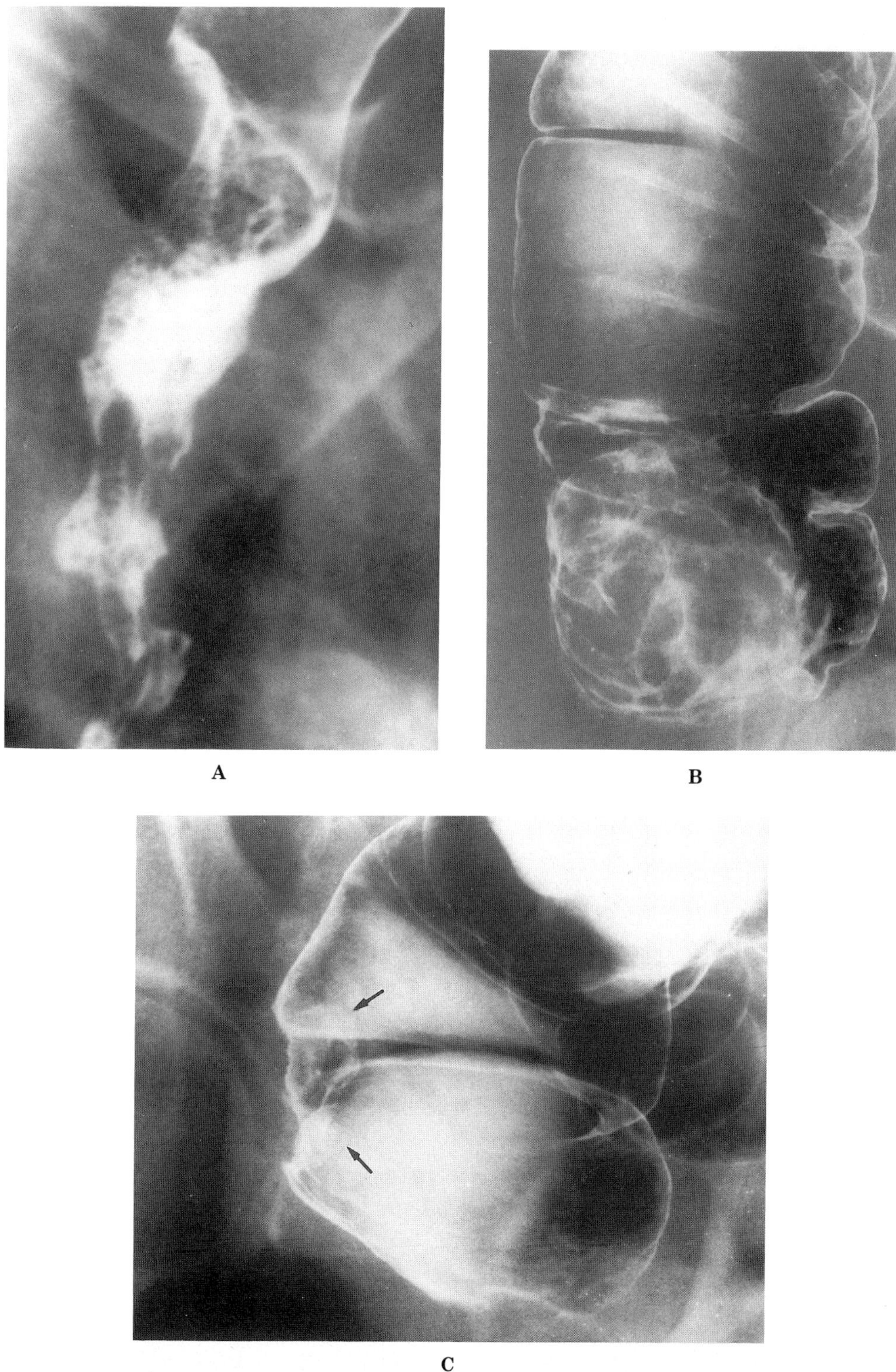

Figure 3.34. Polypoid carcinoma (A) in the esophagus; (B) in the cecum; and (C) in the rectum (arrows).

Table 3.1. Features of Alimentary Canal Stenoses

Feature	Benign	Malignant
Mucosal relief	may be preserved	destroyed, masses may protrude into the lumen
Tumor	regular (inflammatory, granuloma)	neoplasms are irregular tissue masses
Transition into normal wall	gradual	abrupt, overhanging margins, "shouldering"
Pliability of wall	partially preserved	often completely missing
Length of stenosis	long sections	short
Proximal dilatation	marked	moderate, less pronounced
Poststenotic dilatation	pseudodiverticular near scarred areas	due to destruction of intramural neuronal network

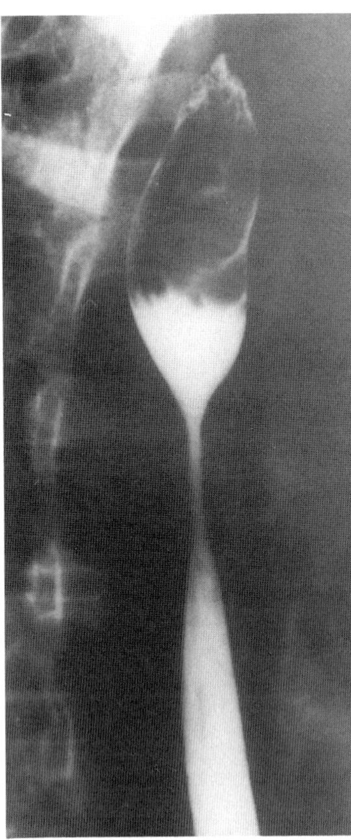

Figure 3.35. Congenital esophageal stenosis with benign characteristics. Gradual transition of the narrowed segment into the normal wall. No signs of mucosal destruction in the stenosed area.

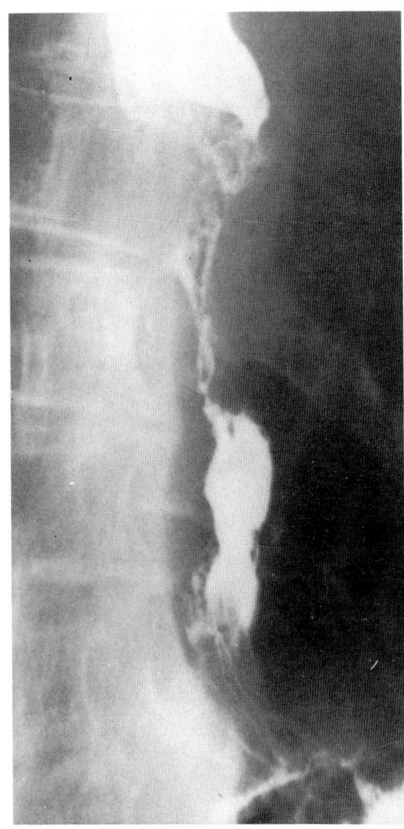

Figure 3.36. Malignant esophageal stricture. Abrupt transition from the stenosed segment to normal wall with "shouldering." Tumor masses protrude into the esophageal lumen, destroying mucosal relief.

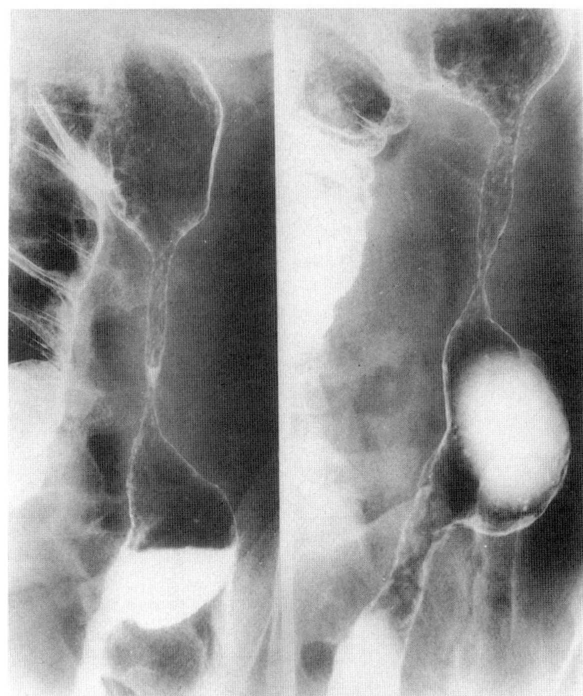

FIGURE 3.37. Stenotic phase of Crohn's disease. Postinflammatory strictures with "pseudoaneurysmal" dilatation of the intervening descending colon. Narrowed segments have lost compliance.

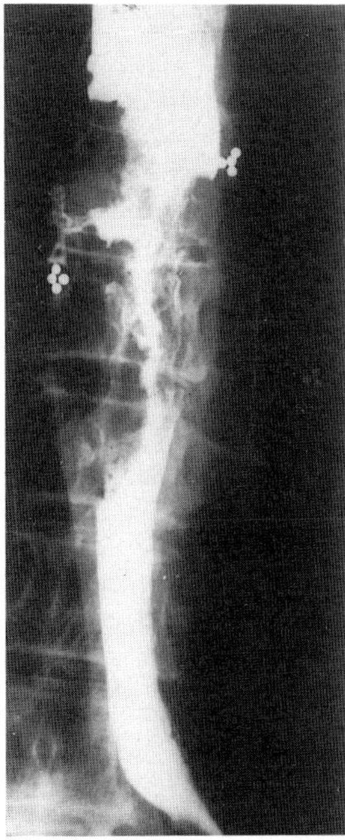

FIGURE 3.38. Esophageal carcinoma. Radiopaque markers for radiation therapy field.

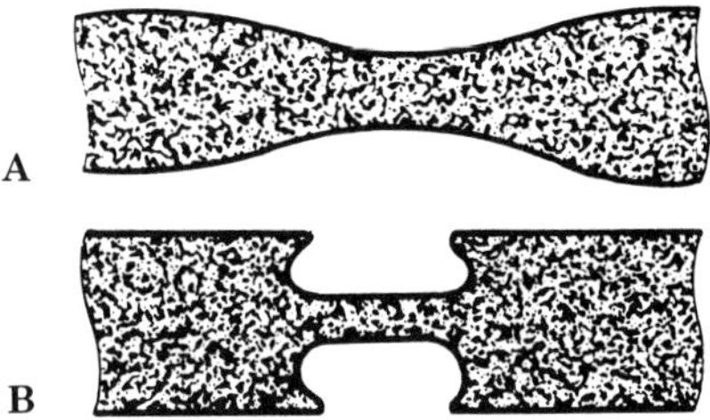

DIAGRAM 3.6. Stenoses of the alimentary canal. (A) Benign. Gradual transition from normal to stenosed section. Preserved mucosal relief in the region of the stenosis. (B) Malignant. Abrupt transition from normal wall to the stenosed section with overhanging margins ("shouldering"). Destruction of mucosal relief in the region of the stenosis. Compliance of the wall is decreased in both (A) and (B).

fect which corresponds to an ulcer (Diagram 3.5, Figs. 3.39 and 3.40). Malignant gastrointestinal neoplasms may originally appear as ulcers.

Carcinomas are the most common malignant neoplasms of the alimentary canal. On the

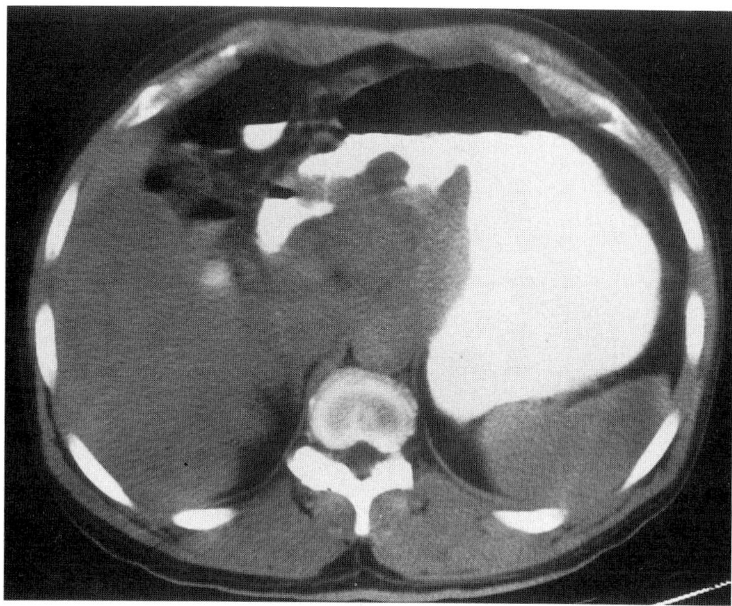

FIGURE 3.39. CT of ulcerated gastric carcinoma.

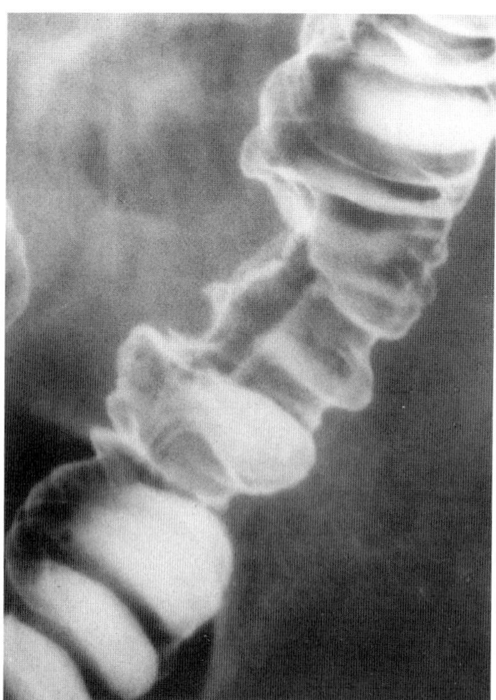

FIGURE 3.40. Ulcerated carcinoma of the colon.

basis of macroscopic appearance, they may be classified into several categories (Diagram 3.5). However, there is no correlation between macroscopic features and histologic tumor type. *Polypoid* carcinomas grow predominantly into the lumen (Figs. 3.34 and 3.41). The surface of the tumor may be ulcerated so as to resemble a volcano (Figs. 3.40 and 3.42). Mucinous carcinomas are soft and pliable and occur predominantly in the stomach and colon. *Scirrhous carcinomas* appear in any section of the alimentary canal. These tumors are hard and grow circumferentially as an annular carcinoma narrowing the lumen and causing rigidity of the wall; thus the organ appears smaller (Figs. 3.43 and 3.44). Carcinoma may also present as an *ulceration.*

Carcinoma in situ, an intraepithelial noninvasive carcinoma, is confined to the epithelium and does not penetrate the basement membrane. Any carcinoma penetrating through the basement membrane is termed invasive.

Early and superficial carcinomas extend no deeper than the submucosa but an early carcinoma may affect quite a large area. An early carcinoma is one that is recognized early, and is most likely curable in this phase; a superficial

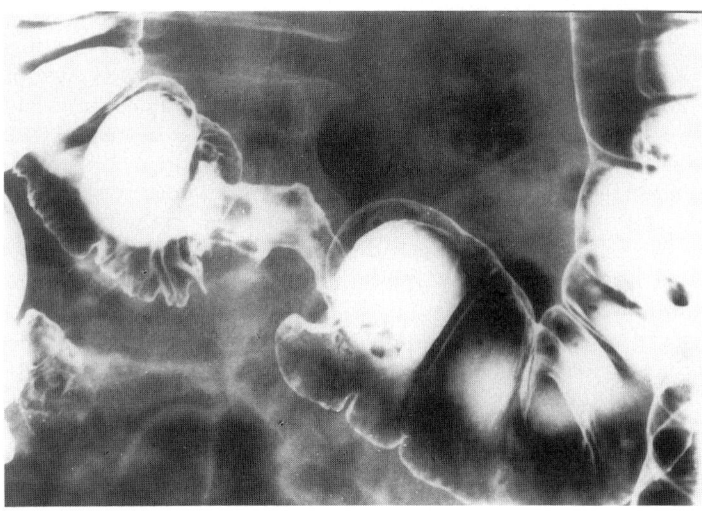

Figure 3.41. Apple-core lesion of transverse colon, demonstrating carcinoma.

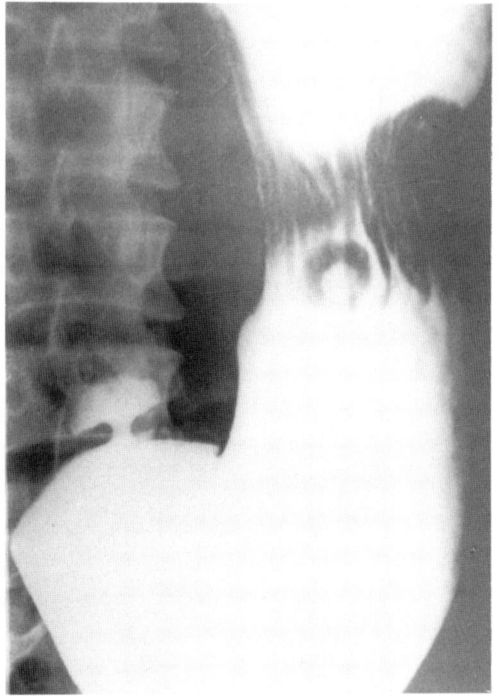

Figure 3.42. Target lesion of the stomach. Although mesenchymal neoplasms or metastatic diseases (particularly malignant melanoma) may give such an appearance, spasm of the gastric wall suggests a peptic ulcer surrounded by edema.

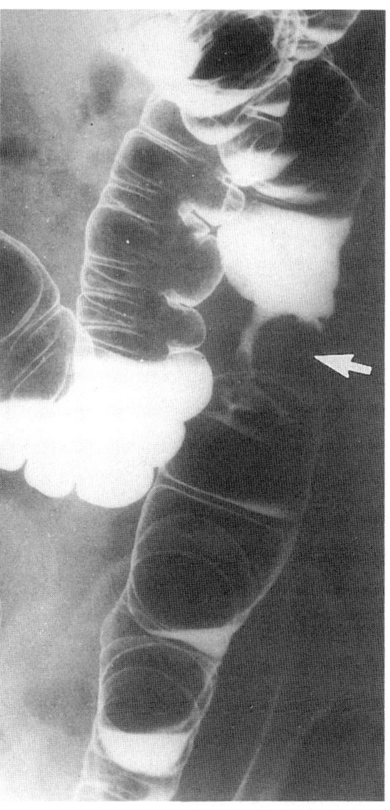

Figure 3.43. Annular, scirrhous carcinoma of the descending colon (arrow).

carcinoma is one that has spread superficially. Early carcinomas of various organs are classified differently with regard to metastases in regional lymph nodes. Diagnosis of a gastric carcinoma as early is not necessarily a contradiction, even with invasion of regional lymph nodes, or lymph and blood vessels, or in the presence of multifocal primary tumor. The 10-year survival rate does not differ significantly whether metastases in the regional lymph nodes are present or not. In contrast, there is a significant difference between early and superficial carcinomas of the esophagus. Neither penetrates the principal muscular coat but early carcinoma excludes involvement of lymph nodes. The prognosis for superficial esophageal carcinoma with involvement of regional lymph nodes is the same as for advanced esophageal carcinoma.

Carcinoid tumors grow preferentially in the ileocecal area. These are neuroectodermal neoplasms. The mucosa overlaying a carcinoid is often intact and the malignant potential of a carcinoid is less than that of a carcinoma.

Neoplasms derived from *smooth muscles* originate either from a principal muscular layer or from the muscularis mucosae. They are distributed in the alimentary canal in the following proportions: stomach (66%), small intestine (24%), esophagus (7%), and large intestine (3%). Approximately 60% grow in the submucosa and 35% in the subserosa. The remaining 5% grow bidirectionally and are dumbbell shaped.

Leiomyomas are benign, spherical or oval, hard, and well-demarcated neoplasms. Occasionally, necrotic changes within the neoplasm cause ulceration. Leiomyomas detected by radiography average 5 cm in diameter. One-third of these tumors are leiomyoblastomas, epitheloid leiomyomas. Leiomyosarcomas are usually irregular in shape. They grow as exophytic masses. Among malignant tumors of the stomach, small intestine, and large intestine, *leiomyosarcomas* represent 1%, 20% and 0.1%, respectively.

Both benign and malignant mesenchymal neoplasms represent only 1% of the total num-

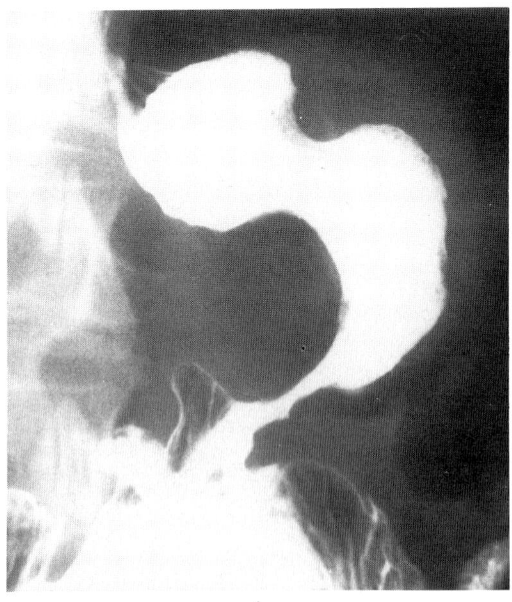

A

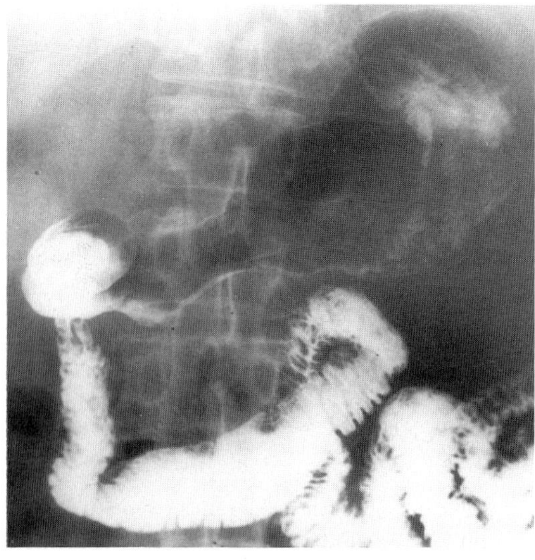

B

Figure 3.44. Scirrhous carcinoma of the stomach. In (A) the entire stomach is affected. In (B) the distal portion of the body and antrum is affected.

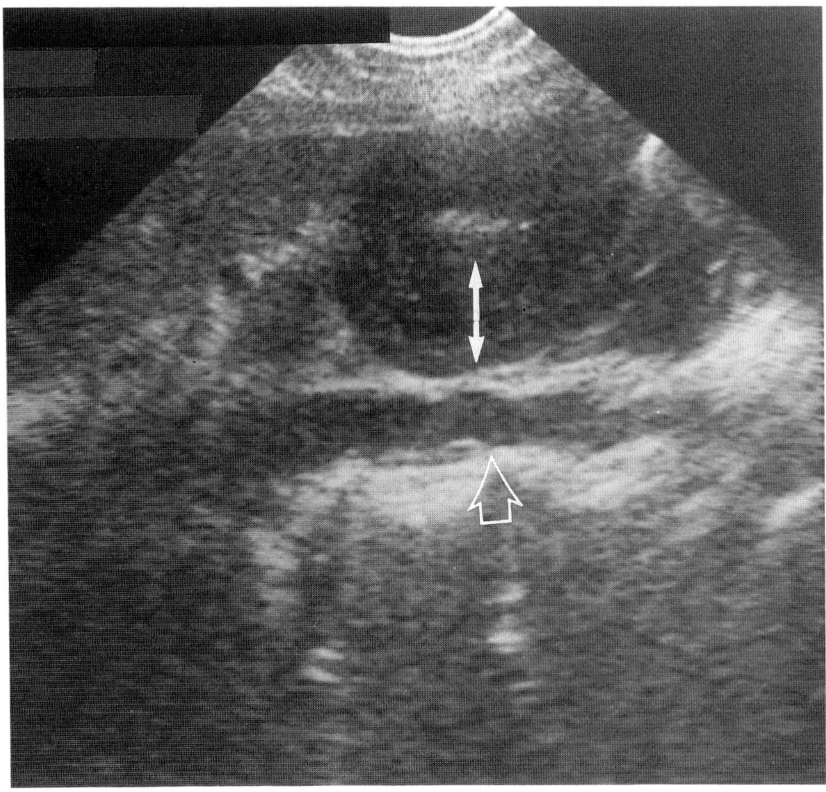

Figure 3.45. Ultrasound of gastric lymphoma. Diffuse thickening of gastric wall (closed arrow). Aorta (open arrow). (Courtesy of W.L. Wells, M.D., Louisiana State University, New Orleans.)

ber of alimentary canal neoplasms. *Sarcomas* are malignant neoplasms which may originate from any mesenchymal constituent of the alimentary canal. They often assume large dimensions and affect long sections of the digestive tube. The radiologic appearance corresponds to intraluminal or intraparietal infiltrative masses. *Lymphomas* are malignant neoplasms of lymphoid origin. They arise in the submucosa and spread toward the mucosa and/or serosa (Fig. 3.45).

Staging of malignant neoplasms is possible according to the TNM classification, where T pertains to the primary tumor, N denotes the presence or absence of the tumor cells in regional lymph nodes, and M corresponds to the presence or absence of distant metastases. Malignant transformation of adenomatous polyps, and premalignant conditions such as ulcerative colitis or Crohn's disease, are discussed in chapter 12.

Bibliography

Bond MR, Roberts JBM. Intussusception in the adult. Br J Surg. 1964;51:818.

Dreyfuss JR, Benacerraf B. Saddle cancers of the colon and their progression to annular carcinomas. Radiology. 1978;129:289.

Ebert PA, Zuidema GD. Primary tumors of the small intestine. Arch Surg. 1965;91:452.

Herlinger H. Recognition of exogastric tumors. Br J Radiol. 1966;39:25.

Kelly RB, Mahoney PD, Johnson JF. CT demonstration of an unusual enteric duplication cyst. J Comput Assist Tomogr. 1986;10:506.

Kressel HT, Glick SN, Laufer I, Banner M. Radiologic features of esophagitis. Gastrointest Radiol. 1981;6:103.

Megibow AJ, Balthazar EJ, Hulnick DH, Naidich DP, Bosniak MA. CT evaluation of gastrointestinal leiomyomas and leiomyosarcomas. AJR. 1985; 144:727.

Morson BC, Konishi F. Contribution of the pathologist to the radiology and management of colorectal polyps. Gastrointest Radiol. 1982;7:275.

Op den Orth JO, Dakker W. Gastric erosions: Radiologic and endoscopic aspects. Diagn Imag. 1976; 45:88.

Schatzki R, Hawes LE. The roentgenologic appearance of extramucosal tumors of the esophagus. AJR. 1942;48:1.

Takeshita K, Habu H, Yaegash K, Hirayama R, Miyanaga T, Hoshik K, Menjo M, Aoki N. A long-term postoperative result of early gastric cancer–prognostic analysis on extent of dissection. Nippon Gekke Gakkai Zasshi. 1980;81:724.

Vandertoll DJ, Beahrs OH. Carcinoma of rectum and low sigmoid. Arch Surg. 1965;90:793.

Chapter **4**

Radiologic Examination of the Alimentary Canal

PRINCIPLES

Indications for radiologic examination of the alimentary canal and plain abdominal radiography are signs of diseases which can be detected radiologically. They may vary from functional disturbances to alarming circumstances such as an acute abdomen or active bleeding from the alimentary canal. Radiologic examination enables insight into morphology and, to a lesser extent, into physiology.

Before performing any alimentary canal examination, it is important to correlate previous radiologic examinations and other medical procedures, especially surgery. While fluoroscopy is the most important method of alimentary canal examination (Fig. 4.1), detailed evaluation of mucosal surfaces is only possible by analysis of roentgenograms. Each segment of the alimentary canal should be presented in its maximal length and in every projection which contributes to the diagnosis (Figs. 4.2 and 4.3).

Radiologic examinations are not without hazards, such as those related to ionizing radiation and to iodinated contrast media. The risk-benefit ratio has to be taken into account.

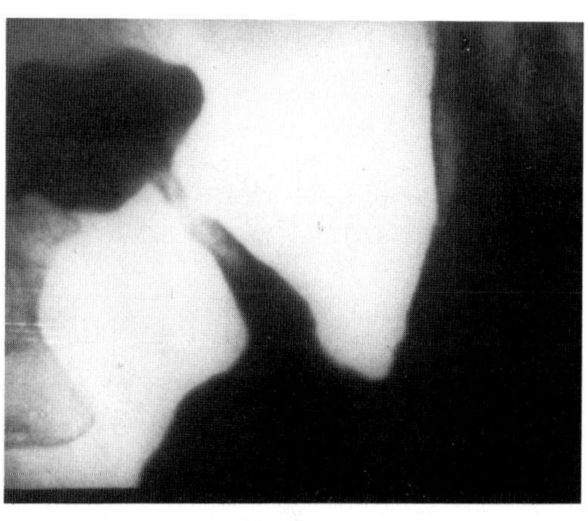

A

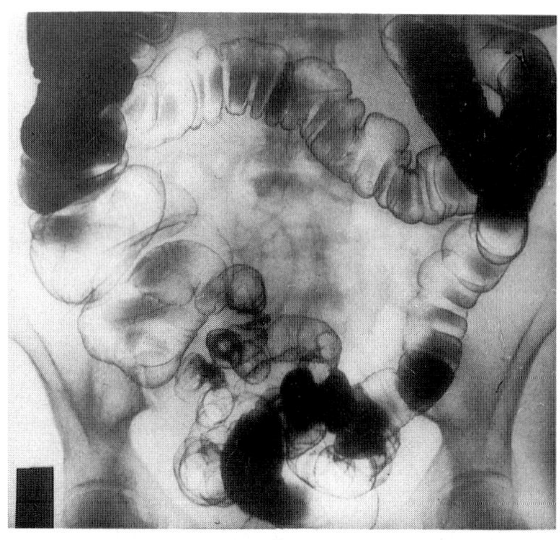

B

FIGURE 4.1. The fluoroscopic image is "negative" compared to films. (A) Hypertrophic pyloric stenosis in an adult. (B) Double-contrast barium enema study, in supine P-A position.

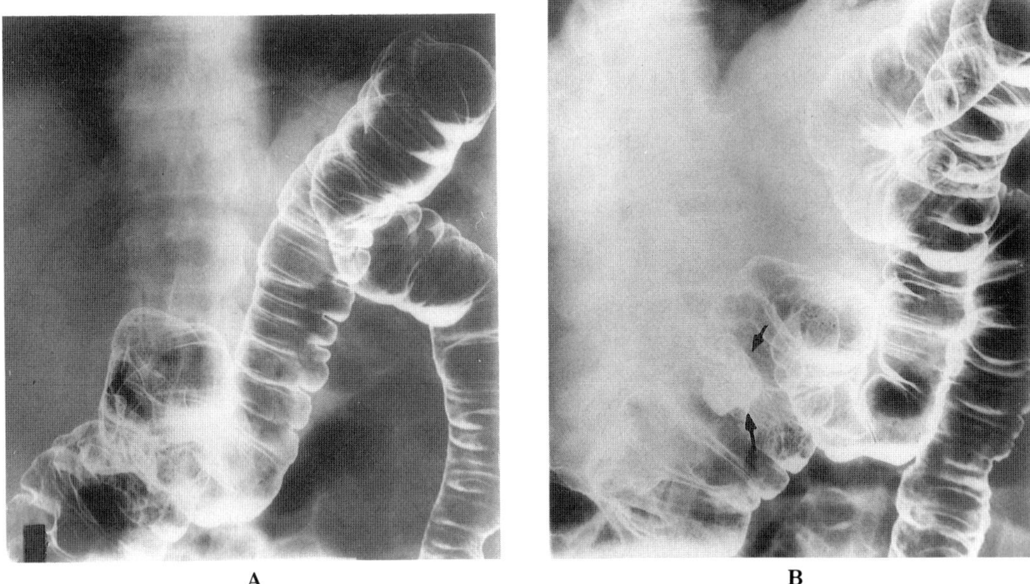

A B

Figure 4.2. Double-contrast barium enema. (A) P-A projection without obvious pathology. The colon is elongated and redundant. (B) Right anterior oblique projection demonstrates carcinoma (arrows).

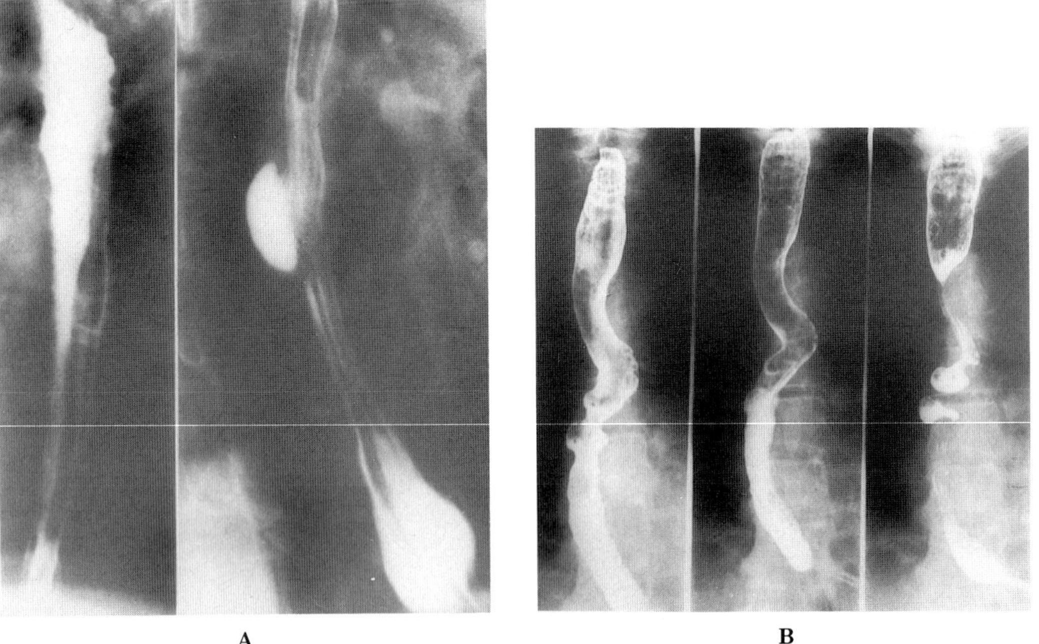

A B

Figure 4.3. (A) Left esophagogram without significant pathologic changes evident. By changing projection (right), a large pulsion diverticulum is seen. (B) Esophageal diverticula are best demonstrated during the course of esophageal peristalsis.

PLAIN ROENTGENOGRAPHY OF THE ABDOMEN

Plain radiographs or scout films of the abdomen register the density of electrons in organs through which X-rays have passed. Organs within the peritoneal cavity and retroperitoneal space absorb X-rays almost equally. However, the absorption of X-rays is less in gas and adipose tissues. Differences in X-ray absorption allow structures to be seen.

Analysis of the scout film should include: the gas pattern of the alimentary canal, possible free gas in the peritoneal cavity and retroperitoneal space, other radiolucent areas, and calcification (Fig. 4.4). In addition to intraperitoneal and retroperitoneal organs, the position and contour of the diaphragm, psoas muscles, and bones have to be analyzed.

Gas in the lumen of the alimentary canal (Figs. 4.5 and 4.6A) is clearly demarcated on plain abdominal roentgenography. The dis-

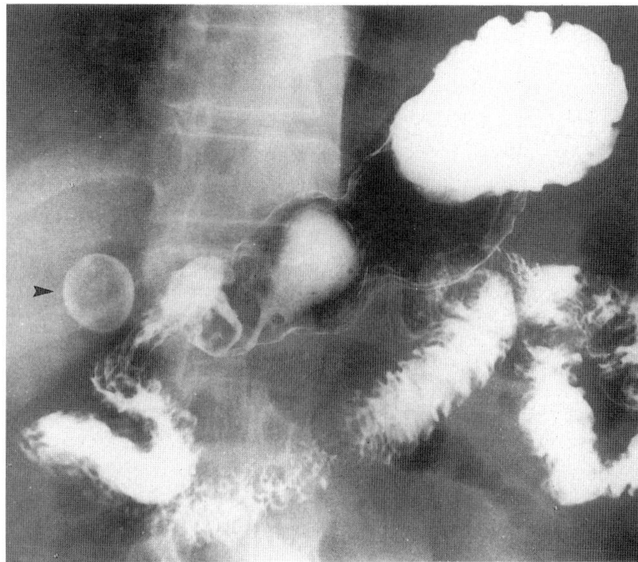

FIGURE 4.4. Large radiopaque gallstone (arrowhead). Barium studies of upper gastrointestinal tract demonstrate atypical course of a nonfixated, mobile duodenum.

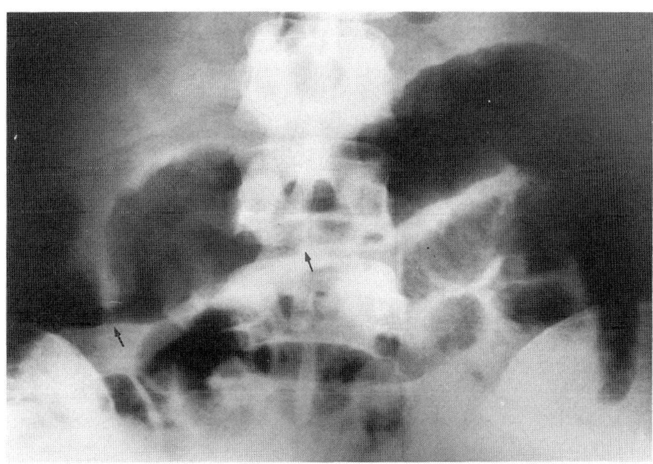

FIGURE 4.5. Toxic megacolon in Crohn's disease with significant stenoses (arrows) and regenerating mucosal formations (pseudopolyps) protruding into the lumen.

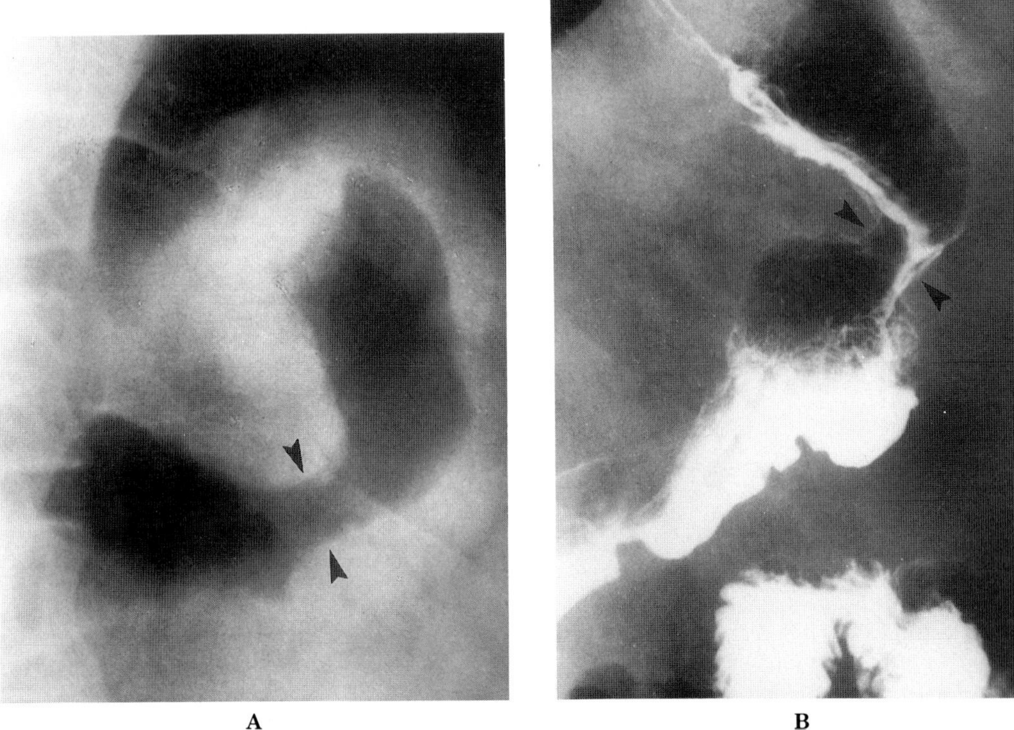

Figure 4.6. Annular carcinoma of the stomach (arrow heads). (A) Plain abdominal film. (B) Barium examination (arrowheads).

tance between gas in the fundus of the stomach and air in the lungs usually equals 15–30 mm. This allows estimation of the diaphragm and gastric fundus wall thickness. Luminal narrowing and widening can be noticed in organs containing gas. Tumors (Fig. 4.6) and swelling of the mucosa can be seen as protrusions in the organ lumen. Free peritoneal gas collects under the diaphragm in the upright position and has to be distinguished from subphrenic abscesses, emphysematous gastritis or cholecystitis, intestinal pneumatosis, liver and splenic abscesses, and Chilaiditi's interposition of the colon (Figs. 4.7 and 4.8). Scout films can also demonstrate pneumobilia (Fig. 4.9).

Intra-abdominal fluid collections and solid viscera create shadows of equal density. The presence of fluid within the alimentary canal can be recorded only when gas is simultaneously present. In the standing position free fluid accumulates in the inferior segment of the peritoneal cavity, absorbing more X-rays than fluid-free areas above.

The most common calcifications within the alimentary canal are enteroliths. Calcifications in costal cartilages project over the hypochondriac regions. The commonest abdominal calcifications outside the alimentary canal are phleboliths, arterial calcifications (Fig. 4.15), and calcified lymph nodes (Fig. 4.10). Renal and biliary calculi encrusted with inorganic salts are demonstrable on plain abdominal roentgenographs. Dead parasites like *Echinococcus* (Fig. 4.11) and *Cysticercus* often undergo calcification. Calcium salts are precipitated in chronic inflammations such as "porcelain" gallbladder (Fig. 4.12) and pancreatitis (Fig. 4.13), and in tissues undergoing necrosis, such as myoma of the

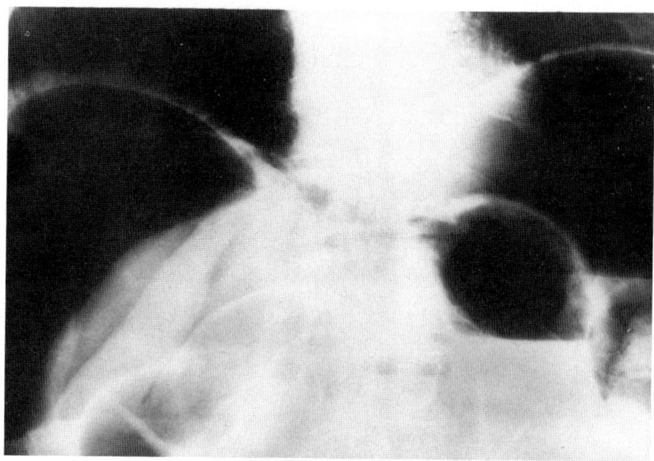

FIGURE 4.7. Pneumoperitoneum with accumulation of large amount of gas.

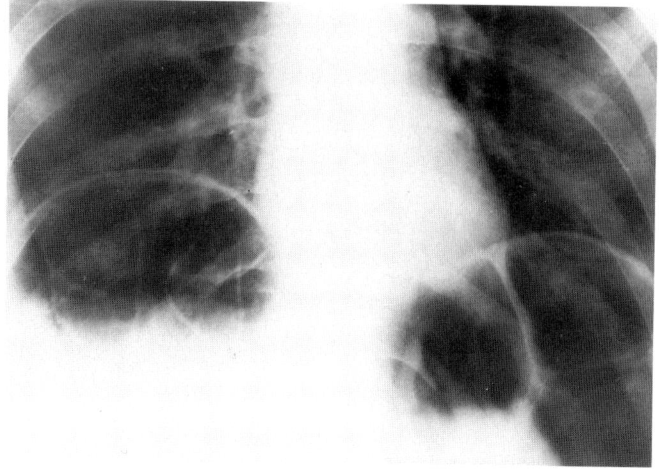

FIGURE 4.8. Chilaiditi's syndrome. Interposition of colon between the liver and right hemidiaphragm. Ectopic colon is also seen below the left hemidiaphragm. Haustral markings with semilunar folds are clearly visible.

uterus. Phleboliths, tuberculous foci (Fig. 4.14), and lesions caused by *Brucella* in the spleen can also undergo calcification. Atherosclerotic calcifications of abdominal arteries are often seen (Figs. 4.15 to 4.17). Calcifications can pervade tumors. They are seen on plain roentgenograms in 50% of neuroblastomas and 12% of Wilm's tumors in children. Mucinous carcinoma of the stomach and colloid carcinoma of the colon may also appear calcified. Tumors of the urinary bladder can also undergo calcification. Nephrocalcinosis in the kidneys, calcifications in segments of the male and female genital tract, and abdominal wall calcifications

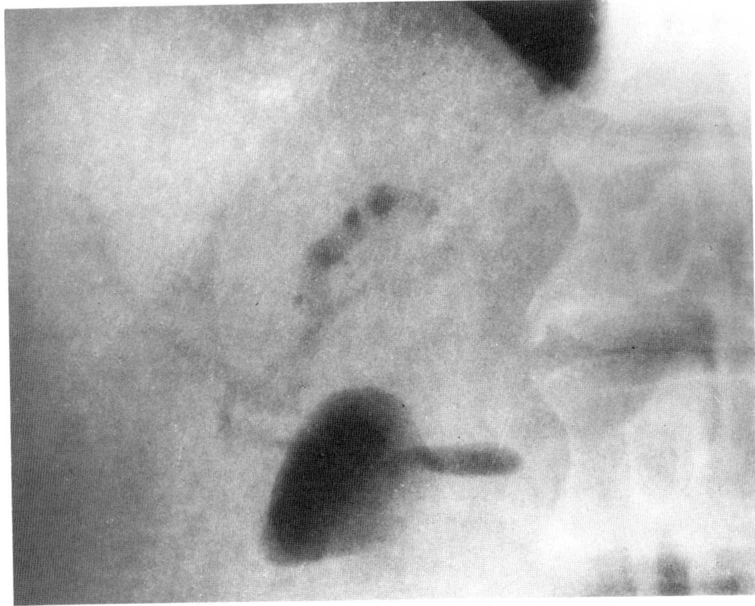

FIGURE 4.9. Pneumobilia, gas in the biliary system, after choledochojejunostomy.

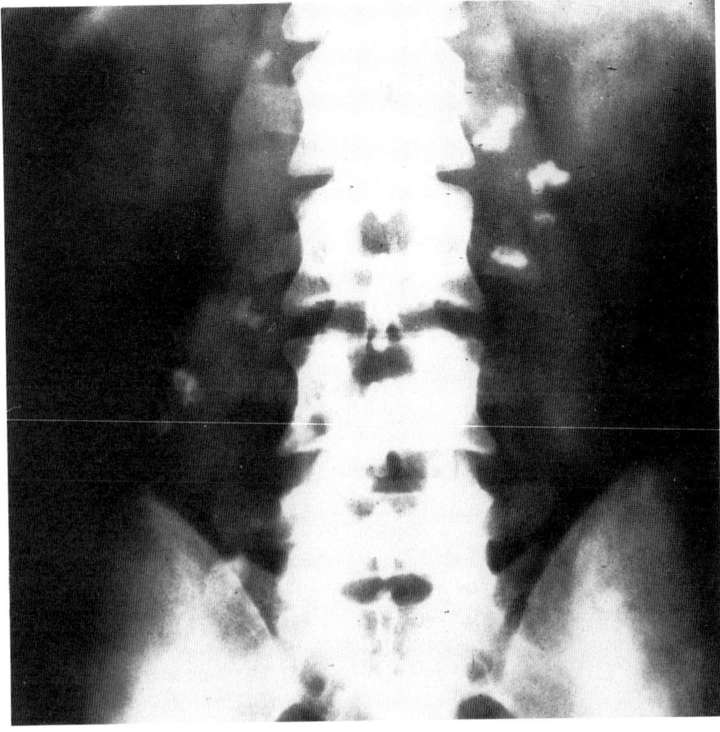

FIGURE 4.10. Calcifications of mesenteric lymph nodes.

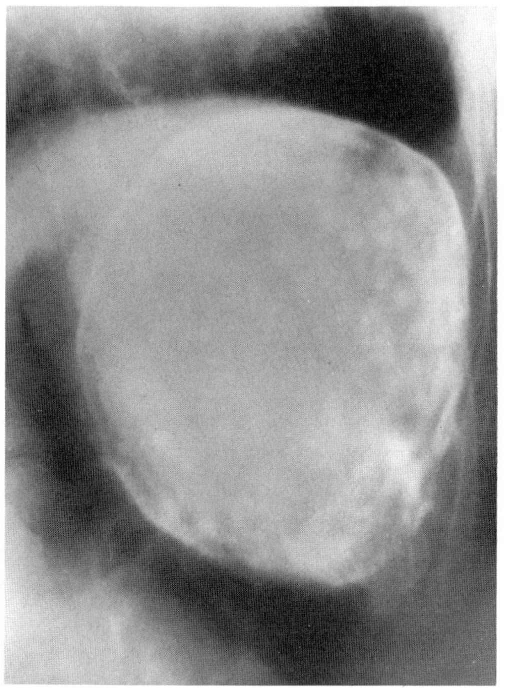

Figure 4.11. Calcified echinococcal cyst in the spleen.

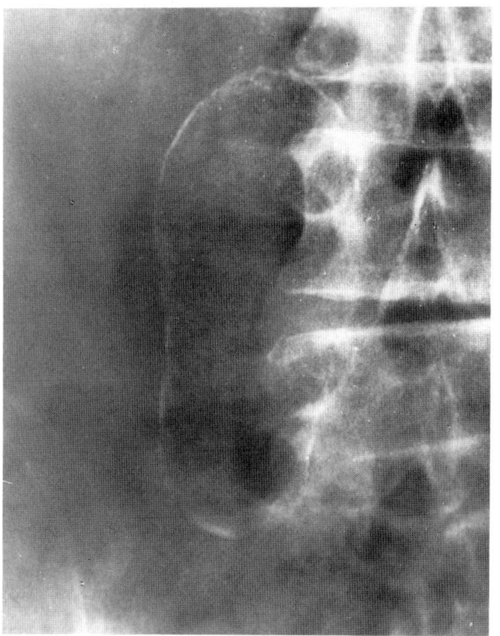

Figure 4.12. Porcelain gallbladder.

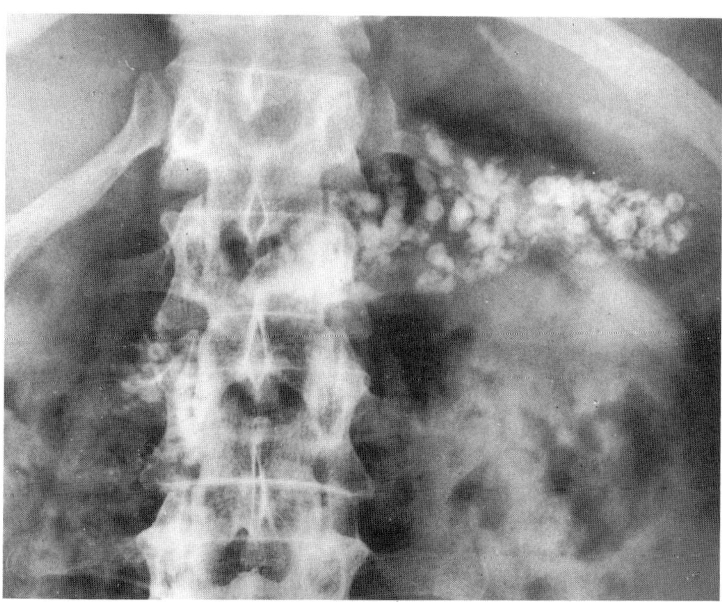

Figure 4.13. Calcifications of the pancreas.

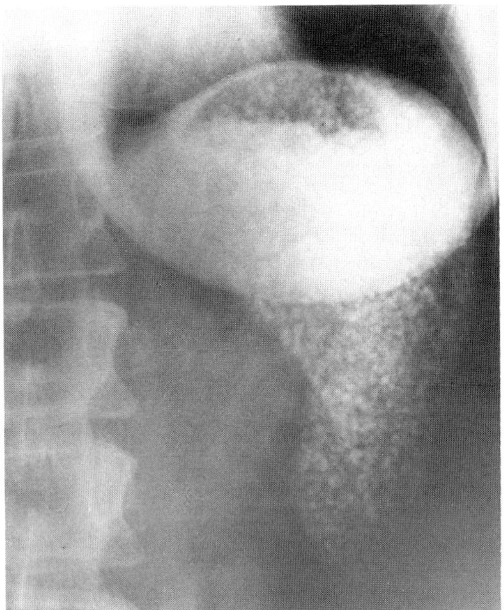

FIGURE 4.14. Calcified tuberculomas in the spleen.

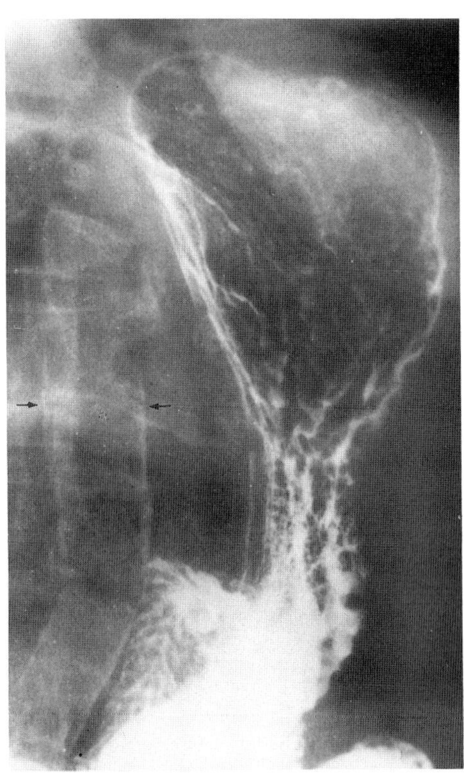

FIGURE 4.16. Calcification of abdominal aorta (arrows) seen on upper gastrointestinal barium studies.

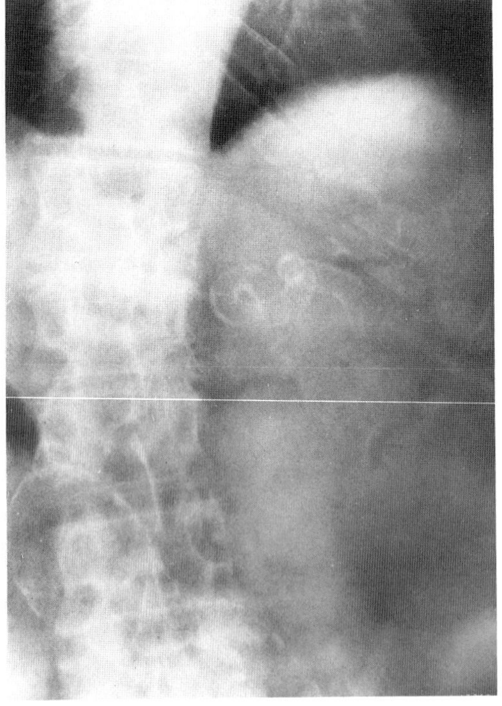

FIGURE 4.15. Calcified walls of the abdominal arteries.

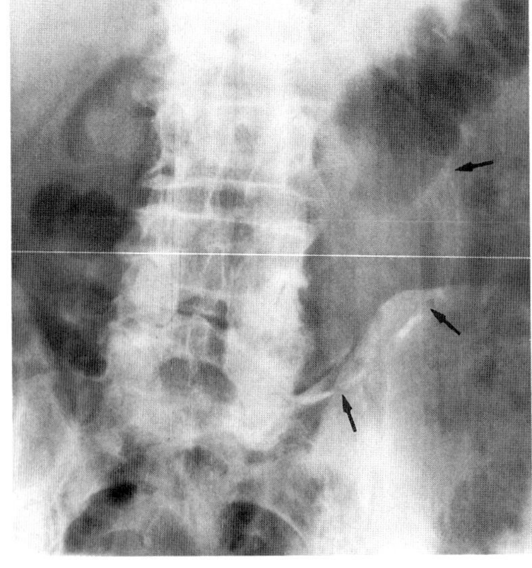

FIGURE 4.17. Calcification of abdominal aortic aneurysm wall (arrows).

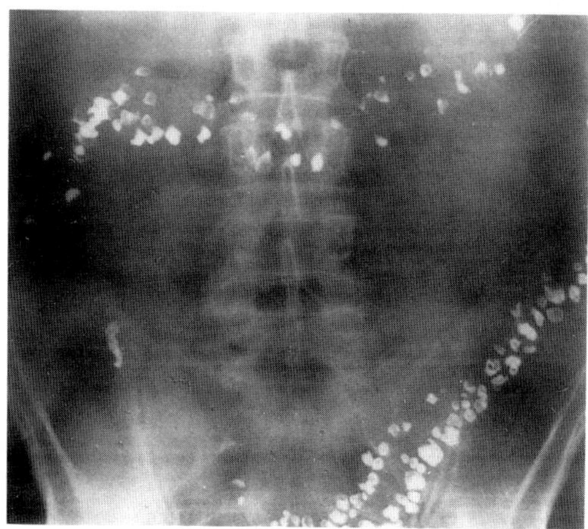

FIGURE 4.18. Barium in colonic diverticula and appendix five days after barium enema examination.

are also seen. In addition, contrast medium remaining from previous radiologic examinations can cast similar calcific density (Fig. 4.18).

GAS IN THE ALIMENTARY CANAL

Gas is found in the stomach and colon, but is not seen under normal conditions in the small intestine, except for the proximal duodenum and the terminal ileum. Gas may be present without pathologic significance in the small intestine of infants and bedridden patients. In such instances the intestine is not dilated as with obstruction.

When the transit of bowel contents is significantly slowed or obstruction is present, gas is liberated from bowel contents into the small intestine just as normally occurs in the large intestine. Disturbances of blood flow in the arter-

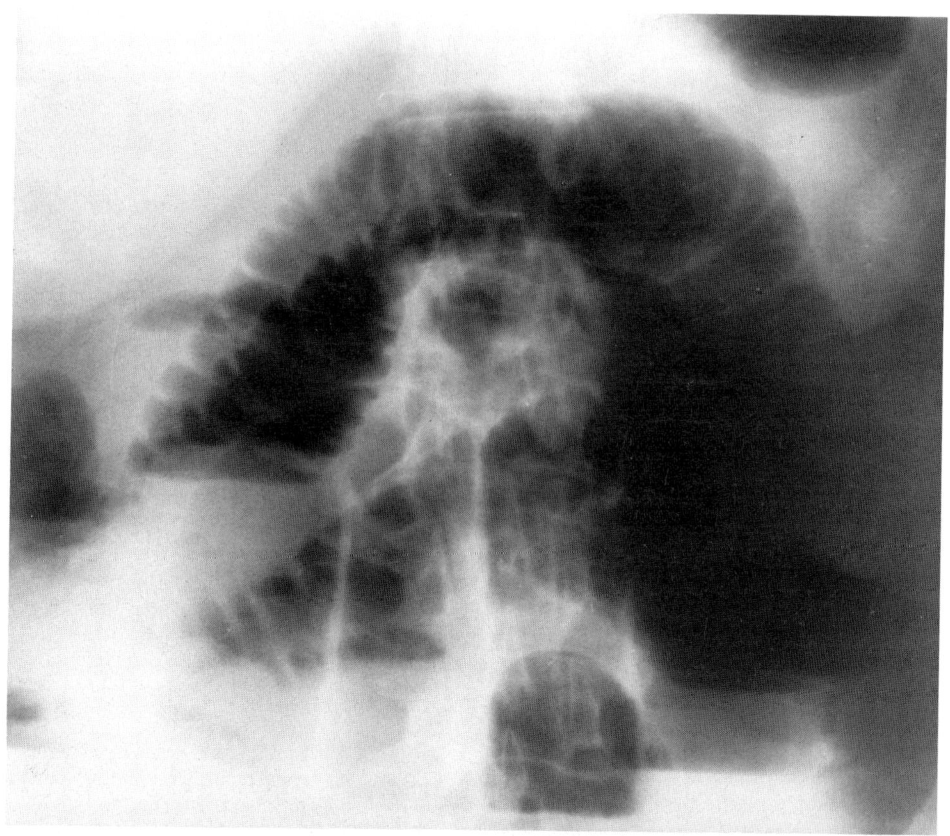

FIGURE 4.19. Mechanical obstruction of the distal large intestine, with proximal dilatation and gas-fluid levels in the dilated small and large bowel loops resembling an inverted "U."

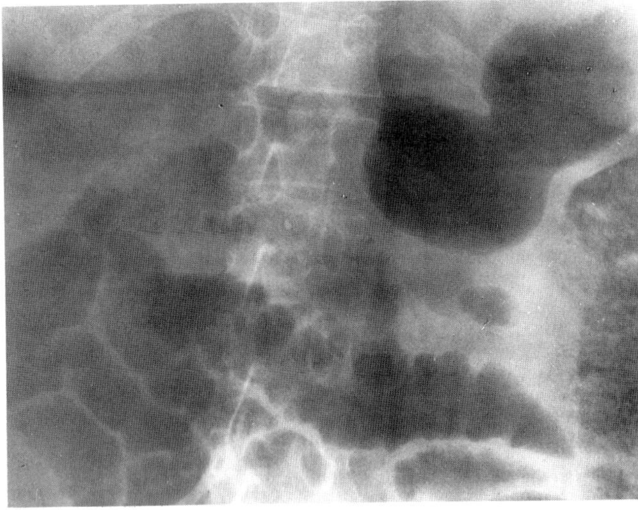

FIGURE 4.20. Adynamic, paralytic ileus. Gas present in the stomach, small bowel, and large bowel.

ies diminish gas absorption, resulting in bowel dilatation (Figs. 4.19 and 4.20).

All types of severe pancolitis can result in toxic dilatation of the colon where the lumen of the large intestine is very distended with gas. When the diameter of the transverse colon exceeds 5 cm in the supine position, there is an accompanying threat of perforation (Figs. 4.5 and 11.37).

GAS-FLUID LEVELS IN THE ALIMENTARY CANAL

A horizontal line dividing liquid and gas within the alimentary canal, a gas-fluid level, can be recorded on films taken with the patient in the upright or decubitus position with cross-table radiography (Figs. 4.21 and 4.22). Air-fluid levels are often a pathologic sign but can be normal in the stomach, duodenal bulb, and cecum, and, as a transitory phenomenon, in the terminal ileum. They are present without obstruction in patients with metabolic disorders like uremia, diabetic ketoacidosis, and low levels of serum potassium. Gas-fluid levels are also incidentally seen with acute diarrhea and following a water enema. In these instances, the alimentary canal lumen is not dilated. However, gas-fluid levels, with various heights and dilatation of intestinal loops resembling an upside down letter "U," are characteristic of obstruction. Such gas-fluid levels are more common with obstruction than with paralytic ileus.

A double gas-fluid level in the left hypochondrium is a sign of gastric volvulus or obstruction of the duodenum distal to the superior

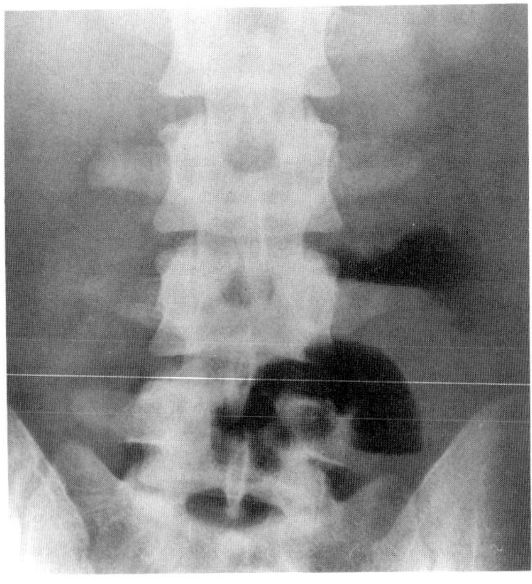

FIGURE 4.21. Gas-fluid levels in moderately dilated small bowel loops. The finding may be interpreted as incidental gas-fluid formation or as an early phase of obstruction. A follow-up film in one hour would be helpful.

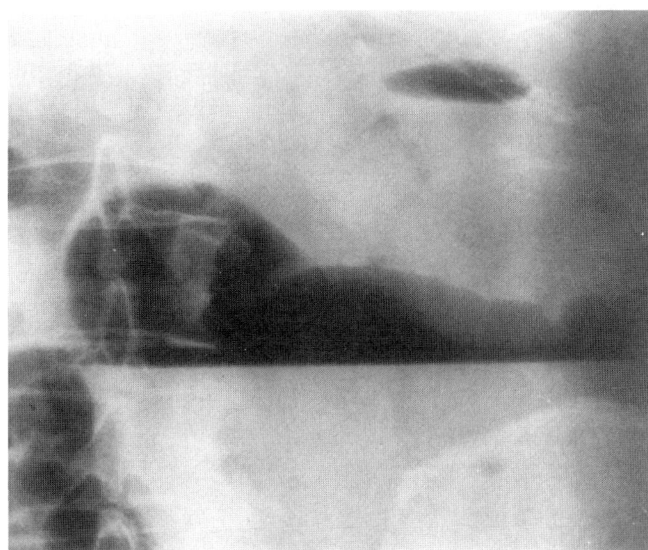

Figure 4.22. Gas-fluid level in the transverse colon.

flexure due to atresia, mesenteric bands, annular pancreas, or superior mesenteric artery syndrome.

Pneumoperitoneum

Gas is normally confined to the alimentary canal lumen. Free gas in the peritoneal cavity (pneumoperitoneum) accumulates in the nondependent portions. If pneumoperitoneum is not recorded on the initial supine scout film of the abdomen or on erect chest films, a patient with suspected alimentary canal perforation is to lie for 10–15 minutes in the position in which he will be next x-rayed. This enables free gas to accumulate (Fig. 4.23) in the superior aspects of the peritoneal cavity. A prominent pneumoperitoneum, with simultaneous presence of gas in the alimentary canal, identifies the outer and inner surfaces of the wall and provides an estimation of its thickness.

Spontaneous pneumoperitoneum can result from perforation of an alimentary canal organ containing gas, or from rupture of gas-inflated cysts, such as in intestinal pneumatosis. *Iatrogenic pneumoperitoneum* is a common finding after abdominal surgery and gynecological manipulations.

The average rate of absorption of air from the abdominal cavity is approximately 100 mL/day. However, carbon dioxide will disappear from the peritoneal space in only a few minutes.

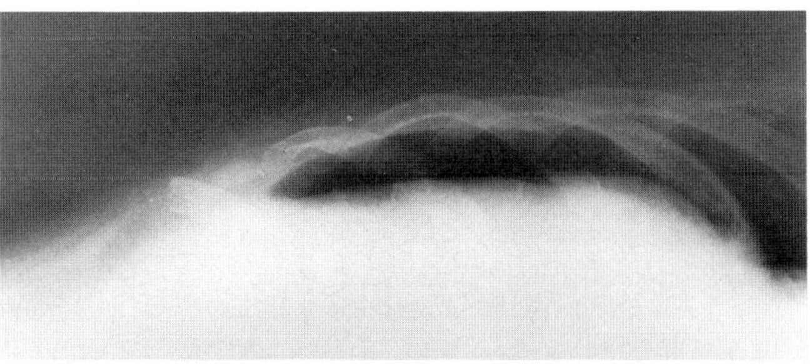

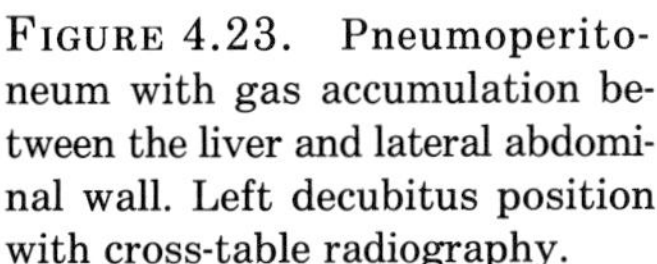

Figure 4.23. Pneumoperitoneum with gas accumulation between the liver and lateral abdominal wall. Left decubitus position with cross-table radiography.

Free Fluid in the Peritoneal Cavity

The composition of ascites cannot be determined radiographically. Transudate, exudate, hemorrhagic, or chylous ascites create opacities of equal density. However, CT may, by measuring attenuation, establish the density of ascites. Computed tomography is capable of demonstrating even very small amounts of peritoneal fluid. Only relatively large amounts of free liquid in the peritoneal cavity can be demonstrated on plain films of the abdomen. With a patient standing erect, fluid tends to accumulate in lower segments of the abdomen, producing generalized opacity.

FLUOROSCOPY

Fluoroscopy, the observation of X-ray exposed portions of the body on the monitor of a fluoroscopic apparatus, may be performed without or with the addition of contrast medium. In comparison with conventional roentgenographs, the fluoroscopic image appears as a negative image (Fig. 4.1). Fluoroscopy is performed to analyze the morphology and motor functions of alimentary canal organs, and spot films are taken during the procedure.

Most diagnoses are pursued during fluoroscopy. However, static roentgenographs enable detection of minute pathologic lesions such as erosions, aphthoid ulcers, plaques on mucosal surfaces, and polyps. In addition, roentgenographs document a radiologic examination. Abnormalities should be initially observed during fluoroscopy and the optimal positions for spot filming are then chosen. Positioning of the patient can greatly influence the demonstration of a pathologic process (Figs. 4.2 and 4.3).

Fluoroscopy enables evaluation of graded compression of a particular organ. One minute of abdominal fluoroscopy approximately equals the total radiation dose absorbed while obtaining a single roentgenograph (dimensions 35 × 35 cm) of the abdomen. However, one minute of such directed fluoroscopy can be more useful than several roentgenographs of the same area. The fluoroscopic field should be limited as much as possible.

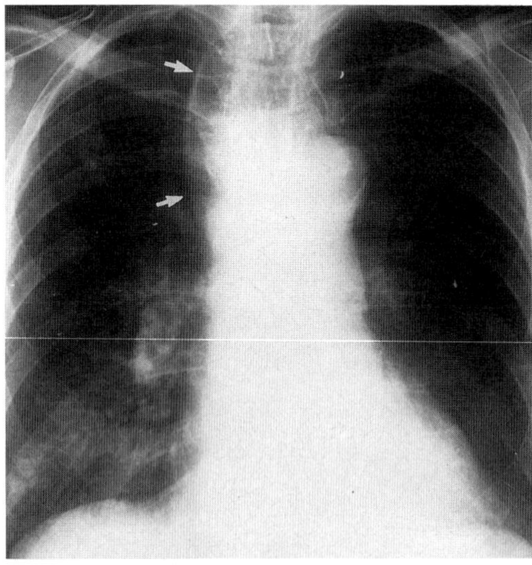

Figure 4.24. Achalasia of the lower esophageal segment. Widening of the upper mediastinum (arrows) and aspiration pneumonia in the right lung base.

ROENTGENOGRAPHY OF THE CHEST

Chest roentgenographs can also be useful in digestive tract diagnoses.

The right mediastinal contour may be widened in *achalasia* by a dilated esophagus (Fig. 4.24). An air-fluid level may be seen within a widened esophagus. The interstitial pulmonary pattern of the lungs is accentuated in one-quarter of patients with *progressive systemic sclerosis. Aspiration pneumonia* can result from altered transportation of esophageal contents. A large *esophageal diverticula* may contain a gas-fluid level (Fig. 4.25).

Widening of the mediastinum, with displacement of the trachea and the mediastinal pleura in front of the azygos vein, may be caused by *esophageal carcinoma*. Similar changes can be caused by a large esophageal diverticulum, enlarged left cardiac atrium, lymph node mass, or posterior herniation of the right lung after pneumonectomy. *Gastric hiatus hernia* can exhibit a gas-fluid level in herniated portions of the alimentary canal in the retrocardiac region (Fig. 4.26).

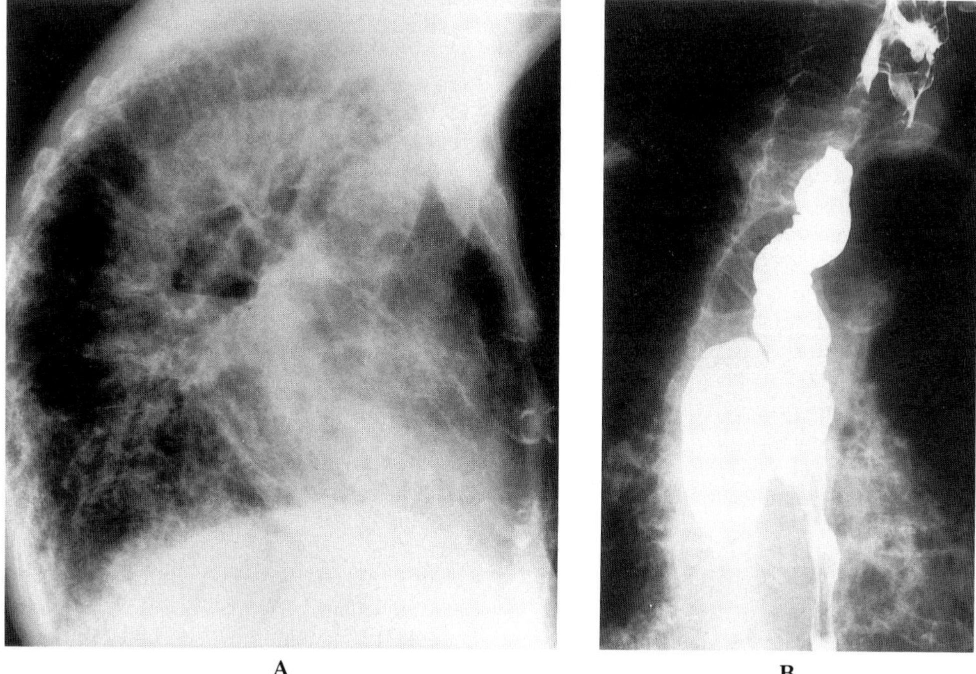

A B

FIGURE 4.25. (A) Gas-fluid level in the mediastinum. (B) Large pulsion esophageal diverticulum on barium series.

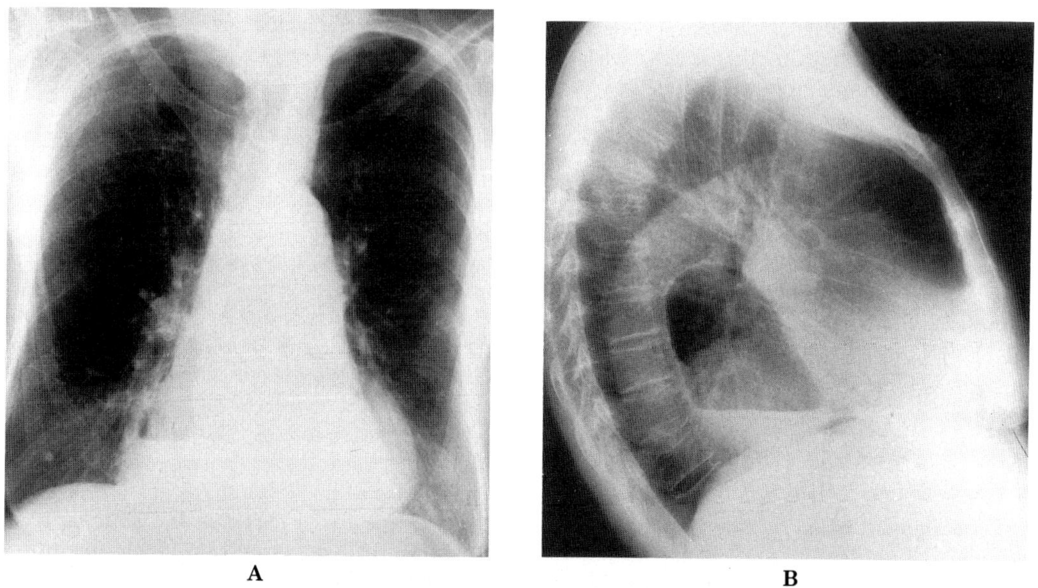

A B

FIGURE 4.26. (A) Widening of the mediastinum just above the diaphragm with a gas-fluid level. (B) Gas and fluid accumulation in an entrapped hiatus hernia of the stomach.

Malignant tumors of the alimentary canal can metastasize to the lungs. Colorectal carcinoma may result in lymphangitic and hematogenous pulmonary metastases. Approximately one-half of colonic and 64% of rectal carcinomas metastasize to the lungs by the time they have reached advanced stages.

Segmental and subsegmental plate-like pulmonary atelectases and fluid in the left pleural cavity are found in 50% of patients with *pancreatitis*. Large *pancreatic pseudocysts* can extend into the mediastinum through the esophageal hiatus and other normal or pathologic openings in the diaphragm.

Pneumoperitoneum can be readily diagnosed on chest radiographs. A gas-fluid level within the cavity of a *subphrenic abscess* can be accompanied by an accumulation of pleural fluid, and elevation and immobility of the ipsilateral leaf of the diaphragm.

RADIOLOGIC MANAGEMENT PRECEDING A BARIUM MEAL

A short interview about patient symptoms and information about previous radiologic examinations, surgical interventions, and medication may be helpful. Chest roentgenogram may reveal a cause for hemoptysis which could have been confused with hematemesis. Oral administration of barium or water-soluble contrast medium is contraindicated in patients with intestinal gangrene, complete obstruction of the bowel, or toxic megacolon. However, with mechanical bowel obstruction, barium enema may be performed.

Contrast medium remaining after previous radiologic examinations or deposition of mineral salts in abdominal organs can interfere with an examination. Conversely, subsequent barium filling may overlay abnormalities which might be visible on plain films.

RADIOGRAPHIC CONTRAST MEDIA FOR ALIMENTARY CANAL STUDIES

On plain abdominal radiograms and at fluoroscopy, alimentary canal organs cannot always be readily discriminated from adjacent anatomical structures which absorb X-rays almost equally. When a segment of the alimentary canal is filled with negative contrast medium, for example, gas, it becomes visible since fewer X-rays are absorbed. Positive contrast media absorb more X-rays than normal soft tissues, facilitating visualization of the internal surface of alimentary canal organs.

Negative contrast media are most commonly administered in combination with positive contrast media. "Double contrast" is a name for such methods of examination. Suitable negative contrast media are air and carbon dioxide.

Positive Contrast Media

Positive contrast media can be insoluble in water, such as barium sulfate, or water-soluble, such as triiodinated compounds of aminobenzoic acid.

Barium Sulfate. Barium sulfate is suitable for examination of all segments of the alimentary canal. It is of negligible solubility in body fluids and water, and eventually should be completely eliminated after the examination. In commercial form, some of the particles are of colloidal dimensions and the remainder are coarsely dispersed, forming a nontransparent suspension.

Colloid solutions, sols, can be lyophobic or lyophilic. Lyophobic sols are characterized by an absence of attraction between the dispersant phase and the dispersal medium and have a tendency to separate. Like electrical charges on the surface of particles prevent aggregation and sedimentation. The dispersant phase and the medium of lyophilic sols attract each other. Changes in the properties of lyophilic and lyophobic sols are gradual, and most systems have intermediate properties.

Flocculation is the irreversible sedimentation of lyophobic sols. It results from a loss of electrical charge, most frequently after addition of small amounts of electrolytes. Except for this effect on electric charge, the solvent, an additive in barium suspensions which adheres to particles of barium sulfate, has stabilizing properties. Smaller particles and a higher concentration of barium sulfate result in slower flocculation. Protective additives, in as low a concentration as 1%, interpolate between particles of barium and water. In this way lyophobic sols are transformed into lyophilic sols and the suspension becomes resistant to the effect of electrolytes, enabling the use of high concentrations of barium sulfate without flocculation. When the acidity changes, particles of protective additives can be exchanged for others not possessing these properties, thus increasing the flocculation tendency. Consequently, a suspension of barium sulfate of high quality has to be resistant to changes in acidity since gastrointestinal fluids can vary from very acid gastric juice to alkaline contents of the small bowel.

Additives (adjuvants) further refine the properties of barium sulfate suspensions. *Suspending additives* are big organic molecules which slow down the sedimentation of barium sulfate and contribute to increased viscosity of the suspension. Gelatin, carboxymethylcellulose, gum arabic, kaolin, pectin, starch, and sorbitol have such properties. Suspending additives allow the more intimate adherence of barium, a property of particular importance in double-contrast examinations. *Dispersing agents* are sodium citrate and sodium carboxymethylcellulose. Simethicone prevents the formation of *bubbles* during gas liberation from an effervescent agent, or insufflation of air for double-contrast enema (Fig. 4.27). Citric acid and sodium bicarbonate influence the *acidity* of a suspension. Potassium sorbate prevents *growth of bacteria*. *Flavoring agents* added to barium suspensions are sucrose, vanillin, levulose, dextrose, and chocolate. The single most important requirement of a barium suspension is good adherence to the mucosa. The thickness of the barium layer coating the mucosa, and consequently the quality of roentgenograms, depends on the concentration of barium sulfate particles and the viscosity of the suspension. A very thin layer of barium tends to disintegrate, particularly when feces and mucus are present.

Flocculation of barium sulfate may result from excessive mucus (Fig. 4.28). Segmentation of barium is a sequel of flocculation and presents as discontinuity of the barium column and lumping of particles, forming clusters (Fig. 4.29). An increase in barium sulfate concentration lessens the tendency for flocculation caused by gastric juice.

Barium suspensions of low viscosity and high concentration are suitable for double-contrast examinations. A decrease in viscosity can be obtained by increasing the number of large particles. Such a suspension adsorbs less wa-

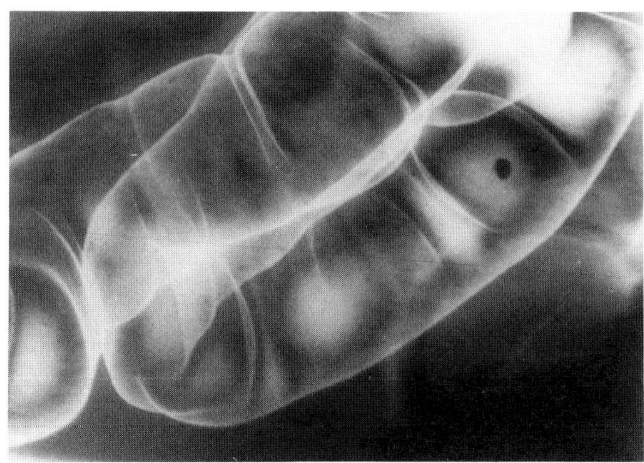

A

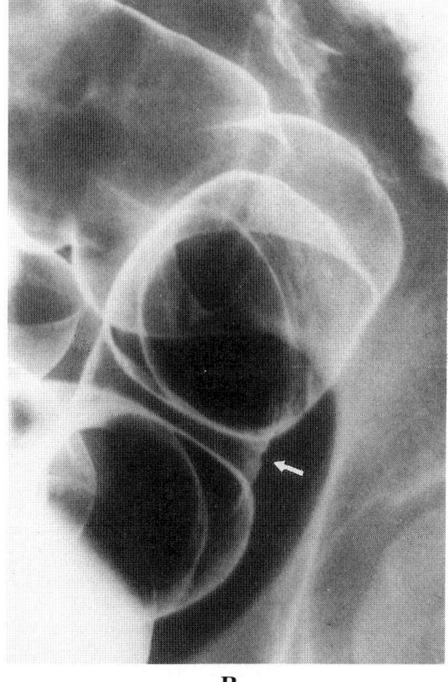

B

FIGURE 4.27. (A) Small colonic polyp mimics an air bubble on double-contrast enema studies. (B) After rotation and additional air insufflation, the lesion persistently alters colonic contour (arrow). Endoscopy confirmed the diagnosis.

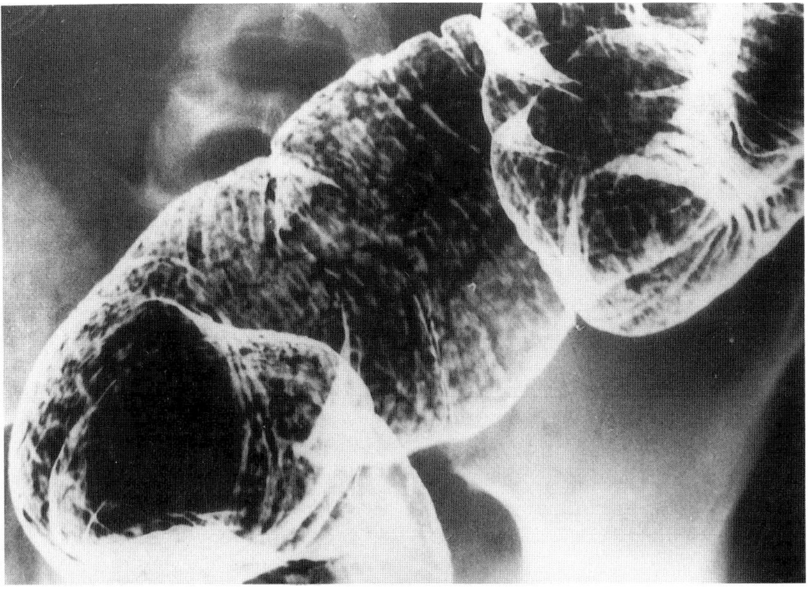

FIGURE 4.28. Flocculation of barium sulfate suspension during double-contrast enema.

ter. The quantity of barium sulfate in the suspension may be expressed in weight/weight (wt/wt) or weight/volume (wt/vol) ratio.

While an alimentary canal examination using only barium is termed a single-contrast examination, a double-contrast examination is performed by adding a negative contrast medium such as air. The latter method allows satisfactory penetration of X-rays through the thin layer of barium sulfate necessary for demonstration of mucosal surface detail. In single-contrast examinations, graded compression attenuates the barium column (Fig. 4.30) and increased kilovoltage allows better X-ray penetration of the barium column. The larger the lumen of an organ, the more dilute the suspension of barium sulfate that would be suitable.

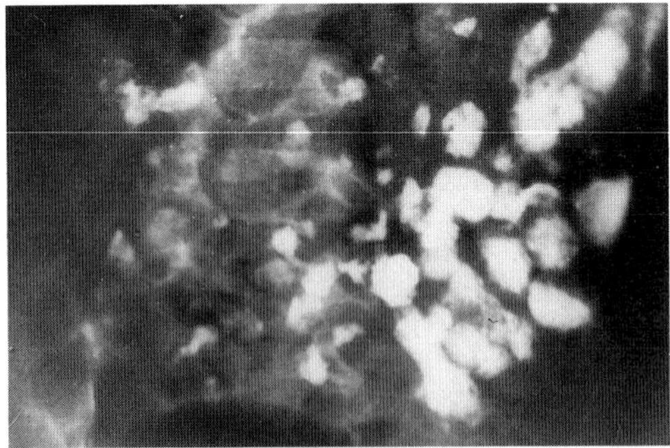

FIGURE 4.29. Segmentation of barium column in the small bowel. Flocculated barium accumulates in clusters.

Barium sulfate has few side effects and the majority are not significant. When aspirated, barium sulfate is eliminated from the tracheobronchial tree very slowly by the action of macrophages. Granulomas and adhesions can develop after barium enters the peritoneal cavity. Deep ulcerations as in ulcerative colitis can allow entrance of barium into draining veins, resulting in embolism.

No more than 106 cases of *hypersensitivity* reactions to barium sulfate have been described as of 1987. Approximately 62% of the reactions were manifest as a skin rash. Respiratory complaints accounted for 8% and loss of consciousness for 8%. The remaining 22% were of various forms. Hypersensitivity reactions could not be classified as to type. Less than half of the patients reacted during or immediately after an upper gastrointestinal series. The remainder

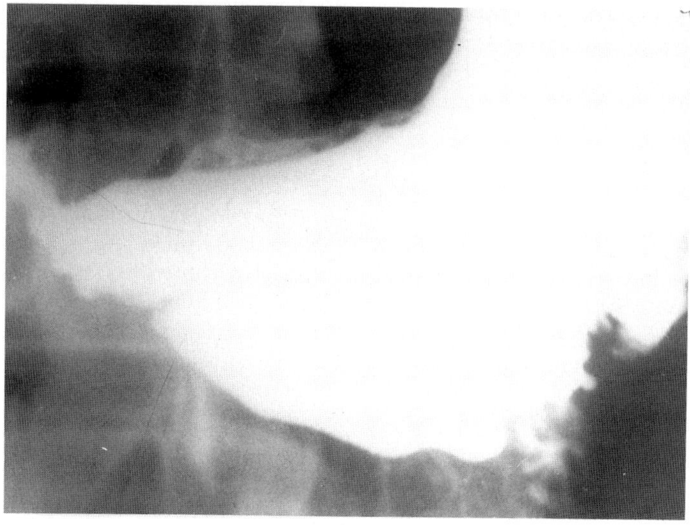

A

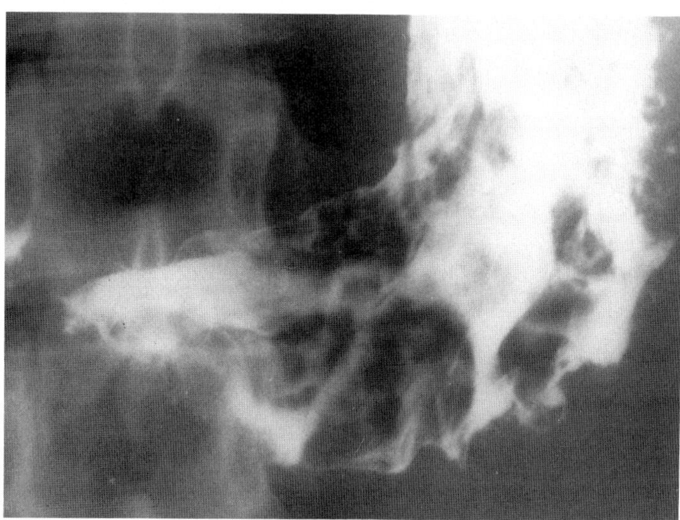

B

FIGURE 4.30. (A) Stomach filled with high-concentration barium suspension demonstrates irregularities of the greater curvature. (B) Graded compression reveals a large polypoid carcinoma occupying the distal segment of the gastric body and antrum.

reacted during or following barium enema examination, the majority of which were double-contrast enemas. The reactions occurred in one of 750,000 barium examinations. The effect of a hypotonic agent also cannot be discounted. Reactions are more likely caused by additives than by the barium suspension itself. The majority of reactions occurred with double-contrast examinations where the role of effervescent agents needs to be considered. Allergic reactions to glucagon can be anticipated in one out of a million applications. Double-contrast enema may also result in bacteremia, but the role of such an event in provoking a hypersensitivity reaction is not fully understood. Mild forms of hypersensitivity reactions disappear without treatment, while more serious forms require medication. In the case of a true anaphylactic reaction, epinephrine, antihistaminic agents, aminophylline, and corticosteroids have to be administered.

Water-Soluble Contrast Media. Water-soluble contrast media are indicated whenever alimentary canal perforation or fistula are suspected, such as after surgery, in Hirschprung's disease, and in meconium ileus. Hyperosmolar water-soluble contrast media, in contrast to iso-osmolar media, undergo dilution in the small intestine as well as concentration in the colon. Sodium meglumine amidotrisoate (76%) (Gastrografin) is not significantly absorbed from the alimentary canal. Its osmolarity is five times that of blood plasma, and therefore it has to be diluted when used in children. Precipitation may occur if there is slow gastric emptying. The sediment may cause irritation of the gastric mucosa with erosions and bleeding.

Low osmolarity contrast media such as metrizamide (Amipaque) or ioxaglate (Hexabrix) are suitable for examinations in children. They are isotonic with body fluids and are therefore not diluted within the alimentary canal. Only 1% of orally administered metrizamide is absorbed from the alimentary canal. Aspiration does not cause alarming symptoms since iso-osmolar solutions do not cause pulmonary edema or significant irritation of pneumocytes. Barium aspiration in newborns may result in respiratory distress with cyanosis, atelectasis, pneumonia, and fibrosis. Aspirated hypertonic solutions such as Gastrografin can cause hypovolemic shock. Fatalities have been reported following barium and Gastrografin aspiration.

A water-soluble contrast medium which can also be safely used is diatrizoate sodium (Hypaque). However, when used for an enema, a 10- to 100-fold increase in serum iodine can be measured one hour after administration. Concern for iodine hypersensitivity is therefore important. Iohexol (Omnipaque) is an excellent iso-osmolar, nonionic contrast medium with minimal side effects.

Transitory eosinophilia can be anticipated in 20% of patients after intravenous application of iodinated water-soluble contrast media.

The following criteria should be considered when selecting a contrast medium: toxicity, quality of opacification of alimentary canal, simplicity of use, absorption from the alimentary canal, and cost.

PHARMACORADIOLOGY

Barium examinations provide diagnostic information regarding alimentary canal anatomy as well as function. The rate of barium evacuation from the stomach may depend on the type of barium product utilized, and is proportional to the quantity of ingested suspension. Sympathomimetic activity results in slow evacuation of barium from the stomach and the duodenum, while cholinergic activity stimulates alimentary canal motility.

Transportation of barium can be accelerated or slowed. The transit of barium through the esophagus is slowed in the horizontal position. Small bowel transit is shortened by walking. Such actions are, however, limited to certain segments of the alimentary canal and are not always successful. Alimentary canal hypotonia with decrease or cessation of peristalsis, or an increase in tone along with peristaltic activity, can help estimate wall pliability. Demonstration of pathologic lesions in dilated organs is enhanced by hypotonia. Although a shortened small intestine transit time is desirable to preserve diagnostic properties of a barium suspension, hypotonia is welcomed when barium reaches the ileocecal valve.

Pharmacological agents are used to modify tone, peristalsis and secretion of the alimentary canal, thus enabling distinction between functional and structural changes, enhancing gaseous distension, and improving adherence of barium to mucosal surface.

Spasmolytics

Spasmolytic agents, either neurotropic or musculotropic, cause smooth muscles to relax. *Papaverine* is musculotropic and has a direct action on smooth muscles. Since effects are expressed mainly on blood vessel muscles, it is used only rarely in pharmacoradiography of the alimentary canal. *Oxyphenonium bromide* (Antrenyl) is a neurotropic agent, a parasympathetic blocking agent. It has been widely used for hypotonia in duodenography. Contraindications for its use are ischemic heart disease, glaucoma, and extreme myopia. *Atropine sulfate* is also a neurotropic anticholinergic preparation, which acts by blocking parasympathetic ganglia. It has a powerful effect on the peripheral autonomic nervous system, and acts as a spasmolytic while inhibiting gastric secretion. Atropine competes for the same receptors as acetylcholine. It relaxes smooth muscles, and lowers the tone of the alimentary canal, inhibiting small bowel and colonic motility. *Hyoscine butylbromide* (Buscopan) manifests its spasmolytic activity within a few minutes of parenteral application. It can be injected intravenously or intramuscularly. The therapeutic effect lasts about 20 minutes. In addition to the anticholinergic action, it blocks autonomic nervous system ganglia and has properties similar to those of curare. Buscopan inhibits gastric secretion and alimentary canal motility, but is contraindicated in patients with prostatic adenoma, tachycardia, megacolon, and advanced atherosclerosis of the cerebral arteries. In patients with glaucoma, pilocarpine eye drops have to be administered prior to Buscopan. *Propantheline bromide* (Probanthine) blocks nerve impulses in autonomic ganglia and parasympathetic tissue receptors, interfering with acetylcholine. If administered intravenously or intramuscularly, action occurs within five to eight minutes, with therapeutic and side effects lasting up to one hour. It has been widely used in hypotonic duodenography, but causes dry mouth, prolonged blurred vision, tachycardia, and urinary retention. Use of propantheline bromide has been said to cause fatalities (Dr. R.E. Miller, oral communication, May 1982). All anticholinergic drugs can cause visual disturbances.

Hormones of the gastrointestinal tract are spasmolytics that act upon the esophagus, stomach, and intestines.

Glucagon is secreted by alpha cells of the pancreatic islets. It causes hypotonia of the esophagus and can provoke gastroesophageal reflux in 8% of individuals in whom reflux was not previously evident. Immediately after intravenous application of 0.25 mg of glucagon, the stomach and duodenum dilate and peristaltic activity ceases for about 10 minutes. The pylorus opens, allowing barium to pass into the duodenum when the patient is turned to the right side from the supine position. By increasing the dose, the hypotonia will last longer, but will not become more pronounced.

Glucagon is the most reliable hypotonic drug for upper gastrointestinal double-contrast examinations. Even small doses of glucagon (0.025–0.125 mg) decrease motility of the stomach but do not increase distensibility, as with barium sulfate suspension. Its influence on the pyloric sphincter is negligible. Visualization of the duodenum is significantly improved after application of glucagon, in contrast to the situation with the stomach. However, some feel that visualization of the stomach can be improved by use of glucagon. Hypotonic duodenography can be easily performed without a tube by using glucagon.

For use during a barium enema examination, doses of at least 0.5 mg glucagon are administered intravenously. Doses of 0.25–1.5 mg do not cause side effects. Doses of 2 mg or higher may provoke nausea and vomiting. Glucagon is contraindicated in patients with adenoma of the prostate, insulinoma, and pheochromocytoma. A hypotonic effect of glucagon on the mesenteric small intestine has also been verified.

Glucagon may be administered before or during a barium meal. In contrast, neurotropic drugs are contraindicated before contrast medium reaches the duodenum. Application of 1 mg of glucagon does not significantly improve the sensitivity or specificity of a double-contrast enema. However, glucagon is a more suitable spasmolytic than hyoscine butylbromide and propantheline bromide because its therapeutic effects are more pronounced, and its side effects are fewer and less intense.

Cholecystokinin (pancreozymin) is secreted by the mucosa of proximal portions of the small intestine after contact with fats and proteins. Except for contraction of the gallbladder, it causes shortening of small bowel transit time so that the terminal ileum can often be visualized in less than 20 minutes. Cholecystokinin has a mild spasmolytic effect on the stomach and the colon.

Secretin is released into the blood stream by cells of the duodenal and jejunal mucosa. Its effects on the smooth muscles of the alimentary canal are similar to those caused by glucagon, that is, intravenous injection decreases their motility. Depending on the dose, hypotonia can last for 8–14 minutes. Increased pancreatic secretion provoked by secretin does not affect the coating of mucosa with barium for hypotonic duodenography.

Prostaglandins have a considerable hypotonic effect on smooth muscles of the alimentary canal but are not routinely used in pharmacoradiographic barium studies.

Spasmolytics are used to distinguish organic from functional narrowing of the alimentary canal. Since they cause hypotonia of the stomach, thus preventing the rapid transition of barium into the duodenum, overlapping of the stomach with the duodenum can be avoided. They are routinely used in performing hypotonic duodenography but can also make a barium enema more comfortable and assist in relieving bowel spasms.

Accelerating Procedures

Rapid transit of barium through the small bowel is desirable. The most physiologic and simplest method is to give a large volume of barium (400–600 mL). A similar effect can be obtained by examining the stomach with 300 mL of iced barium suspension. The large volume and chilling effect stimulates peristalsis. Hyperosmolar contrast media like Gastrografin cause distension of the small intestine, producing a vagal reflex stimulation which results in accelerated transit. Some feel that an empty colon allows more rapid small bowel transit and recommend colon cleansing as preparation.

Parasympathomimetics. Parasympathomimetics increase the transit rate of barium. *Mecholyl* is an anticholinesterase drug. It provokes painful contractions of the esophagus in patients with achalasia. *Prostigmin* increases gastric peristalsis and emptying of the stomach and small bowel. *Metoclopramide* is an antiemetic drug of unknown mode of action. It relieves pylorospasm and accelerates small bowel transit. Metoclopramide does not affect the secretion of gastric glands and does not diminish gastric secretion. Given in a dose of 20 mg intravenously or in tablets, it increases gastric emptying but does not improve adherence of barium sulfate to mucosal surfaces. Metoclopramide increases the resting tone of the lower esophageal segment. It has virtually no side effects. A single dose, prior to introduction of the intestinal tube, improves results of enteroclysis by shortening small bowel transit time. *Serotonin* injected in a dose of 10 mg also shortens small intestine transit time.

Both cimetidine and pirensepine improve the visibility of areae gastricae. Unlike cimetidine, pirensepine decreases the quantity of gastric secretions during fasting. This indicates that factors other than the volume of gastric juice affect the quality of mucosal surface demonstration. Although *sodium bicarbonate* decreases the viscosity of gastric mucus, making the mucus layer thinner, premedication does not significantly affect the visualization of mucosal surfaces during double-contrast upper gastrointestinal series.

Effervescent preparations are used for distension of upper gastrointestinal organs with gas. They appear in various forms, such as granules, powder, crystals, and tablets. The liberated carbon dioxide causes prompt distension and is soon absorbed. Simethicone is an effective antifoaming agent often added to effervescent preparations. However, if bubbles are accidentally formed, they should be destroyed by rotating the patient around the longitudinal body axis in the horizontal position. Otherwise, air bubbles can resemble polyps.

SINGLE-CONTRAST EXAMINATIONS

Single-contrast examinations demonstrate defects in the contrast medium column. Positive defects created by depressed lesions such as ulcers or diverticula create an abnormal accumulation of contrast medium outside of the organ contour. Negative defects are caused by protruding lesions and manifest as radiolucent areas within the contrast column (Diagram 3.1 and Figs. 3.1 and 3.2).

Upper Gastrointestinal Tract

In the last several years the number of upper gastrointestinal barium studies in the United States decreased by one-third because of the wide use of endoscopy. While radiologic examination can be partially replaced by endoscopic procedures, an endoscope cannot always reach certain portions of the alimentary tract. This is certainly true for segments distal to stenoses, for gastric volvulus, and for almost the entire small intestine. Very elongated segments of the alimentary canal such as dolichocolon, and sharp angulations, can make endoscopy difficult or impossible.

Since the upper gastrointestinal tract extends from the oral part of the pharynx to the duodenojejunal junction, the entire upper gastrointestinal tract needs to be examined radiographically. However, each segment may also be examined separately by the use of fluoroscopy and spot filming. Each pathologic lesion must be roentgenographed in at least two projections, and during various stages of relaxation and contraction of the organ wall. A double-contrast examination can give detailed insight into discrete changes in the mucosal surface.

Patient Preparation. Solid food must not be taken for eight hours or liquids for four hours prior to upper gastrointestinal examination. Analysis of a plain abdominal roentgenograph or short preliminary fluoroscopy of the abdomen can reveal information such as the presence of pneumoperitoneum, obstruction, or abnormal calcification. The chest roentgenograph can show widening of the mediastinum or the presence of pleural fluid and metastatic disease.

The Pharynx. Examination of the pharynx lies within the domain of direct endoscopy. However, morphologic changes can be examined by radiologic methods. Radiologic examination can analyze the act of swallowing, which is not possible, or is more difficult, by other methods such as manometry.

The pharynx should be examined in at least two projections. For demonstration of soft tissues of the pharynx, roentgenographs with a tube-to-film distance of 2 m are taken while the patient is breathing continuously and performing a Valsalva maneuver. Air in the lumen of the pharynx as a negative contrast medium facilitates visualization of soft tissues (see Fig. 1.3).

Soft tissues of the pharynx, cervical spine, tongue, hyoid bone, inner surface of the pharyngeal walls, larynx, palate, and vocal cords should be analyzed during swallowing and phonation, starting with the lateral position.

Profile roentgenographs demonstrate the base of the tongue with the valleculae and larynx. Retropharyngeal tissue thickness and protrusions into the lumen should be analyzed. Prevertebral soft tissues of the hypopharynx in normal adults can be up to 5 mm thick. In the epipharynx this value should not exceed 3 mm. However, greater thickness can be seen in normal children particularly in the epipharynx. For locating foreign bodies, additional oblique roentgenographs are helpful and tomography may be necessary.

The inner surface of the oral and laryngeal segments of the pharynx are shown in detail by the use of barium. Rapid movement of barium makes it difficult for static roentgenographs of the contrast-filled pharynx to be taken. Movement of the contrast bolus can be slowed by positioning the patient supine in the Trendelenburg position. After the contrast bolus has passed, the surface of the mucosa often remains coated with barium. Simultaneous presence of air enables double-contrast study with detailed presentation of the mucosal surface. In lateral and oblique projections the epiglottic vallecula is seen as an anterior outpouching of contrast medium. Pyriform sinuses are symmetrically filled with contrast medium when low viscosity barium is swallowed. However, thick barium sulfate suspensions may flow mainly into one pyriform sinus and this should not be mistaken for contralateral pharyngeal palsy. When examined fluoroscopically in the P-A position the patient is instructed to hold a mouthful of barium and swallow after raising the chin. While x-raying in the lateral and oblique projections, superimposition is avoided by lowering the patient's shoulders.

The following is a brief outline recommended as an X-ray sequence:

1. Sagittal and lateral roentgenograms of the pharynx filled with contrast medium (Fig. 4.31). It is not easy to obtain such roentgenographs at the right moment because of the fast-moving bolus.
2. P-A and lateral double-contrast roentgenographs.

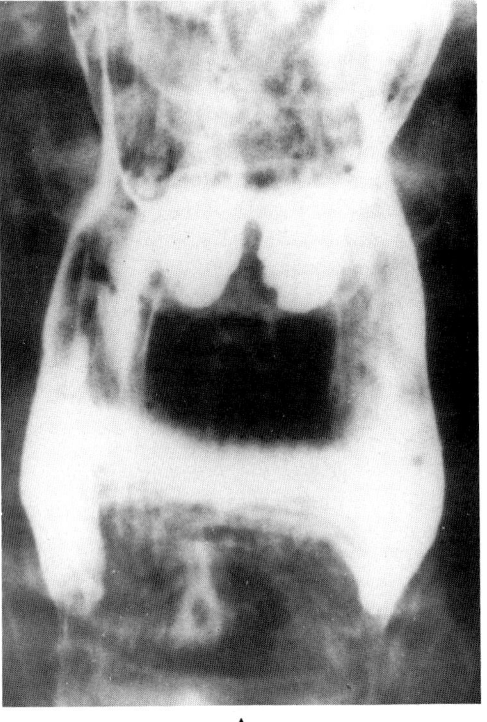

A

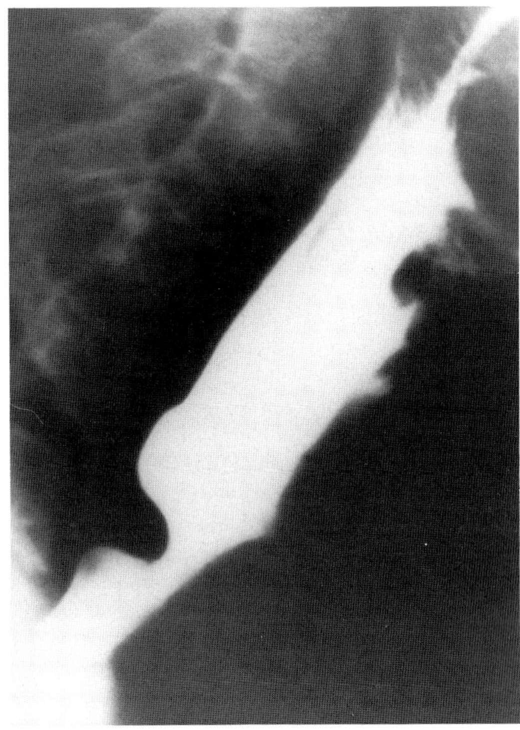

B

FIGURE 4.31. Barium studies of the hypopharynx. (A) Normal finding in P-A projection. (B) Profile film of the hypopharynx demonstrates impression on the posterior wall by the lower esophageal constrictor. "Irregularities" of the upper anterior aspect of the wall are caused by normal structures.

3. P-A roentgenogram while performing a Valsalva maneuver.
4. Oblique double-contrast roentgenographs.

Morphology and activity of the tongue, palate, pharynx, epiglottis, and lower pharyngeal constrictor need to be analyzed and the type of esophageal peristalsis determined. For detailed insight into the pharyngeal phase of swallowing, fluoroscopy should be recorded on videotape or rapid sequence roentgenography. Each frame needs to be studied separately.

Specific Procedures. In severely ill patients 10–15 mL of dilute barium suspension is given. Gastrografin should be avoided because of the possibility of respiratory distress if aspirated. Iso-osmolar water-soluble contrast media can be used.

While motility disturbances usually alter swallowing of liquids, a more solid contrast bolus is occasionally needed when there are structural changes in the pharynx, since swallowing of a solid bolus can be abnormal when swallowing liquids is not. *Video-manometry* provides correlation between motility observed during fluoroscopy and variations in intraluminal pressure.

Contrast pharyngolaryngography can be performed in patients with malignant neoplasms of the pharynx so that both the magnitude of the process and extent of pharyngeal involvement are demonstrated. Propiliodone suspension is injected through a tube inserted down to the root of the tongue while the patient inhales under local anesthesia. On inspiration of the contrast medium, the pharynx and larynx are demonstrated with double contrast. The roentgenographs are taken during phonation of the letter "e," quiet breathing, and a Valsalva maneuver. Thin section CT with 3-D reconstruction or magnetic resonance imaging (MRI) can now provide similarly detailed imaging.

The Esophagus. Initially, the region of the esophagus is analyzed on chest roentgenograms or during fluoroscopy without contrast medium. The patient, standing flat against the upright table of a fluoroscopic apparatus, holds a cup of barium suspension in the left hand. He is instructed to take one large swallow of barium, then turns about 45 degrees to the left, to prevent overlapping the esophagus with the spine and the heart, and drinks one more large swallow. Another swallow can be taken after complete relaxation of the esophagus (Fig. 4.32). The table is then lowered to the horizontal position and the patient is rotated 360 degrees to the left in order to facilitate evaluation of the esophagus in various projections. Additional barium may be given in the horizontal position. The recumbent position slows transport of the contrast bolus and provides better filling of any narrow-necked diverticula. Spot films should be taken during the course of fluoroscopy.

Longitudinal folds, mucosal relief, and the type and degree of peristalsis are studied during swallowing. During the phase of relaxation, the smooth walls of the normal esophagus are demonstrated with double contrast. The contrast bolus may be temporarily delayed in the region of the gastroesophageal vestibule. However, stoppage at any other place should be considered abnormal until proven otherwise.

The search for a gastric hiatus hernia is performed after the stomach is filled with at least 250 mL of barium suspension. For examination of the esophagus, suspensions of various concentrations and viscosities may be used, although suspensions of lower viscosity are more suitable for double-contrast studies. More viscous suspensions are used when the speed of the bolus needs to be slowed or when the adherence of barium on the mucosal surface has not been satisfactory.

Detailed analysis of the esophagus by repeated large swallows of barium can be per-

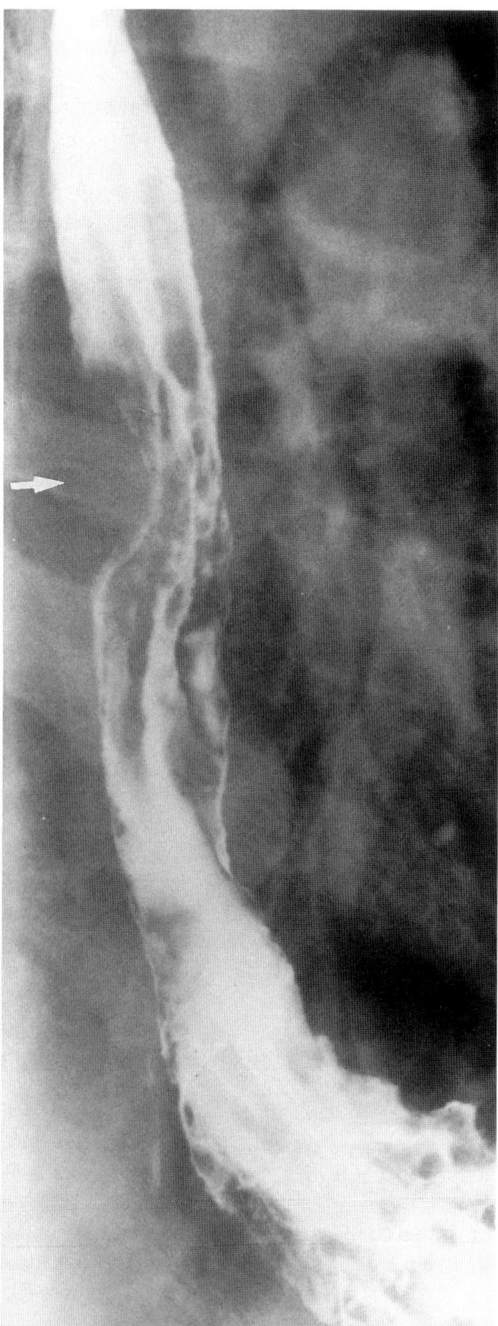

Figure 4.32. Barium examination of the esophagus in right anterior oblique position. Hiatus hernia of the stomach. Reflux esophagitis and leiomyoma of the posterior wall of the esophagus (arrow).

formed at the end of the upper gastrointestinal study. In that way, excesses of barium will not interfere with examination of the stomach and duodenum. When the possibility of aspiration is suspected, isotonic water-soluble contrast media should be utilized.

Analysis during fluoroscopy and on static roentgenograms includes examining the position, contours, and width of the lumen, compliance of the wall, type of peristalsis, indentations by adjacent structures, and mucosal relief. Several techniques can be utilized for double-contrast esophagography.

Specific Procedures. *Esophageal varices* are optimally demonstrated when pressure is increased in the abdomen and decreased in the chest. Deep inspiration in the horizontal or Trendelenburg position can facilitate filling of varices. Deep inspiration or Valsalva maneuver is performed after swallowing a contrast bolus, while lying prone, and with a slightly elevated right side (prone right posterior oblique). However, the patient should not swallow after coating the esophagus with barium to allow filling of the varices with blood prior to spot filming. Pharmacoradiography is used when suspected varices cannot be visualized by these maneuvers. Buscopan or glucagon gives good results.

In cases with *insufficient innervation*, such as achalasia, Mecholyl causes painful contractions.

Accurate measurement of a restricted *esophageal diameter* is possible by using wax globules filled with barium. The diameter of the globule should be about the same as the width of the stenosed area. If the globule becomes impacted the wax readily melts without causing prolonged obstruction.

In patients with early reflux esophagitis an *acidified suspension* of barium (prepared by adding 0.5 mL of 37% HCl to 100 mL of barium suspension) may be used. The swallowing of such a suspension causes tertiary esophageal contractions in 90% of patients with reflux esophagitis. After the acidified suspension, the patient should be given an antacid to drink.

Functional Tests of the Esophagus. Barium examination and esophagoscopy discover morphologic lesions of the esophagus. However, they may be insensitive in estimation of motor functions. Although the majority of the esophageal diseases affect function, that is, distal transportation of a bolus, evaluation of function is primarily reserved for patients without organic lesions. In testing esophageal function, the rate of distal advancement of a bolus is measured. Functional abnormalities are manifested by slowing of the distal transportation of esophageal contents.

Esophageal function can be studied by several means. Manometry is uncomfortable, time consuming, and labor intensive for the primary examiner. Interpretation problems are common. Transport of water labeled with technetium 99m (99m Tc) estimates esophageal function by nuclear medicine techniques. In children, satisfactory results can be similarly obtained by krypton 81m-labeled glucose, administered orally or by an intravenous route. The latter method delivers significantly less radiation exposure than a barium swallow.

When measuring transport of a barium-filled capsule during fluoroscopy in the supine position, peristalsis remains the only significant factor determining the speed of the bolus. A barium-filled capsule should reach the stomach in six seconds.

The Stomach and Duodenum. Impressions caused by adjacent anatomical structures, motility and elasticity of the gastric wall, stenoses, and the rate of evacuation of the contrast medium from the stomach can all be clearly identified by single-contrast examination. It is performed using 150 mL or more of barium suspension. Portions of the stomach that are readily accessible to palpation and compression are easier to examine. Mucosal relief is demonstrated by rotating the patient in the horizontal plane around the longitudinal body axis. Air present in the stomach enables limited double-contrast examination (Fig. 4.33A). However, delicate pathologic lesions, such as tiny polyps, may be missed.

The examination starts with small amounts of a high-density barium suspension (at least 130% wt/vol) to provide good mucosal coating. However, low-density barium (not more than 30% wt/vol) should be used for continuation of the examination.

The examination is best performed with the following sequence:

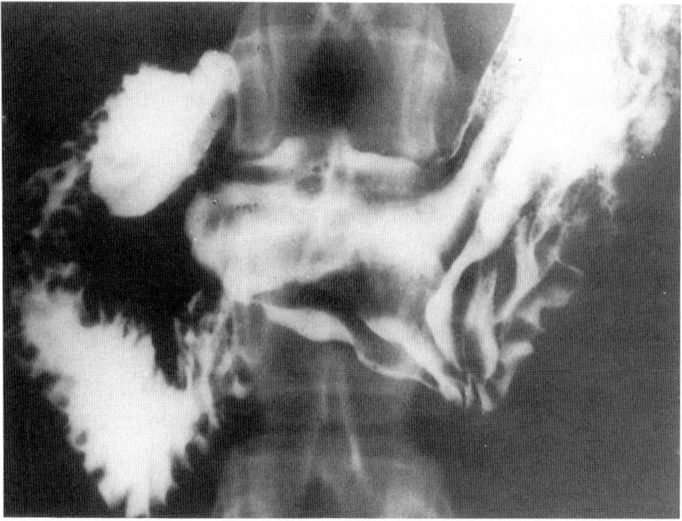

A

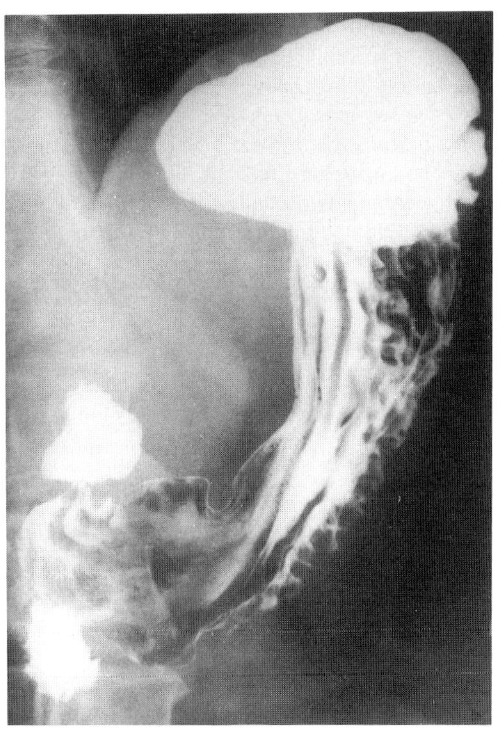

B

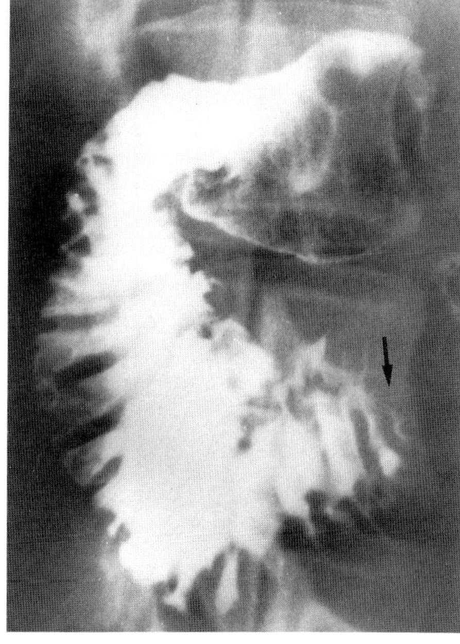

C

FIGURE 4.33. (A) Distal portion of the gastric body, antrum, and duodenum demonstrated with barium, in the P-A position. Thickening of duodenal folds of duodenitis with erosions. (B) Mucosal relief of the gastric antrum and duodenal bulb in the supine right anterior oblique position. (C) Compression of the third duodenal segment by superior mesenteric artery (arrow) with proximal dilatation. Same position as (B).

1. The patient stands with his back leaning against the upright table of a fluoroscopic apparatus, holding the cup with barium in his left hand. The table is tilted 20–30 degrees so that the head of the patient is away from the examiner (Diagram 4.1A). After rotating the patient 30–40 degrees to the left, one large bolus (approximately 30 mL) of barium is swallowed and the patient takes a deep breath so as to hold barium in the distal segment of the esophagus. Emptying of this first contrast bolus into the stomach is observed in this position. Barium should enter into the stomach as a single stream with the anterior and posterior walls of the stomach presented in profile (Diagram 4.1B). The superior segment of the duodenum, which is directed posteriorly, shows its greatest length, and the anterior wall of the duodenal bulb is identified.

2. The table is then lowered to the horizontal position and the patient is rotated toward the left onto his abdomen without fluoroscopy. In the prone position the lesser and greater curvatures of the stomach and duodenum can be evaluated and mucosal relief of the gastric fundus is displayed (Diagram 4.1A).

3. The patient then turns to his right side, spot films are taken (Diagram 4.1C), and then he continues to rotate beyond the supine position until his right side becomes elevated 20–40 degrees from the table assuming a supine right anterior oblique position. Mucosal relief of the antrum and duodenal bulb can be analyzed in this position (Diagram 4.1B and Fig. 4.33B and C).

4. The patient turns back onto his right side and continues to rotate until the anterior aspect of his trunk and the table form an angle of 60 degrees. In this prone left posterior oblique position, the cardia and peristalsis of the stomach are best analyzed, and the anterior and posterior wall of the stomach are seen in profile. Holding this position, the patient is instructed to drink an additional 50–100 mL of barium suspension through a straw.

5. The patient then turns over his right side onto his back, assuming the same position as in the third phase of the examination (Diagram 4.1B).

6. When the fluoroscopic apparatus is raised back to the vertical position, the gastric fundus and duodenal bulb are evaluated in oblique projections (Diagram 4.1B and C; Figs. 4.34 to 4.36). The entire duodenum should also be analyzed throughout the course of the upper gastrointestinal tract examination.

Any abnormal appearance of gastric or duodenal morphology should be scrutinized by graded compression, palpation, or gaseous distension. Only segments of the stomach which are not overlapped by the costal margin are accessible to palpation. The addition of a hypotonic agent may improve results of the examination.

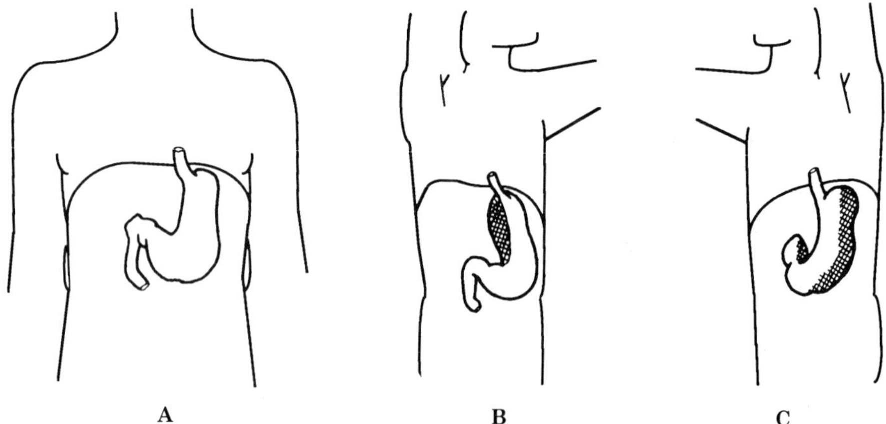

DIAGRAM 4.1. (A to C) Visibility of particular portions of the stomach and duodenum depend on projection at upper gastrointestinal series.

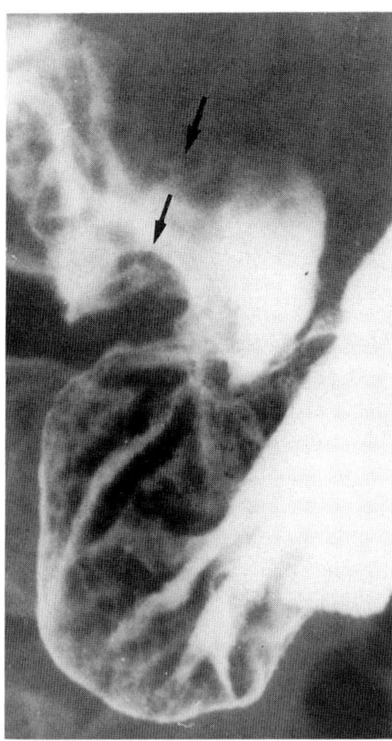

FIGURE 4.34. Gastric antrum and duodenal bulb in semierect left anterior oblique position. Anterior wall of the stomach and duodenum are on the left and posterior wall on the right (see Diagram 4.1C). Linear defect of the bulb is caused by a dilated common bile duct (arrows).

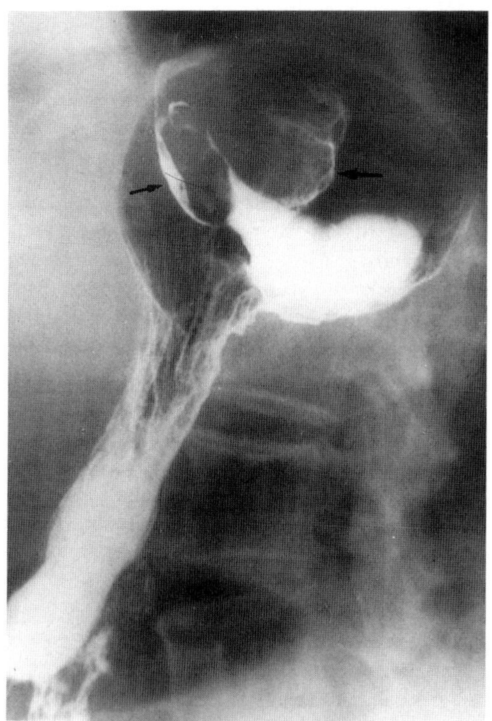

FIGURE 4.35. Profile roentgenogram of the stomach in standing position. Barium and air double-contrast demonstrates a leiomyosarcoma of the fundus.

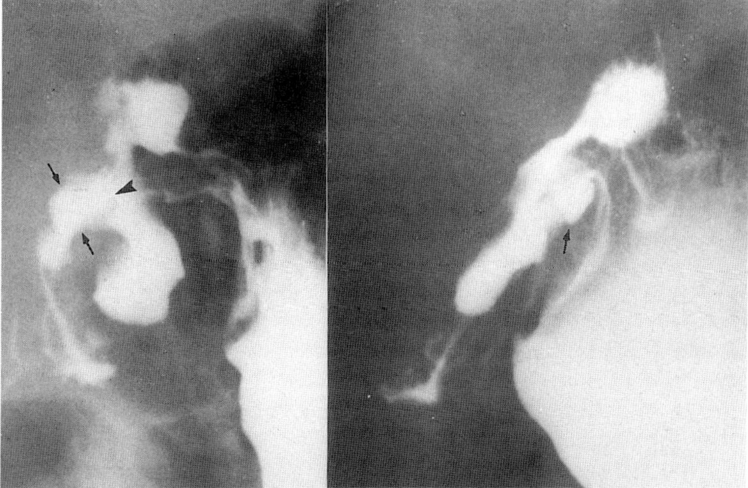

FIGURE 4.36. Peptic ulcer of the posterior wall of the duodenal bulb (arrowhead and arrows). P-A projection cannot reveal location (left figure). Left anterior oblique (right figure) demonstrates posterior wall ulceration (arrow).

Graded compression with the cone mounted on the fluoroscopic apparatus or with a separate hand-held palpator enables a good estimate of mobility of the stomach and pliability of the gastric wall (Fig. 4.37). *Palpation* using a leaded rubber glove can be performed for the same reason, but is not recommended because the hand of the examiner cannot be fully shielded from direct beam radiation. In the erect posture the stomach is palpated and compressed against the spine. When the patient is prone, peristaltic waves appear near the cardia in contrast to the erect position, where they originate adjacent to the angular notch. The prone position, therefore, allows analyses of the pliability of the more proximal segments of the gastric wall. Gaseous distension is used to estimate compliance of those portions which cannot be palpated and are without peristalsis, such as the gastric fundus.

Single-contrast fluoroscopic examination of the upper gastrointestinal tract should not exceed five minutes. However, specific circumstances can result in more prolonged evaluation.

Specific Procedures. In patients with *a cascade stomach*, contrast medium tends to hold up in the gastric fundus. Flexion of the waist in a bowing posture allows contrast medium to move distally. The same effect can be achieved by placing the patient in the prone position.

Delayed filling of the duodenal bulb prolongs an examination of the upper gastrointestinal tract. This can often be overcome by placing the patient recumbent onto the right side. If the bulb does not fill with barium entirely on a single-contrast examination, deformities of the bulb cannot be evaluated. This is not the case for double-contrast examinations. Palpation may enhance the propulsion of barium into the duodenum.

Highly concentrated barium suspensions of relatively low viscosity can demonstrate the areae gastricae. The gastric antrum should be *compressed* so that rugae are on an even plane with sulci. High kilovoltage (100–120 kV) and shortened exposures (0.10 sec or less) are recommended. However, double-contrast examination is the method of choice for demonstration of areae gastricae. Indeed, by this method areae gastricae can be demonstrated throughout the entire stomach (Fig. 4.38).

Prolonged *spasm* of the pylorus or duodenal bulb can be relieved by using spasmolytics (see pp 78–80).

The examination of a patient with an *acute*

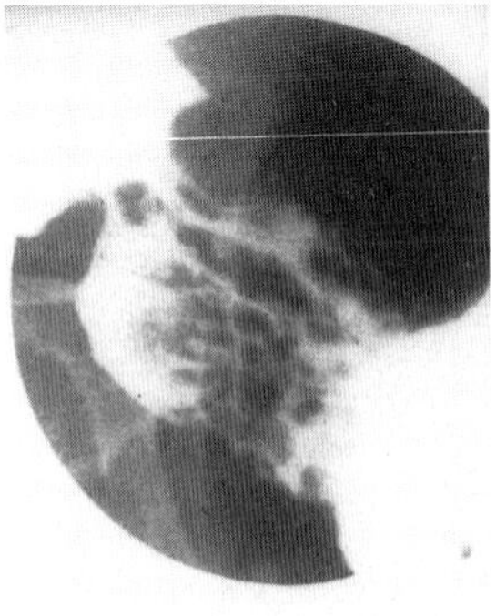

Figure 4.37. Enlarged areae gastricae and hyperplastic polyps in the stomach demonstrated by controlled compression.

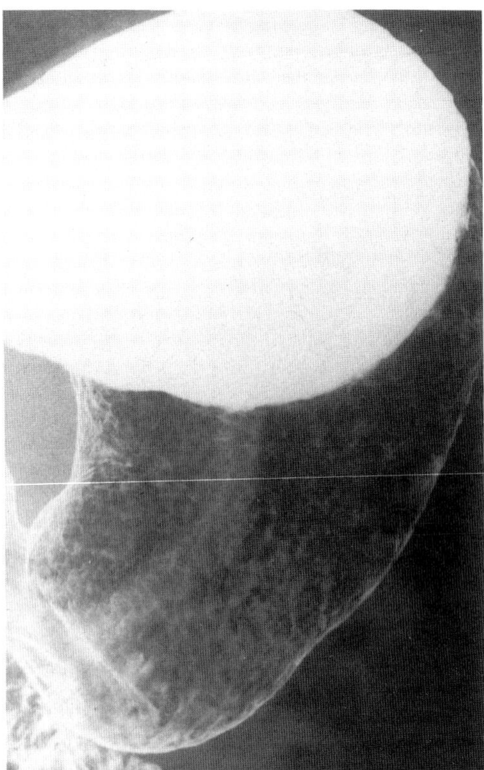

Figure 4.38. Normal areae gastricae demonstrated by double-contrast barium examination of the stomach.

abdomen is described in sections on plain abdominal roentgenograms (see pp 63–69) and the acute abdomen (see chapter 5).

In order to diagnose a *hiatal hernia*, the stomach has to be filled with a large amount of barium. The Trendelenburg position is not recommended since the majority of patients do not usually find themselves in such a posture. In the majority of patients, hiatal hernia will become evident in the prone position. It is essential to determine if the herniated stomach slides back into the abdomen in the upright position, and to show gastroesophageal reflux. However, demonstration of reflux esophagitis and its complications are also of utmost importance.

Gastroesophageal reflux is evaluated while the patient is prone or recumbent with the left side elevated from the examination table. The density of barium suspension should be 1.4–1.8 g/mL since this concentration simulates conditions under which reflux usually appears. In the majority of other examinations this density and viscosity of barium suspensions would be too high. A large amount of barium suspension should fill the stomach. With the gastric fundus filled with barium, swallowing of saliva or water can demonstrate reflux better than swallowing of additional contrast medium. Since nonopaque liquids absorb X-rays in a fashion similar to adjacent structures, the examiner is readily able to identify the origin of contrast medium in the lower esophageal segment. The entrance of barium from the stomach into the esophagus is most likely to occur during swallowing. Reflux of gastric contents occurs when the pressure gradient exceeds the resting tone of the lower esophageal segment. However, gastroesophageal reflux is not directly linked to tone of the lower esophageal sphincter alone. Hence, measuring of pH in the esophagus, testing peristaltic clearance of the esophagus, prolonged manometry, and testing response to perfusion with an acidified liquid can be performed in addition to radiologic examinations and radionuclide studies. Decrease in lower esophageal segment tone may also be stimulated by taking food or drinking water. Gastroesophageal reflux may be stimulated by body posture and increased intra-abdominal pressure. *Passive reflux* (preprandial) is examined in the horizontal position while the patient coughs or performs a Valsalva maneuver. *Active reflux* (stimulated by food) is examined with the patient supine, prone, and recumbent on the left side. The presence and degree of reflux can be monitored after the patient chews and swallows food such as bread with butter. In examination for both passive and active reflux, the patient swallows barium. This test should be considered positive whenever a stream of barium running from the stomach into the esophagus extends at least 5 cm proximal to the cardia.

Some patients should be examined by *provocative studies* so as to evaluate specific symptoms. The posture of a patient's body, or a particular type of food or drink may provoke symptoms. If a conventional examination is not successful, the patient should be allowed to reproduce whatever activity causes symptoms.

A site of *bleeding* from the upper gastrointestinal tract may be shown by barium studies. The most common lesion that causes hemorrhage is a peptic ulcer. A "no touch" technique of examination should be used, because firm compression of the stomach may enhance bleeding. Radiographic signs of bleeding include:

1. Clot in the ulcer crater or adjacent to the site of bleeding.
2. Defect at the bottom of the crater caused by the bleeding artery.
3. Disturbance in barium suspension flow above the site of bleeding.

However, endoscopy is the method of choice for the diagnosis and treatment of bleeding from the upper gastrointestinal tract. Arteriography may show the site of bleeding and provide access for vasopressin infusion, which has a high rate of success in stopping gastrointestinal bleeding. Radionuclides may also demonstrate a gastrointestinal bleeding site.

Postoperative examination should be performed one week following gastric surgery using water-soluble contrast media, especially if an anastomotic leak is suspected. A partially resected stomach is best examined with small amounts of barium. Indeed, the best results are accomplished by a double-contrast examination.

When suspecting *superior mesenteric artery syndrome* the patient can be placed in the knee-chest position. Resultant displacement of the vessel and the mesentery will result in disappearance of the ribbon-like defect caused by the superior mesenteric artery.

THE SMALL BOWEL

Patient Preparation. Solid food should not be taken for eight hours, and liquids for four hours, before the examination. Cleansing of the large intestine can improve small bowel barium examination by shortening transit time. The small intestine is long, with an extremely large surface area. Chyme is not always completely evacuated and mucus may enhance the tendency of barium to flocculate. Water is normally absorbed from distal portions of the ileum resulting in increased concentration of barium.

Indications for radiological examination of the small intestine are:

1. Prolonged diarrhea and steatorrhea.
2. Mid-abdominal pain of unexplained etiology.
3. Bleeding, the cause of which cannot be found in other segments of the alimentary tube.
4. Suspicion of chronic inflammatory or neoplastic disease of the small intestine.

In patients with intestinal gangrene or perforation, administration of any contrast media is contraindicated.

Examination should establish the position, lumen caliber, mucosal relief pattern, mobility, and points of tenderness. Barium normally fills the small intestine in a continuous column. Segmentation of the barium column may be a normal or abnormal phenomenon.

The small intestine may be examined by oral application of barium, or through a tube placed in the proximal segment of the first loop of the jejunum. Barium may also be administered in a retrograde manner through an incompetent or hypotonized ileocecal valve during the course of a single-contrast barium enema examination.

Follow-through Examination. Following examination of the upper gastrointestinal canal, the mesenteric small intestine can be examined by an additional quantity of barium. The total amount should not be less than 350 mL. However, up to 700 mL of barium suspension can be given to assure a satisfactory rate of distal progression. The barium suspension should be about 45% wt/vol. However, if high-density barium was used for examination of the upper gastrointestinal tract, a more dilute suspension should be given. If a dedicated small bowel study is performed, 500–600 mL of barium is given without examining the upper gastrointestinal tract. Fluoroscopy is performed with compression three times in the first hour and later at half hour intervals, with fluoroscopic findings determining the number of spot and overhead films. Films are taken in supine, prone, and Trendelenburg positions, and this should minimize superimposition of bowel loops (Figs. 4.39 and 4.40).

Transit time is calculated from the moment barium enters the duodenum until it reaches the colon. The normal range is between 30 minutes and 6 hours. *Evacuation time* is measured from the moment barium enters into the duodenum until all barium leaves the small intestine; it usually lasts nine or more hours. The dynamics of barium evacuation may be useful in distinguishing patients with partial obstruction from those with paralytic ileus.

Shortened Transit Time. Accelerated evacuation of the small bowel improves the quality of a barium examination, since barium has less time to undergo change. Functional studies performed to analyze the rate of small bowel

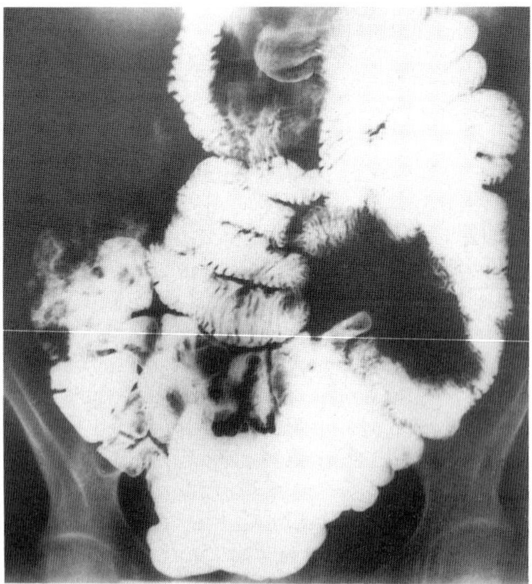

FIGURE 4.39. Follow-through (peroral) barium examination of the small bowel. Jejunal loops swing around a mass in the left iliac region.

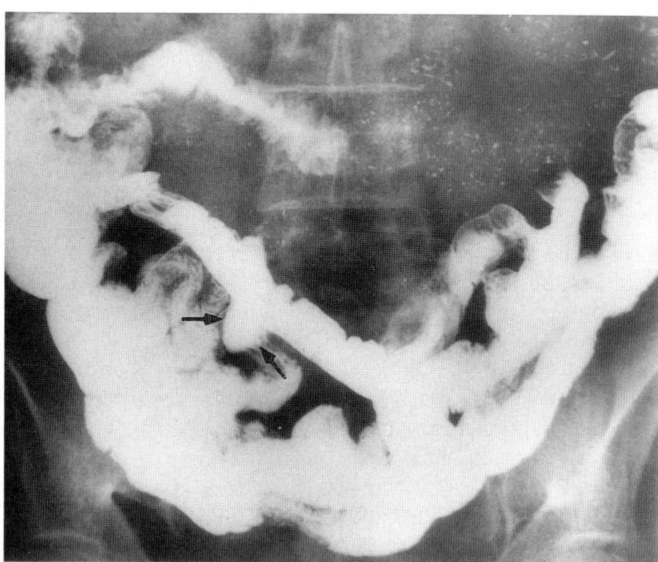

Figure 4.40. Meckel's diverticulum (arrows) demonstrated by peroral barium small bowel series.

motility are of negligible merit because the range of normal values is wide and is affected by volume, consistency, temperature, barium particle size, and characteristics of any additives.

Except for provoking a gastroileal reflex, a large amount of ingested barium increases buffer capacity of the suspension and facilitates a high quality small bowel examination. After the first dose of barium is administered, addition of another 100 mL after 30 minutes not only accelerates the movement of barium, but improves presentation of the terminal ileum as well. Fractionated ingestion of smaller amounts of barium suspension should be avoided because prolonged exposure of barium to the gastric and intestinal environment results in poor coating of intestinal mucosa.

Transit time can be shortened by taking 200 mL of ice-cold water at the end of the first hour after all of the barium has been administered. A light meal taken after most of the barium has left the stomach may stimulate small intestine peristalsis by distension of the gastric antrum.

Accelerating pharmacological agents are described in the section on pharmacoradiology (see pp 78–80). Best results may be achieved by using metoclopramide. Similar effects are produced by cholecystokinin, prostigmin and acetylcholine. Adding sorbitol to the barium suspension may also shorten the transit time to less than 60 minutes. Gastrografin, taken after barium sulfate, accelerates movement of small bowel contents significantly but should not be used because large amounts cause pronounced dilution of barium.

Specific Procedures. Small intestinal loops situated in the pelvis may be moved cephalad by manual compression of the lower abdomen during forced expiration. Good hydration without voiding will cause the urinary bladder to push intestinal loops out of the pelvis. In patients suspected of having disaccharidase deficiency, the addition of a particular sugar to the barium suspension will result in the provocation of symptoms.

Enteroclysis. Enteroclysis is infusion of contrast medium into the small intestine and is also referred to as a small bowel enema.

Patient preparation is important for performing single-contrast enteroclysis. The large intestine has to be cleansed as for a barium enema of the large bowel. However, water cleansing enemas should be omitted, since water can propagate large bowel contents retrograde through an incompetent ileocecal valve into the ileum. Patients with Crohn's disease, severe diarrhea, and intestinal obstruction should be spared from laxatives. Patients are not to eat eight hours prior to the examination.

A 12-gauge radiopaque catheter 135 cm long is placed through the nose or the mouth with the patient sitting. A tube with six side holes and a closed end is preferred. The head should be extended until the tip of the catheter reaches the oropharynx. The catheter is then swallowed and advanced by the patient. When the catheter tip is in the mid-esophagus, the passing of the catheter is facilitated, particularly along the greater curvature of the stomach, by having the patient stand. With the tube in the stomach, the patient is placed supine on a fluoroscopic table for controlled positioning of the catheter. A metal guide-wire is then introduced into the catheter, and the tip is placed at least 3 cm from the distal end. The guide-wire acts as a stiffener inside the catheter. The flexible tip of the catheter is advanced through the pylorus and proximal duodenum into the ascending portion of the duodenum or preferably into the jejunum. However, the guide-wire tip should remain proximal to the pylorus. The tube can be orientated in the correct direction and propelled forward from the antrum by rotation of the guide-wire under fluoroscopic control.

Once the catheter is in place, a 20% (wt/vol) barium suspension, at a temperature of 5-15°C, is gravity instilled continuously from an enema bag suspended 1-1.5 m above the fluoroscopic table. The recommended rate of infusion is about 75 mL/min. Too slow an infusion rate will not distend the intestine adequately. If the application is too fast, overdistension and paralysis of the jejunum can result. Vomiting can also result from too fast an infusion rate. A total of 500-1000 mL is given. When the head of the contrast medium column reaches the terminal ileum, water should be added to the enema bag.

Propagation of the barium column is monitored by short intermittent fluoroscopy. Roentgenographs should be obtained after application of 300 mL and 600 mL of suspension, using high kilovoltage technique (100-120 kV) (Fig. 4.41).

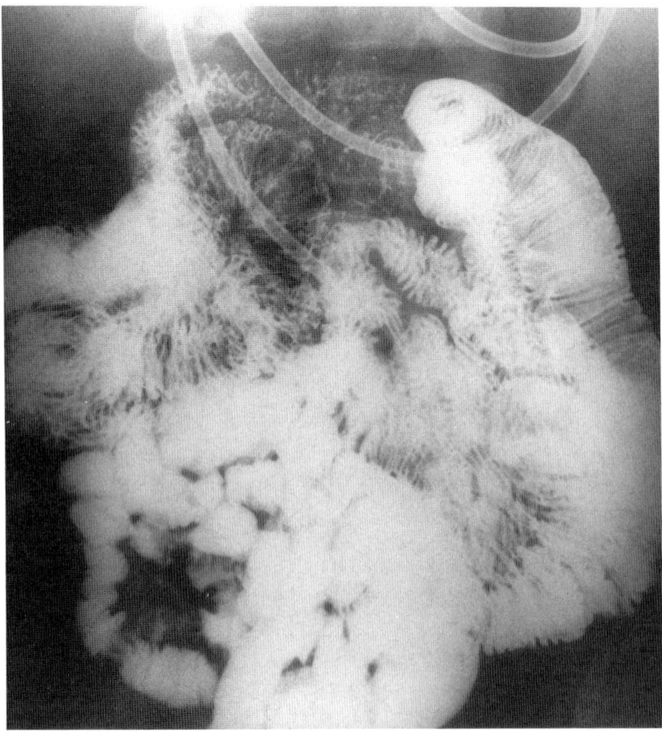

FIGURE 4.41. Single-contrast enteroclysis.

The small intestine should be compressed during filming. Several modifications of enteroclysis have been described. Metoclopramide in doses of 20 mg, given by either IM or IV routes, may shorten the small intestine transit time and make the examination more comfortable. If contrast medium transport is greater than 10 minutes, 300–600 mL of physiologic solution should be added over a matter of minutes. A mechanical pump can be employed when contrast suspensions of higher viscosity are utilized.

A soft rubber tube is used in examination of children. A total volume of 100 mL of barium suspension is administered, and the suspension has to be more dilute than for adults. For adolescents, 250 mL of contrast medium is diluted in the same manner as for adults.

Enteroclysis provides better visualization of adhesions, tumors, and Crohn's disease lesions, compared to orally administered contrast medium examinations. It is indicated when the terminal ileum is insufficiently outlined by orally administered contrast medium or when results are not diagnostic. There are fewer false negative results. Better visualization of lesions in Crohn's disease makes enteroclysis the method of choice in these patients. However, it is disadvantageous in patients with malabsorption syndromes. Introduction of the intestinal tube is contraindicated in patients with duodenal peptic ulcer. Enteroclysis does not alter the electrolyte status of blood plasma.

In comparing single-contrast enteroclysis with conventional follow-through examination, radiation exposure is five times greater with enteroclysis. Enteroclysis is also more time-consuming. The sensitivity of enteroclysis is 94% and specificity 89%, compared to 92% and 94% respectively, for peroral study in diagnosing Crohn's disease, adhesions and small intestine metastases. Meckel's diverticulum and adhesions are better visualized by enteroclysis. The main advantage of enteroclysis is optimal distension of the small bowel.

Examination by Use of Miller-Abbott Tube. A Miller-Abbott tube may be used to examine patients with small intestine obstruction. Contrast medium can be injected when the tip of the tube reaches the site of the obstruction. Secretions, blood, gas, and any excess of barium may also be aspirated. An intestinal tube should not be used in patients with peptic ulcer of the stomach and duodenum.

Retrograde Small Intestine Examination. After cleansing of the colon as for a barium enema and fasting as for a peroral examination, atropine and calcium gluconate are injected to relax the ileocecal valve. However, better relaxation of the ileocecal valve can be obtained by injecting 1 mg of glucagon. Retrograde administration of 3000–4500 mL of barium 20% wt/vol suspension by rectum is followed by a physiologic solution, or water, until the duodenum is reached. This method allows demonstration of discrete lesions. However, it is uncomfortable for the patient and has never been widely accepted. Indeed, it has been largely replaced by enteroclysis.

Retrograde Ileography. Application of glucagon prior to double-contrast barium enema was associated with reflux into the terminal ileum in 73% of patients, whereas reflux occurred in only 29% of the control group. Retrograde ileography can successfully demonstrate the terminal ileum with double-contrast technique (Fig. 4.42).

Reflux Examinations Via an Ileostomy. Contrast medium can be advanced into the small intestine via an ileostomy. A balloon catheter

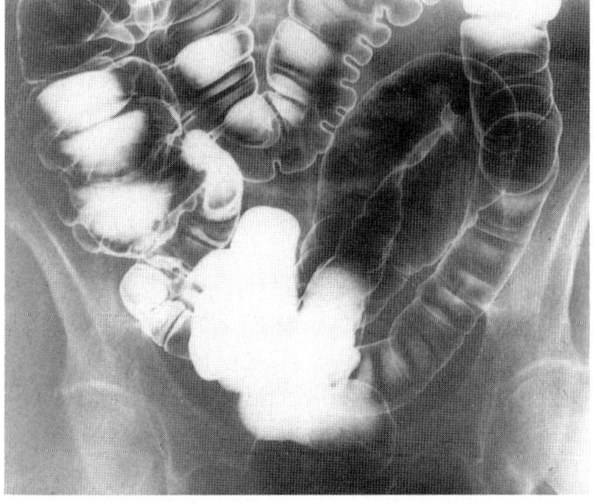

Figure 4.42. Retrograde hypotonic ileography during a double-contrast barium enema examination.

is introduced and the balloon insufflated when it is proximal to the stoma. Prior to insertion the balloon may also be insufflated to a dimension almost that of the stoma, with the rest of the air being added after the catheter is placed into the intestinal lumen. Barium sulfate 30% wt/vol suspension is used to fill the small intestine in a retrograde manner. If air is given after the barium, a double-contrast examination can be obtained (Fig. 4.43).

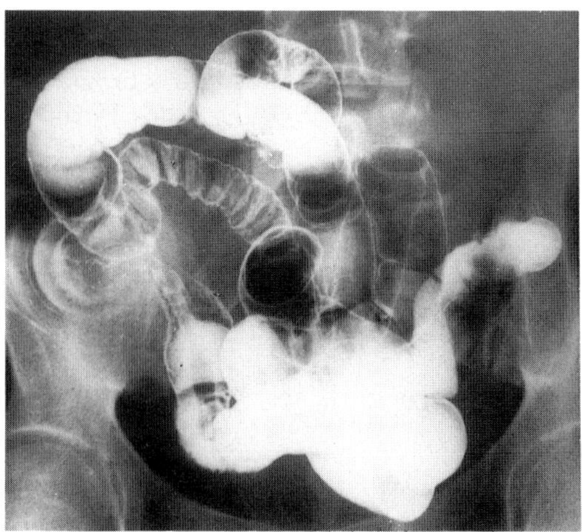

Figure 4.43. Small bowel examination via an ileostomy.

Herniography. Some external hernias (inguinal, femoral, and obturator) which could not be diagnosed by physical examination can be demonstrated by herniography.

The urinary bladder should be empty. The peritoneal cavity is punctured in the left lower quadrant adjacent to the lateral margin of the rectus abdominal muscle with the patient supine. Gastrografin in a dose of 80 mL is injected and washed among the small intestinal loops. The patient is rotated several times around the longitudinal body axis. Abdominal films are taken with the patient performing a Valsalva maneuver. However, these studies may be replaced by less invasive abdominal CT.

The Colon

Patient Preparation. A thoroughly cleansed colon is an essential prerequisite for a successful examination. Preparation should make the colon free of feces and mucus. Although a clear liquid diet is given for 24–48 hours, diet is the least significant aspect of the preparation.

Magnesium citrate or sulfate in the dose of 7.5 g, or senna extract, is usually given 12–24 hours prior to the examination. However, castor oil (30–60 mL) more effectively evacuates small and large bowel contents. In addition, bisacodyl tablets are given the evening before and one bisacodyl suppository is given on the morning of the examination.

Hydration consisting of 2–3 L of fluids 6–8 hours prior to the examination prevents absorption of water from the barium suspension in the colon. A cleansing water enema (2 L) given two hours before the examination removes all remnants from the colon.

Barium Enema. *Indications* for single-contrast barium enema examinations are:

1. Determining patency of the colon.
2. Demonstrating large, stenotic, or polypoid lesions.
3. Examinations in elderly patients and others in poor mental or physical condition.
4. Diverticulitis without perforation.
5. Congenital megacolon.
6. Reduction of intussusceptions.
7. Studies in infants and young children in general.

In patients with congenital megacolon single-contrast barium enema is the examination of choice because it clearly demonstrates the aganglionic segment. However, more proximal portions of the colon can be, with great caution, examined using double-contrast enema for the demonstration of discrete mucosal lesions due to prolonged stasis of bowel contents. Indeed, air is more easily evacuated from the colon than a barium suspension.

When localized perforation of the colon is suspected, a single-contrast enema using water-soluble contrast media is indicated. However, with free perforation into the peritoneal cavity, any form of enema is contraindicated. Fistulae accompanying diverticulitis, Crohn's disease, or malignancies are best demonstrated using a water-soluble single-contrast enema, because positive contrast is better than air for demonstration of a thin sinus tract.

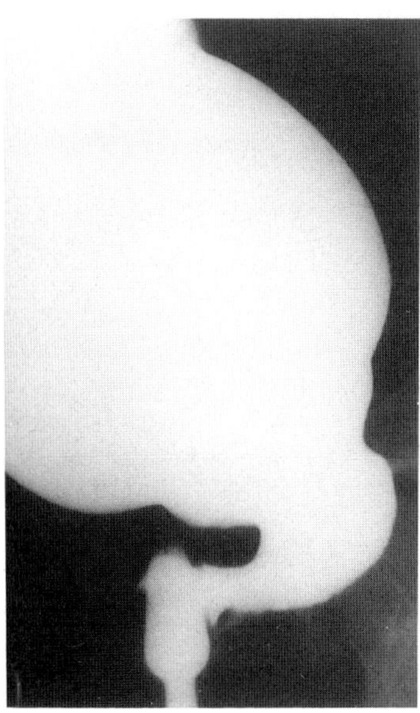

FIGURE 4.44. Single-contrast barium enema in congenital megacolon, Hirschprung's disease.

Analysis of the abdominal scout film offers estimation of the proper preparation for barium enema examination. However, plain roentgenograms of the abdomen do not always reveal important information regarding cleansing of the colon.

For single-contrast barium enema 1500–2000 mL of barium suspension 15–25% wt/vol is used. Using gravity, filling of the colon with contrast medium is enhanced by changing the patient's position and by inclination of the fluoroscopic table. Barium is administered from a plastic bag placed one meter above the table with the patient prone or recumbent on the left side. The table is tilted in a moderate Trendelenburg position and the examination is cautiously monitored by fluoroscopy. After the rectum and sigmoid colon are filled with barium the patient turns from the prone position onto his back and rotates to oblique positions to show the sigmoid colon in its greatest length. The descending colon is filled in the supine position, with the table still in the Trendelenburg position. The splenic flexure of the colon is filled with barium and demonstrated by rotating the patient from the supine position to the right side, where filling of the transverse colon is also enhanced. The hepatic flexure of the colon is best demonstrated with the patient in the supine position and turned so that the right side of the trunk is elevated from the table. Filling of the ascending colon and the cecum is facilitated by bringing the fluoroscopic table into the vertical position.

Spot films are taken during fluoroscopy. The rectum is filmed in profile (Fig. 4.44). Roentgenograms of the sigmoid colon are taken in oblique projections before the cecum is filled with contrast medium, thus avoiding superimposition. In the same manner flexures are filmed in oblique projections and the cecum is filmed with the patient supine. Compression during fluoroscopy and spot roentgenography thins the contrast column, enhancing demonstration of small lesions. Overhead films, demonstrating the entire large bowel, should be taken (Fig. 4.45) using at least 90 kV to assume adequate penetration. Postevacuation roentgenograms (Fig. 4.46) do not offer important data and need not be performed routinely.

Contraindications for single-contrast barium enema include suspicion of free perforation of the colon, toxic megacolon and fulminating in-

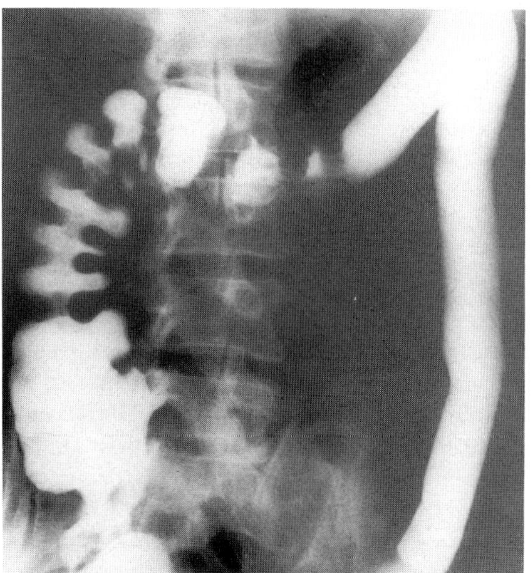

FIGURE 4.45. Single-contrast barium enema in early ulcerative colitis. Distal half of the transverse colon lacks haustral markings. The spine can be identified through a diluted barium suspension.

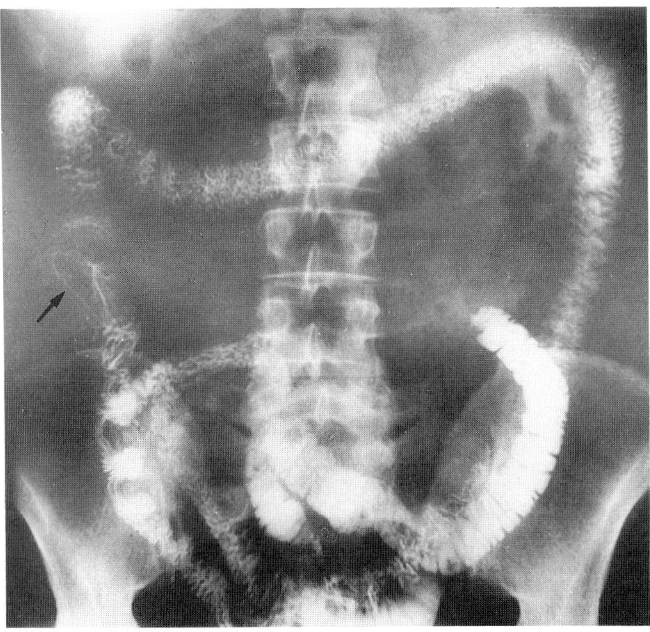

Figure 4.46. Postevacuation roentenogram of a single-contrast barium enema. Polypoid carcinoma of the ascending colon (arrow) showed unexpectedly. A feathery pattern of colonic mucosa, and reflux of barium into the terminal ileum are both evident.

flammatory disease of the large intestine, deep biopsy of the colon within the preceding four days, and concern for the discovery of small lesions. However, a patient can be examined after superficial biopsy, and barium enema can be safely performed four to six days following deep biopsy or polypectomy. The majority of transcolonoscopic biopsies are superficial but transproctoscopic biopsies can be deep. Rectal introduction of contrast medium is contraindicated in patients with perforation or toxic megacolon. Entrance of barium into the venous system of patients with ulcerative colitis can result in cardiac arrest. Deep ulcers resulting from necrosis of the intestinal wall may perforate during the course of a barium enema. However, the presence of gas in the portal vein during a barium enema in patients with ulcerative colitis does not cause clinical symptoms and, in contrast to spontaneous occurrence, should not be considered ominous. Of utmost importance is the fact that a single-contrast barium enema can miss small pathologic lesions.

Specific Procedures. *Incontinent*, uncooperative, or unconscious patients can be examined using a catheter with a balloon tip; however, a balloon catheter should be used only in patients with a normal digitorectal exam. Initially a small quantity of barium is instilled which allows fluoroscopic monitoring of balloon insufflation. The balloon should be placed just proximal to the anal canal. If barium leaks out, the patient is placed in the prone position and asked to contract the gluteal muscles, and the table is then placed in the Trendelenburg position. Alternatively, approximation of the gluteal muscles can be assisted with firmly applied adhesive tape.

Examination via a *colonostomy* can be performed with a funnel-like device through which a soft catheter is introduced. Spillage of barium can be prevented by packing bandages around the soft catheter or using a catheter with a balloon. After the balloon is insufflated to the approximate size of the stoma, the catheter is introduced into the colon through the colostomy by the patient. Then, more air can be added. After placement of the catheter, a single-contrast enema examination is performed.

Defecography. Abnormalities of anorectal functions, such as incontinency and incomplete emptying of the rectum, are examined by defecography. The patient sits on a special chair fitted with a receptacle, while highly concentrated barium paste is instilled into the rectum under fluoroscopic control. The patient is then asked to strain and cough without evacuation of bowel contents so that the anal sphincter is contracted. Then the patient defecates with films taken in the lateral projection. The anorectal angle is measured. This angle normally varies between 90 and 100 degrees.

EXAMINATION OF CHILDREN UNDER FOUR YEARS OF AGE

Once a child turns four years of age, the alimentary canal can be examined as in adults as long as there is proper concern for radiation and other safety factors. However, in younger children some specifics of the examinations have to be appreciated. Ionizing radiation exposure should be reduced to a minimum. Fluoroscopy has to be short, with a well-collimated X-ray beam and a minimal number of exposures. A highly concentrated barium suspension of relatively low viscosity should be used. Iso-osmolar nonionic water-soluble contrast media are important in small children and infants because, if aspirated, they do not cause lung edema. Gastrografin and other water-soluble hyperosmolar contrast media should be avoided except as an enema in patients with meconium ileus where they have therapeutic implications (assisting in the release of impacted meconium).

Since chest pathology may mimic some abdominal diseases, a chest roentgenogram may offer useful information prior to administering contrast medium. Infants who need to be examined in the vertical position are placed in an immobilizator which enables examination without the need for a parent to hold the child.

The Upper Gastrointestinal Tract

A child is not to eat or drink for four hours before the examination. Contrast medium may be given from a nursing bottle or through a thin soft catheter introduced into the stomach. In children, gastroesophageal reflux can be demonstrated by a *water siphon test* whereby the child is given 120–140 mL barium suspension and is then put supine and rotated 25 degrees to the right. After that, 30–120 mL of water is given. As nonopaque water opens the gastroesophageal junction, opaque barium may reflux to a varying degree. If the stream of barium reaches the level of the carina or more proximally, the test is considered positive. In comparison with the measurement of pH and pressures of the LES, the water siphon test is a more suitable examination in patients with clinical symptoms or findings. However, the rate of false-positive results is relatively high.

The stomach and the duodenum are examined by rotating the child so as to obtain optimal roentgenograms in as many projections as necessary. In infants, the pylorus is often directed posteriorly so that lateral positioning of the patient is required for optimal identification.

The Small Bowel

The small intestine can be examined as a continuation of an upper gastrointestinal series. More barium is added and the film sequence determined by intermittent short fluoroscopy. Barium examination does not always confirm the diagnosis of malabsorption syndromes since flocculation and segmentation of the barium column and dilatation of the intestine can be normal findings in infants and young children.

The Colon

Small children and infants with obstipation are best examined without preparation. Otherwise, a water cleansing enema can be administered three to four hours before a barium enema. It is best that the patient not eat during this period. Laxatives are given only in obstipated children. If small lesions are of concern, the colon must be thoroughly cleansed and a double-contrast enema performed with great caution. If colon cleansing is not initially satisfactory, repeated filling and emptying of the colon with dilute barium may clean the colon adequately for diagnostic roentgenograms.

In children with Hirschprung's disease, the flow of barium should be terminated as soon as the aganglionic segment is demonstrated because barium is poorly evacuated from more proximal portions of the colon.

DOUBLE-CONTRAST EXAMINATIONS

All segments of the alimentary canal can be examined by a double-contrast method in which the mucosal surface is coated with a thin layer of barium and the lumen distended with air or other gas. The thin layer of barium allows adequate penetration of X-rays for analyzing superimposed segments of the alimentary canal. The mucosal surface is superbly demonstrated and portions of the alimentary canal inaccessible to palpation can be thoroughly examined. For double-contrast examinations, highly concentrated barium suspensions of relatively low viscosity enable satisfactory mucosal coating. The organs are dilated by gas released from effervescent preparations or by the insufflation of air. Distension of the lumen should not be extreme because such a distension causes discomfort, may flatten or efface discrete pathologic protruding lesions, and can damage pathologically altered bowel wall.

In double-contrast studies, analysis of subsequent roentgenograms is used to diagnose discrete mucosal lesions. Fluoroscopy is used mainly to monitor filling with barium and distension of the organ by gas, and to select projections for spot filming. However, pathologic lesions can be seen at fluoroscopy.

Interpretation of double-contrast studies differs from single-contrast examinations. Appearance on double-contrast roentgenograms depends on the type of lesion, its position on the dependent or nondependent wall, and the accumulation of a pool of barium on the dependent wall.

There are two fundamental types of pathologic lesions in the alimentary canal. Depressed lesions, like diverticula or ulcers, create a defect in continuity of the wall. Protruding lesions such as tumors project into the organ lumen. Normal structures, regardless of the location, have a similar appearance throughout the alimentary canal. Mucosal folds protrude into the lumen, and the spaces between folds accumulate barium as depressed lesions. A depressed lesion shows as a collection of barium on the dependent wall, but on the nondependent wall, it manifests as a ring shadow because barium empties from the defect (Fig. 4.47). Protruding lesions on the dependent wall are seen as transparent, lucent (black) filling defects. However, a protruding formation on the nondependent wall has white margins (Figs. 4.48 and 4.49). These distinctions, not evident in single-contrast examination, help to identify whether the lesion is on the anterior or posterior wall. However, it must be emphasized that even large lesions on the nondependent wall can be missed when they reveal only a thin white line. Compression of the protruding lesion on the nondependent wall against barium accumulation on the dependent wall allows estimation of a lesion's protrusion into the lumen and the dimensions of the elevated area. While small protrusions and excavations can be obscured by the barium accumulation, alterations in body posture can change barium pooling and reverse the dependent-nondependent wall relationship.

However, too great an enthusiasm for double-contrast examinations may not be justified. Analysis of data on the diagnosis of peptic ulcer and carcinoma of the stomach, duodenal ulcer, and polyps of the colon shows that the double-contrast method was superior to single-contrast examination only in patients with polyps of the colon. Single-contrast technique with proper fluoroscopy, graded compression, and

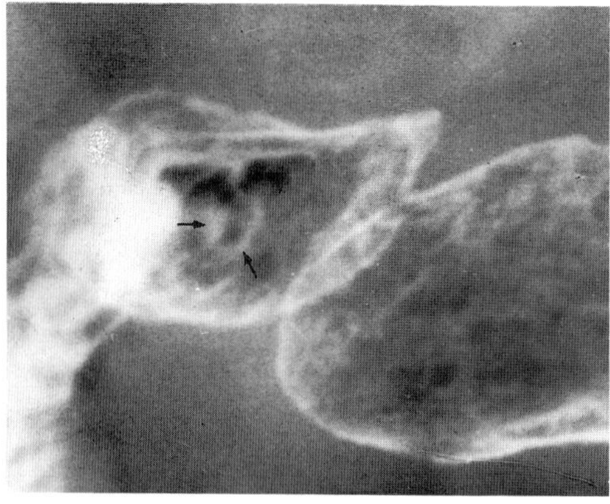

Figure 4.47. Nondependent wall peptic ulcer of the duodenal bulb empties barium, resulting in a ring-like appearance.

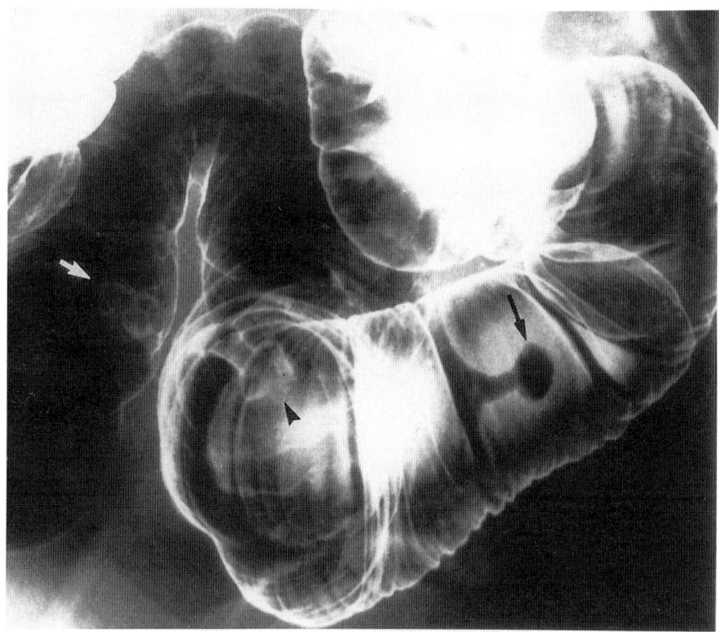

Figure 4.48. Double-contrast enema demonstrates polyps in the sigmoid colon. Accumulation of barium on the dependent wall (black arrow) creates a negative defect (black). Polyps on the nondependent wall are outlined by barium (white) protruding into the lumen (white arrow and arrowhead).

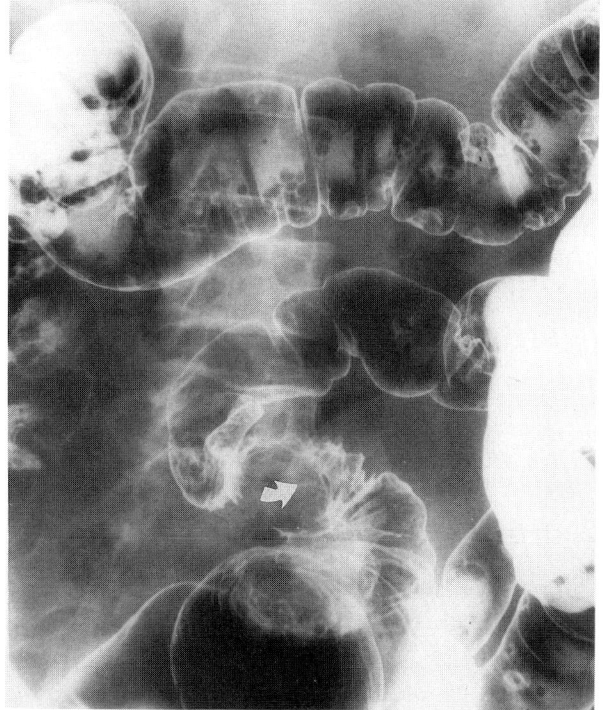

Figure 4.49. Double-contrast barium enema in familial polyposis. Dependent wall polyps are radiolucent and the nondependent wall is covered with barium. Carcinoma of the sigmoid colon is evident (arrow).

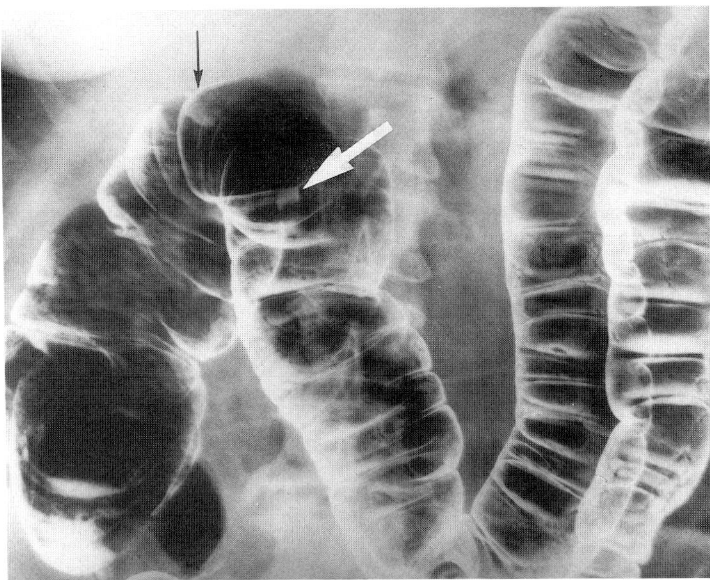

Figure 4.50. Double-contrast barium enema examination. Stalactite phenomenon, a drop of barium hanging from a nondependent wall, may mimic a polyp or diverticulum (arrows).

palpation reveals a majority of lesions if they are not very small. Contrary to double-contrast techniques, where *en face* views are essential, *profile projections* may often be conclusive in single-contrast studies. With appropriate manipulation of the patient, any excess of barium can be removed and gastric mucosal relief demonstrated in a single-contrast study. With the use of high voltage, dilute barium suspensions, and compression, protruding lesions as small as 7 mm can be demonstrated during a single-contrast barium enema.

If not properly recognized, artifacts on double-contrast studies may cause interpretation problems. Fecal residue adherent to the mucosa may mimic polypoid lesions. Radiopaque structures superimposed on segments of the alimentary canal and coated with a thin layer of barium may simulate pathologic lesions. A drop of barium suspension hanging from the nondependent wall, the stalactite phenomenon, may resemble a collection of barium within a pathologic lesion (Fig. 4.50). Large pathologic lesions are not likely to be missed by single-contrast examination. However, they can be easily missed on double-contrast roentgenograms if on the nondependent wall. By combin-

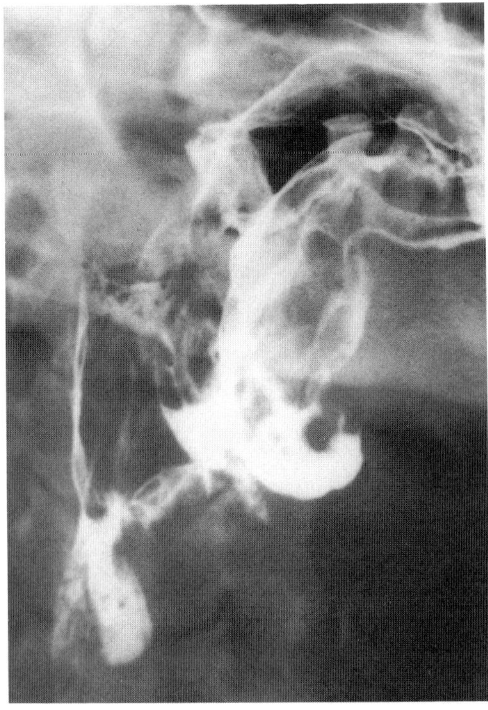

Figure 4.51. Double-contrast pharynography demonstrating Kaposi's sarcoma of the pharynx.

Figure 4.52. Double-contrast esophagography. (A) Early achalasia. (B) Reflux esophagitis. (C) Moniliasis. (D) Ulcerated leiomyosarcoma.

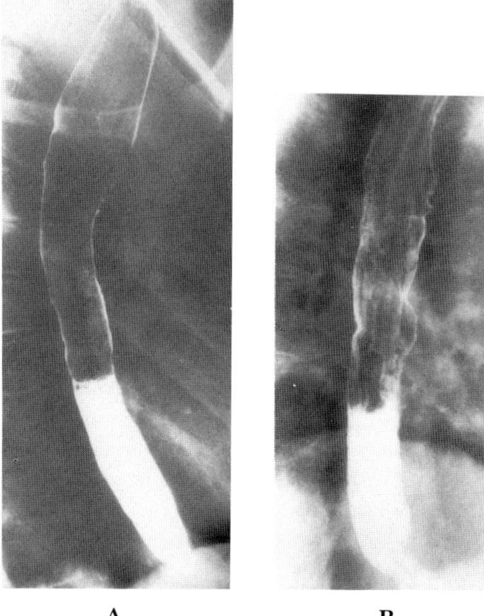

A B

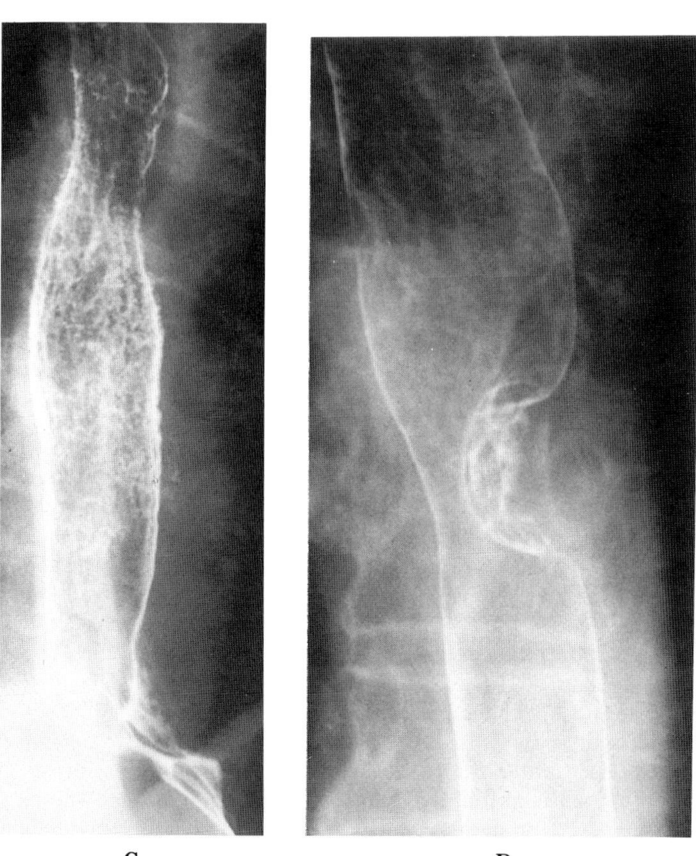

C D

ing principles of both single- and double-contrast techniques, the number of false-positive and false-negative results can be significantly decreased.

The Mesopharynx and Hypopharynx

The middle and lower portions of the pharynx are readily evaluated by double-contrast techniques. A patient standing with his or her back against the upright fluoroscopic table swallows one bolus of barium suspension (150–200% wt/vol). The pharynx is coated with barium while air previously present in the pharynx allows a double-contrast examination. Roentgenograms are taken in the P-A and lateral projection. For oblique views, proper projections are best chosen at fluoroscopy (Fig. 4.51).

The Esophagus

A majority of the techniques for double-contrast esophagography are performed with the patient standing. However, single-contrast examination of the esophagus is best performed with the patient recumbent. The esophagus may be examined by double-contrast technique simply by swallowing air or saliva after ingestion of a barium bolus of 40–50% wt/vol concentration. The patient ingests barium while standing in a right anterior oblique position. Double-contrast spot esophagograms are then taken.

Double-contrast esophagography can be performed by regurgitation of gas liberated from effervescent granules or powder. After IV administration of 0.2 mg of glucagon and ingestion of an effervescent agent, the patient is instructed to swallow small portions of contrast medium suspension while lying in a left lateral position. This causes reflux of gas from the stomach, with appropriate definition of the inner surface of the esophagus (Fig. 4.52).

As an alternate method for double-contrast examination of the esophagus, the patient, standing in a right anterior oblique position, chews and swallows 15–20 mL of thick barium suspension under fluoroscopic observation. Then the patient rapidly ingests 200 mL of 100% hydroxypropylmethylcellulose and films are obtained. Without the use of effervescent granules, this procedure is free of intraluminal bubbles.

Instead of gas, foam with similar absorption values may be used for double-contrast examination of the esophagus. The esophagus becomes distended after ingesting a spoonful of barium followed by a foamy mixture. Good demonstration of the esophagus by a double-contrast method can also be obtained when a special tube with a pump is used.

Although the images may be more pleasing, double-contrast methods do not significantly improve detection of esophageal lesions. Diagnostic accuracy is not improved because it is accompanied by a larger number of false-positive interpretations which lower the specificity of the method.

Reflux esophagitis, previously diagnosed by endoscopy, has been confirmed in 80% of patients by double-contrast esophagography (Fig. 4.52B). Esophagitis was detected in 77% of these patients by a single-contrast method. Using both methods, the accuracy increased to 90%. A double-contrast method is superior in diagnosing esophagitis only if the mucosa contains granularities or if erosions exist.

Just as in double-contrast examinations of other parts of the alimentary canal, roentgenographs need to be carefully analyzed. In addition, the flow of positive and negative contrast media and movement of the esophageal wall should be fluoroscopically monitored.

The Stomach

All portions of the stomach can be visualized in excellent detail by double-contrast examination.

Fasting for eight hours is recommended. The stomach is distended with 300–400 mL of gas released from an effervescent preparation taken with a small amount of water. Larger amounts of water may interfere with coating of the mucosa.

The diameter of the fundus of a satisfactorily dilated stomach should be 10 cm, of the middle portion of the body, 7 cm, and of the duodenum, 4 cm. Glucagon or Buscopan can make the examination easier to perform and improve visualization of the duodenum. Since resultant hypotonia prevents filling of the duodenum by peristalsis, the duodenum is filled by rotating the patient. The patient, standing in the right anterior oblique position to avoid overlapping the esophagus with the spine and heart, drinks 50–100 mL of barium suspension (150–200% wt/vol). Spot films of the esophagus with double contrast are first obtained. The table is then tilted to the horizontal position and the patient is instructed to rotate over the left side onto the stomach and back over to the left side several times, to facilitate coating of the mucosa. Turning to the right side is not allowed at that point because consequent filling of the duodenum would overlap and obscure the gastric antrum. After a spot film of the stomach is obtained in the right posterior oblique position, the patient again turns onto his stomach, then to his right side in the supine position, and finally, turns once more, to the supine right anterior position (Figs. 4.53 and 4.54). Spot films of the antrum and the duodenum are then taken. The patient now turns to his left side, rotates into the left posterior oblique prone position, and drinks 200–300 mL of barium suspension (15–20% wt/vol) through a straw. Full-column films of the upper gastrointestinal tract can be obtained. Evaluation of gastroesophageal reflux is performed in this position or in either a flat prone or supine position. The table is then elevated and compression films are obtained. Repeated washing of the mucosa with barium results in improved coating. Spot films of the gastric fundus can be taken in various oblique projections (Fig. 4.55).

When compared to endoscopy, single-contrast upper gastrointestinal examination results in 20–30% false interpretations and the double-contrast method in 7%. Single-contrast

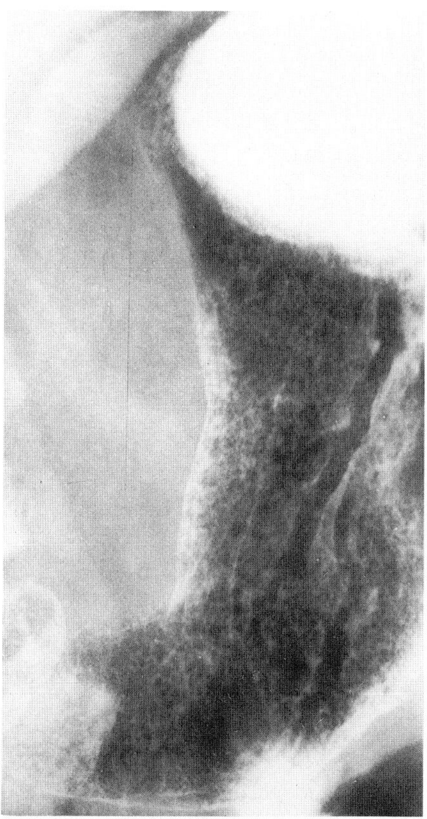

Figure 4.53. Double-contrast examination of the stomach.

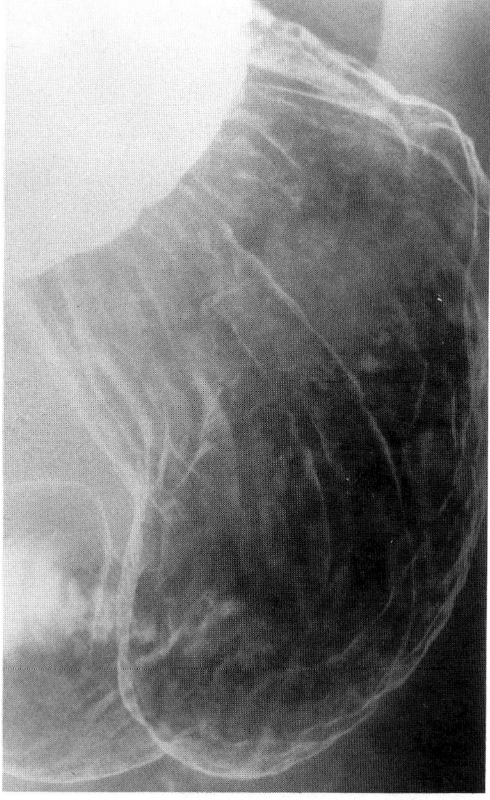

Figure 4.54. Double-contrast study demonstrates thickened rugae in gastric lymphoma.

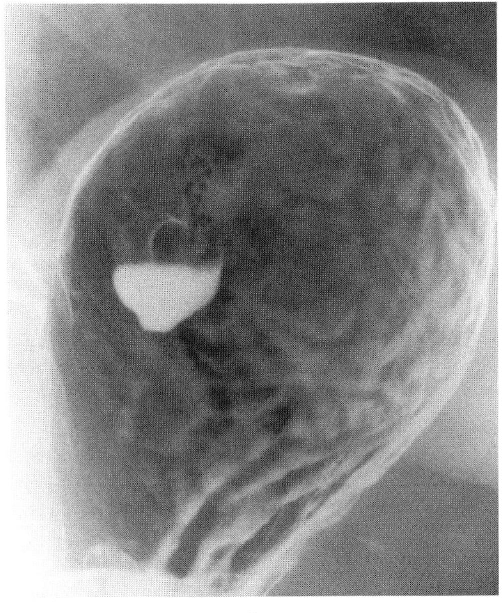

A

Figure 4.55. Double-contrast demonstration of gastric diverticulum adjacent to the cardia. (A) P-A projection. (B) Oblique projection.

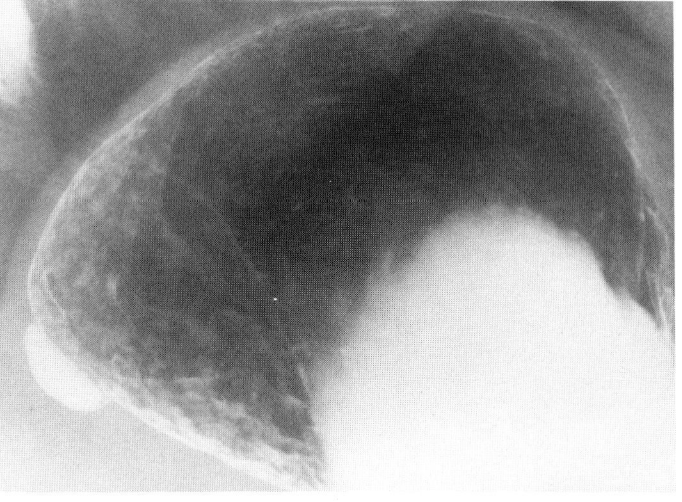

B

examination using small amounts of barium and compression results in 20–70% sensitivity. However, the number of false-positive results is high. The rate of false-negative findings on double-contrast examination of the upper gastrointestinal tract is 5.2%; the most common pathological findings missed were duodenal ulcer and gastric erosions. Common causes of radiologic errors are inappropriate examination technique and problems of interpretation. Technical difficulties are encountered in old, immobile, and obese patients.

Double-contrast examination is more difficult following gastric surgery. Double-contrast studies are more accurate. Except for the possibility of leakage around the anastomosis there are no contraindications for the use of hypotonia or gaseous distension.

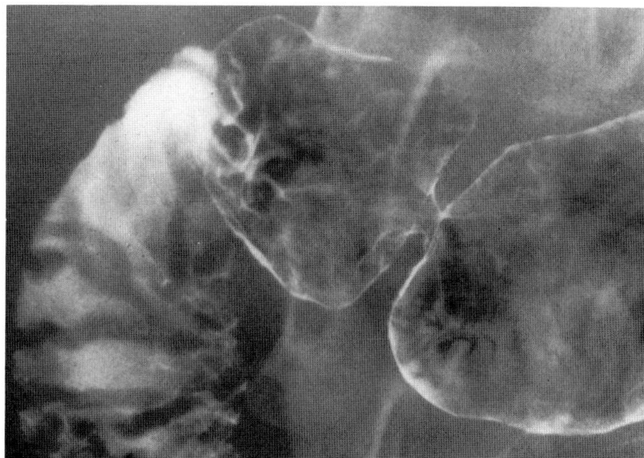

FIGURE 4.56. Double-contrast study demonstrates several erosions of the distal portion of the duodenal bulb.

THE DUODENUM

The duodenal bulb is examined during an upper gastrointestinal series. It is demonstrated by double-contrast technique after being coated with barium and distended by gas from the stomach (Fig. 4.56). Distension of the stomach by gas displaces the bulb into a sagittal plane. If it becomes obscured, the superior duodenal segment can be examined after the gas is partially absorbed or eructated. Other segments of the duodenum can be examined by hypotonic duodenography.

Hypotonic Duodenography. Pathologic changes of the duodenum and pancreas can be demonstrated in an aperistaltic and gas-distended duodenum.

Anatomical details such as the minor duodenal papilla are shown (Fig. 4.57). As with other double-contrast examinations, there are certain limitations to hypotonic duodenography. When properly performed and appropriately combined with a single-contrast examination, hypotonic duodenography can demonstrate all types of duodenal pathology (Fig. 4.58). It has been shown, however, that the majority of pancreatic carcinomas demonstrated by this technique were already inoperable.

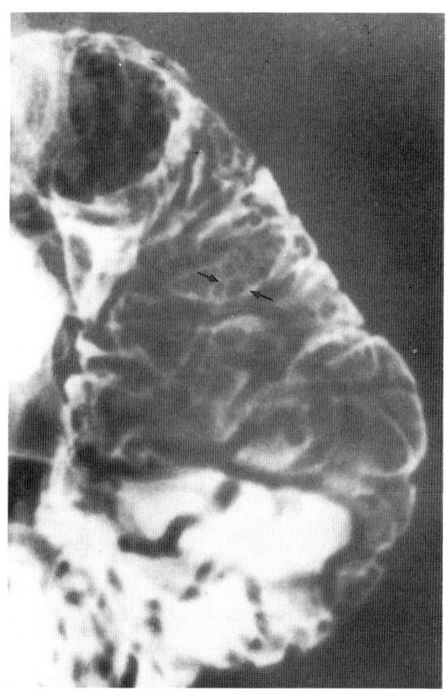

FIGURE 4.57. Hypotonic duodenography demonstrates the minor duodenal papilla (arrows). The patient is prone.

Hypotonic duodenography can be performed with or without an intestinal tube. When a tube is used, it is advanced into the descending portion of the duodenum, 30 mL of barium suspension is introduced, and the duodenum is made hypotonic by intravenous glucagon or Buscopan. More barium can be added or any excess removed. After peristalsis ceases, air is

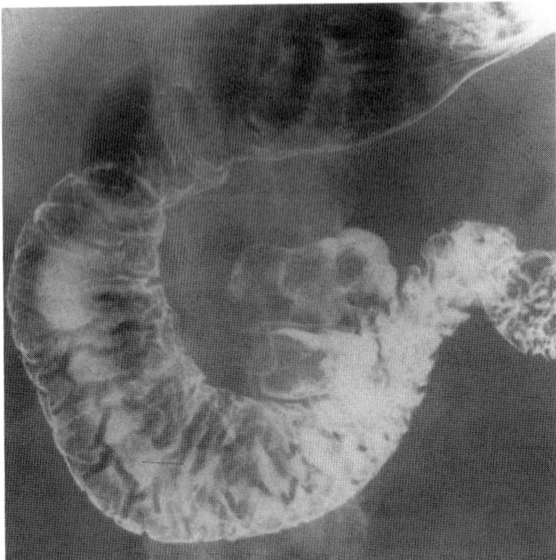

FIGURE 4.58. Double-contrast study of the duodenum demonstrates large diverticulum of the ascending segment filled with food remnants.

instilled to dilate the duodenum. Spot films are taken in the sagittal and oblique projections.

Hypotonic duodenography is performed without a tube after routine examination of the upper gastrointestinal tract. After at least 20 mL of barium suspension have been swallowed, the patient lies on his right side to facilitate filling of the duodenum with barium. A spasmolytic, glucagon or Buscopan, is then injected intravenously. Gas released from an effervescent preparation in the stomach is driven into the duodenum by rotating the patient to his left side and then to his back.

While hypotonic duodenography reveals lesions originating in the duodenal wall and extrinsic compression defects, ultrasound and CT are more sensitive for diagnosing pancreatic neoplasm. Ductal and periductal tumors can be best diagnosed by endoscopic retrograde cholangiopancreatography (ERCP). While hypotonic duodenography identifies pancreatitis in 48% of affected patients, ERCP is diagnostic in 83% of patients without jaundice in whom chronic inflammatory disease of the pancreas is suspected.

Radiologic examination of the upper gastrointestinal tract and endoscopy are complementary methods. While proper use of double-contrast technique can decrease the number of endoscopies necessary for evaluation, too aggressive a radiologic approach may result in a high number of false-positive results.

THE SMALL BOWEL

A series of direct and indirect procedures can provide double-contrast demonstration of the small bowel. However, small intestine double-contrast technique may call for barium and effervescent preparation to be followed by application of a hypermotility agent such as serotonin, acetylcholine, or pancreozymin (Table 4.1).

In another technique, after the head of the barium column reaches the distal portion of the ileum, the patient is given two doses of effervescent preparation within 10 minutes and is instructed to lie on his left side. Films are taken in supine and prone positions (Fig. 4.59). Dila-

TABLE 4.1. DOUBLE-CONTRAST EXAMINATION OF THE SMALL INTESTINE

Indirect Methods
Swallowing barium and effervescent agent
Peroral pneumocolon (for terminal ileum)
Retrograde ileography
Direct Methods
Double-contrast enteroclysis
Double-contrast examination via an ileostomy

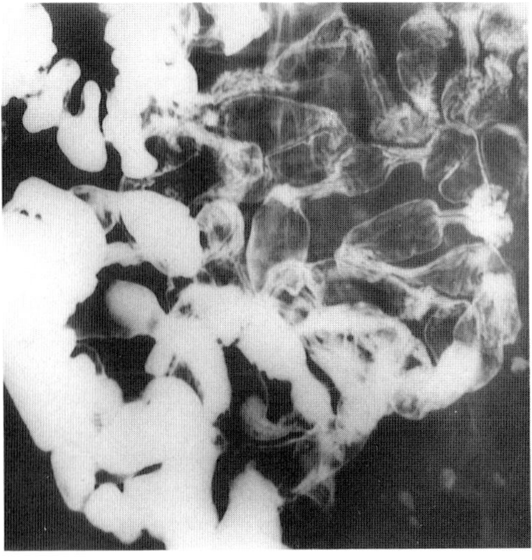

FIGURE 4.59. Double-contrast examination of the small bowel after oral administration of two doses of effervescent agent.

tation of the intestinal lumen by this method is never as successful as in enteroclysis.

In yet another technique, barium and capsules containing an effervescent preparation which liberates gas in the small bowel are administered orally. Distal segments of the small intestine may also be demonstrated with double contrast by using a peroral pneumocolon technique or retrograde ileography.

The Peroral Pneumocolon. Indications for peroral pneumocolon are:

1. Inadequate demonstration of the terminal ileum by a conventional follow-through study.
2. A normal-appearing terminal ileum in a patient with clinical suspicion of chronic inflammatory bowel disease.
3. Abnormalities of terminal ileum and cecum warranting further examination.

The colon should be prepared as for a barium enema but the patient needs to fast for eight hours prior to the study. After ingesting 250–400 mL of barium, the head of the barium column is followed to the ascending colon. Air is then insufflated into the rectum until the colon and terminal ileum are dilated. If the air does not enter into the small intestine, glucagon may help relax the ileocecal valve. Spot films are taken with graded compression. This method is useful in demonstrating pathologic processes in the ileocecal region, particularly in children.

Enteroclysis. Patient preparation is the same as for single-contrast enteroclysis. Intubation of the first jejunal loop is followed by introduction of 350–500 mL of barium suspension (concentration 60% wt/vol) from an enema bag at the rate of 70–80 mL/min. After barium has reached the cecum, 800–1000 mL of air is injected. If fluoroscopy reveals that the small intestine is not sufficiently distended, intravenous glucagon or Buscopan may be of assistance. Spot films with compression are taken if any abnormality is observed. Otherwise, prone and supine views of the entire abdomen will suffice (Fig. 4.60).

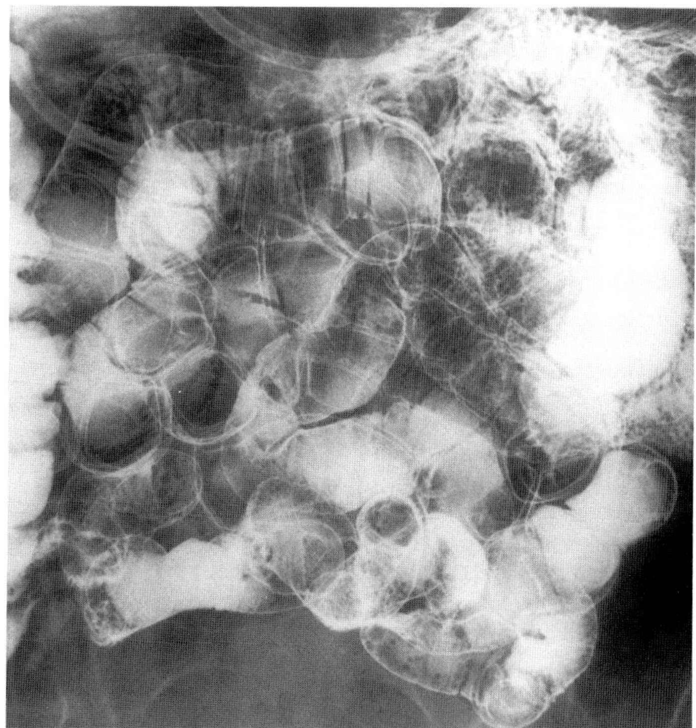

FIGURE 4.60. Air contrast enteroclysis.

Instead of air, barium sulfate can be followed by 800–1200 mL of 0.5% methylcellulose infused at 90–110 mL/min. Infusion of methylcellulose is preferable to water because it decreases small intestine motility and reduces diffusibility into the barium suspension. Filming is the same as for the air-contrast enteroclysis.

Double-contrast examination of the small intestine can also be performed by injecting barium and air through an ileostomy.

Barium Enema

A double-contrast barium enema is the method of choice for examination of the entire large bowel. It is preferred over a single-contrast barium enema whenever there is rectal bleeding, suspicion of carcinoma or polyps, and whenever discrete mucosal lesions need to be demonstrated. Patient preparation is the same as for single-contrast examination.

With an inflatable balloon catheter introduced in the rectum, the patient is placed either prone or supine, or on his left side in the Trendelenburg position. The colon is filled from an enema bag placed 1–1.5 m above the tabletop. Dense barium of relatively low viscosity is allowed to flow up to the distal segment of the transverse colon. Barium flow is then stopped and the patient placed on his or her right side to passively fill proximal segments of the transverse colon. The table is then elevated and the enema bag lowered in order to drain barium from the distal portions of the large intestine. The table is then again lowered and air insufflated with the patient again lying on his or her right side. When the cecum is filled with barium pushed proximally by air, the patient is placed supine and the tabletop is elevated to an angle of 45 degrees. Additional air is insufflated to obtain adequate distension of the co-

Table 4.2. Radiographic Sequence for Double-Contrast Enema

With the Table Horizontal
P-A of large intestine
Sigmoid colon in right anterior oblique position (spot film)
Large intestine in profile
A-P of large intestine
Cross-table right decubitus
Cross-table left decubitus
With the Table Vertical
P-A of large intestine
Hepatic flexure in right anterior oblique position (spot film)
Splenic flexure in left anterior oblique position (spot film)
With the Table Horizontal
Prone cross-table of the rectum without catheter

A

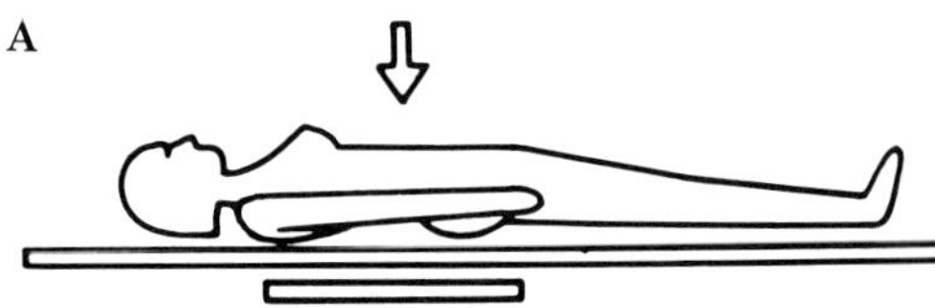

Diagram 4.2. Radiography for double-contrast enema. (A) Supine position. (*Diagram continued throughout Fig.* 4.61.)

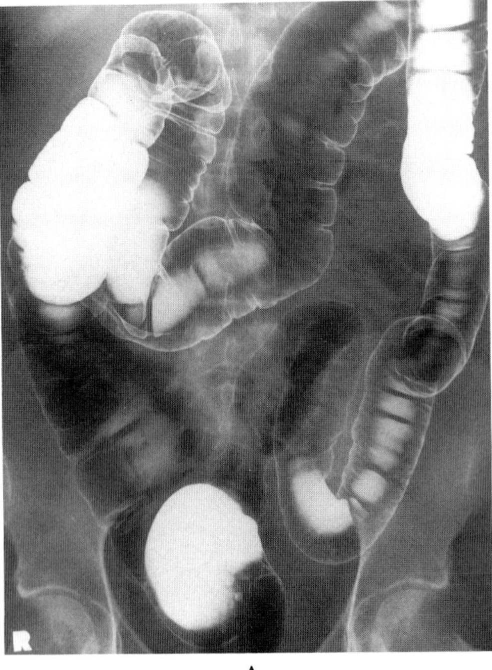

A

Figure 4.61. Radiography of a double-contrast enema. (A) A-P, supine of the entire large bowel. (See Diagram 4.2A.) (*Figure continued on pp.* 109–111.)

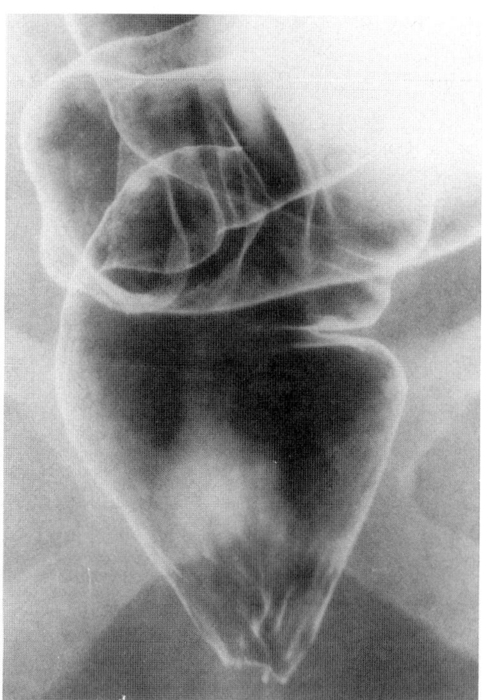

B

lon as monitored by fluoroscopy. If coating of the mucosa is not satisfactory, the patient can be rotated one or two revolutions in a clockwise direction while the table is flat. With the table elevated, spot films are taken of both flexures in oblique projections. Oblique spot films of the sigmoid colon are taken in the horizontal position.

A sequence of overhead and spot films is presented in Table 4.2 and illustrated with Diagram 4.2 and Fig. 4.61. Filming should be

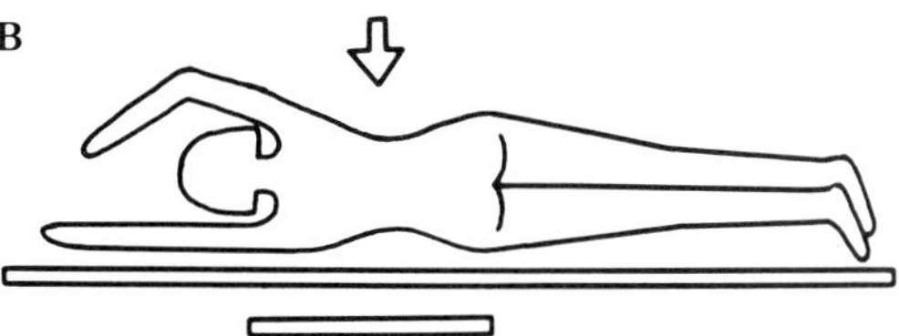

DIAGRAM 4.2 *continued.* (B) Lateral projection.

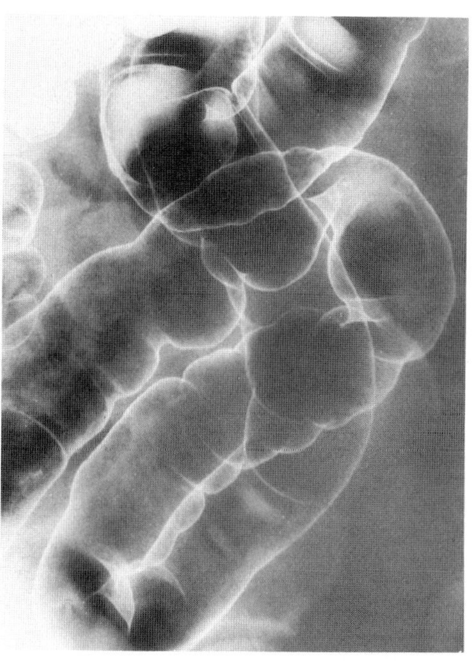

C

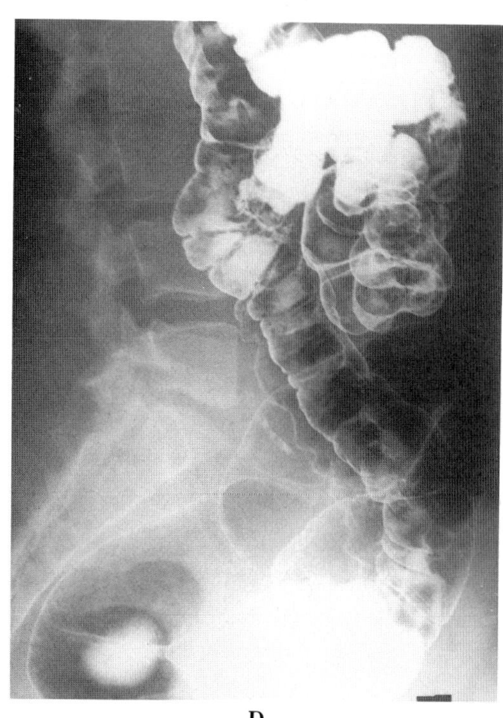

D

FIGURE 4.61 *continued.* (B) P-A, supine of the rectum. (C) Spot film of the sigmoid colon in oblique projection. (D) Profile decubitus projection of large intestine. (See Diagram 4.2B.)

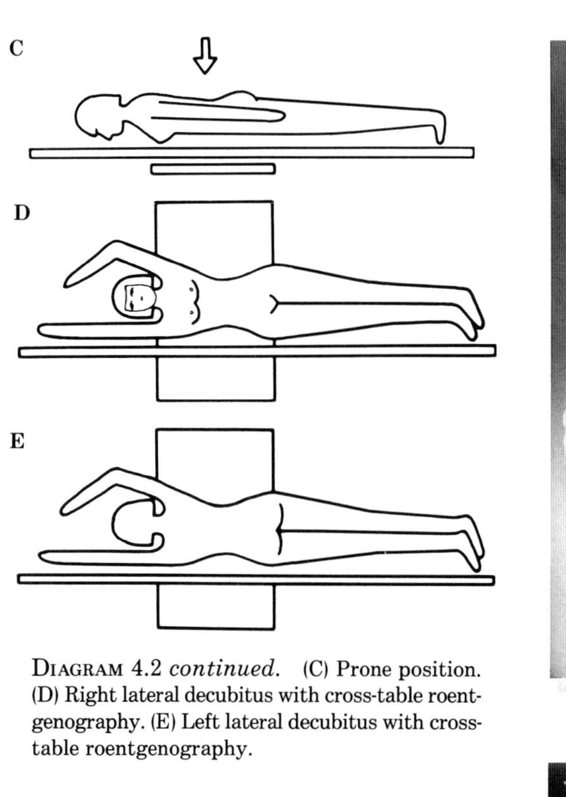

DIAGRAM 4.2 *continued.* (C) Prone position. (D) Right lateral decubitus with cross-table roentgenography. (E) Left lateral decubitus with cross-table roentgenography.

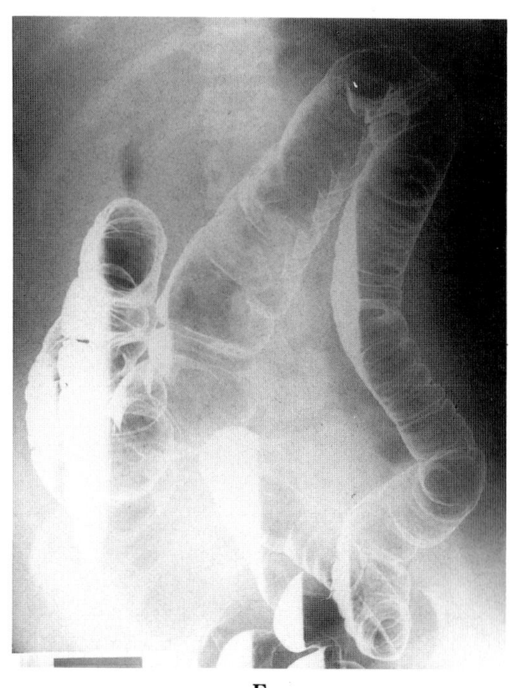

F

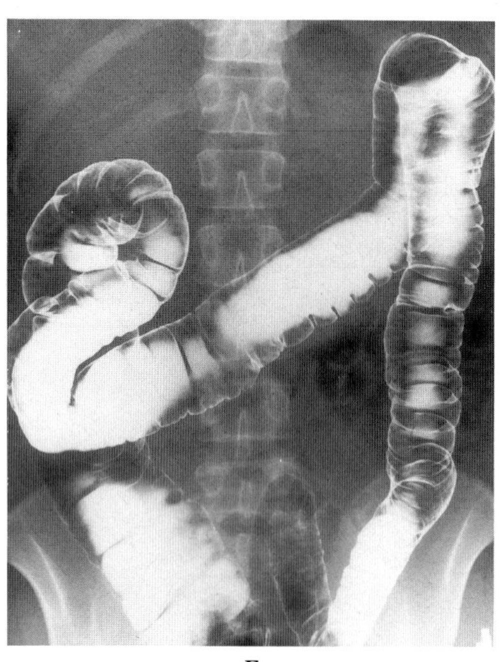

E

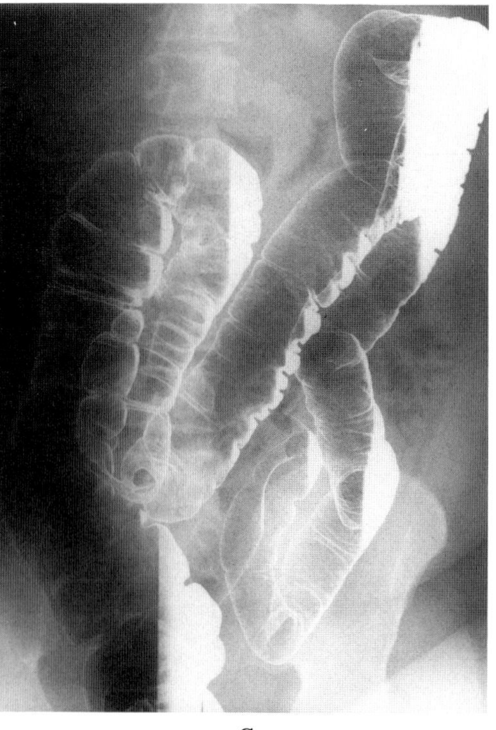

G

FIGURE 4.61 *continued.* (E) P-A, prone. (See Diagram 4.2C.) (F) Cross-table right decubitus. (See Diagram 4.2D.) (G) Cross-table left decubitus. (See Diagram 4.2E.)

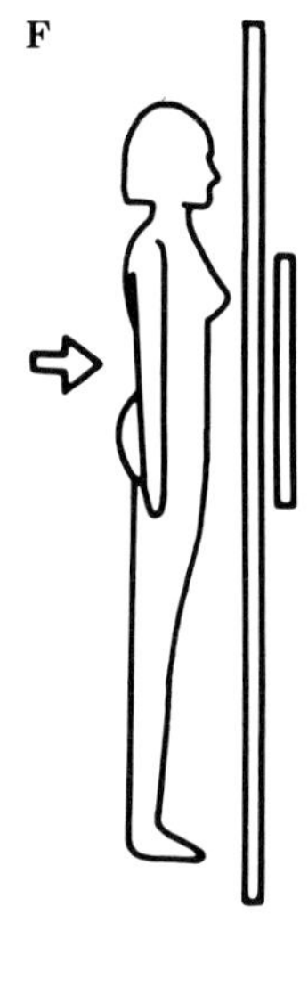

DIAGRAM 4.2 *continued.* (F) Upright.

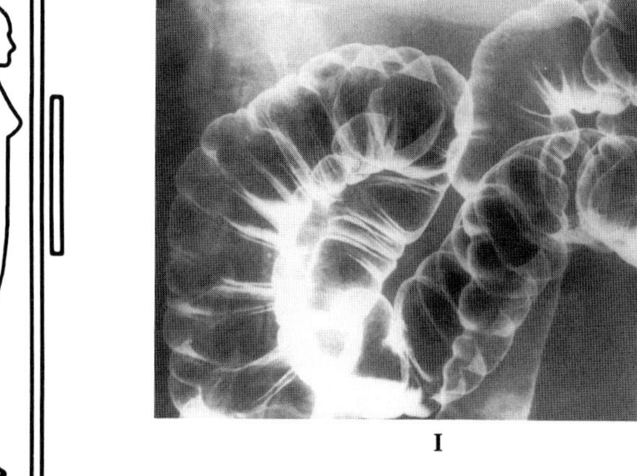

I

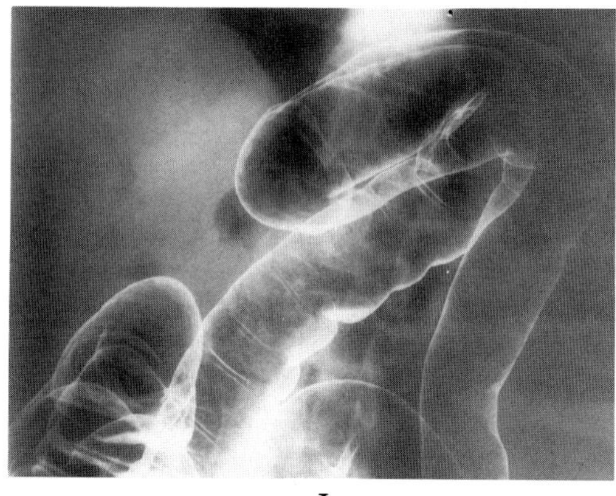

J

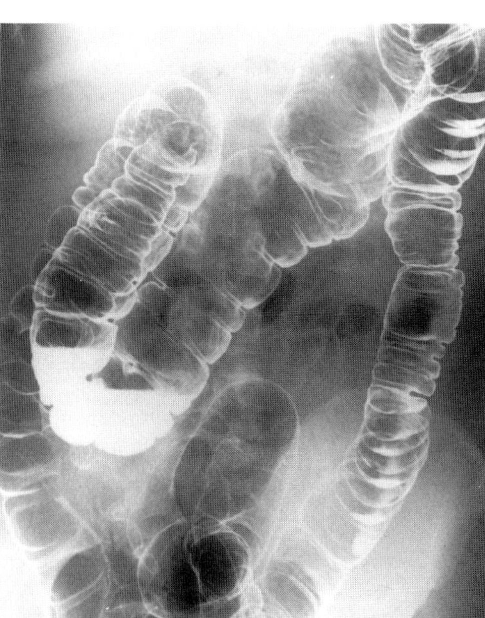

H

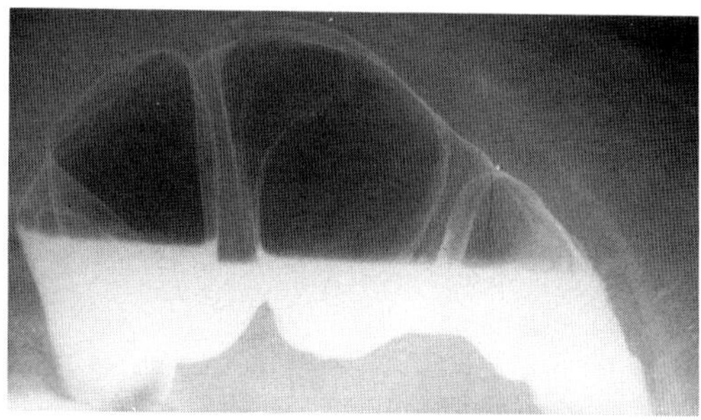

K

FIGURE 4.61 *continued.* (H) P-A in vertical position. (See Diagram 4.2F.) (I) Right anterior oblique spot film of hepatic flexure. (J) Left anterior oblique spot film of splenic flexure. (K) Prone cross-table of the rectum.

done in at least five projections. If any segment of the colon remains obscured, additional spot or overhead films with an angled X-ray tube are taken. Detailed fluoroscopy with controlled compression should be performed only in those sections of the colon where large collections of barium persist.

Endoscopy performed prior to double-contrast barium enema should not interfere with the feasibility of performing the enema if the barium suspension is diluted more than for a usual double-contrast barium enema. The patient should be spared from a double-contrast barium enema for least 48 hours, but preferably six days, following deep biopsy or polypectomy. Biopsy of the rectal mucosa can cause rectal ulcers of various depth. However, surface irregularities of mucosa at the biopsy site are more common.

Contraindications for double-contrast enema are similar to those for single-contrast examination.

Double-contrast barium enema is superior to single-contrast examination in detecting discrete mucosal lesions. Lesions as small as 5 mm can be discovered by double-contrast enema (Fig. 4.62). Double-contrast and single-contrast examinations can provide equally good results in detecting carcinomas proximal to the sigmoid colon. Double-contrast enema is superior in detecting polyps, and may reveal faceted mucosal protrusions representing colonic dysplasia in the quiescent phase of ulcerative colitis.

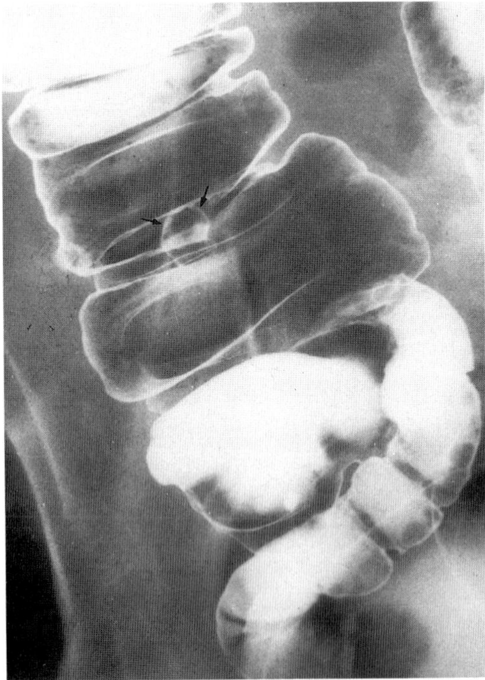

FIGURE 4.62. Double-contrast study shows an ascending colon polyp.

False-positive results in interpreting double-contrast enemas increase while searching for tumors smaller than 1 cm in diameter. False-negative results are mainly the result of perception errors.

Double-contrast barium enema examination and colonoscopy are complementary methods. Even most modern endoscopes have "blind spots" caused by sharp angulations of the intestine. Fibroscopes cannot reach portions of the colon proximal to significant narrowings. However, a double-contrast enema shows all segments of the large intestine.

Specific Procedures. If insufflated air reaches proximal segments of the colon that are not filled with barium, *air block* can prevent further filling with barium. Evacuation of the bowel and reapplication of barium suspension with the patient in a dependent position usually allows proximal progression of barium. If this maneuver fails the colon can then be easily filled with a diluted barium suspension.

When insufflation of air does not *advance* barium to the tip of the cecum, 1 L of diluted barium can be added. After evacuation of excess barium, additional air is insufflated resulting in a diagnostic presentation of the right colon (Fig. 4.63).

An excess of rectal barium can be evacuated by elevating the table to approximately 45 degrees with the patient prone and placing the enema bag on the floor with open drainage. If this maneuver fails, the catheter is pushed anteriorly to enable better evacuation. With the table sufficiently elevated, insufflated air is not likely to leave the colon even when a balloon catheter is not used.

EXAMINATIONS FOLLOWING A POSITIVE HEMOCCULT TEST

Early detection of colorectal carcinoma is essential for any improvement in therapy. In positive hemoccult test patients, the prevalence of colorectal carcinoma is 3–10% and of adenomatous polyps with various degrees of dysplasia, 20%. Right colon carcinomas bleed more frequently than colon carcinomas elsewhere, and

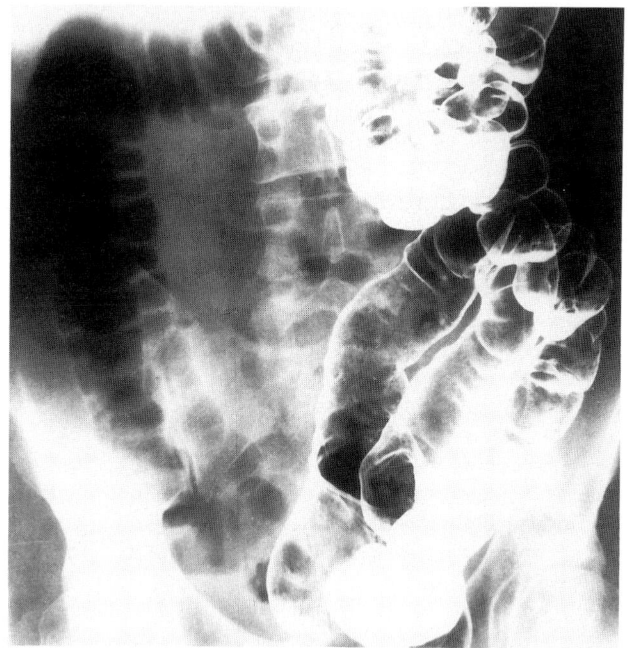

A

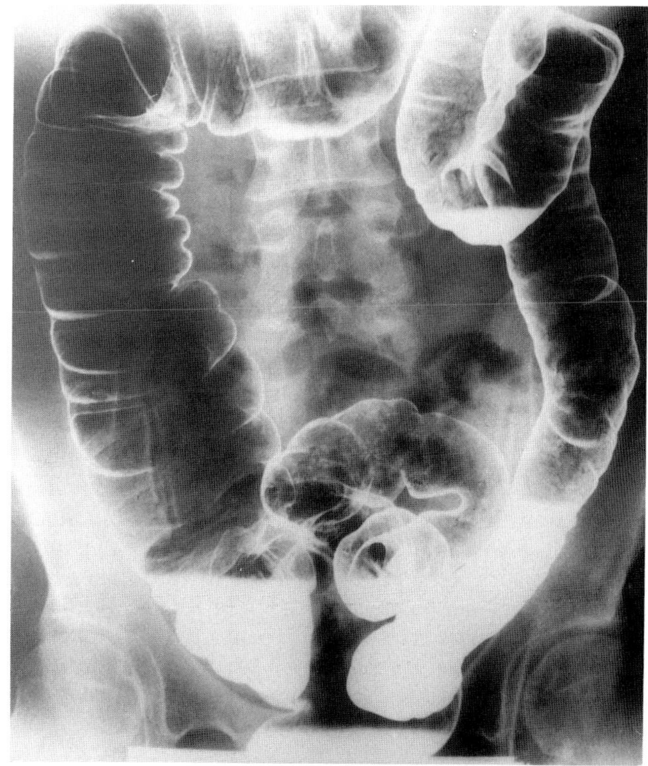

B

Figure 4.63. (A) Double-contrast barium enema. Insufflated air did not succeed in propelling barium proximally. (B) Double-contrast barium enema. After administration of dilute barium suspension, evacuation of excess barium, and reinsufflation of air, a diagnostic roentenogram has been produced.

are more likely to be detected. A negative hemoccult test can obviate the need for more expensive procedures such as double-contrast barium enema and colonoscopy.

The accuracy of a double-contrast barium enema is close to that of colonoscopy. However, colonoscopy is not always successful in examining the entire colon, particularly in patients with dolychocolon. It also carries a higher risk than a barium enema. The method of choice in examining patients with a positive hemoccult test, therefore, is double-contrast barium enema which may be followed by colonoscopy in selected situations.

Pathological changes in the upper gastrointestinal tract are not likely to result in a positive hemoccult test since enzymes within pancreatic secretions deactivate hemoglobin peroxidase. Only large amounts of blood from the upper gastrointestinal tract will result in a positive hemoccult test.

MULTIPHASIC GASTROINTESTINAL EXAMINATIONS

Some authors consider multiphasic gastrointestinal examination and double-contrast examination synonymous while others distinguish between them. The multiphasic examination consists of both double-contrast and single-contrast phases in sequence. *Mucosal relief* of the organ can be shown during the single-contrast phase. By rotating the patient in the horizontal position and by changing the table elevation, barium is moved away so that air in the stomach demonstrates mucosal relief. By controlled compression of the abdomen, mucosal relief of the distal stomach, duodenum, major segments of the small intestine, and portions of the colon and cecum can be demonstrated.

In examining *the esophagus* multiphasically, a portion of the double-contrast technique is first performed. A full-column examination is performed with the patient prone or in the prone left posterior oblique position. The LES is optimally demonstrated recumbent while most double-contrast techniques are performed in the upright position. Barium mucosal relief of the esophagus is then demonstrated by swallowing saliva.

More detailed examination of the esophagus during upper gastrointestinal series is performed after completion of the upper gastrointestinal study; otherwise an excess of barium may hide pathologic lesions in the stomach and duodenum. If a hypotonic agent is used in examination of the esophagus, the single-contrast phase should precede the double-contrast phase in order to analyze esophageal motility.

After single-contrast examination of the *stomach* with compression, and demonstration of mucosal relief by patient rotation, effervescent agents allow further double-contrast demonstration. However, the double-contrast phase may precede single-contrast examination.

A single-contrast technique with compression and demonstration of mucosal relief is used in the initial phase of multiphasic examination of *the duodenum* in the same manner as with the gastric antrum. The patient turns to the supine position and then 45 degrees leftward. Air present in the stomach fills the antrum and, after relaxation of the pylorus, the superior segment of the duodenum. Hypotonia and gas released from an effervescent agent in the stomach enable demonstration of the entire duodenum.

The small bowel can be examined by multiphasic enteroclysis if single-contrast barium application is followed by at least two doses of effervescent agent. Multiphasic enteroclysis is similar to double-contrast enteroclysis. Methylcellulose, air, or water can be used in the double-contrast phase.

Multiphasic examination of the *colon* consists of a single-contrast barium enema followed by air insufflation. In the single-contrast phase the colon should be filled with the smallest possible quantity of diluted barium. Highly concentrated barium, especially when of high viscosity, can be difficult to evacuate from the colon, and may result in incomplete double-contrast demonstration. Since barium pools may obscure pathologic processes, application of barium is carefully monitored and compression spot films are taken. Excess barium is then evacuated and air insufflated before typical spot and overhead roentgenograms are taken.

ULTRASOUND EXAMINATION

The stomach and the bowel can be examined by ultrasound (US) (Fig. 4.64). Thickening of the pyloric muscle in hypertrophic pyloric ste-

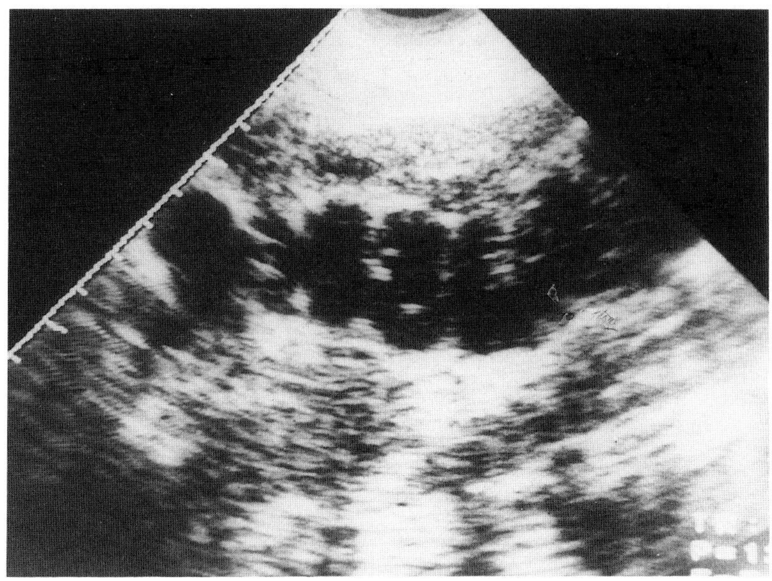

Figure 4.64. Normal ultrasound appearance of the transverse colon after water enema administration.

nosis can be readily demonstrated (Fig. 4.65A). Diffuse thickening of the gastric wall and gut may be demonstrated by US (Fig. 4.65). Gastric neoplasms, as well as spread into adjacent structures and ascites, are identifiable. Ultrasound may also show neoplasms of the small and large intestine. Neoplasms involving the gut are generally demonstrated by ultrasound

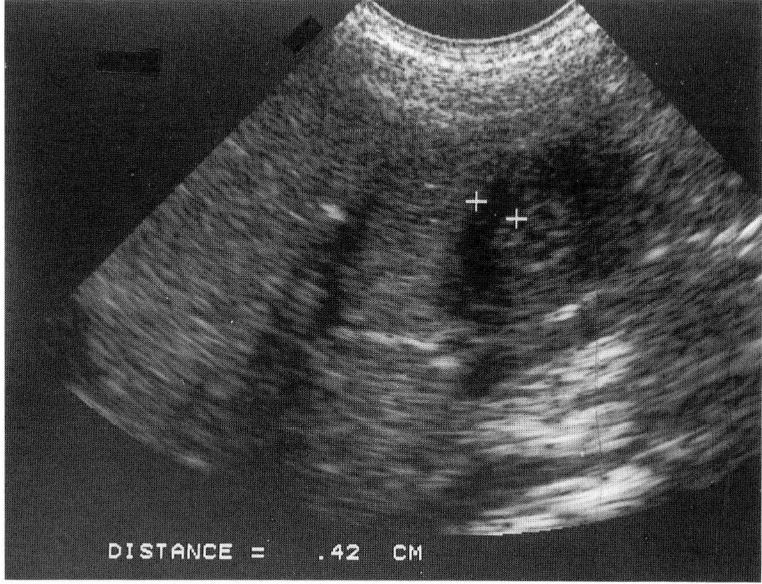

Figure 4.65. (A) Sonographic demonstration of hypertrophic pyloric stenosis in a child. (Courtesy of W.L. Wells, M.D., Louisiana State University, New Orleans.) (*Figure continued on overleaf.*)

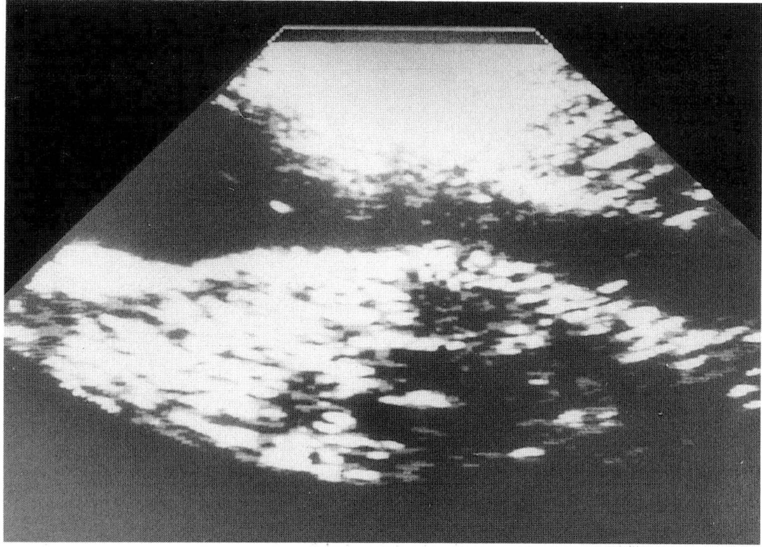

Figure 4.65. (B) Descending colon stenosis demonstrated by ultrasound.

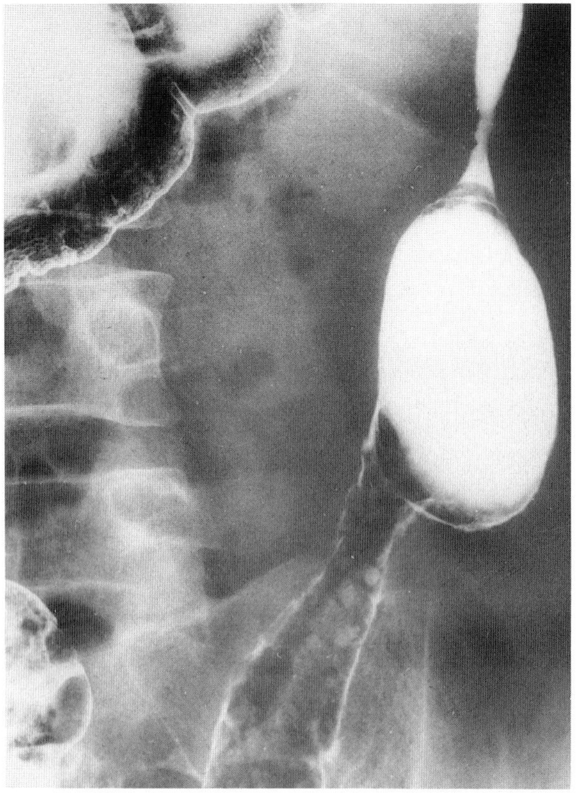

Figure 4.65. (C) Double-contrast barium enema in the same patient.

as a solid hypoechoic mass with a wall thicker than 10 mm, whereas in normal subjects the thickness of the gut wall does not exceed 5 mm. If the gastric wall is not thickened, or if the tumor is situated in the proximal portion of the stomach, it cannot be clearly shown by ultrasound. Duodenal hematoma and its natural course can be followed by US, and even demonstration of intestinal intussusception is possible.

Real-time US visualizes infiltration of the terminal ileum and cecum in Crohn's disease. Thickening of the wall is presented by a sonolucent halo surrounding a dense central echo creating a "bull's eye" phenomenon. Thickening may also appear as an elongated tubular structure (Fig. 4.65B). Carcinoma of the colon can also be demonstrated by echosonography (Fig. 4.66).

Processes that result in thickening of the wall of the stomach or bowel, such as neoplasm, inflammation, intussusception, and ischemia, may create a "pseudokidney" sign. The structure roughly resembles a kidney but does not have all of the morphologic properties of a kidney. The bowel lumen is an echogenic center surrounded by a sonolucent rim created by the thickened wall.

Ultrasound demonstrates abdominal cavity abscesses and allows their drainage. The normal bowel wall is readily compressed by the ultrasound transducer. A thickened wall is found in appendicitis and the noncompressible appendix can be directly visualized (Fig. 12.78); ileus can be demonstrated with rupture of an appendiceal abscess. Ultrasound combined with controlled compression identifies enlarged mesenteric lymph nodes. Changes in imperforate anus can be evaluated by real-time sonography.

SPECIFIC PROCEDURES

The alimentary canal can be *distended with water* for better ultrasonic demonstration. *Transrectal examination* may enhance presentation of masses originating from the rectal or perirectal areas. Masses situated up to 12 cm proximal to the anus, such as carcinoma of the rectum, perirectal abscesses and endometriosis, dermoids, and angiomas in the rectal wall, may be identified. Neoplastic infiltration of adipose tissue and lymph nodes is readily diagnosed. Endosonographic examination and CT are equally accurate in diagnosing rectal and extrarectal tumors.

COMPUTED TOMOGRAPHY

Computed tomography has proved to be of considerable clinical value in the diagnosis of a wide range of gastrointestinal disorders. Although air contrast barium studies remain the

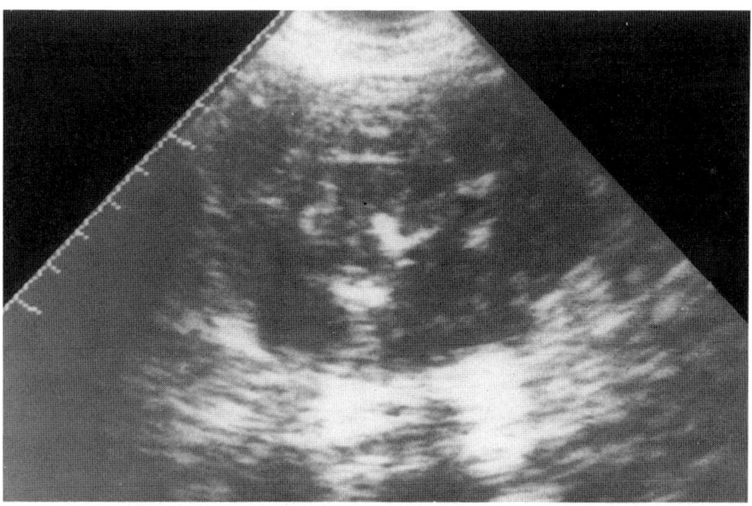

FIGURE 4.66. Ultrasound appearance of an annular transverse colon carcinoma.

procedure of choice in the evaluation of mucosal abnormalities, CT greatly facilitates the diagnosis of many alimentary tract lesions by directly imaging the bowel wall, mesentery, and adjacent viscera. In selected patients, CT provides unique diagnostic information unavailable with conventional radiographic studies alone.

Careful attention to CT technique is essential for optimal diagnosis of many gastrointestinal lesions. The use of both oral and intravenous contrast is often essential to identify and characterize both visceral and alimentary lesions. To visualize mural abnormalities, the lumen of the gut should be distended with positive contrast agents (dilute solution of either barium 1.5–2% or "iodinated contrast" 2–3%) or negative contrast agents (air or fat emulsions). Intravenous contrast enhancement administered as a bolus often enables characterization of the vascularity and solid or cystic nature of the underlying lesion.

Although plain abdominal radiographs are essential for the initial assessment of patients with acute gastrointestinal abnormalities, they are often nonspecific, and fail to adequately characterize the underlying pathologic process. Even when plain abdominal radiographs are positive, CT may aid the clinical management by guiding percutaneous therapy or defining the anatomical relationship of the lesion to visceral, vascular, and other vital structures in the abdomen. Occult gastrointestinal perforation may be diagnosed by CT on the basis of ectopic gas bubbles or extravasated oral contrast (Figs. 4.67 and 4.68). In patients with unusual forms of gastrointestinal obstruction, CT may clearly identify areas of intussusception, since invaginated mesenteric fat can be diagnosed due to its characteristically low CT numbers (−80 to −120 HU) (Fig. 4.69). Obstructive small bowel masses from metastatic tumor, or other unusual forms of small bowel obstructions such as internal hernias, gallstone ileus, or closed loop obstruction may be diagnosed by CT (Figs. 4.70 and 4.71).

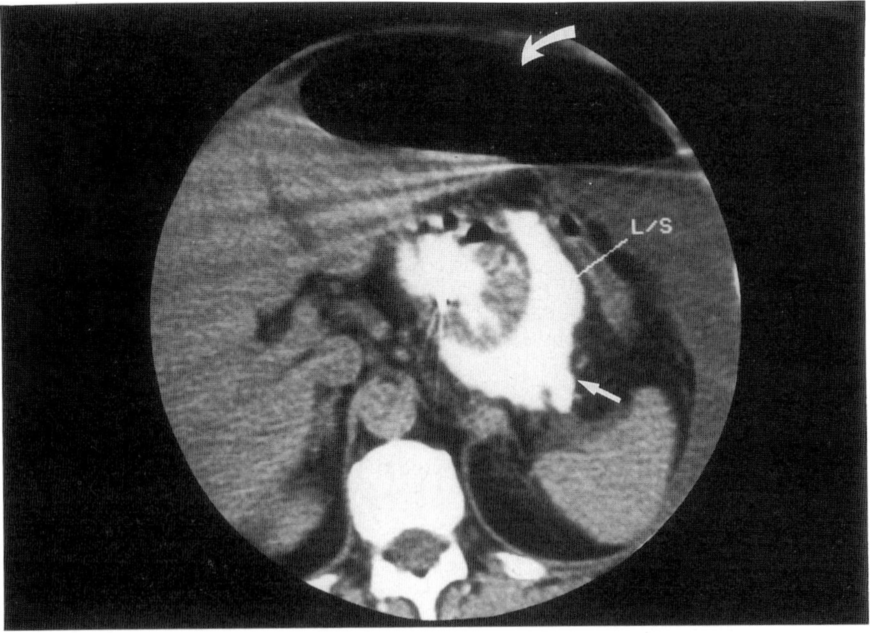

Figure 4.67. Perforated gastric ulcer. High-density contrast (arrow) is noted in the lesser sac (LS) from a posterior penetrating gastric ulcer. Note the large hydropneumoperitoneum (curved arrow). (Reprinted with permission from Jeffrey RB Jr. CT and sonography of the acute abdomen, Chapter 6, The gastrointestinal tract. New York: Raven Press; 1989.)

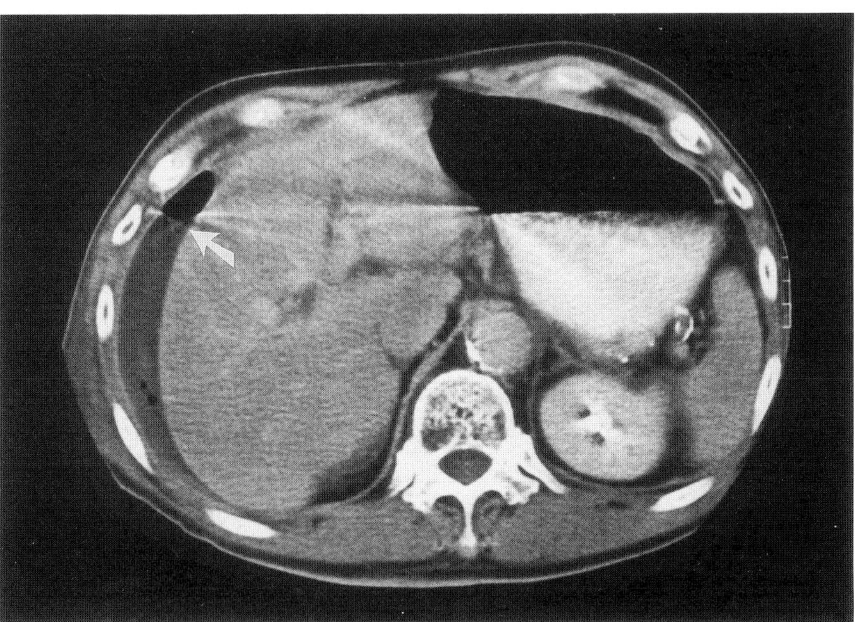

Figure 4.68. Perforated duodenal ulcer. Hydropneumoperitoneum is noted adjacent to the liver (arrow). (Reprinted with permission from Jeffrey RB Jr. CT and sonography of the acute abdomen. Chapter 6, The gastrointestinal tract. New York: Raven Press; 1989.)

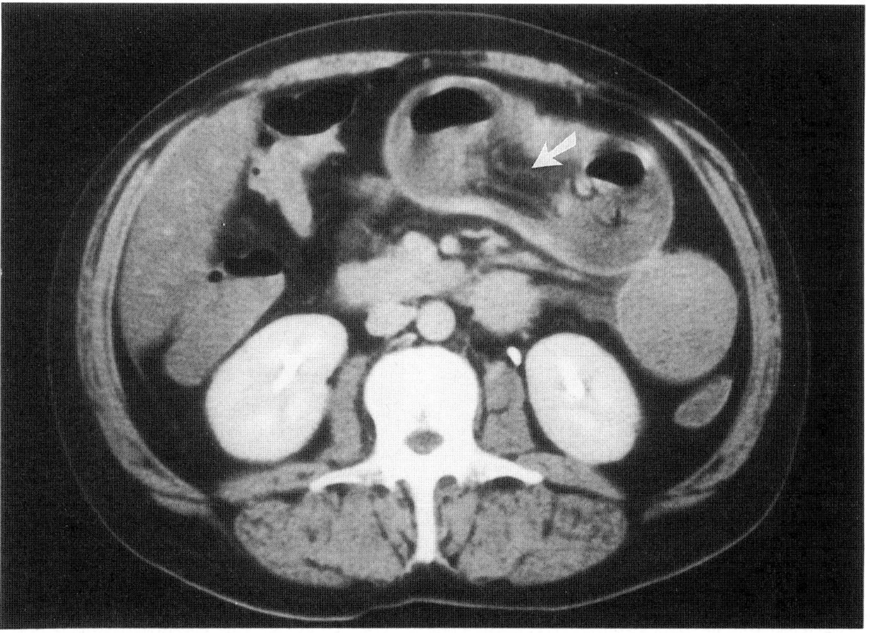

Figure 4.69. (A) Jejunojejunal intussusception. A focally dilated loop contains mesenteric fat and enhances mesenteric vasculature (arrow). (*Figure continued on overleaf.*)

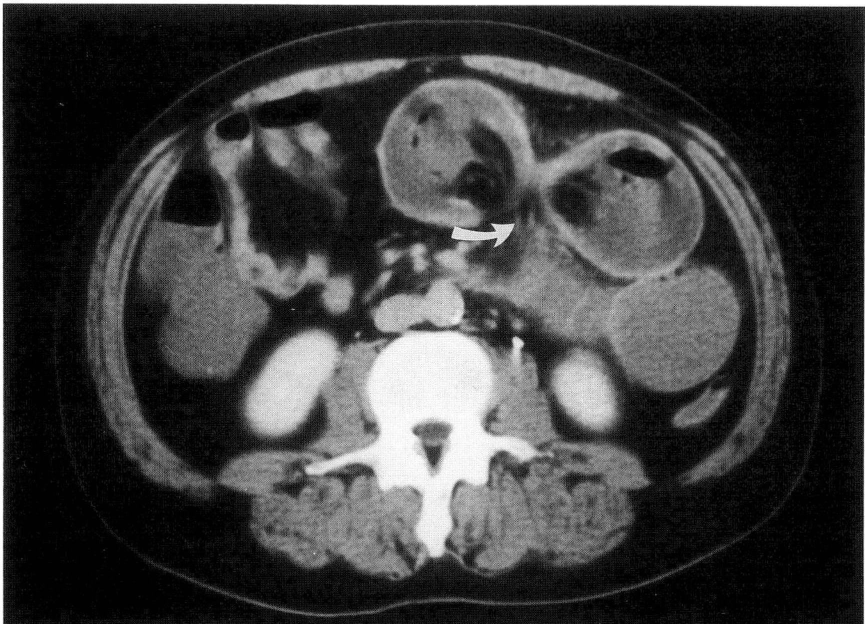

Figure 4.69. (B) Jejunojejunal intussusception. The site of invagination of the intussusceptum (arrow) is demonstrated. (Reprinted with permission from Jeffrey RB Jr. CT and sonograhy of the acute abdomen, Chapter 6, The gastrointestinal tract. New York: Raven Press; 1989.)

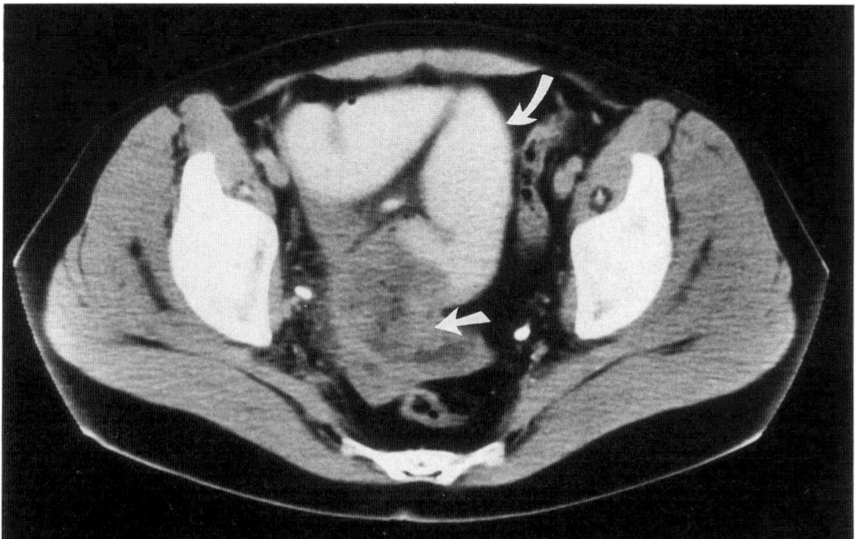

Figure 4.70. Small bowel obstruction from metastatic lung carcinoma. A dilated loop of bowel (curved arrow) is noted in the pelvis with obstructing soft tissue mass (arrow). This was proven at surgery to be a metastatic lesion from carcinoma of the lung. (Reprinted with permission from Jeffrey RB Jr. CT and sonography of the acute abdomen, Chapter 6, The gastrointestinal tract. New York: Raven Press; 1989.)

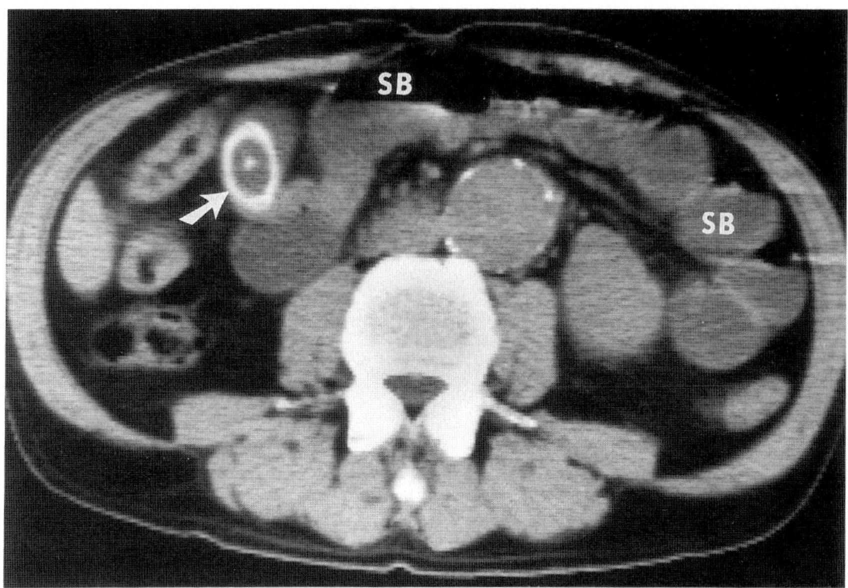

FIGURE 4.71. Small bowel obstruction from gallstone ileus. A high-density gallstone (arrow) is seen within the terminal ileum, resulting in proximal small bowel obstruction (SB = small bowel). (Reprinted with permission from Jeffrey RB Jr. CT and sonography of the acute abdomen, Chapter 6, The gastrointestinal tract. New York: Raven Press; 1989.)

Although gastrointestinal angiography is often required for definitive assessment of small bowel infarction, CT may be of value in excluding other diagnoses such as hemorrhagic pancreatitis or in demonstrating highly suggestive features of small bowel infarction such as intramural gas, portal venous gas, focal bowel wall thickening, or direct visualization of a thrombus in the superior mesenteric artery or vein. Although the exact sensitivity of CT in early small bowel infarction is unknown, in more advanced cases a constellation of CT findings may suggest the diagnosis (Figs. 4.72 to 4.74).

Blunt trauma to the bowel is often not suspected clinically as extravasation of small bowel contents rarely results in early peritonitis. The CT demonstration of focal bowel wall thickening, adjacent mesenteric hematoma, and extravasated air or contrast is highly specific for gastrointestinal lesions in the setting of blunt abdominal trauma. Isolated mesenteric hematomas, or small intramural hematomas without evidence of extravasation or hemoperitoneum, are treated conservatively and thus CT may aid in the clinical management of these patients (Figs. 4.75 and 4.76).

One of the main clinical indications for abdominal CT is the search for an abscess, which is often due to enteric perforation such as appendicitis or diverticulitis. Characteristic features of an abscess on CT are a low-density lesion demonstrating mass effect, and surrounding edema and infiltration of adjacent soft tissue planes. In some patients, there are gas bubbles or air-fluid levels in the presence of an enteric fistula. Computed tomography may be of particular value in direct percutaneous therapy, either for definitive cure or as a temporizing measure (Fig. 4.77). Focal inflammatory lesions cause both thickening of the bowel wall and soft tissue infiltration in adjacent mesenteric omental fat (Fig. 4.78). In patients with inflammatory bowel disease, acute exacerbation of symptoms is often related to abscess formation within the mesentery and this is readily diagnosed by CT (Figs. 4.79 and 4.80).

Although CT has not been used as a primary screening modality to detect alimentary tract neoplasms, it may be useful in identifying

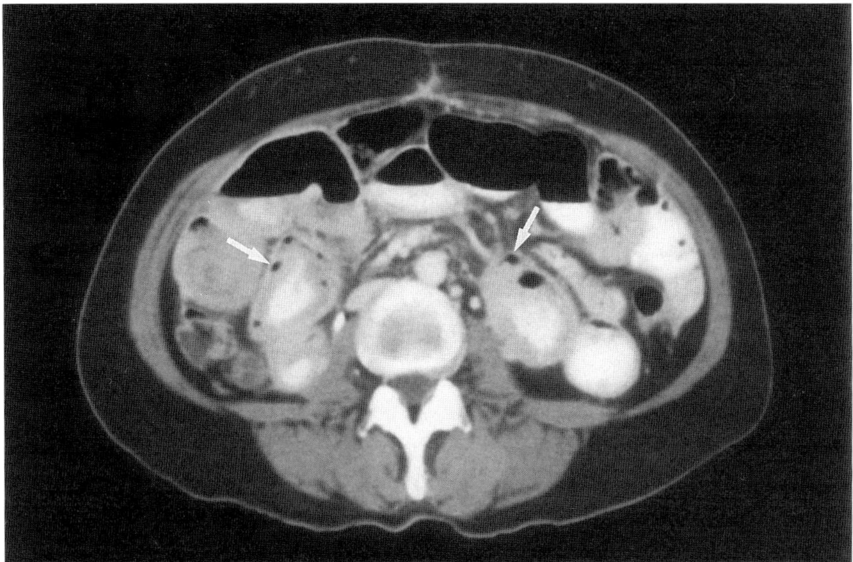

FIGURE 4.72. Small bowel infarction. Numerous thickened loops of small bowel are identified with intramural gas (arrows). Laparotomy confirmed small bowel infarction. (Reprinted with permission from Jeffrey RB Jr. CT and sonography of the acute abdomen. Chapter 6, The gastrointestinal tract. New York: Raven Press; 1989.)

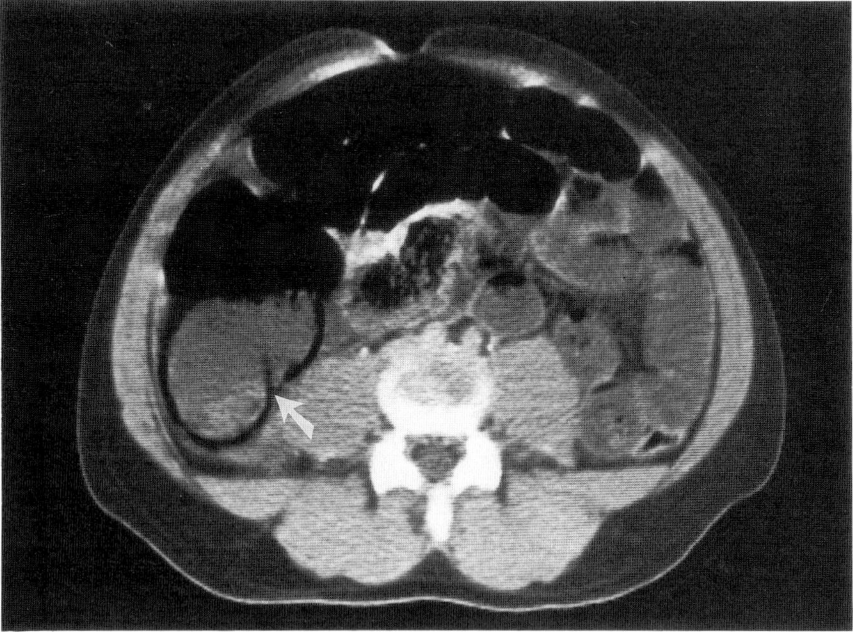

FIGURE 4.73. Infarction of the right colon. The right colon is dilated and demonstrates extensive intramural gas (arrow) from infarction. (Reprinted with permission from Jeffrey RB Jr. CT and sonography of the acute abdomen. Chapter 6, The gastrointestinal tract. New York: Raven Press; 1989.)

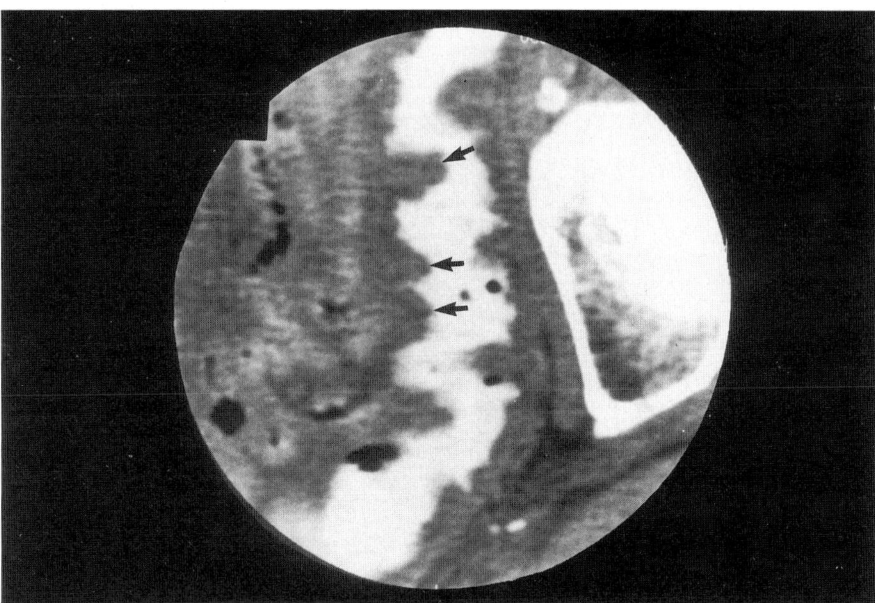

FIGURE 4.74. Ischemic colitis. CT performed with rectal contrast demonstrates marked thickening of the wall of the rectosigmoid, with areas of "thumbprinting" (arrows) secondary to submucosal hemorrhage from ischemic colitis. (Reprinted with permission from Jeffrey RB Jr. CT and sonography of the acute abdomen. Chapter 6, The gastrointestinal tract. New York: Raven Press; 1989.)

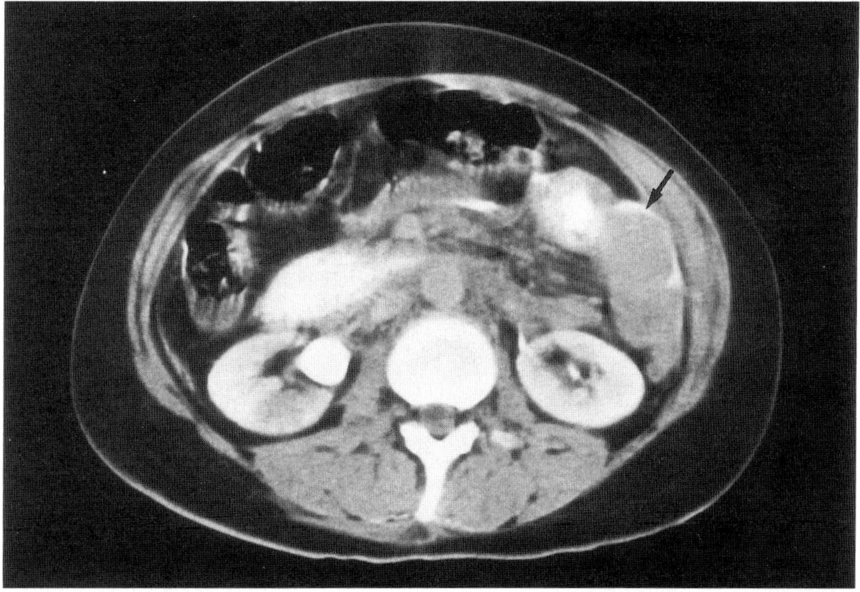

FIGURE 4.75. Laceration of the jejunum from blunt trauma with resulting perforation. Focal thickening is noted at the wall of the proximal jejunum, with extravasation of oral contrast medium into the left paracolic gutter (arrow) from laceration. (Reprinted with permisson from Jeffrey RB Jr. CT and sonography of the acute abdomen. Chapter 6, The gastrointestinal tract. New York: Raven Press; 1989.)

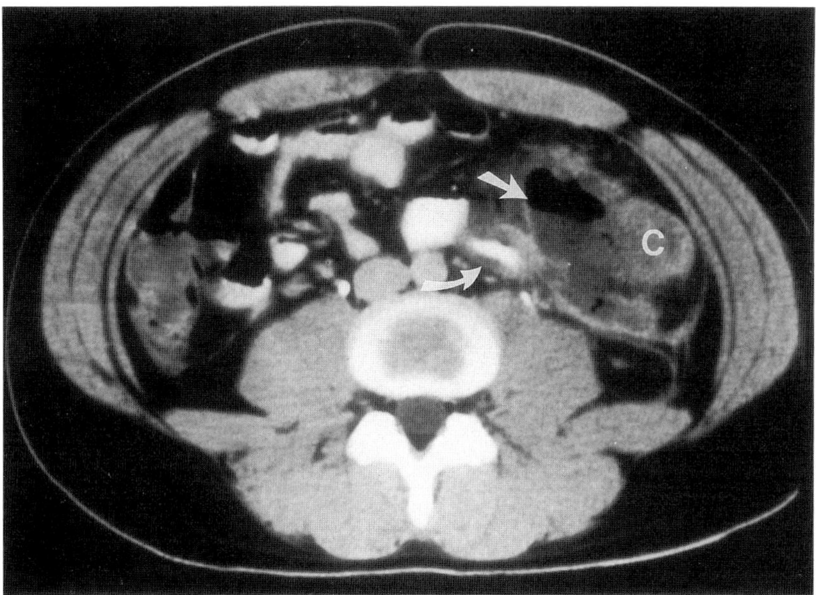

Figure 4.76. Laceration of the descending colon and jejunal hematoma. Focal thickening of the jejunum is noted from an intramural hematoma (arrow). A gas-fluid level is seen adjacent to the thickened portion of descending colon (curved arrow) secondary to perforation at this site. (Reprinted with permission from Jeffrey RB Jr. CT and sonography of the acute abdomen, Chapter 6, The gastrointestinal tract. New York: Raven Press; 1989.)

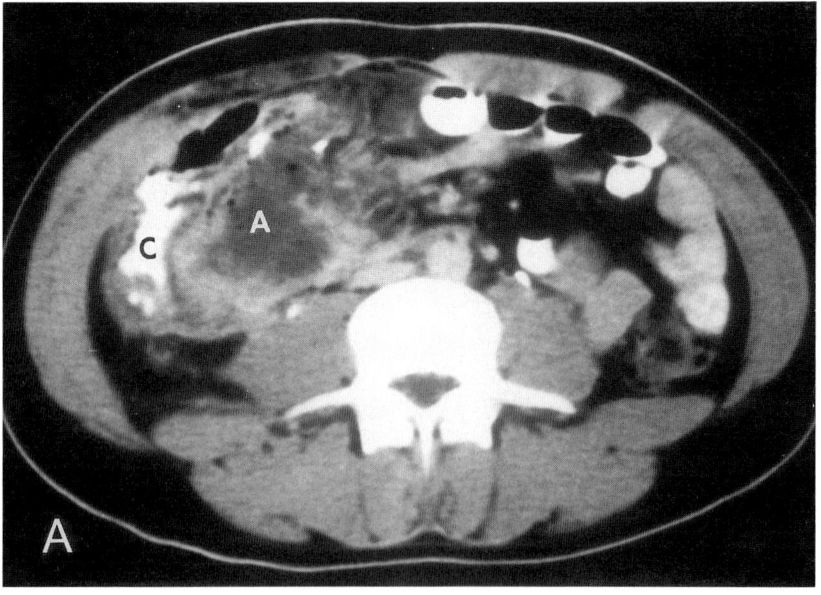

Figure 4.77. (A) CT-guided drainage of a periappendiceal abscess. Low-density abscess cavity [A] is adjacent to the cecum [C].

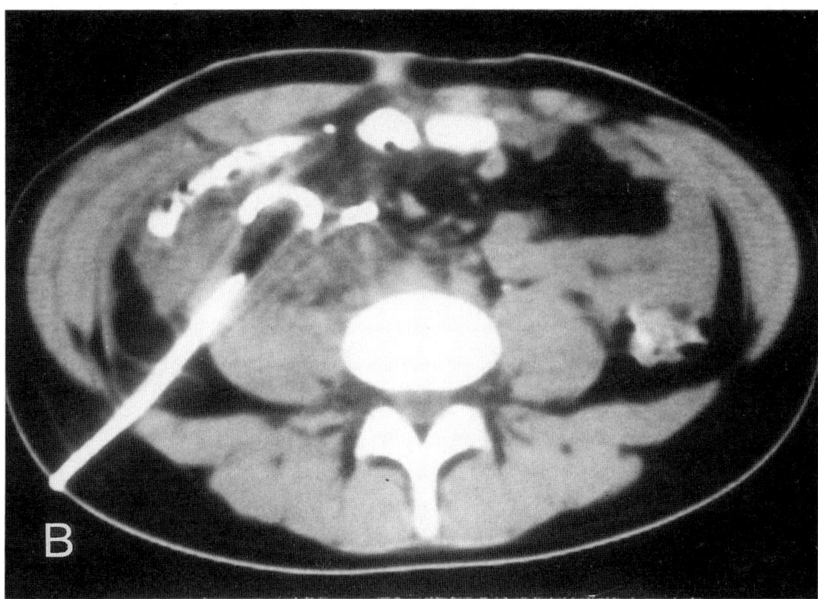

Figure 4.77. (B) Under CT guidance, a catheter was placed into the lesion with complete evacuation of the abscessed cavity. (Reprinted with permission from Jeffrey RB Jr. Abdominal abscesses: The role of CT and sonography. In: McGahan JD, ed. Interventional Ultrasound, p 134. © 1990, the Williams and Wilkins Co., Baltimore.)

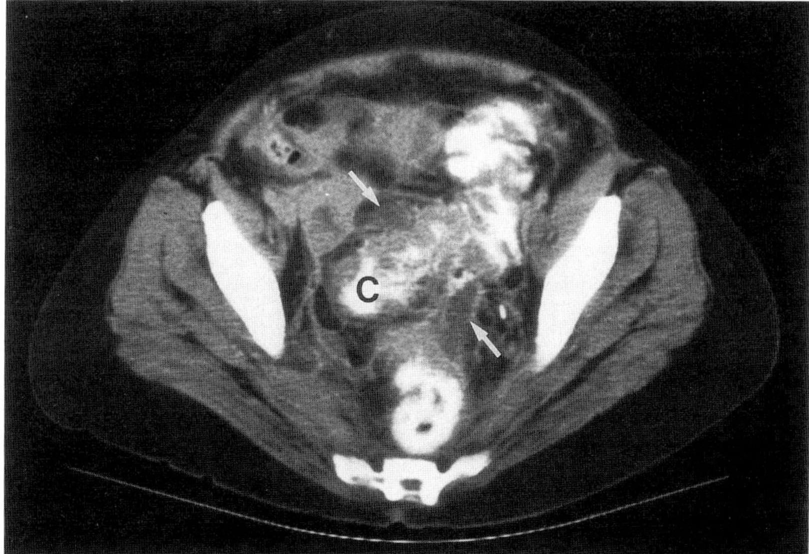

Figure 4.78. CT of acute diverticulitis. CT with rectal contrast demonstrates marked thickening of the rectosigmoid colon (C) with inflammatory changes in the sigmoid mesocolon. Small adjacent fluid collections are noted from paracolonic abscesses (arrows). (Reprinted with permission from Jeffrey RB Jr. CT and sonography of the acute abdomen. Chapter 6, The gastrointestinal tract. New York: Raven Press; 1989.)

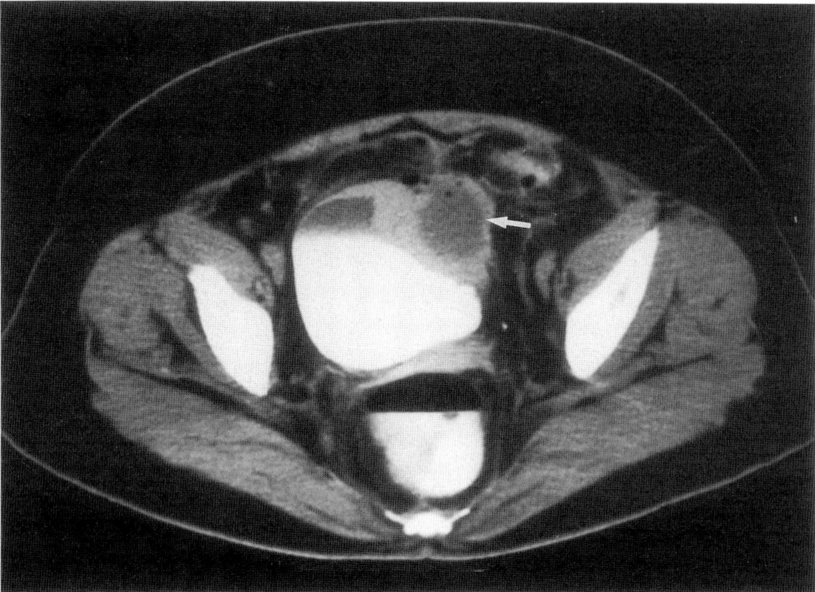

FIGURE 4.79. CT diagnosis of diverticular abscess. Diverticular abscess (arrow) is seen adjacent to focal thickening of the bladder wall. This abscess was successfully drained percutaneously, preventing the development of colovesicle fistula. (Reprinted with permission from Jeffrey RB Jr. CT and sonography of the acute abdomen, Chapter 6, The gastrointestinal tract. New York: Raven Press; 1989.)

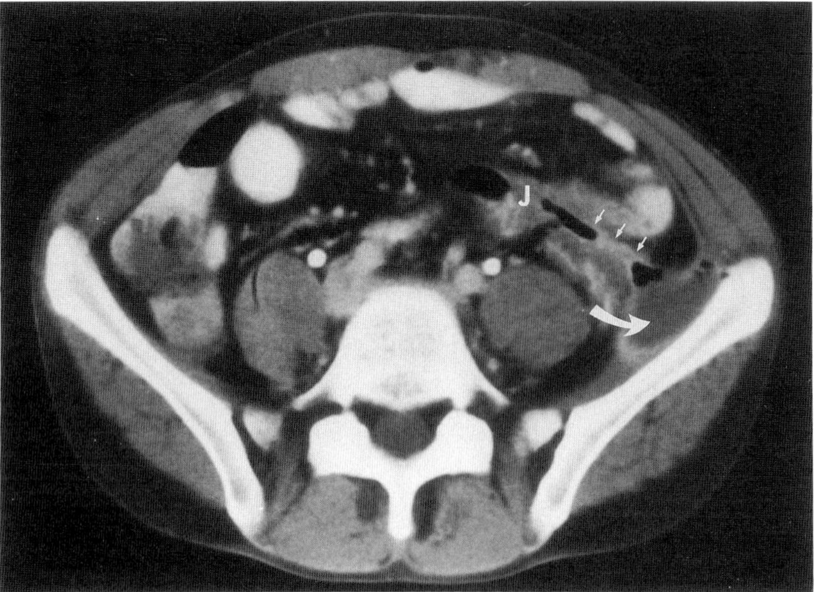

FIGURE 4.80. (A) Crohn's disease with small bowel perforation and iliac fossa abscess. (A) Focally thickened segment of jejunum is evident. (J = jejunum.) A fistulous tract extends to the iliac fossa (arrow) with adjacent abscess (curved arrow).

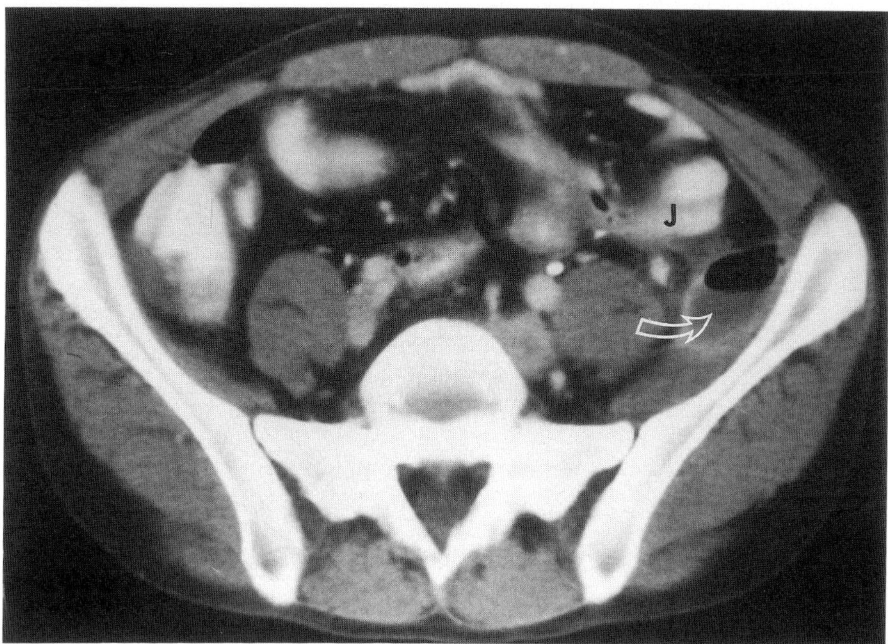

FIGURE 4.80. (B) A gas-fluid level appears within the iliac fossa abscess (curved arrow = abscess cavity, J = jejunum).

hepatic metastasis, direct local invasion, or evidence of peritoneal carcinomatosis. Gastrointestinal tract malignancies appear as nonspecific focal bowel wall thickenings that may contain ulceration and adjacent lymphadenopathy (Fig. 4.81). There may be considerable overlap in the appearance of either inflammatory or neoplastic conditions as shown by CT; thus biopsy is always required to confirm the presence of an underlying neoplasm (Figs. 4.82 to 4.85). Computed tomography is not reliable in identifying metastases to normal size mesenteric nodes.

MAGNETIC RESONANCE IMAGING

Magnetic resonance imaging (MRI) serves as a complementary modality for demonstration of selected alimentary canal lesions. Neoplasms of the parapharyngeal space are better visualized by MRI than by CT because of:

1. More distinct tumor contour.
2. Better visualization of blood vessels in the neck without contrast medium.
3. Identification of tumor vascularity.
4. Advantageous direct sagittal and coronal imaging (Fig. 4.86).

The digestive tube is not easily distinguished from adjacent solid structures by MRI. Nevertheless, the stomach and the duodenum can be fairly well presented after administration of an effervescent agent and IV injection of glucagon. A collapsed stomach or duodenum may appear as if the walls are thickened. A duodenal hematoma with characteristic MRI signal is described in chapter 9.

Separation of intestinal loops is not easy by MRI or CT. Namely, the difference in contrast between the bowel and surrounding structures is not significant. In addition, both position and configuration of the bowel are subject to great variation. To facilitate reference, the bowel is filled with positive or negative contrast medium prior to CT examination. Paramagnetic substances, for the same reason, can be administered prior to MRI examinations. They are nontoxic and provide clear demarcation of the alimentary canal from surrounding

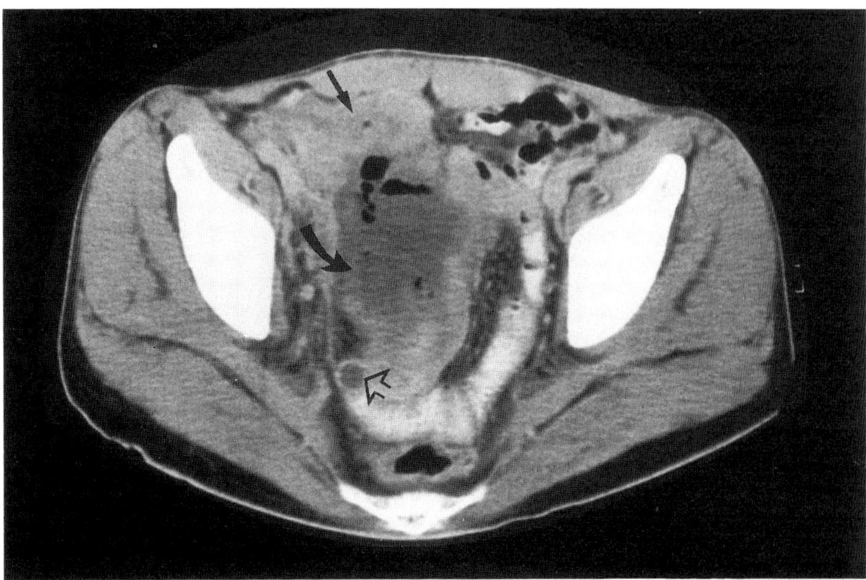

FIGURE 4.81. Pelvic abscess from perforation of cecal lymphoma. A soft tissue mass (arrow) is seen in the right hemipelvis (arrow). The mass has a nonspecific appearance on CT and was proved to be a cecal lymphoma. Note adjacent abscess cavity with gas bubbles (curved arrow) by the abscessed cavity.

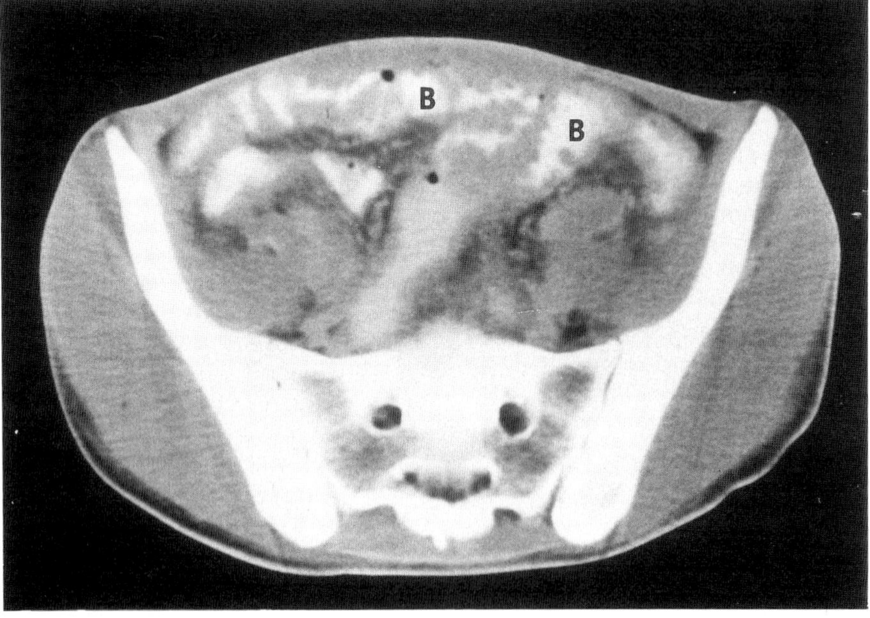

FIGURE 4.82. Cytomegalovirus enteritis in a patient with AIDS. Marked thickening of the entire small bowel (B) is noted from opportunistic infection related to cytomegalovirus in a patient with AIDS. (Reprinted with permission from Jeffrey RB Jr, Nyberg DA, Bottles K, et al. Abdominal CT in acquired immunodeficiency syndrome. AJR. 1986;146:7, © American Journal of Roentgenology.)

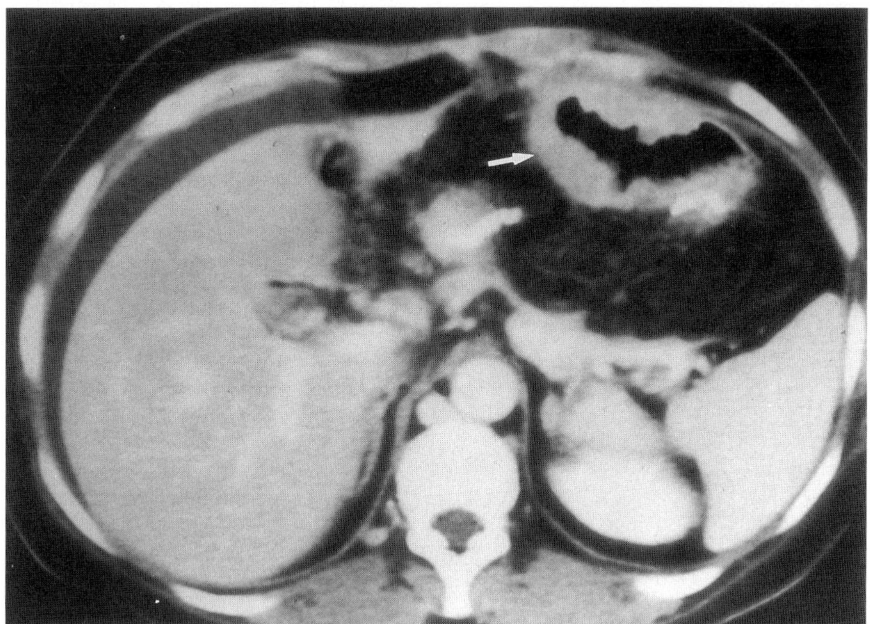

FIGURE 4.83. Gastric carcinoma. CT demonstrates focal thickening that proved to be a carcinoma (arrow).

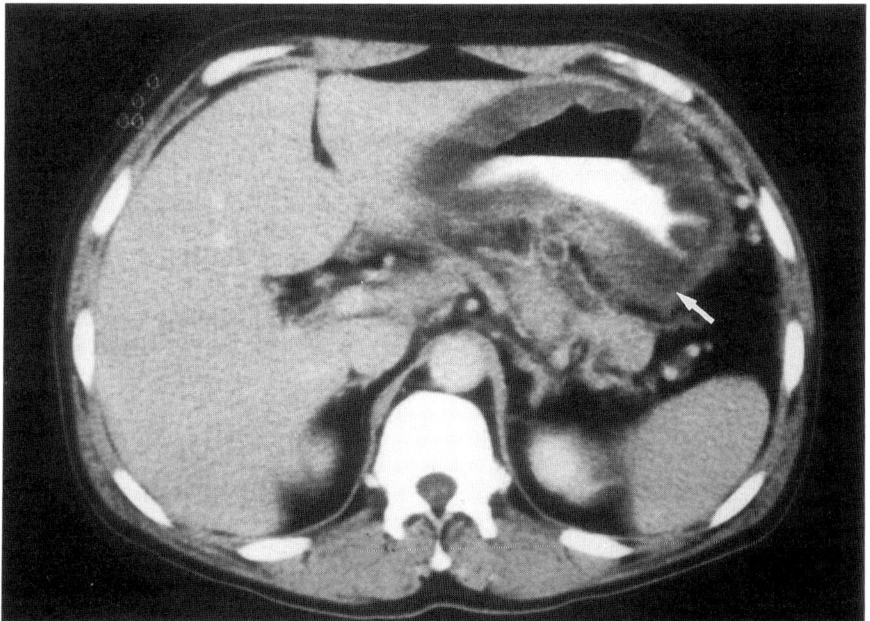

FIGURE 4.84. Diffuse gastritis on CT simulating neoplasm. The gastric wall is diffusely thickened (arrow). However, it is very low in attenuation. Repeated biopsies demonstrated only gastritis and no evidence of neoplasm.

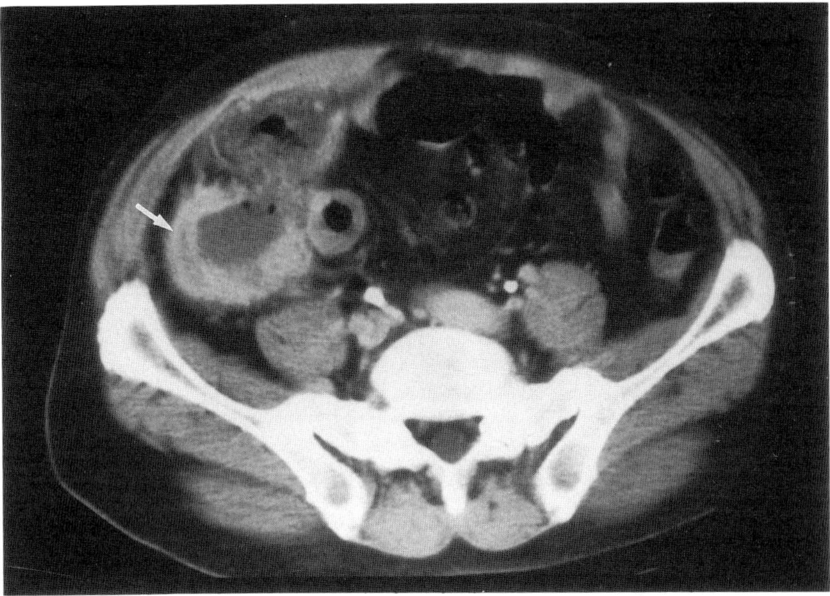

Figure 4.85. CT of cecal carcinoma. Marked thickening of the wall of the cecum (arrow) is nonspecific, but proved to be a cecal carcinoma at endoscopy.

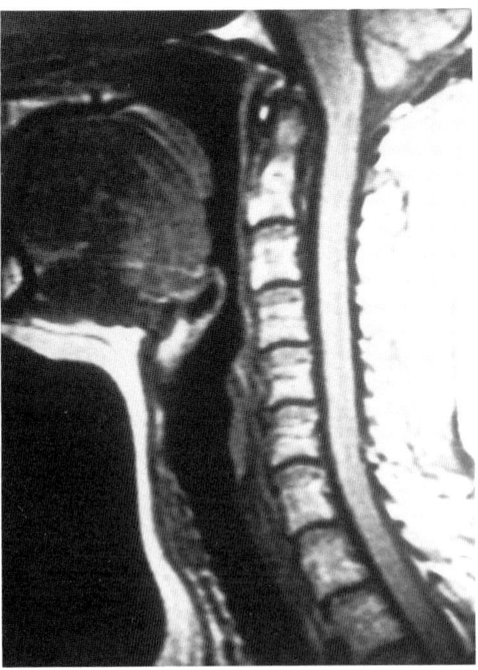

Figure 4.86. MRI-proton density study of structures of the pharynx and the neck shows normal findings.

anatomical structures. Paramagnetic compounds that may be used as positive contrast agents in the gastrointestinal tube are oral solutions of ferric ammonium citrate, ferric sulfate heptahydrate or gadolinium. Negative contrast media for gastrointestinal tract MRI are perfluoroctylbromide organic compounds. Intestinal gas is a welcomed negative contrast, since it provides no signal. The dominant abnormality detected by MRI is thickening of the alimentary canal wall. Inflammatory processes demonstrate increased signal intensity on T2-weighted images. Most carcinomas have, in general, prolonged T1 relaxation times and also demonstrate increased signal interaction on T2-weighted images. However, some other specificities occur.

Colonic carcinoma can be visualized by MRI (Fig. 4.87). Rectal carcinoma can be staged by MRI. Perirectal fat invasion by carcinoma is best seen on T1-weighted images. A carcinoma may be impossible to differentiate from perirectal fat on T2 images. However, muscle invasion is demonstrated on T2-weighted images since a neoplasm will have a higher signal than muscle. Both CT and MRI are capable of visualizing a primary neoplasm in the rectal wall as

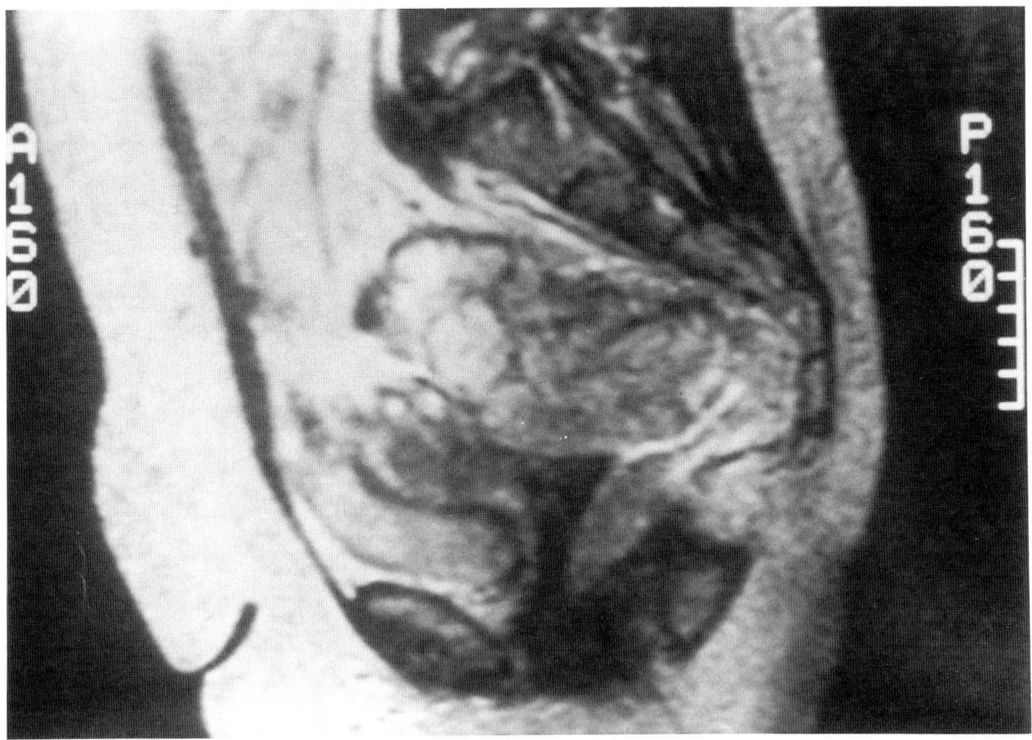

FIGURE 4.87. T2-weighted image of a large sigmoid carcinoma.

well as invasion of perirectal adipose tissue and adjacent organs. However, when infiltration of lymph nodes is not associated with enlargement, it often cannot be recognized by either CT or MRI.

The large intestine should be prepared for MRI examination in the same fashion as for double-contrast enema. Neoplasms and intraluminal feces have similar patterns on MRI. Magnetic resonance imaging is now the method of choice for optimal detection of metastases to the liver.

ARTERIOGRAPHY

Arteriography is capable of demonstrating a bleeding site in the alimentary canal or vascularization of a neoplasm. Selective catheterization is necessary for satisfactory visualization. Contrast medium extravasates with blood into the lumen of the gut in patients who are actively bleeding (Fig. 4.88). Angiography is advantageous when compared with barium examination because it provides precise localization of bleeding and permits immediate therapy. The one and only criterion for diagnosis is extravasation of contrast medium. In one study of patients with gastric bleeding, 98% had only one site of extravasation. The proximal stomach accounts for 90% of gastric bleeding, 85% within the pool of the left gastric artery. In patients with endoscopically proven multiple bleeding sites, angiography showed solitary extravasation in each. Angiography is the modality of choice in revealing obstructive lesions of blood vessels. Also, angiodysplasias may be demonstrated by selective arteriography (Fig. 4.89).

Malignant neoplasms of the alimentary canal vary in vascular patterns. Gastrointestinal lymphomas and gastric adenocarcinomas, in contrast to adenocarcinoma of the colon, are avascular. Leiomyomas, carcinoids and sarcomas have plentiful vascular networks.

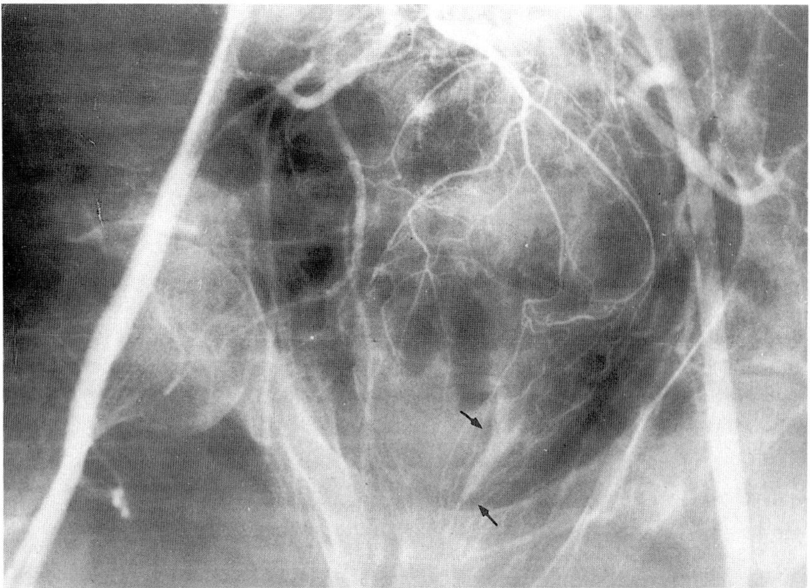

FIGURE 4.88. Hemorrhage into the sigmoid colon (arrows). Selective inferior mesenteric arteriography.

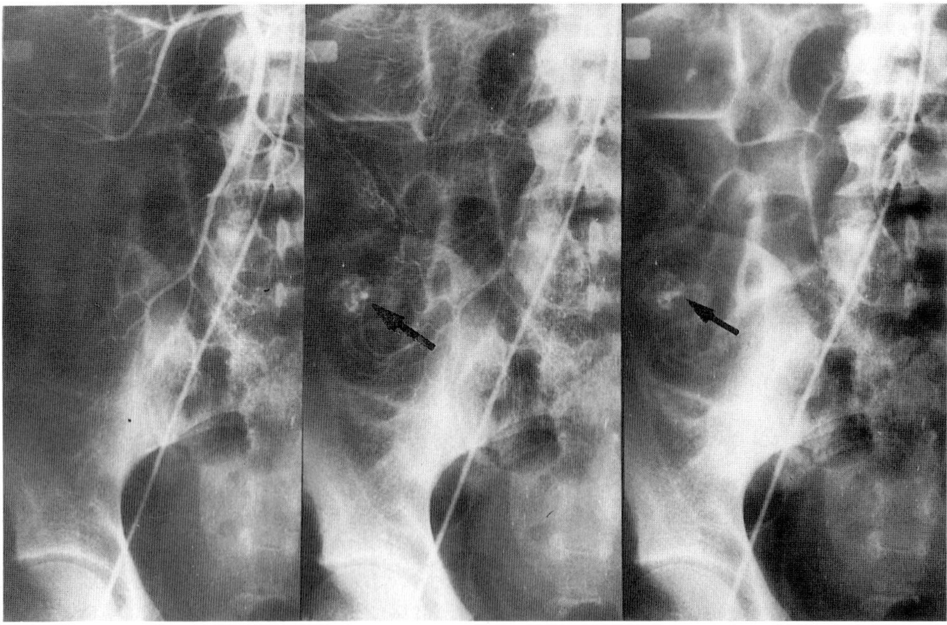

FIGURE 4.89. Angiodysplasia of the ascending colon. Selective arteriography of the superior mesenteric artery. (Courtesy of S. Simunic, M.D., University of Zagreb, Yugoslavia.)

LYMPHANGIOGRAPHY

Lymphangiography is seldom applied to diagnose alimentary canal diseases. Regional metastases of rectal carcinoma produce constriction of afferent lymph vessels. Neoplasms may displace lymph vessels or grow into them. Occasionally, collateral lymphatic circulation compensates for lymphostasis.

SCINTIGRAPHY

Information obtained by GI nuclear scintigraphy mainly concerns organ function and, to a lesser extent, structure.

These noninvasive methods provide quantitative data. Table 4.3 lists conditions and characteristics that can be evaluated by nuclear GI procedures currently applied in most medical centers.

Esophageal motility is assessed by peroral administration of technetium 99m (99m Tc) sulfur colloid or 99m Tc pertechnetate. The patient swallows a small bolus in either an erect or supine position in front of a gamma camera. The bolus first fills the upper third of the esophagus, being briefly delayed at the base of the heart. In the second phase the bolus rapidly fills the remainder of the esophagus, under gravity. The bolus traverses the gastroesophageal junction in the third phase. Both diffuse esophageal spasm and achalasia can be well demonstrated as can fistulae and perforations.

TABLE 4.3. CONDITIONS AND CHARACTERISTICS THAT CAN BE EVALUATED BY RADIONUCLIDE EXAMINATIONS OF THE ALIMENTARY CANAL

Esophageal motility
Gastroesophageal reflux
Gastric emptying
Gastric secretion
Meckel's diverticulum
Bleeding
Inflammation
Neoplasm

In the evaluation of *gastroesophageal reflux* 99m Tc sulfur colloid is introduced via a stomach tube. Recording is performed over a period of 20 to 60 minutes. Gastroesophageal reflux is graded either subjectively or quantitatively. Gastroesophageal reflux is not considered significant within the first six minutes after administration of the radionuclide, but reflux that continues in an intermittent fashion thereafter is regarded as abnormal. Sensitivity of gastroesophageal scintigraphy amounts to 75–90% as compared to cine-esophagography and endoscopy which are 50–60% and 40%, respectively. However, structural abnormalities of the esophageal wall associated with gastroesophageal reflux are detected either by a barium meal or by endoscopy.

Gastric emptying is evaluated after the ingestion of 99m Tc sulfur colloid attached to various solids, from paper particles to chicken livers. Fluid evacuation is recorded with 99m Tc-labeled DTPA (diethyltriaminopentaacetic acid). Evacuation of fluids appears to vary exponentially with time, while emptying of solids is more closely approximated by a linear function of time. Both gastric emptying rate and gastric emptying half-time are extrapolated from curves. In normal subjects, results may vary according to the volume and caloric content of the meal. The radiation dose from gastric scintigraphy is considerably lower than conventional barium studies.

Gastric secretion is evaluated by use of 99m Tc pertechnetate, an anion secreted by parietal cells. The rate of secretion correlates with that of hydrochloric acid. Pentagastrin is given prior to administration of pertechnetate to stimulate gastric secretion. Secretory rates are reduced in patients with pernicious anemia, gastric carcinoma, and gastric ulceration, whereas this parameter is increased in patients with duodenal ulcer.

Ectopic gastric mucosa with a *Meckel's diverticulum* can be demonstrated approximately 40 minutes after administration of 99m Tc pertechnetate, 2.9 μBq per kg body weight (Fig. 4.90). The method has a sensitivity of 75% and a specificity of 100%, and is indicated when unexplained bleeding from the alimentary canal and/or anemia is found in children.

Gastrointestinal bleeding, particularly from

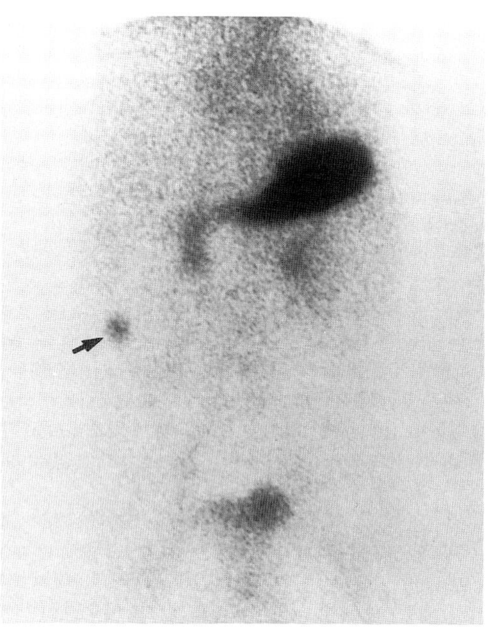

Figure 4.90. Meckel's diverticulum (arrow). Scintigraphy after administration of 99m Tc-pertechnetate. (Courtesy R.J. Campeau, MD, Tulane University, New Orleans.)

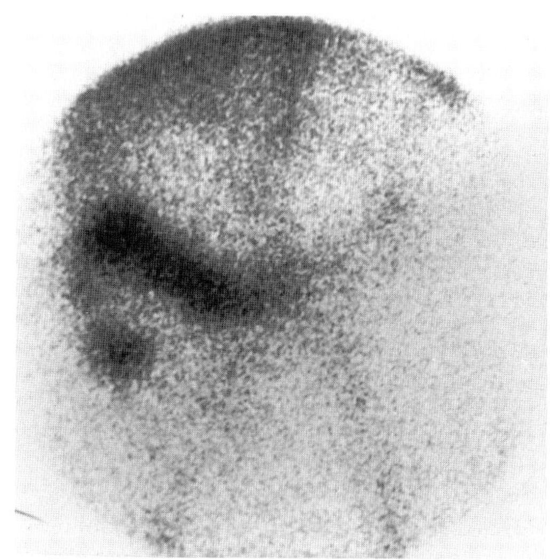

Figure 4.91. Scintigraphy of acute cecal hemorrhage demonstrated 99m Tc-labeled erythrocytes.

distal alimentary canal sections, may be detected and localized by intravenous administration of 99m Tc sulfur colloid. The site of bleeding corresponds to a "hot spot" that appears against a relatively low-activity background. Active gastrointestinal bleeding can be visualized within 10 to 15 minutes, but the bleeding episode must be active at the time of recording. Furthermore, the lesion must be separated from spleen and liver, which normally accumulate this radiotracer. More prolonged blood pool activity is provided by 99m Tc- or 111 In-labeled red blood cells or 99m Tc-labeled human serum albumin (Fig. 4.91). Scintigraphic studies have shown greater sensitivity for the detection of gastrointestinal bleeding than either double-contrast radiography or angiography. Scintigraphy is advantageous in that it is less invasive, whereas angiography offers the added possibility of therapy using vasopressin or embolization.

Inflammation of the alimentary canal may be demonstrated by scintigraphy. There is no significant difference in 99m Tc-DTPA accumulation between normal subjects and patients with ulcerative colitis and Crohn's disease. 111 In-labeled leucocytes have been reported to successfully identify *infarcted bowel* segments. A nonspecific cancer imaging agent, gallium (67 Ga) accumulates in certain *neoplasms*. However, since it normally accumulates in the colon, its application to abdominal scintigraphy is limited.

INTERVENTIONAL RADIOLOGY

A balloon catheter introduced into the esophagus may be insufflated under fluoroscopic control in order to *dilate* a benign stricture. This may be applied to congenital stenoses, corrosive, postoperative and postinflammatory strictures and achalasia. Dilatation by use of a balloon catheter yields better results than the use of bougies in children. Sedation without general anesthesia is usually sufficient. Improvement occurs after the first dilatation with a balloon catheter in 77% of patients with congenital and acquired esophageal stenoses. The asymptomatic interval lasts nine months for stenoses treated by bougie whereas it is four times longer in patients dilated by a balloon catheter. Repeated dilatations with the balloon catheter can be a palliative procedure in patients bearing malignant stenoses. Perforations have not been reported as a complication.

Fluoroscopy is often utilized during *extraction* of foreign bodies from the esophagus. Sharp foreign bodies, or those potentially caustic and toxic, such as discoid alkaline batteries, have to be immediately removed. Smooth surfaced foreign bodies spontaneously pass through the alimentary canal in most cases. Evacuation may be facilitated with glucagon. Besides endoscopy, foreign bodies may also be removed by use of a balloon catheter under fluoroscopy. The balloon is inflated distal to the impacted foreign body. With the balloon inflated, the foreign body may be extracted with the catheter. Basket extraction is another method for foreign body removal from the esophagus. Both methods remove foreign bodies that have no sharp edges and have not been in the esophagus longer than two weeks. This type of extraction is contraindicated in the case of previously existing pathologic changes in the esophagus.

Ileocolic intussusception in young children may be reduced by hydrostatic pressure created by a column of barium suspended 1.5 m above the table. If invagination has been present more than 12 hours, it may be more safely treated surgically. Shock, peritonitis, and gangrene with perforation are contraindications for hydrostatic reposition by barium enema. A patient under the age of six months, and signs of obstruction are relative contraindications. Successful reposition can be facilitated by administration of atropine sulfate, avoiding surgery in almost 80% of patients. Glucagon does not improve results of the first attempt for reduction. It neither increases the success rate nor provides faster reposition. It may be useful in the third attempt, when the first two attempts without glucagon have failed.

Reflux of barium into the iluem after reduction of an ileocolic intussusception is regarded as a sign of success. However, it has been proved that barium can enter the ileum even with partial reduction. Therefore, compression studies need to performed to exclude the presence of persistent ileal loop in the large intestine.

In patients with incomplete or complete sigmoid volvulus, the sigmoid colon is filled with a large volume of gas. *Decompression* is often successful after careful introduction of a fibroscope via the rectum. Not only can the cause of the volvulus be demonstrated, but surgical intervention is usually avoided.

After demonstrating the site of *gastrointestinal bleeding* by selective arteriography, vasopressin may be administered by infusion of 0.2 unit/min over the course of 20 to 30 minutes. If the bleeding stops, infusion of vasopressin can be continued in the intensive care unit. Selective infusion of vasopressin is inefficient if the bleeding site is supplied by more than one artery. In this case, systemic infusion into all supplying arteries yields better results. Hemostasis should be attempted by vasopressin infusion because embolization of small arteries could lead to infarction.

In selected patients with acute gastrointestinal bleeding in whom surgery is contraindicated, embolization may be the method of choice. Bleeding from esophageal varices can be treated by transhepatic catheterization and gelfoam embolization or by implantation of steel coils. This was reported to be effective in seven out of eight patients. Embolization of the left gastric artery by gelfoam is efficient when bleeding is from the stomach. In high-risk patients, it is indicated in endoscopically proved gastric bleeding without apparent leakage at angiography in order to prevent repeated bleeding. Both gelfoam embolization and metal coil implantation give good results. Duodenal bleeding has been successfully treated by selective embolization of the posterior pancreaticoduodenal artery. Transcatheter embolization succeeds in 50% of children bleeding from gastric erosions, duodenal peptic ulcer, and vascular malformations.

Arteries supplying diverticula, arterio-venous malformations, and other potential sites of bleeding from the large bowel are embolized with success. Distal portions of the superior rectal artery may be selectively embolized in patients with angiodysplasia as an alternative to surgery. Ischemic stenoses have been reported following therapeutic arterial embolizations.

Tapeworm may be eliminated from the bowel after Gastrografin application via a duodenal tube.

Prednisolone can be infused into the superior and inferior mesenteric arteries of patients with severe ulcerative colitis nonresponsive to medical therapy and in patients with toxic megacolon. This has been shown to improve 57% of the patients. There is a positive correlation between the diameter of the inferior mesenteric artery and successful intervention.

A periappendicular abscess or phlegmon will develop in 2% of patients with appendicitis. Contrast-enhanced CT enables distinction between these two pathologic processes. Percutaneous access and drainage of a periappendicular abscess is possible under CT control. Distinction between an abscess and phlegmon is important, since a phlegmon is amenable to antibiotic therapy, whereas an abscess should be aspirated or drained.

Percutaneous biopsy of the presacral space is indicated in grading rectal carcinomas and in diagnosing postoperative recurrences. It is also needed to diagnose patients bearing inoperable rectal carcinomas. Both metastases and recurrences may be detected by percutaneous biopsy. The puncture is performed under the control of CT, US or fluoroscopy, in the same way as drainage of an abscess in the peritoneal cavity or retroperitoneal space.

Principles utilized in *angioplastic techniques* may be applied to widen stomas created by alimentary canal surgery, when strictures develop. Dilatation of stomas is successful following gastric, gastroenteric, jejunal, ileal, and Roux's operations.

Percutaneous gastrostomy and gastrojejunostomy are techniques that are alternatives to surgically or endoscopically performed procedures (Fig. 4.92). A patient with an intact small bowel may be fed in this manner. Gastrostomy is indicated in patients with severe disorders of deglutition who aspirate pharyngeal content. Percutaneous gastrostomy is indicated in patients with esophageal obstruction. After the stomach is inflated with air so that it can be easily observed at fluoroscopy, it is punctured by a special needle and a tube is introduced into the first jejunal loop.

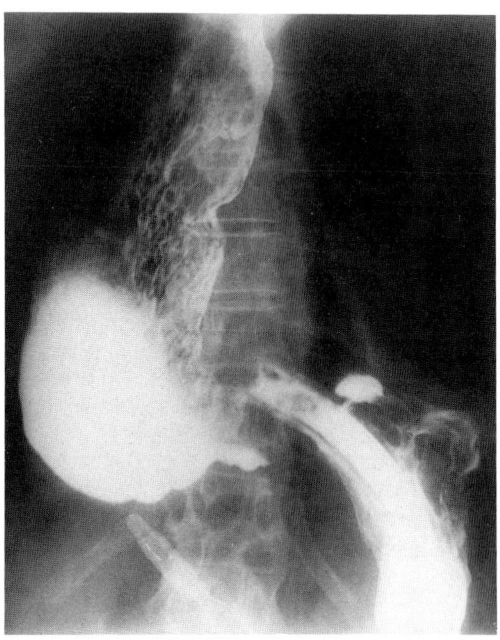

FIGURE 4.92. Percutaneous gastrostomy for achalasia of the LES and ulcerated carcinoma of the gastric fundus.

ERRORS IN THE PROCESS OF RADIOLOGIC DIAGNOSIS

Errors threatening to interfere with radiologic diagnosis of alimentary canal diseases may occur in any phase of the diagnostic process—from patient preparation for the examination to dictation and transcription of the radiologic report.

Patient preparation is necessary for the majority of radiographic examinations of the alimentary canal. Inadequate fasting leaves food remnants which interfere with proper demonstration of the upper gastrointestinal tract. Inadequate preparation for a barium enema makes both exclusion and confirmation of pathologic changes difficult. Moreover, errors may occur within the domain of the technologist, such as an inappropriate preparation of the contrast suspension, inadequate concentration, or undesirable suspension temperature. The radiologist should review plain chest and abdominal roentgenographs or at least exclude obvious abnormalities by short fluoroscopy. Barium remnants from preceding examinations may interfere with proper visualization of the alimentary organ.

If unaware of the optimal technique, a radiologist can make a series of errors, ranging from administering too large a volume of barium to failing to take advantage of pharmacoradiographic adjuncts. Inadequate radiographic technique yields roentgenographs of poor quality which compromise analysis and interpretation. Pathologic changes may be missed during fluoroscopy or on roentgenographs because of common perceptional errors such as unrecognized pathologic signs, examiner fatigue, or lack of attention.

Moreover, inability to discriminate between normal and pathologic findings of the alimentary canal may lead to misinterpretation. Error may also occur during transcription of the radiologic report. It is therefore necessary to carefully review all reports before signing.

RADIOLOGIC REPORTS

A radiologic report should consist of the following key features: first, a list of the most important observations, then an impression or concluding diagnosis, and finally, discussion or comment. The impression should be short and expanded only when recommendations are appended. Occasionally, an entire report is confined merely to an impression on the nature and extent of a pathologic lesion. Brevity, pertinence, and clarity are essential regardless of the style one selects for organizing a formal report. An ideal report states all positive findings and a few pertinent negatives.

Attention should be paid to the following:

1. Clarity and brevity
2. Complete sentences in a narrative style
3. Division into as many paragraphs as necessary, for example, to separate abnormal from normal findings
4. Present tense for observations from the films, and past tense for method of examination
5. Specific answers to clinical requests regarding the diagnosis in question, with the most important pathologic finding(s) stated first
6. Recommendations.

Not all incidental observations are worth reporting. Some might be overinterpreted by the attending physician. The degree of certainty has to be clear; it is often inversely proportional to the number of differential diagnostic possibilities. Purely radiologic terms, such as Carman's or Frostberg's signs, should be avoided and descriptive words used instead.

Finally, reports should be reviewed. This practice has two advantages: significant errors are identified and corrected, and brevity can be encouraged. Two-thirds to three-fourths of errors are typographic. Significant errors occur when, for instance, the side of the patient's body is reversed or when a negation is omitted.

EVALUATION OF RADIOLOGIC DIAGNOSTIC METHODS

The most important feature of a particular diagnostic procedure is the capability of detecting pathologic lesions. Inadequate evaluation of a procedure may compromise or invalidate conclusions.

The results of any diagnostic test may be either true-positive (TP), true-negative (TN), false-positive (FP) or false-negative (FN).

When evaluation of a radiologic procedure is performed by comparison with a reference procedure, the latter is called the "gold standard." If two alternative diagnostic procedures are evaluated and compared, neither of them should be taken as the "gold standard." One would inevitably invalidate the results of the other. If the reference examination is considered infallible, the diagnostic method compared to it is always shown to produce inferior results. When, for instance, comparing a radiologic with an endoscopic examination, another procedure such as surgical or autopsy finding should be considered as the "gold standard."

A series of quantitative parameters have been designed to evaluate the efficacy of a radiologic diagnostic procedure.

Sensitivity states the probability of detecting an existing lesion, that is, effectiveness of an examination in a diseased person. It is defined as:

$$\text{sensitivity} = \frac{\text{TP}}{\text{TP} + \text{FN}}$$

$$= \text{fraction of existing lesions detected.}$$

Sensitivity also shows what proportion of disease will remain unrecognized by a particular method and is therefore the most useful parameter of an imaging method. It is also the most applicable in comparing alternative methods.

Specificity states the probability of recognizing normal cases. It is defined as:

$$\text{specificity} = \frac{TN}{TN + FP}$$

$$= \text{fraction of normal subjects identified.}$$

Specificity also shows the proportion of healthy individuals who will be unnecessarily subjected to further examinations increasing both expense and discomfort to the patient.

Both sensitivity and specificity are inherent to the method and do not vary with prevalence of the disease in a population, because the former includes only diseased and the latter only normals. Therefore, these parameters may be reasonably used for comparisons of different diagnostic modalities.

The *predictive value of a positive (PPV) or negative result (NPV)* expresses the likelihood that a positive or negative radiologic diagnosis is correct and is defined as:

$$PPV = \frac{TP}{TP + FP}$$

$$= \text{fraction of positive diagnoses that are correct}$$

$$NPV = \frac{TN}{TN + FN}$$

$$= \text{fraction of negative diagnoses that are correct.}$$

Predictive values are calculated from the prevalence of disease and from the sensitivity and specificity of the method.

Diagnosticians are primarily concerned with the likelihood that a particular patient is diseased or not, based on the result of a diagnostic procedure. This likelihood is defined by predictive values. Being greatly affected by the variable proportion of normals, predictive values are of no value in comparing the results of one investigation to those of another. The positive predictive value is always high when disease prevalence is high. Under typical clinical conditions, negative predictive values are less variable with disease prevalence.

Accuracy is defined as the percentage of correct diagnoses:

$$\text{Accuracy} = \frac{TP + TN}{TP + TN + FP + FN}$$

$$= \frac{\text{correct diagnoses}}{\text{all diagnoses}}$$

$$= \text{fraction of correct diagnoses.}$$

As it is highly influenced by the proportion of normals in the population studied, it is of virtually no value in comparing results of alternative examination methods.

Bibliography

Aardenne YT, Winter WA, Verdegaal WP, Taconis WK. Detection of inflammatory bowel disease with 99 m Tc DTPA. Diag Imag. 1980;49:344.

Abrams JS. A second look at colonoscopy: Indications failures and costs. Arch Surg. 1982;117:913.

Adler O, Rosenberg A. Selective arterial embolization in duodenal bleeding. Clin Radiol. 1976;45:413.

Alavi A, McLean GK. Studies of GI bleeding with scintigraphy and the influence of vasopressin. Sem Nucl Med. 1981;9:216.

Amaral NM. Radiographic diagnosis of shallow gastric ulcers; a comparative study of technique. Radiology. 1978;129:597.

Anderson W, Harthill JE. Barium sulphate preparations for use in double contrast examination of the upper gastrointestinal tract. Br J Radiol. 1980;53:1150.

Balfe DM, Koehler RE, Karstaedt N, Stanley RJ, Sagel SS. Computed tomography of gastric neoplasms. Radiology. 1981;140:431.

Balthazar EJ, Megibow AJ, Hulnick D, Gordon RB, Naidich DP, Beranbaum ER. CT of appendicitis. AJR. 1986;147:705.

Barakos JA, Jeffrey RB, Federle MP, Wing VW, Laing FC, Hightower DR. CT in the management of periappendiceal abscesses. AJR. 1986;146:1161.

Barloon TJ, Franken EA. Plasma electrolyte status after small-bowel enteroclysis. AJR. 1986;146:323.

Barnes MR. How to get a clean colon with less effort. Radiology. 1968;9:948.

Bednarek DR, Rudin S, Wong R, Andres ML. Reduction of fluoroscopic exposure for the air contrast barium enema. Br J Radiol. 1983;56:823.

Bilbao MK, Frische LH, Dotter CT, Rosch J. Hypotonic duodenography. Radiology. 1967;89:438.

Billing PR, Bernstein MS. Physicians poor at prevalence and positive predictive value. JAMA. 1985;254:1173.

Blane CE, Di Pietro ME, White SJ, Klein ME, Coran AG, Wesley JR. An analysis of bowel perforation in patients with intussusception. J Can Assoc Radiol. 1984;35:113.

Blane CE, White SJ, Wesley JR, Coran AG. Sonography of ruptured appendicitis. Gastrointest Radiol. 1986;11:357.

Blumhagen JD, Christie DL. Gastroesophageal reflux in children: evaluation of water siphon test. Radiology. 1979;131:345.

Bluth EJ, Merritt CRB, Sullivan MA. Ultrasonic evaluation of the stomach, small bowel and colon. Radiology. 1979;133:677.

Bookstein JJ, Naderi MJ, Walter JF. Transcatheter embolization for lower gastrointestinal bleeding. Radiology. 1978;127:345.

Bull MJ, Kaye B. Portal vein gas following double-contrast barium enema. Br J Radiol. 1985;58:1129.

Butch RM, Stark DD, Wittenberg J, Tepper JE, Saini S, Simeone JF, Mueller PR, Ferucci JT Jr. Staging rectal cancer by MR and CT. AJR. 1986; 146:1155.

Campbell JB, Foley LC. A safe alternative to endoscopic removal of blunt esophageal foreign bodies. Arch Otolaryngal Head Neck Surg. 1983;109:323.

Carsen GM, Finby N. Hypotonic duodenography with glucagon. Radiology. 1976;118:529.

Casscells W, Schoenberger A, Graboys T. Interpretation by physicians of clinical laboratory results. N Engl J Med. 1978;299:999.

Cassel DM, Anderson MF, Zboralske FF. Double-contrast esophagograms – the prone technique. Radiology. 1981;139:737.

Channer KS, Virjee JP. Esophageal function tests: are they of value? Clin Radiol. 1985;36:493.

Christensen T, Thommesen P. Food-stimulated gastroesophageal reflux demonstrated by barium examination. Acta Radiol Diagn. 1986;27:45.

Clark RA. Computed tomography of bowel infarction. J Comput Assist Tomogr. 1987;11:757.

Clark RA, Towbin R. Abscess drainage with CT and ultrasound guidance. Radiol Clin North Am. 1983; 21:445.

Cohen MD. The result of metrizamide (Amipaque) evaluation of the bowel in 75 newborn infants. Ped Radiol. 1984;14:246.

Conces DJ, Lappas JC, Cockerill EM. Bacteremia during double-contrast barium enema examination. Radiology. 1985;155:49.

Creteur V, Thoeni RF, Federle MP, Cello JP, Moss AA, Ominsky SH, Goldberg HI, Axel L. The role of single- and double-contrast radiography in the diagnosis of reflux esophagitis. Radiology. 1983; 147:71.

Crummy AB. The water test in the evaluation of gastroesophageal reflux. Radiology. 1966;78:501.

de Lange EE, Fechner RE, Harold J. Suspected recurrent rectosigmoid carcinoma after abdominoperineal resection: MR imaging and histopathologic finding. Radiology. 1989;170:323.

Derchi LE, Biggi E., Rollandi GA, Cicio GR, Neumaier CE. Sonographic staging of gastric cancer. AJR. 1983;140:273.

De Roos A, Hermans J, Shaw PC, Kroon H. Colon polyps and carcinomas: prospective comparison of the single- and double-contrast examination in the same patients. Radiology. 1985;154:11.

Dick Smireaux C, Hall CM. The use of oral metrizamide in the investigation of the gastrointestinal tract of neonates. Ped Radiol. 1984;14:246.

Dinkel E, Dittrich M, Peters H, Baumann W. Real-time ultrasound in Crohn's disease: characteristic features and clinical implications. Ped Radiol. 1986;16:8.

Donohue JH, Federle MP, Griffiths BG, Trunkey DD. Computed tomography in the diagnosis of blunt intestinal and mesenteric injuries. J Trauma. 1987;27:11.

Donahue JK, Hunter CH, Balch HH. Significance of fluid levels in X-ray films of the abdomen. N Engl J Med. 1958;259:13.

Drane WE, Haggar AM, Engel MA. Glucagon and gastroesophageal reflux. AJR. 1984;142:709.

Dreyfuss JR. On evaluating upper gastrointestinal symptoms by provocative study. Radiol Clin North Am. 1971;9:15.

Du Brow RA, Frank PH. Barium evaluation of anal canal in patients with inflammatory bowel disease. AJR. 1983;140:1151.

Dyet JE, Bennett JR, Buckton G, Ashwarth D. The radiological measurement of the esophageal stricture diameter. Clin Radiol. 1983;34:647.

Eisenberg RL, Hedgcock MW. Preliminary radiography for barium enema examination. Is it necessary? AJR. 1981;136:115.

Eisenberg RL, Hedgcock MW, Shauser JD, Brenner RJ, Gedguadas RK, Marks WM. Iodine absorption from the gastrointestinal tract during Hypaque enema examination. Radiology. 1979;133: 597.

Eisenberg RL, Meyers PC, May ST. Optimum overhead views in double-contrast barium enema examinations. AJR. 1983;140:505.

Ekberg O. Inguinal herniography in adults. Technique, normal anatomy, and diagnostic criteria for hernia. Radiology. 1981;138:31.

Ekberg O, Nylander G, Fork FT. Defecography. Radiology. 1985;155:45.

Fagelman D, Caridi JG. CT diagnosis of hernia of Morgagni. Gastrointest Radiol. 1984;9:153.

Fagelman D, Warhit JM, Reiter JD, Geiss AC. CT diagnosis of fecaloma. J Comput Assist Tomogr. 1984;8:599.

Feczko PJ, Halpert RD. Reassessing the role of radiology in hemoccult screening. AJR. 1986;146:697.

Feczko PJ, Simms MS, Iorio J, Halpert R. Gastroduodenal response to low-dose glucagon. AJR. 1983; 140:935.

Federle MP. Computed tomography of blunt abdominal trauma. Radiol Clin North Am. 1983;21:461.

Federle MP, Chun G, Jeffrey RB, Raymor R. Computed tomographic findings in bowel infarction. AJR. 1984;142:91.

Feldberg MAM, Hendriks NJ, van Waes PFGM. Role of CT in diagnosis and management of complications of diverticular disease. Gastrointest Radiol. 1985;10:370.

Ferrucci JT Jr, Benedict KT Jr. Anticholinergic-aided study of the gastrointestinal tract. Radiol Clin North Am. 1971;19:23.

Figiel SJ, Figiel LS, Rush DK. High-kilovoltage spot compression technique. JAMA. 1958;166:1269.

Fischer A. Uber eine neue rontgenologische Untersuchungsmethode des Dickdarms: Kombination von Kontrasteinlauf und Luftaufblahung. Klin Wschr. 1923;2:1595.

Fisher JK. Computed tomography of colonic pneumatosis intestinalis with mesenteric and portal venous air. J Comput Assist Tomogr. 1984;8:573.

Fisher R, Malmud LS, Roberts GS, Lobis IF. Gastroesophageal scinti-scanning to detect and quantitate GE reflux. Gastroenterology. 1976;70:301.

Fitch SJ, Magill HJ, Benator RM, Parvey LP, Hixon SD. Pseudoreduction of intussusception: is ileal reflux the end point? Gastrointest Radiol. 1985; 10:181.

Flickinger F. Location of active lower GI bleeding by technetium 99m sulphur colloid scan. J Nucl Med. 1981;22:38.

Fork FT, Lindstrom C, Ekelund G. Double-contrast examination in carcinoma of the colon and rectum (a prospective clinical series). Acta Radiol Diagn. 1983;24:177.

Frank PH, Riddell RH, Feczko PJ, Levin B. Radiological detection of colonic dysplasia (precarcinoma) in chronic ulcerative colitis. Gastrointest Radiol. 1978;3:209.

Fraser GM. The double-contrast barium meal in patients with acute upper gastrointestinal bleeding. Clin Radiol. 1978;29:625.

Fraser GM, Earnshaw PM. The double-contrast barium meal. A correlation with endoscopy. Clin Radiol. 1983;34:121.

Friedman PJ. Radiologic reports – structure and review – reply. AJR. 1984;142:648.

Fries M, Mortensson W, Robertson B. Technetium pertechnetate scintigraphy to detect ectopic gastric mucosa in Meckel's diverticulum. Acta Radiol Diagn. 1984;25:417.

Froelich JW, Juni J. Glucagon in the scintigraphic diagnosis of small bowel hemorrhage by 99m Tc labeled red blood cells. Radiology. 1984;151:239.

Funaro AH, Ring EJ, Freiman DB, Oleaga JA, Gordon RL. Transhepatic obliteration of esophageal varices using the stainless steel coil. AJR. 1979; 133:1123.

Gedguadas RK, Torres WE, Colvin RS, McClees EC, Baron MG. Thoracic findings in gastrointestinal pathology. Radiol Clin North Am. 1984;22: 563.

Gelfand DW. High-density, low-viscosity barium for fine mucosal detail on double-contrast upper gastrointestinal examinations. AJR. 1978;130:813.

Gelfand DW, Ott DJ. Single- versus double-contrast gastrointestinal studies: critical analysis of reported statistics. AJR. 1981;137:523.

Gelfand DW, Ott DJ. Decline in upper gastrointestinal studies. AJR. 1984;143:431.

Gelfand DW, Ott DJ. Methodologic considerations in comparing imaging methods. AJR. 1985;144:1117.

Gelfand DW, Ott DJ. Technical note. Double-contrast enema: a simplified method for filling the colon. AJR. 1990;154:279.

Gerson DE, Lewicki AM, McNeil BJ, Abrams HL, Korngold E. The barium enema: evidence for proper utilization. Radiology. 1979;130: 297.

Gold RP, Seaman WB. The primary double-contrast examination of the postoperative stomach. Radiology. 1977;124:297.

Goldberg HJ, Gore RM, Margulis AR, Moss AA, Baker EL. Computed tomography in the evaluation of Crohn's disease. AJR. 1983;140:277.

Goldstein HM, Zboralske FF. Tubeless hypotonic duodenography. JAMA. 1969;210:2036.

Gonzalez JG, Gonzalez RR, Patino JV, Garcia AT, Alvarez CP, Pedrosa CSA. CT findings in gastrointestinal perforation by ingested fish bones. J Comput Assist Tomogr. 1988;12:88.

Grahl KO. Erfahrung mit der hydrostatischen Reposition der Kindlichen Darminvagination – Verbesserung der Ergebnisse unter Atropin-Pramedikation. Radiol Diagn. 1983;24:619.

Gray RR, St Louis EL, Grosman H. Percutaneous gastrostomy and gastrojejunostomy. Br J Radiol. 1987;60:1067.

Greenspon EA, Lentino W. Retrograde enterography: a new method for the roentgenologic study of the small bowel. AJR. 1960;83:909.

Grumbach K, Levin MS, Wexler JA. Gallstone ileus diagnosed by computed tomography. J Comput Assist Tomogr. 1986;10:146.

Gutierrez JG, Chey WY, Shah A, Holzwasser G. Use of secretin in hypotonic duodenography. Radiology. 1974;113:563.

Halpert RD, Dubin L. Feczko PJ, Weitz J. Air-contrast tube esophagogram – technique and clinical examples – technical notes. J Can Assoc Radiol. 1984;35:58.

Halvorsen RA, Magruder-Habib K, Foster WL, Roberts L, Postlethwait RW, Thompson WM. Esophageal cancer staging by CT: long-term follow-up study. Radiology. 1986;161:147.

Ham HR, Piepsz A, Georges B, Delaet MH, Rodesch P, Guillaume P, Cadranel S. Evaluation of esophageal transit in children and infants by means of Krypton 81m. Ped Radiol. 1985;15:161.

Hamlin DJ, Burgner A, Sichy D. New technique to stage early carcinoma by computed tomography. Radiology. 1981;141:539.

Hampton AO. A safe method for the roentgen demonstration of bleeding ulcers. AJR. 1937;38:565.

Harned RK, Williams SM, Maglinte DDT, Hayes JM, Paustian FF, Consigni M. Clinical application of in vitro studies for barium enema examination following colorectal biopsy. Radiology. 1985;154: 319.

Hulnick DH, Megibow AJ, Balthazar EJ, Naidich DP, Bosniak MA. Computed tomography in the evaluation of diverticulitis. Radiology. 1984;152: 491.

Hunter TB. Radiologic reports—structure and review. AJR. 1984;142:647.

Husband JE, Hodson NJ, Parsons CA. The use of computed tomography in recurrent rectal tumors. Radiology. 1980;134:677.

James WB, Hume R. Action of metoclopramide on gastric emptying and small bowel transit time. Gut. 1986;9:203.

Janower ML. Hypersensitivity reactions after barium studies of the upper and lower gastrointestinal tract. Radiology. 1986;161:139.

Jeffrey RB, Federle MP, Wall SD. Value of computed tomography in detecting occult gastrointestinal perforation. J Comput Assist Tomogr. 1983;7:825.

Johnsen A, Ingemann L, Mauritzen K. Balloon dilatation of esophageal strictures in children. Ped Radiol. 1986;16:388.

Johnson CD, Carlson F, Taylor WF, Weiland LP. Barium enemas of carcinoma of the colon: sensitivity of double- and single-contrast studies. AJR. 1983; 140:1143.

Jones B, Kramer SS, Donner MW. Dynamic imaging of the pharynx. Gastrointest Radiol. 1985;10:213.

Jones B, Ravich WJ, Donner HW, Kramer SS. Pharyngoesophageal interrelationships: observations and work concepts. Gastrointest Radiol. 1985; 10:225.

Kaftori JK, Pery M, Kleinhause U. Ultrasonography in Crohn's disease. Gastrointest Radiol. 1984; 9:137.

Kantor JL. Regional (terminal) ileitis. Its roentgen diagnosis. JAMA. 1934;103:2016.

Karause P, Schilling H. Die rontgenologische Untersuchung zur Darstellung des Magendarmkanals mit besonderer Berucksichtigung des Kontrastmittels. Forschr Rontgenstr. 1912;20:455.

Kelemouridis V, Athanasoulis CA, Waltman AC. Gastric bleeding sites: an angiographic study. Radiology. 1983;149:643.

Kellett MJ, Zboralske FF, Margulis AR. Peroral pneumocolon examination of the ileocecal region. Gastrointest Radiol. 1977;1:361.

Kelvin FM, Gedguadas RK, Thompson WM, Rice RP. The peroral pneumocolon: its role in evaluating terminal ileum. AJR. 1982;139:115.

Kewenter J, Jensen J, Boijsen M, Lycke G, Tylen M. Perception errors with double-contrast enema after a positive guaiac test. Gastrointest Radiol. 1987;12:79.

Kinnunen J, Totterman S. Kaila R, Pietila J, Linden H, Tervahariala P. Effect of sodium bicarbonate pretreatment on barium coating of mucosa during double contrast barium meal. Fortschr Rontgenstr. 1983;139:199.

Koblik PD, Hornof WJ. Gastrointestinal nuclear medicine. Veterin Radiol. 1985;26:138.

Koehler RE, Weyman PJ, Oakley HF. Single- and double-contrast techniques in esophagitis. AJR. 1980;135:15.

Kreel L. Pharmaco-radiology in barium examinations wtth special reference to glucagon. Br J Radiol. 1975;48:691.

Kressel HY, Callen PW, Montagne JP, Korobkin M, Goldberg HJ, Moss AA, Arger PH, Margulis AR. Computed tomographic evaluation of the disorders affecting the alimentary tract. Radiology. 1978;129:451.

Kressel HY, Evers KA, Glick SN, Laufer I, Herlinger H. The peroral pneumocolon examination. Radiology. 1982;144:414.

Kundel HL. Disease prevalence and radiological decision making. Invest Radiol. 1982;17:107.

Kutzen B, Radcliffe RV, Carrier JW. Double-blind evalution of cimetidine as an adjunct to the routine double-contrast upper gastrointestinal examination. Radiology. 1980;134:766.

Lappas JC, Miller RE, Lehman GA, Eskridge JM, Morton GA. Postendoscopy barium enema examinations. Radiology. 1983;194:655.

Laufer I, Mullens JE, Hamilton J. The diagnostic accuracy of barium studies of the stomach and duodenum—correlation with endoscopy. Radiology. 1975;115:569.

Laufer I, Hamilton J, Mullens JE. Demonstration of superficial gastric erosions by double contrast radiography. Gastroenterology. 1975;68:387.

Laufer I. A simple method for routine double contrast study of the upper gastrointestinal tract. Radiology. 1975;117:513.

Lee KR, Levine E, Moffat E, Bigongiari LR, Hermreck AS. Computed tomographic staging of malignant gastric neoplasms. Radiology. 1979;133: 151.

Levine MS, Kressel HY, Laufer I, Herlinger H, Goren R. The tube esophagogram—a technique for obtaining a detailed double-contrast examination of the esophagus. AJR. 1984;142:293.

Lindell MM, Hill CA, Libshitz HJ. Esophageal cancer: Radiographic chest findings and their prognostic significance. AJR. 1979;133:461.

Lloyd GAS, Phelps PD. The demonstration of tumors of the parapharingeal space by magnetic resonance imaging. Br J Radiol. 1986;59:675.

Lukes PJ, Rolny P, Nilson AE, Gamklon R. Hypotonic duodenography and endoscopic retrograde pancreatography in the diagnosis of pancreatic disease. Acta Radiol Diagn. 1981;22:145.

Maglinte DDT, Caudill LD, Krol K, Brown D. The use of small dose of glucagon in upper gastrointestinal radiography. Gastrointest Radiol. 1980;5:383.

Maglinte DDT, Miller RE. A simplified method for imaging of the anterior gastroduodenal wall by double-contrast study. AJR. 1983;141:971.

Maglinte DDT, Miller RE. Salvaging the failed pneumocolon – a simple maneuver. AJR. 1984;142:719.

Maglinte DDT, Miller RE. Decline in upper gastrointestinal studies – reply. AJR. 1984;143:432.

Maglinte DDT. Double-contrast imaging of anterior gastroduodenal wall – reply. AJR. 1984;143:431.

Malmud LS, Fisher RS. The evaluation of gastroesophageal reflux before and after medical therapies. Sem Nucl Med. 1981;9:205.

Margulis AR. Is double-contrast examination of the colon the only acceptable radiographic examination? Radiology. 1976;119:741.

Mayes GB, Zornoza J. Computed tomography of colon carcinoma. AJR. 1980;135:43.

McNeil BJ, Keller E, Adetstern SI. Primer on certain elements of medical decision making. N Engl J Med. 1975;293:211.

Meradji M. Sonographic diagnosis of intussusception – a report of 40 cases. Ped Radiol. 1984;14:255.

Merine D, Fishman EK, Jones B, Siegelman SS. Enteroenteric intussusception: CT findings in nine patients. AJR. 1987;148:1129.

Meyerovitz FM, Fellows KE. Angiography in gastrointestinal bleeding in children. AJR. 1984;143:837.

Miller RE. Barium sulfate suspensions. Radiology. 1965;84:241.

Miller RE. Complete reflux small bowel examination. Radiology. 1965;84:457.

Miller RE, Chernisch SM, Shucas J, Rosenah B, Rodda BE. Hypotonic colon examination with glucagon. Radiology. 1974;113:555.

Miller RE, Lehman G. The barium enema: is it obsolete? JAMA. 1976;235:2842.

Miller RE, Peterson GH. Drainage of the rectum: a simple maneuver to improve the accuracy of colon examinations. Radiology. 1978;128:506.

Miller RE, Sellink JL. Enteroclysis: the small bowel enema. How to succeed and how to fail. Gastrointest Radiol. 1979;4:269.

Miller RE. Solution for the "air block" problem during fluoroscopy. AJR. 1979;132:1020.

Millward SF, Chapman A, Somers S, Stevenson GW. Rectal biopsy as a cause of rectal ulceration. Radiology. 1985;156:42.

Momoshima S, Kohda E, Hiramatsu K, Asakura H. Intra-arterial prednisolone infusion therapy in ulcerative colitis. AJR. 1985;145:1057.

Montagne JP, Moss AA, Margulis AR. Double-blind study of single- and double-contrast upper gastrointestinal examinations using endoscopy as a control. AJR. 1978;130:1041.

Montali G, Croce F, De Para L, Sobbiati L. Intussusception of the bowel: a new sonographic pattern. Br J Radiol. 1983;56:621.

Morris DC, Nichols DM, Connell DG, Burhenne HJ. Embolization of the left gastric artery in the absence of angiographic extravasation. Cardiovasc Intervent Radiol. 1986;9:195.

Mortensson W, Eklof O, Laurin S. Hydrostatic reduction of childhood intussusception. Acta Radiol Diagn. 1984;25:261.

Moss AA, Schnyder P, Thoeni RF, Margulis AR. Esophageal carcinoma – pretherapy staging by computed tomography. AJR. 1981;136:1051.

Murtagh FR, Sanders MB. Precipitation of water-soluble contrast material (Gastrografin) in the stomach in a case of outlet obstruction. Radiology. 1978;126:386.

Nolan DJ, Cadman PJ. The small bowel enema made easy. Clin Radiol. 1987;38:295.

O'Connor K, O'Connell R, Kaene FB, Byrne PJ, Henessy TPJ. The relationship between technetium 99m pertechnetate gastric scanning and gastric contents. Br J Radiol. 1983;56:817.

Oi H, Nokamura H, Nakabayashi T, Waki K. Method for ejecting cestodes – duodenal tube injection of Gastrografin. AJR. 1984;143:111.

Op den Orth JO, Ploem S. The stalactite phenomenon in double-contrast studies of the stomach. Radiology. 1975;115:275.

Op den Orth JO. Radiologic visualization of the normal duodenal minor papilla. Fortschr Rontgenstr. 1978;128:572.

Ott DJ, Gelfand DW, Wu WC, Kerr RM. Sensitivity of double-contrast barium enema. Emphasis on polyp detection. AJR. 1980;135:327.

Ott DJ, Gelfand DW, Ramquist NA. Causes of error in gastrointestinal radiology. Gastrointest Radiol. 1981;5:99.

Ott DJ, Chen YM, Gelfand DW, Swearingen F, Munitz HA. Detailed peroral small bowel examination vs. enteroclysis, part I: expenditure and radiation exposure. Radiology. 1985;155:29.

Parienty RA, Lepreux JR, Gruson B. Sonographic and CT features of ileocolic intussusception. AJR. 1981;136:608.

Pansdorf H. Die fraktionierte Dundarmfullung und ihre klinische Bedeutung. Fortschr Rontgenstr. 1937;56:627.

Pendergrass EP, Ravdin IS, Johnson CG, Hodes PJ. Studies of the small intestine, II: effects of food and pathological states on gastric emptying and small intestine pattern. Radiology. 1936;26: 651.

Peterson GH, Miller ER. The barium enema: a reassessment looking toward perfection. Radiology. 1978;128:315.

Phatak MG, Doben GD, Asselmeir GH. CT demonstration of scirrhous carcinoma of the stomach: a case report. Comput Radiol. 1982;6:31.

Phatak MG, Frank SJ, Ellis JJ. Computed tomography of bowel perforation. Gastrointest Radiol. 1984;9:133.

Phillips LG. Esophageal perforation. Radiol Clin North Am. 1984;22:607.

Phillips WC, Scott JA, Biascynski G. Statistics for diagnostic procedures, I: how sensitive is "sensitivity"; how specific is "specificity"? AJR. 1983; 140:1265.

Pirkey EL. Double-contrast roentgenograms of the stomach. AJR. 1949;62:70.

Plavsic B, Kuzmanic D, Rotkvic I. Eosinophilia caused by iodinated radiographic contrast media. Clin Radiol. 1983;34:639.

Pracros JP, Tranminh AV, Louis D, Derivoyre V. Imperforate anus—real time sonographic evaluation. Ped Radiol. 1984;14:255.

Puyeart JBCM. Mesenteric adenitis and acute terminal ileitis: US evaluation used graded compression. Radiology. 1986;161:691.

Quint LE, Glazer GM, Orringer MB, Gross BH. Esophageal carcinoma: CT findings. Radiology. 1985;155:171.

Rankin RN, Ford J, Grace DM. Intestinal stomal dilatation. J Can Assoc Radiol. 1984;35:327.

Ratcliffe JF. Glucagon in barium examinations in infants and children: special reference to dosage. Br J Radiol. 1980;53:860.

Ratcliffe JF. The small bowel enema in children: a description of a technique. Clin Radiol. 1983; 34: 287.

Ratcliffe JF. The use of ioxaglate in the pediatric gastrointestinal tract: a report of 25 cases. Clin Radiol. 1983;34:579.

Raushoff DF, Feinstein AR. Problems of spectrum and bias in evaluating the efficacy of diagnostic tests. N Engl J Med. 1978;229:926.

Ravek SC. Letter—dictation of radiologic reports. AJR. 1983;141:210.

Reinig JW, Stanley JH, Schabel SJ. CT evaluation of thickened esophageal walls. AJR. 1983;140:931.

Reinig JW, Dwyer J, Miller DL, White M, Frank JA, Sugarbaker PH, Chang AE, Doppman JL. Liver metastasis detection: comparative sensitivities of MR imaging and CT scannning. Radiology. 1987; 162:43.

Riffkin MD, Karks GJ. Transrectal US as an adjunct in the diagnosis of rectal and extrarectal tumors. Radiology. 1985;157:499.

Robbins AH, Wetzner SM, Landy MD. Ceruletide-assisted examination of small bowel. AJR. 1980; 134:343.

Roberts GM, Roberts EE, Davies L, Evans KT. Observations on the behavior of barium sulphate suspensions in gastric secretion. Br J Radiol. 1977; 50:468.

Rosch J, Keller FS, Kozak B, Niles N, Dotter CT. Gelfoam powder embolization of the left gastric artery in treatment of massive small-vessel gastric bleeding. Radiology. 1984;151:365.

Roseman DM, Kowlessar OD, Sleisinger MH. Pulmonary manifestations of pancreatitis. N Engl J Med. 1960;263:294.

Samuelson L, Hambraeus GM, Mercke CE, Tylen L. CT staging of esophageal carcinoma. Acta Radiol Diagn. 1984;25:7.

Samuelson L, Tylen L. Delineation of the normal esophagus at computed tomography. Acta Radiol Diagn. 1985;26:665.

Saxton HM. Radiology now. Starting the double contrast barium meal. Br J Radiol. 1977;50:610.

Schatzki R. Small intestinal enema. AJR. 1943;50: 743.

Schule A. Uber die Sondierung und Radiographie des Dickdarms. Arch Verd Krankh. 1904;10:111.

Schwartz EE, Glick SN, Foggs MB, Silverstein GS. Hypersensitivity reactions after barium enema examinations. AJR. 1984;143:103.

Sellink JL. Radiologic examination of the small intestine by duodenal intubation. Acta Radiol Diagn. 1974;15:318.

Shapiro J, Jacobsen HG. Oral 76 percent sodium and methylglucamine diatrizoate, a new contrast medium for the gastrointestinal tract. Ann NY Acad Sci. 1959;78:966.

Silverberg E. Cancer statistics, 1985. CA. 1985; 35:19.

Singleton EB. Hydrostatic reduction of intussusception. Pediatr Clin North Am. 1963;10:175.

Solomon A, Michowitz M, Papo J, Yust I. Computed tomographic air enema technique to demonstrate colonic neoplasms. Gastrointest Radiol. 1986; 11:194.

Souranta H, Standertskjold-Nordemstam CG, Lahde S. The value of simethicone in abdominal preparation. Radiology. 1979;133:307.

Starck E, Paolucci V, Herzer M, Crummy AB. Esophageal stenosis: treatment with balloon catheters. Radiology. 1984;153:632.

Stringer DA, Cloutier S, Daneman A, Durie P. The value of the small bowel enema in children. J Can Assoc Radiol. 1986;37:13.

Stringer DA, Sherman P, Lin P, Deneman A. Value

of the peroral pneumocolon in children. AJR. 1986;146:763.

Tash RR, Weingarten M, Geller M. An alternative technique for double-contrast esophagography. AJR. 1986;147:266.

Thoeni RF, Menuck L. Comparison of barium enema and colonoscopy in the detection of small colonic polyps. Radiology. 1977;124:621.

Thoeni RF, Petras A. Detection of rectal and rectosigmoidal lesions by double-contrast barium enema examination and sigmoidoscopy. Radiology. 1982; 142:59.

Thoeni RF, Vandeman F, Wall SD. Effect of glucagon on the diagnostic accuracy of double-contrast barium enema examinations. AJR. 1984;142:111.

Tsoutsanis J. Intravasation of barium sulphate during roentgenography of the colon. Diagn Imag. 1981;50:1.

Vallance R. An evaluation of the small bowel enema based on an analysis of 350 consecutive examinations. Clin Radiol. 1980;31:227.

Vallebona A. Nuovo metodo di esame radiologico del tubo digerente. Radiol Med (Torino). 1926;13:241.

Van Dam A. The gamma camera in clinical evaluation of the gastric emptying. Radiology. 1974;110:157.

Vecchio TJ. Predictive value of a single diagnostic test in unselected populations. N Engl J Med. 1966;274:1171.

Violon D, Steppe R, Potviliege R. Improved retrograde ileography with glucagon. AJR. 1981;136: 833.

Waes FGM, Kohler PR, Feldberg AM. Management of rectal carcinoma: impact of computed tomography. AJR. 1983;140:1137.

Walls WJ. The evaluation of malignant gastric neoplasms by ultrasonic B-scanning. Radiology. 1976; 118:159.

Weber AL, Ott KS, Watts FB. Radiologic examination of the gastrointestinal tract in infants and children under 4 years of age. Radiol Clin North Am. 1971;19:5.

Weinreb JC, Maravilla KR, Redman HC, Nunnally R. Improved MR imaging of the upper abdomen with glucagon and gas. J Comput Assist Tomogr. 1984;8:835.

Welin S. Results of the Malmo technique of colon examination. JAMA. 1967;199:369.

Wesbey GE, Brasch RC, Engelstad BL, Moss AA, Crooks LE, Brito AC. Nuclear magnetic resonance contrast enhancement study of the gastrointestinal tract of rats and a human volunteer using non-toxic oral iron solutions. Radiology. 1983;149: 175.

Winaver SJ. Screening for colorectal cancer: an overview. Cancer. 1980;45:1093.

Winkler ML, Hricak H. Pelvis imaging with MR: technique for improvement. Radiology. 1986;158: 848.

Chapter **5**

The Acute Abdomen

RADIOGRAPHY

The term "acute abdomen" refers to a condition characterized by abdominal pain, rigidity of the abdominal muscles, vomiting, paralytic ileus and/or mechanical obstruction. It results from diffuse peritoneal irritation caused either by chemical action, produced by enzymes and gall, or by the action of microbial agents. Most conditions leading to an acute abdomen require surgical management. Common causes of an acute abdomen are:

1. Obstruction of the alimentary canal
2. Perforation
3. Inflammation
4. Spasm of either intraperitoneal or extraperitoneal tubular organs.

Mechanical injuries and altered blood supply may also be causative factors. In an attempt to immobilize the painful side of the body, homolateral flexion of the spine is seen on the plain abdominal film.

Plain Radiography of the Abdomen

A sequence of alimentary canal contrast examinations, US, CT, scintigraphy, and angiography may be helpful in diagnosing an acute abdomen. Still, a plain abdominal roentgenograph is critical for detection of both obstruction and perforation of the alimentary canal. The area between the lung base and pouch of Douglas should be recorded on upright, supine, and lateral recumbent films with cross-table roentgenography. When pneumoperitoneum is suspected, a chest film is helpful, although a lateral decubitus abdominal film may detect as little as 1 mL of free gas. If the X-ray beam is angled more cranially than for an abdominal film, discrete subdiaphragmatic gas collections can be detected (Fig. 5.1). Chest films yield a 93% accuracy in detection of pneumoperitoneum.

Plain abdominal films in the erect and supine positions, combined with chest roentgenogram, should demonstrate signs of an acute abdomen. Absence of an upright abdominal film may not affect diagnostic accuracy. A supine roentgenogram in a patient with obstruction allows analysis of the mucosal relief of a bowel loop filled with gas, and facilitates identification of the distended intestinal segments (Fig. 5.2).

Both pneumoperitoneum and gas-fluid levels are well demonstrated on lateral decubitus films with cross-table roentgenography (Fig. 5.2C). Free gas in the peritoneal cavity should be differentiated from lucencies in the lateral abdominal wall caused by adipose tissue. Listed in a medio-lateral direction, these are:

1. Subperitoneal
2. Between transverse and internal oblique abdominal muscles
3. Between internal and external oblique muscles
4. Subcutaneous.

The second and the third adipose layers are usually very thin. If demonstration of free gas in the peritoneal cavity is intended, a patient should be in a left decubitus position, since the majority of peptic ulcer perforations are close to the lesser curvature of the stomach and duodenum.

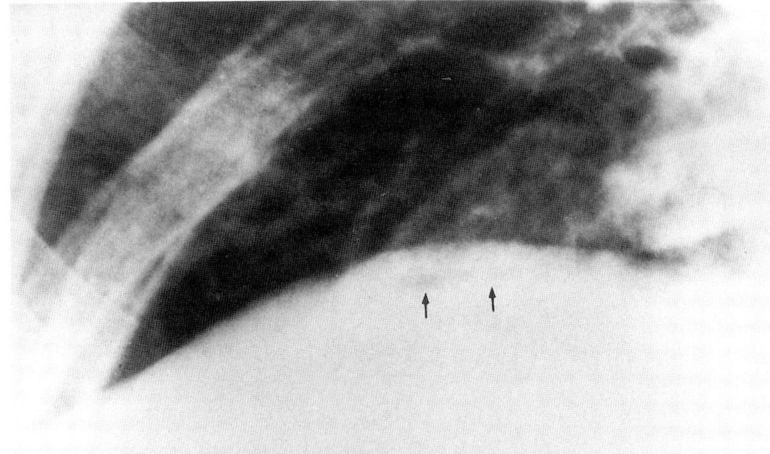

Figure 5.1. Discrete pneumoperitoneum. A small collection of gas is visible below the right leaf of the diaphragm (arrows).

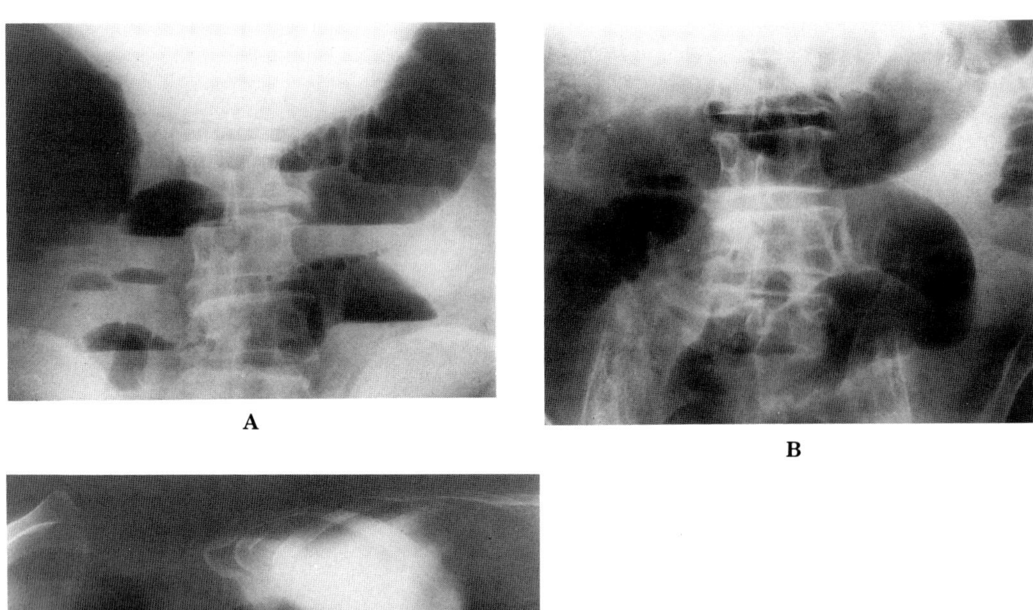

Figure 5.2. Obstruction in the distal colon. (A) This film was taken with the patient in the vertical position, demonstrating gas-fluid levels in distended small and large bowel. A "string-of-beads" appearance also indicates small bowel obstruction. (B) This film was taken with the patient in the supine position, demonstrating gas dilated bowel. (C) Right lateral decubitus film with cross-table roentgenography.

PLAIN RADIOGRAPHY OF THE CHEST

Pathologic processes in the chest may mimic symptoms of an acute abdomen. Such symptoms result from basal pleuropneumonias, pleurisy, pericarditis, and myocardial infarction. Pleural effusion in the thoracic cavity may result from acute pancreatitis. Chest films may also reveal a discrete pneumoperitoneum (Fig. 5.1).

CONTRAST RADIOGRAPHIC EXAMINATION

Barium may be administered orally providing the small bowel is not completely obstructed. It will not turn a partial obstruction into a complete one. A barium enema can be performed when there is large intestine obstruction. In the case of a complete small intestine obstruction, barium should only be given via a Miller-Abbott tube, which allows its removal. Water-soluble radiographic contrast media are contraindicated in patients with obstruction.

Barium is contraindicated when a perforation of a hollow viscus is suspected. However, water-soluble contrast media may be administered. In suspected gastric or duodenal peptic ulcer perforation a patient should remain in right lateral decubitus position for 15 minutes after taking 30–50 mL of a radiographic water-soluble contrast medium, following which an additional 30 mL of contrast medium may be ingested.

OBSTRUCTION

Intestinal obstruction may be either mechanical-dynamic or paralytic-adynamic.

MECHANICAL OBSTRUCTION

Radiologic signs develop three to six hours after complete intestinal obstruction when local homeostatic mechanisms are decompensated. The bowel is distended and filled with gas and fluid proximal to the point of obstruction. Accumulation of fluid results from reduced absorption of intestinal secretions, transudation from the blood, and decomposition of food. Gas is liberated from chyme (70%) and blood (20%), with a minor part generated by bacteria (10%). As an obstruction persists, the quantity of gas increases whereas the quantity of liquid decreases. In chronic obstruction, this ratio tends to be reversed. Simultaneous gas and liquid collections produce gas-fluid levels.

Intestinal loops are distended with gas proximal to the point of obstruction in 70% of cases. Gas-fluid levels are seen within these loops. That portion of the loop containing gas resembles an inverted letter "U" (Fig. 5.3). In the remaining 30% of patients the bowel contains liquid and not gas. These patients may not have an abnormal plain abdominal film. As long as peristalsis persists in trying to overcome an obstruction, gas-fluid levels within the limbs of a loop are at different heights. Intestinal motility can be seen fluoroscopically as changing gas-fluid levels proximal to the point of obstruction. The most accurate radiographic sign of mechanical obstruction is dilatation proximal to the site of obstruction, and abrupt transition to collapsed loops in more distal bowel segments, since bowel contents continue to evacuate. Distal to a site of obstruction, the large intestine is devoid of gas, except when an obstruction is located in the distal colon or in the rectum (Fig. 5.4). Gaseous distended intestine is seen not only in the upright position but also supine. Reversal of peristalsis may be seen proximal to the site of an obstruction.

An obstructed small bowel is considered dilated if its width exceeds 3 cm. Distension of the transverse colon exceeding 5 cm should be regarded as abnormal.

Obstruction in the *upper gastrointestinal tract* produces impressive clinical symptoms, vomiting and reverse peristalsis. Plain radiographic signs may be absent but the diagnosis can be confirmed by use of barium. More distal sites of obstruction demonstrate more distended loops, with gas-fluid levels and clinical symptoms tending to be more chronic. In distal obstruction of the *small intestine*, intestinal loops assume a *stepladder appearance* from the left hypochondriac region to the right iliac fossa (Figs. 5.5 and 5.12). This is due to the position of the mesenteric root. A "*string-of-beads*" appearance of small bowel obstruction depends on the simultaneous presence of a large amount of luminal fluid (Fig. 5.6). Strangulated obstruction of the small bowel may present with a *pseudotumor* and less pronounced proximal

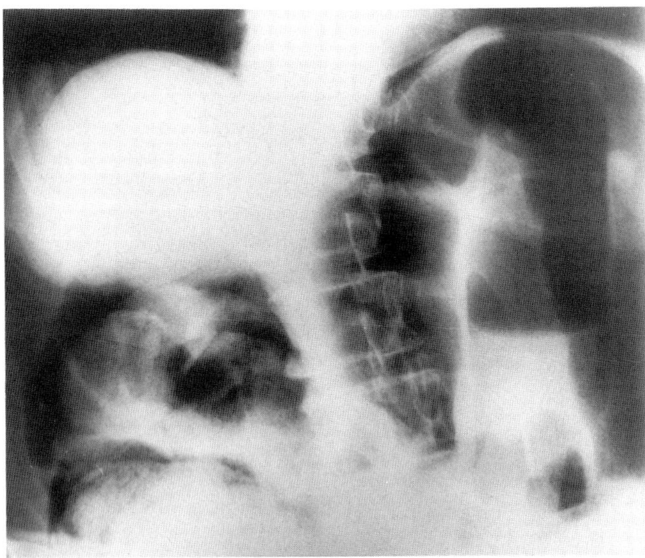

Figure 5.3. Mechanical obstruction results from an annular carcinoma at the transition of sigmoid colon into rectum. The large bowel is distended with gas-fluid levels without signs of small bowel obstruction. The sigmoid colon reaches the diaphragm.

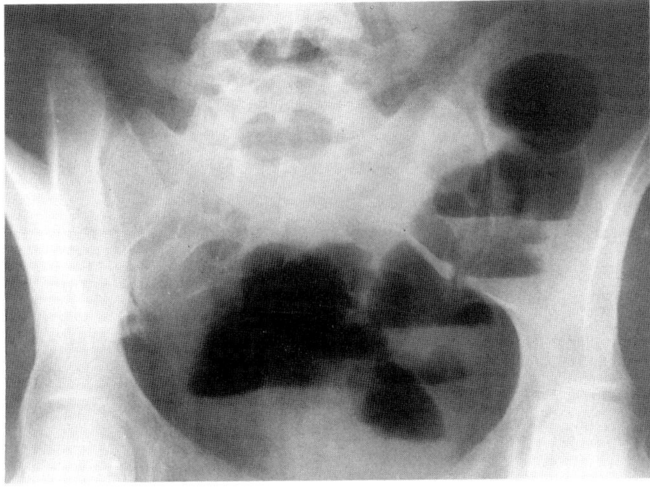

Figure 5.4. Obstruction at the transition of sigmoid colon into rectum presents with gas-fluid levels in the colon and a rectum devoid of gas.

accumulations of gas. In patients who swallow little air or tend to accumulate fluid exclusively, the small intestine may be *devoid of gas* in the presence of mechanical obstruction.

Obstructions of the *large intestine* are commonly located at the rectosigmoid transition or at the transition of the cecum into the ascending colon.

The colon is distended proximal to the site of obstruction and collapsed distally. Prolonged mechanical obstruction results in a superimposed paralytic ileus pattern.

Locating the Site of Obstruction. The point of obstruction is always located distal to the lowest distended loop. A prestenotic, sentinel loop is horseshoe-shaped and may contain a gas-fluid level. It is usually dilated more than other loops (Fig. 5.7). In distal obstructions, the radiographic appearance of the large intestine de-

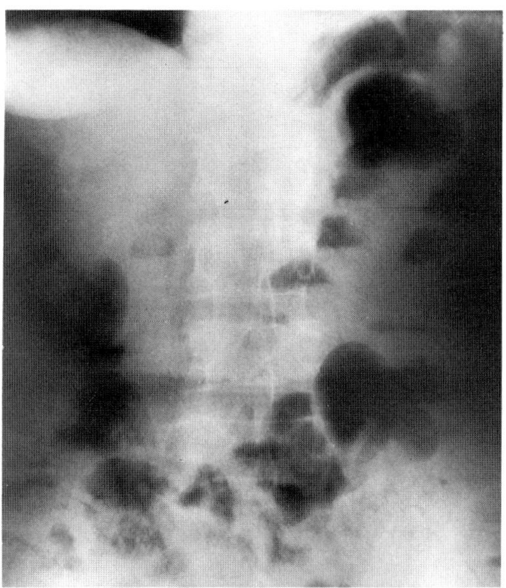

FIGURE 5.5. Long-standing mechanical obstruction from carcinoma of the sigmoid colon. Signs of large and small bowel obstruction include gas-fluid levels in moderately dilated small and large bowel.

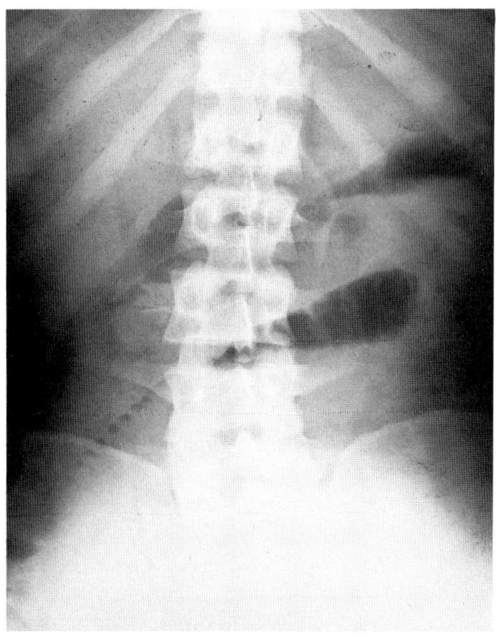

FIGURE 5.6. "String-of-beads" appearance indicates small bowel obstruction.

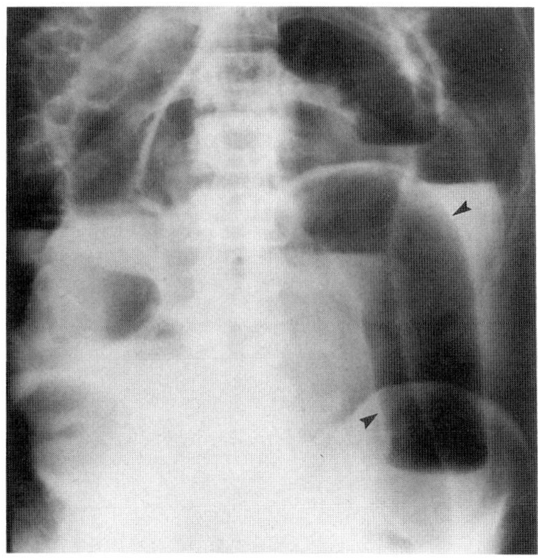

FIGURE 5.7. Mechanical obstruction of the large bowel without signs of small bowel obstruction. A prestenotic sentinel loop (arrowheads) is more distended than others.

pends on ileocecal valve competence. If gas does not fill the small bowel, the entire large intestine is distended, particularly proximal sections (Fig. 5.8). In prolonged obstructions, gas will leak into the small intestine in spite of a competent ileocecal valve. In these cases, besides signs of a distended large bowel, distal portions of the small bowel are shown to be dilated (Fig. 5.9). When the ileocecal valve is incompetent, the small intestine is filled with gas without substantial dilatation of the proximal portion of the large bowel (Figs. 5.10 and 5.11).

Criteria for distinction between obstruction of the small bowel (Fig. 5.12) and the large bowel (Fig. 5.10) are:

1. The small bowel mainly occupies the midportion of the abdomen whereas the large bowel lies in the periphery.
2. Radiographic contours of opposing walls of the small bowel are mutually parallel.
3. There are differences in mucosal pattern between the small and large bowel, that is, the distance between semilunar folds of the colon is greater than between Kerckring's folds. An excessively distended small intes-

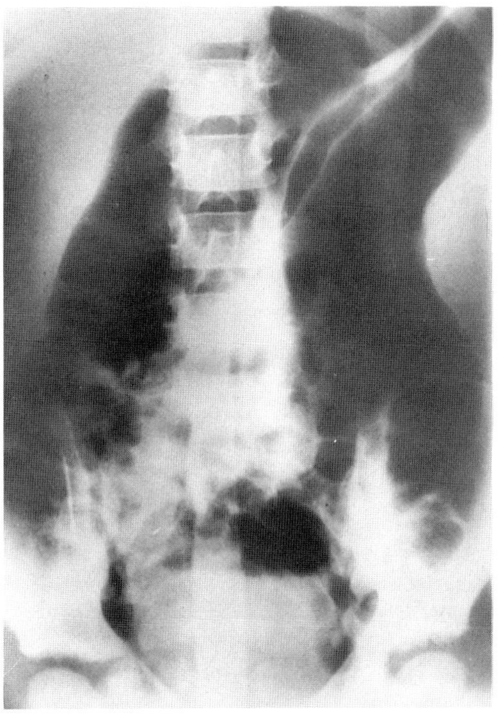

FIGURE 5.8. Obstruction of the distal sigmoid colon after surgery for congenital megacolon. Since the ileocecal valve is competent, signs of obstruction are not seen in the small bowel.

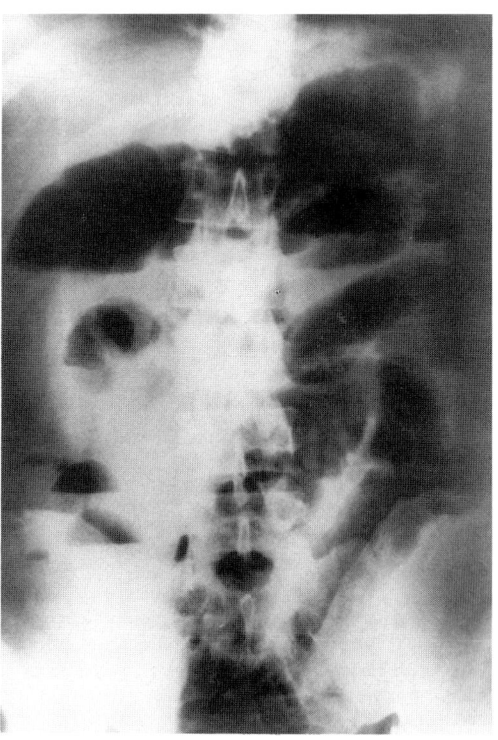

FIGURE 5.9. Long-standing obstruction of the distal rectum by annular carcinoma. The large bowel is more dilated than the small bowel because of a competent ileocecal valve.

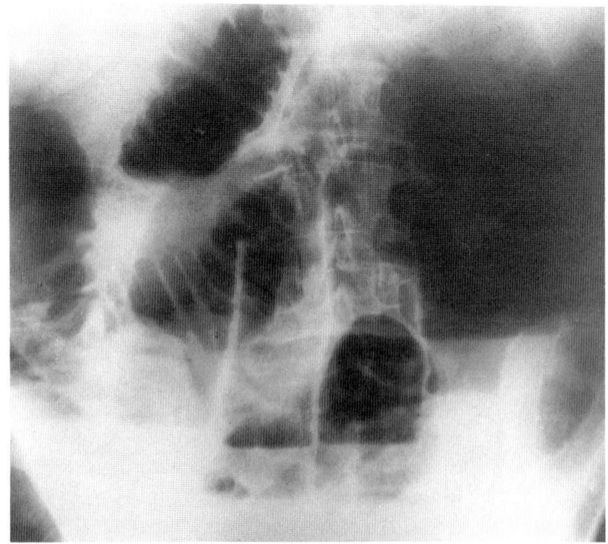

FIGURE 5.10. Mechanical obstruction of the distal colon. As a result of an incompetent ileocecal valve, proximal portions of the large bowel are not markedly distended, but signs of small bowel obstruction are seen.

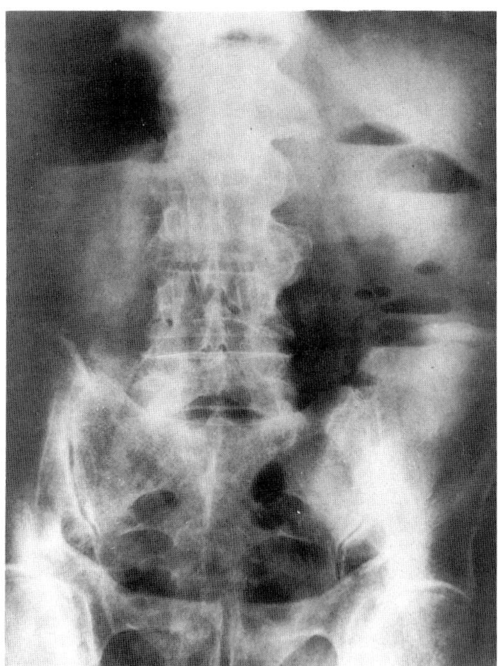

FIGURE 5.11. Incompetent ileocecal valve in transverse colon carcinoma results in insignificant large bowel distension, with signs of small bowel obstruction.

tine may, by its relief, mimic the colon. Namely, overdistension flattens normal mucosal projections in all sections of the small bowel except in the jejunum. When the mucosal surface is to be analyzed, plain abdominal film should be taken in a supine position.

4. Limbs of distended small intestinal loops containing gas-fluid levels are mutually displaced and gas collections are subsequently lower, whereas in the colon they are brought closer to each other and gas columns are higher.
5. Distal obstruction of the small bowel is accompanied by numerous distended loops.
6. Solid feces may be observed in a gas distended colon. In contrast, contents of the small bowel are always liquid.

With abundant distension, intestinal width is of no value in discriminating between the small and large intestine. Widths of normal jejunum and ileum are 2–3 cm and 1.5–2 cm, respectively. The diameter of the large bowel is much greater, even at its narrowest sections. However, because of great distensibility, the small bowel may assume a diameter similar to that of the large intestine, or even greater. As the wall of the large intestine is thick and firm

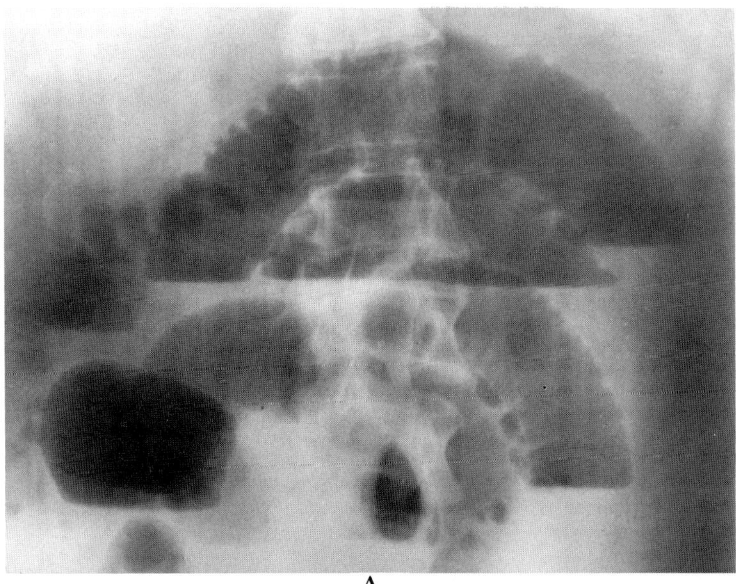

A

FIGURE 5.12. Small bowel obstruction with stepladder appearance. The films were taken with the patient in (A) standing position. (*Figure continued on overleaf.*)

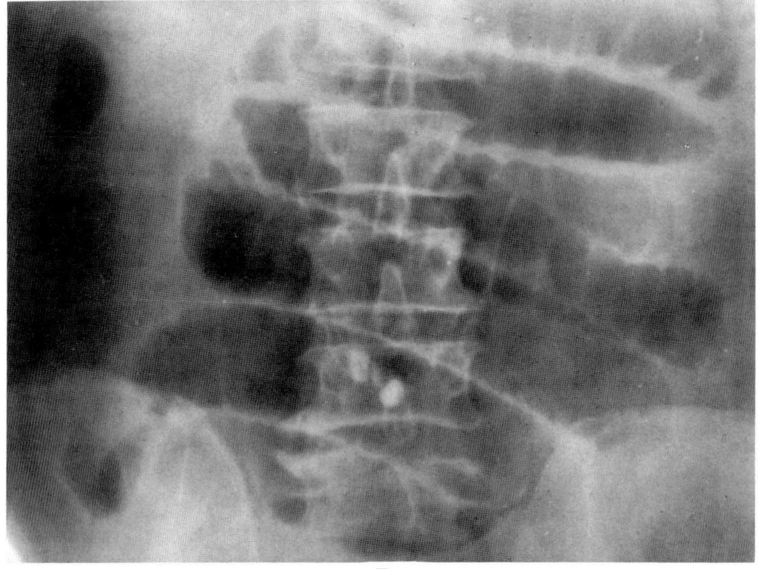

B

Figure 5.12 *continued.* (B) Patient in supine position.

in the distal segments, distal obstructions cause more pronounced distension of the proximal colon.

Strangulation refers to obstructions that compromise intestinal blood supply such as incarcerated hernia, volvulus, intussusception, bands, and other closed-loop obstructions. *Closed-loop strangulation* results from obstruction of both proximal and distal limbs of a bowel loop. A strangulated intestinal loop containing gas, and at times fluid, resembles a coffee bean (Fig. 5.13). The longitudinal denser line corresponds to the thickened intestinal wall. Bowel distension develops proximal to a strangulated loop, but as in other types of strangulation, it is not prominent. Unless surgically treated, strangulations result in intestinal gangrene with a mortality rate of 31%, despite later surgical therapy. Computed tomography can be helpful in confirming the diagnosis.

With any kind of mechanical obstruction, sympathetic activity is stimulated and parasympathetic activity depressed, resulting in inhibition of peristalsis unless the obstruction is relieved. Thus, intestinal obstruction may turn into a paralytic ileus. In addition, progressive proximal dilatation leads to additional intestinal ischemia and secondary ileus.

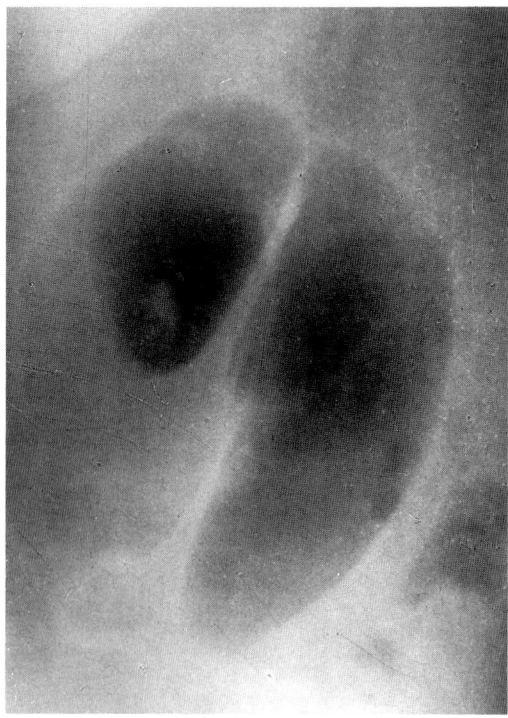

Figure 5.13. Closed-loop obstruction with strangulation, resulting in coffee-bean appearance of an intestinal loop.

Partial Bowel Obstruction. Transport of bowel contents is slowed with partial obstruction. The bowel is dilated and contains gas-fluid levels proximal to the site of partial obstruction. However, unlike complete obstruction, sections distal to partial obstruction contain some gas, particularly in the large intestine (Fig. 5.14).

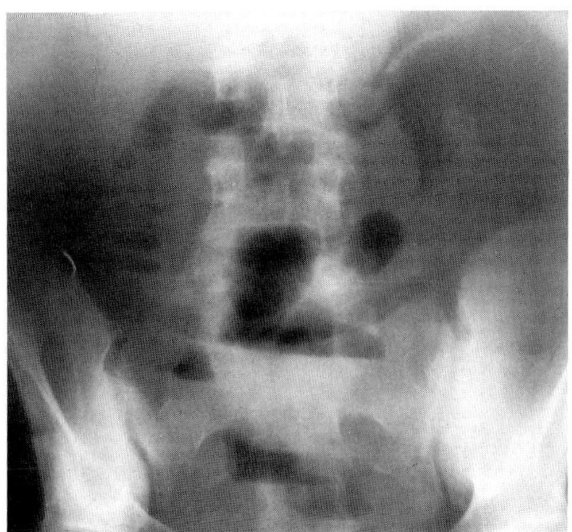

FIGURE 5.14. Partial obstruction of the sigmoid colon with gas-fluid levels proximal and gas distal to the obstruction.

Stenoses of the small and large bowel causing partial obstructions may be diagnosed by giving barium orally. Experimental stenoses of the large intestine in dogs were not converted from partial obstruction to complete obstruction by barium administration. It is therefore believed that barium may be safely applied orally in patients with partial obstructions.

Causes of Mechanical Intestinal Obstruction. The most common causes of small bowel obstruction are adhesion and strangulation of either external or internal hernias. Adhesions provoke strangulation of small intestinal loops but are less likely to do so in the colon. The lumen of the gastrointestinal tract may be occluded by gallstones, matted balls of ascarides, bezoars, or fecaliths. The expulsion of gallstones is often followed by pneumobilia, gas in the biliary tree. Neoplasms, strictures, and impressions from adjacent organs, for example annular pancreas or superior mesenteric artery, may be causes for altered transport of intestinal contents. Intussusception is the most common cause of obstruction in children younger than the age of two. A proximal intestinal segment usually slips into the distal, often in the ileocecal region. The large intestine harbors 20% of the alimentary canal obstructions (Fig. 5.15). Major causes are carcinomas (70%), diverticu-

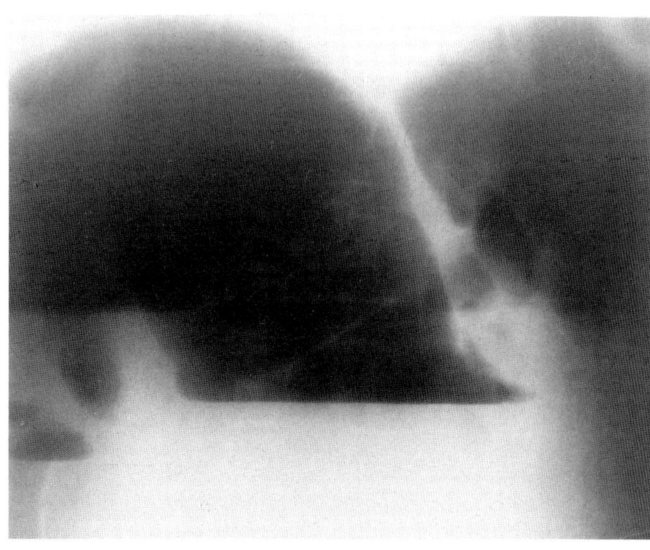

FIGURE 5.15. Mechanical obstruction of descending colon. Plain upright film.

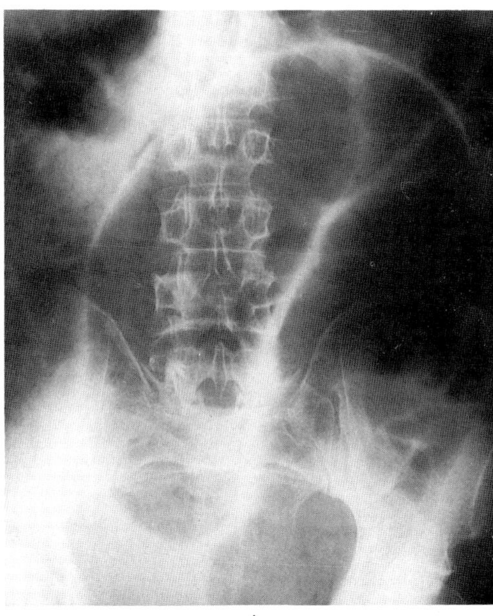

A

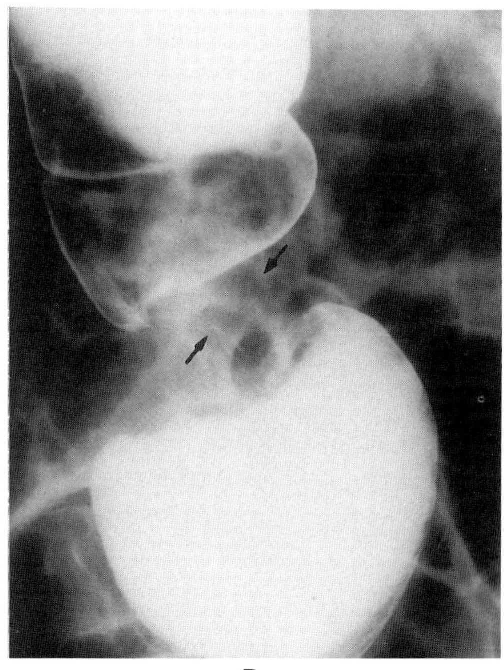

B

FIGURE 5.16. Sigmoid colon volvulus. (A) Plain abdominal film. (B) Barium enema demonstrates the site of torsion (arrows).

litis (15%), fecaliths, adhesions, herniations or foreign bodies (10%), and volvulus (5%). Volvulus preferentially affects the sigmoid colon (Fig. 5.16) with occasional bowel rotation of more than 360 degrees. The right colon is less commonly affected with volvulus.

Both thrombosis and embolism of mesenteric blood vessels are manifested by signs of intestinal obstruction. An ischemic segment is incapable of readily propagating contents resulting in functional obstruction. If a vascular lesion is suspected to be threatening infarction and gangrene, administration of any radiographic contrast medium or cleansing enema is contraindicated.

PARALYTIC ILEUS

Also referred to as adynamic, paretic, functional, and inhibitory ileus, paralytic ileus is prolonged absence of bowel motility. Ileus is characterized by generalized dilatation of the entire alimentary canal distal to the esophagus. The stomach may also be involved by paresis (Fig. 5.17). Ileus develops after peritoneal irritation from any source where cholinergic inhibition and adrenergic stimulation suppress intestinal motility. Diffuse peritoneal affection involves both small and large intestine equally, because solar and sacral plexuses innervate the entire bowel. A reflex arch for the inhibition of intestinal motility starts in peritoneal receptors and is transmitted via splanchnic nerves. Experiments on animals have shown that paralytic ileus may be prevented by simply cutting the splanchnic nerves.

In paralytic ileus, absorption is decreased due to stasis, and gas is liberated from intestinal contents. When peritoneal irritation is local, paresis may involve only a short intestinal section. Paralytic ileus develops after abdominal surgery, but peristalsis often reappears within one hour, unless extensive manipulations of the bowel were performed. Peristalsis recovers approximately three hours after alimentary canal resection.

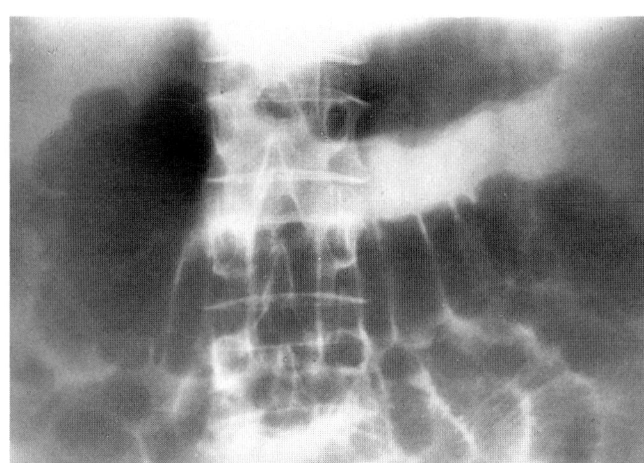

FIGURE 5.17. Paralytic ileus. The stomach, small and large bowel are filled with gas.

Patients with paralytic ileus are unlikely to have numerous gas-fluid levels. The bowel is filled with a considerable volume of gas. As the colon is not evacuated in paralytic ileus, it contains gas; this is not the case in obstructive ileus. Localized intestinal paralysis acts as a functional obstruction.

Distinction between mechanical obstruction and paralytic ileus is of the utmost importance since barium administration is contraindicated in the latter. Mechanical obstruction needs to be relieved surgically while ileus is medically treated. The distinction is possible by radiologic means in typical cases (Table 5.1) However, problems arise in atypical and/or combined forms.

Causes of Paralytic Ileus. After a period lasting a few hours to a few days *mechanical obstruction* has a superimposed paralytic ileus pattern. *Acute inflammation* in the abdomen may lead to intestinal paralysis. *Acute appendicitis* causes paresis of the cecum and the terminal ileum in 50% of patients and can exhibit moderate intestinal dilatation and gas-fluid levels. The degree of intestinal paresis depends on the extent of peritoneal irritation. The earliest described sign of an impending appendicial perforation is gaseous distension of the transverse colon. *Acute cholecystitis* may result in paresis of the duodenum and hepatic flexure. *Acute pancreatitis* often causes duodenal and jejunal ileus with local paralysis, presenting as a "*sentinel loop*" filled with gas. Extension of inflammation into the transverse colon results in local paralysis with obstruction in the region of the splenic flexure, causing an interrupted gas pattern, named the "colon cutoff sign." *Adnexitis* and other inflammations in the peritoneal and retroperitoneal spaces can also cause local ileus of intestinal segments.

Spasms of hollow abdominal viscera resulting in "colicky pain" may alter intestinal motility and cause paralytic ileus. This pertains particularly to biliary and renal colic. Severe pain along with ileus occurs after torsion of a

TABLE 5.1. COMPARISON OF MECHANICAL OBSTRUCTION AND PARALYTIC ILEUS

OBSTRUCTION	ILEUS
Gas distended bowel loops resembling an inverted "U" with gas-fluid levels at different height	Bowel loops distended with equal gas-fluid levels or without fluid
Bowel hypermotility	Bowel motility decreased or absent
Gasless stomach and bowel distal to obstruction	Gas in the stomach, small bowel, and large bowel

pedunculated abdominal tumor such as an ovarian cyst.

Peritonitis is characterized by ileus, fluid in the peritoneal cavity, and reduced motility of the diaphragm. A large volume of fluid separates floating gas-filled intestinal loops in the supine position.

Vascular lesions such as arterial occlusion, bleeding, and ruptures may result in ileus. Aneurysm of the abdominal aorta, particularly aortic dissection, may provoke symptoms of an acute abdomen and can be demonstrated by US, CT, and angiography.

Intestinal obstruction in children needs to be differentiated from *chronic intestinal pseudo-obstruction*, which occurs in children after age one. A discontinuous lack in smooth muscle fibers and myenteric nervous plexus is inherited; the defect is autosomally dominant. Radiographic signs of ileus are found, but the clinical history is chronic. Intestinal motility is segmentally absent or incoordinate.

Toxic megacolon is acute distension of the colon in patients with pancolitis. This can occur most commonly in patients with Crohn's, ulcerative, or ischemic colitis, as well as with diffuse nodular lymphoma of the colon. These patients are in poor general condition. A supine roentgenogram shows transverse colon diameter exceeding 5 cm. Haustra may vanish completely. Occasionally, ulcerations and pseudopolyps protrude into the lumen (Figs. 5.18 and 11.37). An enema or colonoscopy is contraindicated because of a high risk of perforation. Despite colectomy the mortality rate approximates 30%.

Nonobstructive dilatation of the colon must be differentiated from toxic megacolon and mechanical obstruction, since it can be cured endoscopically. It may clinically resemble a mechanical obstruction and occurs two to seven days after surgery in exhausted patients. It may also result from carcinomatous infiltration of the sacral plexus. Intestinal peristalsis, though faint, does not cease completely. The colon is distended by gas, particularly the right colon (Fig. 5.19). The diameter of the cecum may reach 17 cm. When the diameter of the cecum exceeds 10 cm, perforation can occur as the result of ischemia. Simultaneous dilatation of the small intestine is not common. Any type of cleansing or contrast enema is contraindicated in patients with nonobstructive dilatation of the colon.

Disorders of parasympathetic and sympathetic stimuli are possible causes for nonobstructive dilatation of the colon. These may include:

1. Metabolic abnormalities such as uremia and hypokalemia
2. Medications such as opiates, ganglion blockers, vincristine, or bleomycin

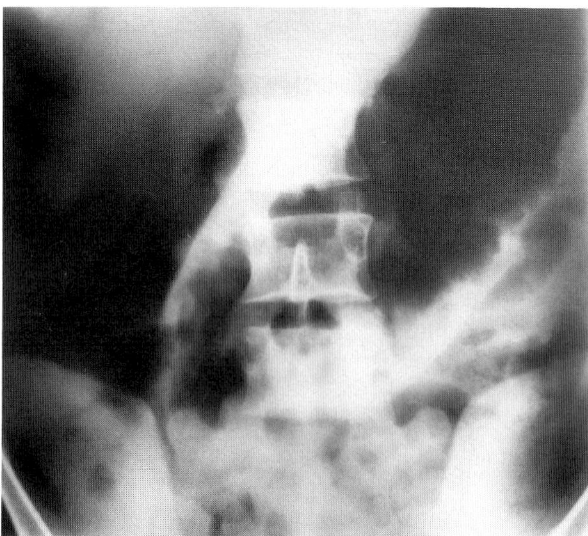

Figure 5.18. Toxic megacolon in ulcerative colitis.

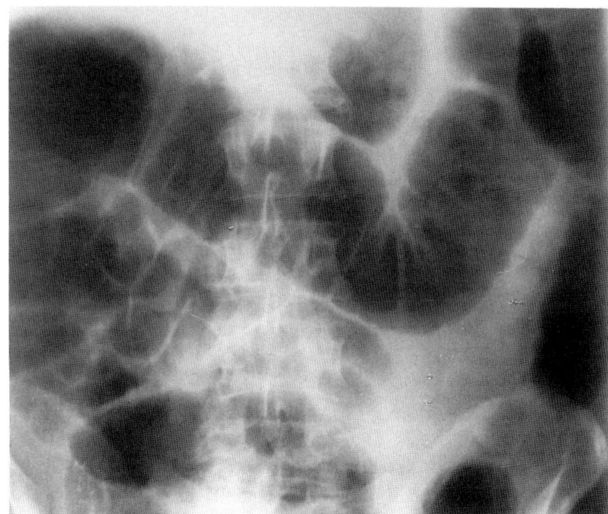

FIGURE 5.19. Nonobstructive colonic dilatation.

3. Inflammation such as pancreatitis, cholecystitis, or appendicitis
4. Injuries such as fractures of the pelvis or spine, and recent surgery

After successful therapeutic colonoscopy or perforation, the distended colon need not collapse at once. This can be explained by the law of Laplace (t = p × r); "t" being the tension of the intestinal wall, "p" intraluminal pressure, and "r" radius. Radius remains unchanged if the tension of the wall and intraluminal pressure drop by the same rate toward the point where collapse begins. However, criteria for a successful colonoscopic decompression include decrease in abdominal distension and cecal diameter.

PERFORATION OF AN ALIMENTARY CANAL ORGAN

Alimentary canal perforations are common causes of an acute abdomen. Pneumoperitoneum (Fig. 5.20) results from perforation of organs containing gas such as the stomach, the duodenum, or the colon. In small intestinal perforations only small amounts of gas may be liberated. However, more gas then enters the peritoneal cavity because of the resultant paralytic ileus. Causes for alimentary canal perforations are peptic ulcers, ulcerated tumors, inflammatory disease such as ulcerative colitis or Crohn's disease, and injuries. Perforated sigmoid diverticula cause pneumoperitoneum only in exceptional cases since perforations are usually limited by adhesions. Ruptures of gas-filled cysts occurring with intestinal pneumatosis or gynecological manipulations may also cause pneumoperitoneum. If fluid is present simulta-

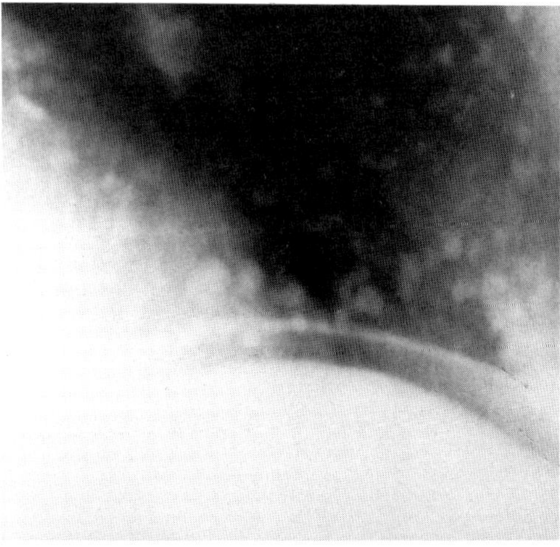

FIGURE 5.20. Pneumoperitoneum. Multiple calcified tuberculous foci are evident in the lung base.

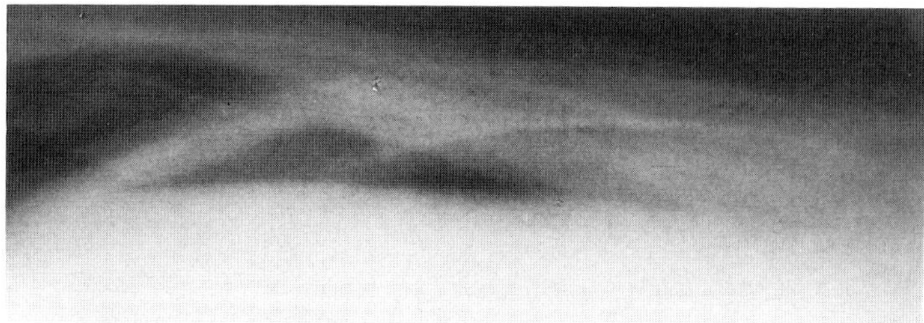

Figure 5.21. Hydropneumoperitoneum. Left lateral decubitus position with cross-table radiography.

neously with gas, hydropneumoperitoneum results (Fig. 5.21).

Gas can be identified within the peritoneal cavity approximately 20 min after a perforation. Radiographic demonstration of free gas is not seen in 7–20% of peptic ulcer perforations. This may be the result of adhesions or lack of gas in the perforated organ. Small subdiaphragmatic gas collections are best demonstrated on films taken at mid-expiration with the X-ray beam at the level of the dome of the diaphragm (Figs. 5.1 and 5.20). A "double-wall sign" is seen on supine abdominal films of patients with abundant pneumoperitoneum and simultaneous presence of gas in the gut lumen. Since it is delineated from both sides by gas, the gut

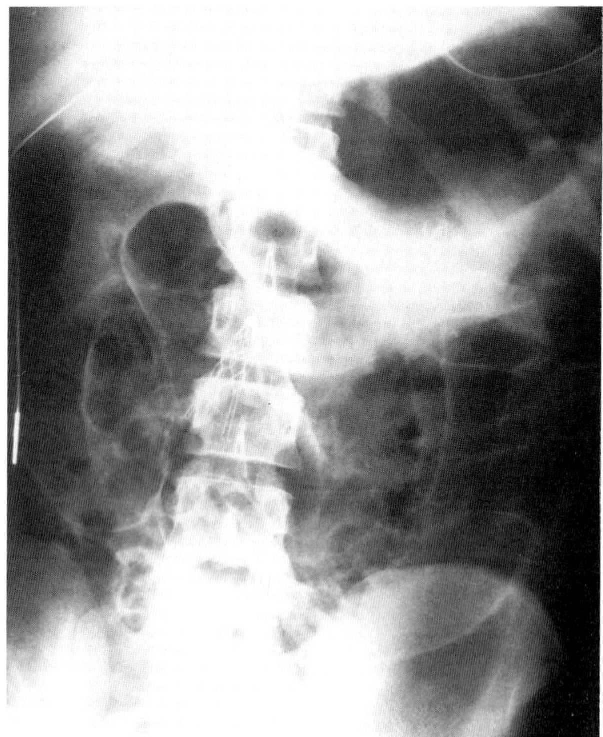

Figure 5.22. Supine roentgenogram shows pneumoperitoneum with simultaneous presence of gas in the bowel lumen resulting in visualization of bowel wall. "Double wall" sign.

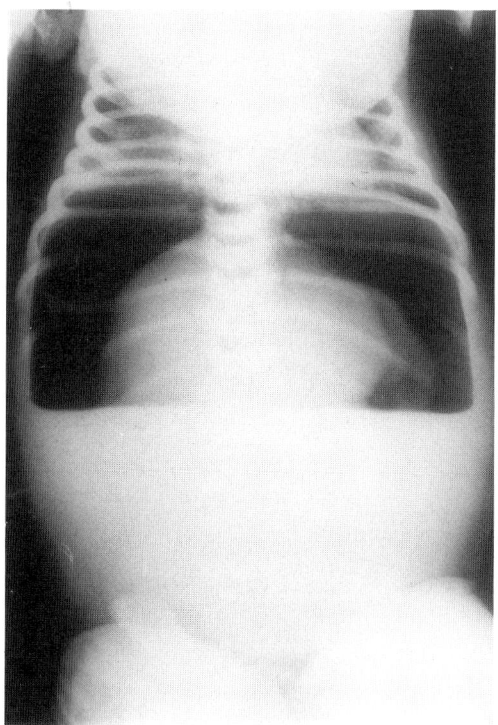

FIGURE 5.23. Massive hydropneumoperitoneum in a child.

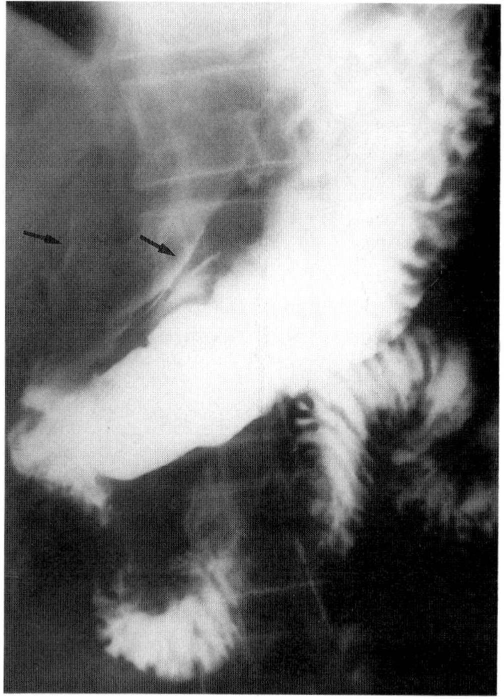

FIGURE 5.24. Perforation of peptic ulcer of the lesser gastric curvature. Water-soluble contrast medium enters the lesser sac (arrows).

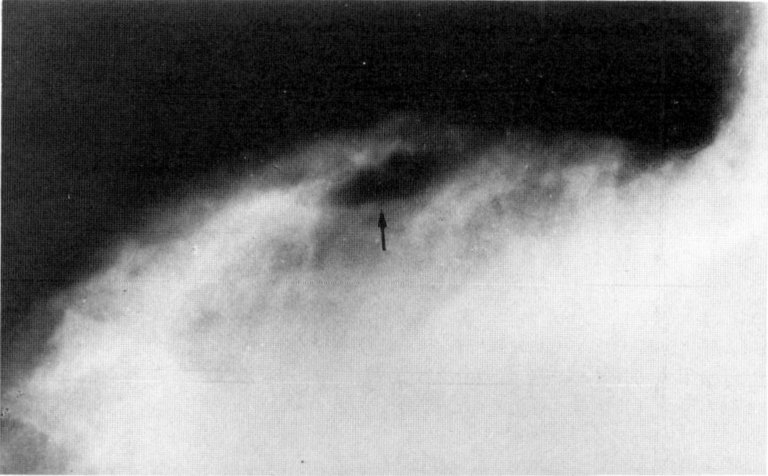

FIGURE 5.25. Subphrenic abscess. The distance between air in the lung and gas in the abscess is greater than with pneumoperitoneum.

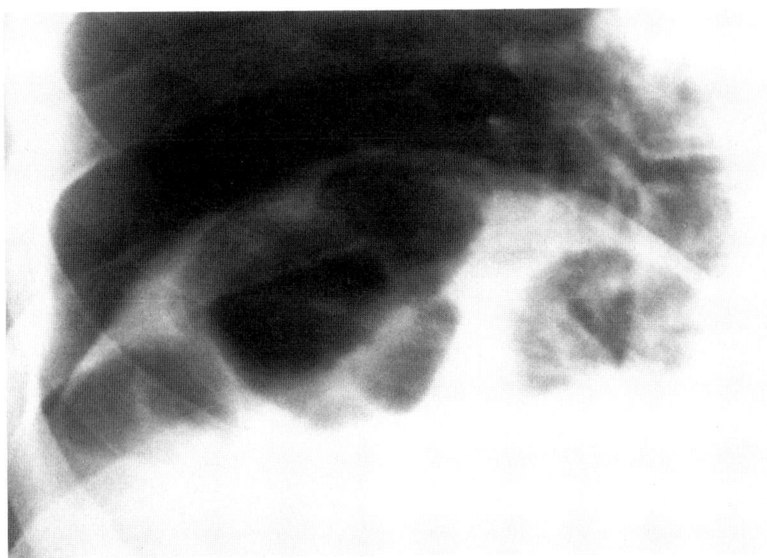

Figure 5.26. Chilaiditi's syndrome. Haustral markings are visible under right leaf of the diaphragm. (See Fig. 4.8.)

wall is seen (Fig. 5.22). Massive pneumoperitoneum can cause the gut to collapse in the midabdomen, particularly in children (Fig. 5.23).

The site of perforation may be visualized with radiographic water-soluble contrast medium (Fig. 5.24). After ingesting 15–100 mL of a water-soluble contrast medium, the patient should be placed in a prone position in order to demonstrate perforated ulcer of the anterior wall of the stomach or duodenum. If not, the patient should then be turned to the right lateral decubitus position to allow demonstration of a perforated ulcer on the lesser curvature. The supine position enhances demonstration of perforated ulcers on the posterior walls of the stomach and the duodenum.

Pneumoperitoneum due to perforation should be distinguished from pneumoperitoneum resulting from other causes, from subphrenic abscesses (Figs. 4.8 and 5.25), and from interposition of the transverse colon between the liver and the diaphragm—Chilaiditi's syndrome (Fig. 5.26). Free air in the abdominal cavity changes position with changes in the patient's posture.

Bibliography

Adrwitz A, Smith DF, Rosenzweig J. The acutely obstructed colon. Am J Surg. 1962;104:474.

Anuras S, Shirazi SS. Colonic pseudo-obstruction. Am J Gastroenterol. 1984;79:525.

Balgey EC, Crabtree H, Fish JC, Miller EB. Volvulus of the right colon. Ann Surg. 1961;154:268.

Balthazar EJ, Schechter LS. Gallstone ileus—the importance of contrast examinations on the roentgenographic diagnosis. AJR. 1975;125:374.

Balthazar EJ, Bauman JS, Megibow AJ. CT diagnosis of closed loop obstruction. J Comput Assist Tomogr. 1985;9:953.

Berliner SO, Burson LC, Lear PE. The mechanical factors in obstructive perforation. Arch Surg. 1961;83:911.

Byrne WJ, Cipel L, Ament MA, Gyepes MT. Chronic idiopathic intestinal pseudo-obstruction syndrome. Diagn Imag. 1981;50:294.

Drapans T, Stewart JD. Acute sigmoid volvulus. Am J Surg. 1963;86:772.

Grossman RJ, Miller WT, Dann RW. Oral barium sulphate in partial large bowel obstruction. Radiology. 1980;136:327.

Hayward MWJ, Hayward C, Ennis WP, Roberts CJ. A pilot evaluation of radiography of the acute abdomen. Clin Radiol. 1984;35:289.

Leonidas JC, Harris DJ, Amoury RA. How accurate is the roentgen diagnosis of acute appendicitis in children? Ann Radiol. 1975;18:479.

McIver MA. Acute intestinal obstruction. Am J Surg. 1933;19:163.

Meyers MA. Colonic ileus. Gastrointest Radiol. 1977;2:37.

Miller RE, Brahme F. Large amounts of orally administered barium for obstruction of small bowel. Surg Gynecol Obstet. 1969;129:1185.

Miller RE, Becker GJ, Slabaugh RD. Detection of pneumoperitoneum: optimum body position and respiratory phase. AJR. 1980;135:487.

Mirvis SE, Young JWR, Keramati B, McCrea ES, Tarr R. Plain film evaluation of patients with abdominal pain: are three radiographs necessary? AJR. 1986;147:501.

Ochsner A. X-ray diagnosis of ileus. Comparison of results obtained by roentgenograms in horizontal and upright positions. Proc Soc Exp Biol. 1931;29:327.

Ogilvie H. Large intestine colic due to sympathetic deprivation. A new clinical syndrome. Br Med J. 1948;2:671.

Shirazi KK, Agha FP, Strodel WE, Amendola MA, Nostrant TT, Dent TL. Non-obstructive colonic dilatation: radiologic findings in 50 patients following colonoscopic treatment. J Can Assoc Radiol. 1984;35:116.

Strodel WE, Nostrant TT, Eckhauser FE, Dent TL. Therapeutic and diagnostic colonoscopy in non-obstructive colonic dilatation. Ann Surg. 1983;197: 416.

Swischuk LE, Hayden CK Jr. Appendicitis with perforation: the dilated transverse colon sign. AJR. 1980;135:687.

Vanek VW, Al-Salti M. Acute pseudo-obstruction of the colon (Ogilvie's syndrome). Dis Colon Rectum. 1986;29:203.

Wanebo H, Methewson C, Conolly B. Pseudo-obstruction of the colon. Surg Gynecol Obstet. 1971;133:44.

Wells C, Rawlinson K, Tinkler L, Jones H, Saunders J. Postoperative gastrointestinal motility. Lancet. 1964;1:4.

Chapter 6

Radiology of the Pharynx

FUNCTIONAL DISORDERS

Disorders of pharyngeal function are most commonly manifested as disorders of swallowing (see chapter 2 on the act of swallowing). Symptomatology is nonspecific. The predominate methods of examination are fluoroscopy with rapid roentgenography or video-recording, and video-manometry. Radiologic examination should exclude primarily neoplasms. In unilateral paralysis or paresis, pharyngeal constrictors push the bolus to the atonic side, resembling a neoplasm on the side with normal motility. A majority of pharyngeal disorders present with dysphagia.

Oropharyngeal dysphagia results from disturbed transport of a bolus from the mouth to the cervical segment of the esophagus. The bolus may be directed toward the larynx or epipharynx, or back toward the mouth. This disorder results from stasis of the bolus due to lack of increase in pharyngeal pressure. The etiology is not completely understood, but this type of dysphagia is frequently a sequel to disturbed function of the lower pharyngeal sphincter, which fails to relax at the correct time or relaxes in a manner uncoordinated with simultaneous contractions of other pharyngeal muscles. Scleroderma and achalasia do not affect striated muscles, thereby sparing the lower pharyngeal constrictor. However, dysphagia does not always result from pharyngeal dysfunction.

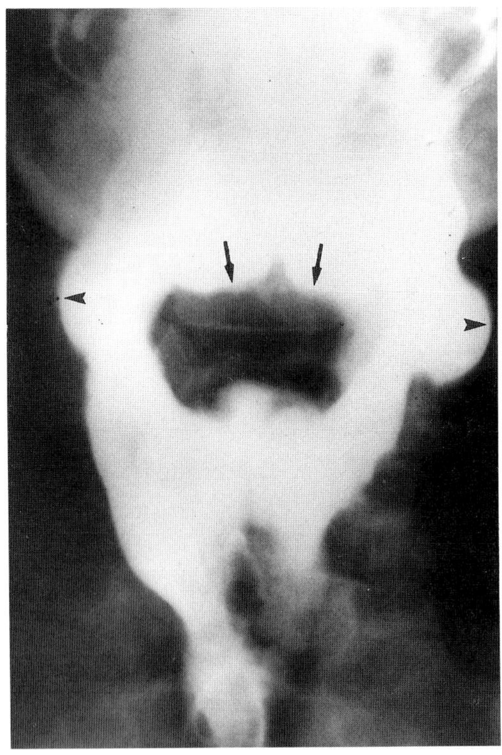

FIGURE 6.1. Paresis of the hypopharynx with swallowing disorder. Dilated lumen of the hypopharynx. The epiglottis is slightly tilted (arrows). Evanescent lateral pharyngeal diverticula (arrowheads). (See Fig. 2.5.)

DISORDERS OF THE PHARYNGEAL PHASE OF SWALLOWING

A deranged pharyngeal phase of swallowing results in symptoms occuring at the onset of deglutition. A prone position leads to the accentuation of radiographic findings. A barium suspension of high viscosity should not be used at the beginning of the examination, since airway obstruction can occur in patients with paresis of constrictors. When aspiration of pharyngeal contents is suspected, water-soluble, iso-osmolar contrast medium might be safer.

Disordered sequence and mode of contraction of muscles engaged in the pharyngeal phase of swallowing result in abnormal deglutition accompanied by dysphagia. This results in radiologic manifestations:

1. Disorders of motility. Disordered pharyngeal motility is the most common sign of an abnormal act of swallowing and the most accurate sign of pharyngeal paralysis. Paresis of pharyngeal muscles results in abnormal width of the lumen, asymmetric passing of the bolus, and oblique positioning of an incompletely closed epiglottis (Figs. 2.5 and 6.1). Muscular contractions are weakened or their sequence is impaired. Contractions may commence too late, or may last too long. A combination of disorders is possible, with complete disruption of the sequence of pharyngeal muscle contraction being the most serious functional abnormality.
2. Stasis of pharyngeal contents. Stasis of barium can be seen in the valleculae and pyriform sinuses after repeated swallowing

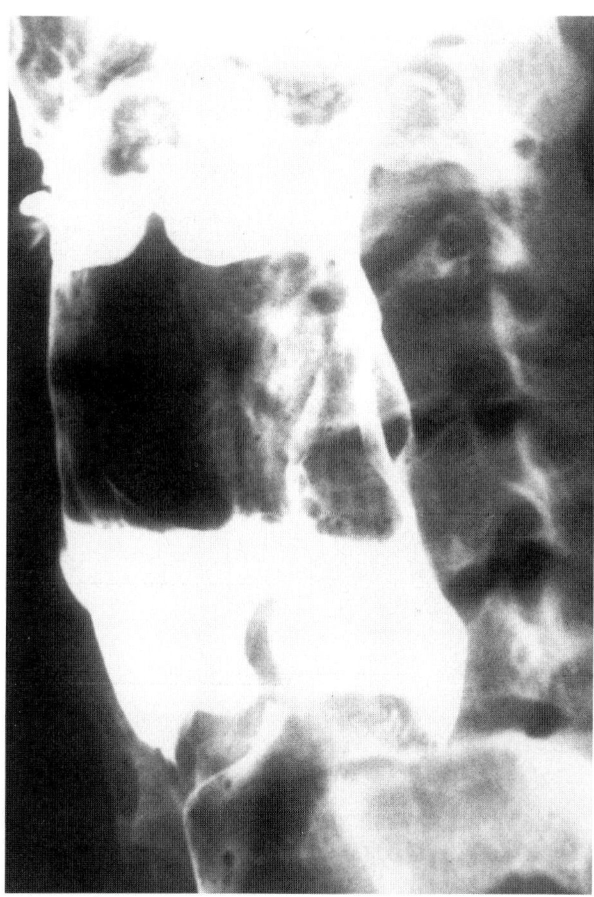

FIGURE 6.2. Barium stagnates in the valleculae and pyriform sinuses after repeated swallowing. Small lateral pharyngeal diverticulum is evident.

(Fig. 6.2). This may result from lowered sensitivity of the pharyngeal mucosa, low muscular tone, or lack of elastic fibers in the pharynx of elderly patients. It may also be related to mechanical obstruction.

3. False directioning of the bolus. Disorders of swallowing can result in inappropriate directioning of the bolus, for example, toward the nasal cavity (Fig. 6.3) or the larynx. In contrast to a liquid bolus which normally flows symmetrically through both pyriform sinuses, a more solid bolus, such as a viscous barium suspension, may normally pass mainly through one pyriform recess. Aspiration is most commonly a consequence of dysfunction of the hypopharynx and the upper esophageal sphincter (Figs. 6.4 and 6.5).

These *neuromuscular diseases* affect the pharyngeal muscles:

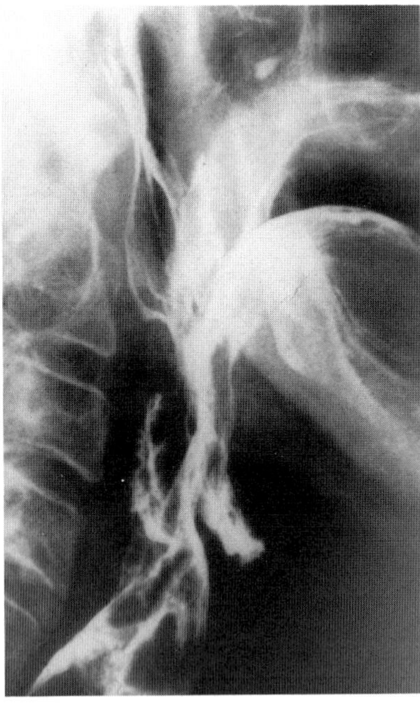

FIGURE 6.3. Reflux of barium into the nasopharynx, nose and trachea during swallowing. Irregularities of the posterior pharyngeal wall with widening of the retropharyngeal space are related to carcinoma of the hypopharynx with abnormal deglutition.

1. Extrapyramidal diseases:
   Parkinson's syndrome
   Huntington's chorea
2. Collagenoses
3. Muscular diseases and myoneuronal junction disorders:
   Myasthenia gravis
4. Demyelinating disease:
   Multiple sclerosis

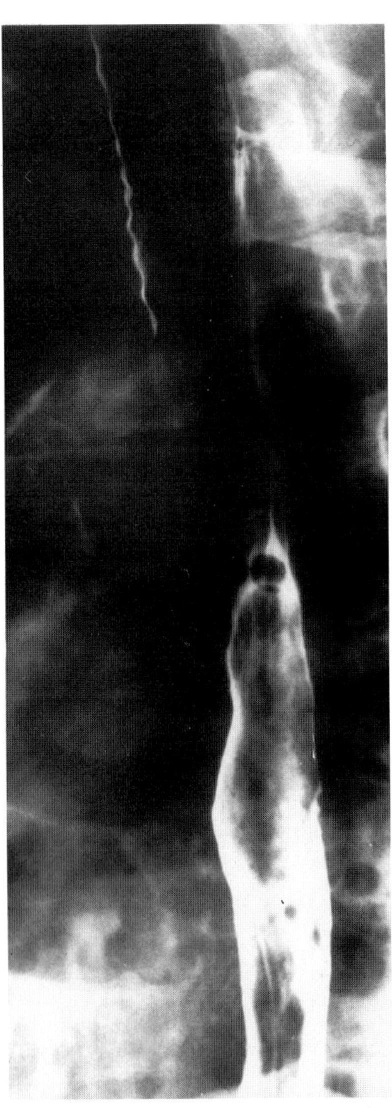

FIGURE 6.4. Discrete aspiration of barium into the trachea results from swallowing disorder.

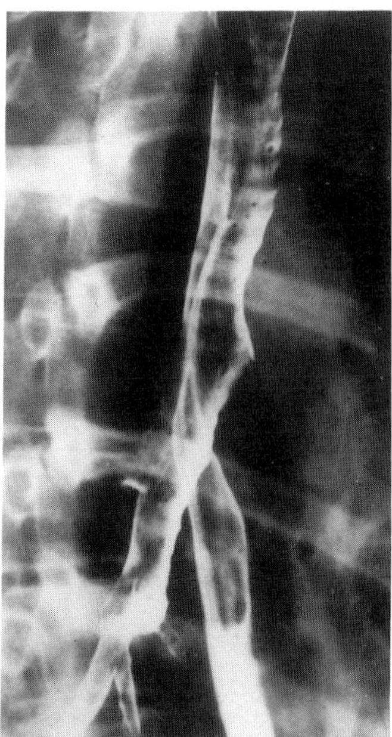

FIGURE 6.5. Prominent aspiration of barium into the trachea and bronchi.

5. Congenital and degenerative disease:
   - Amyotrophic lateral sclerosis
   - Amyotonia congenita
   - Syringobulbia
6. Disorders in the brain stem:
   - Primary or secondary neoplasms
   - Pseudobulbar palsy
   - Tabes dorsalis
   - Poliomyelitis
   - Trauma
7. Disorders of deglutition of unknown etiology:
   - Sideropenic webs (Plummer–Vinson syndrome)
   - Cricopharyngeal hyperactivity

Patients with disordered swallowing may *adapt* to the consistency, viscosity, volume, mass, and temperature of the bolus. Lowering the soft palate can compensate for weakness of the pharyngeal muscles while more pronounced contraction of pharyngeal muscles can compensate for deficient function of the soft palate. When contractions of pharyngeal and lingual musculature are impaired, there is a compensatory backward movement of the larynx. Insufficient epiglottic closure of the larynx is corrected by raising and tilting the larynx forward. Disturbances described under "False directioning of the bolus" (p. 164) result from *decompensation* of compensatory mechanisms. Video-recording of a barium swallow is the method of choice in estimating compensation of pharyngeal functions. When neuromuscular disorders are absent, pharyngeal diverticula, abscesses, and tumors may result in abnormalities of swallowing.

IMPRESSION BY THE INFERIOR PHARYNGEAL CONSTRICTOR

Also referred to as hyperactivity of the inferior pharyngeal sphincter, cricopharyngeal impression manifests as an oval, regularly shaped, sharply demarcated, and inconstant negative defect of the posterior pharyngeal wall at the C6–C7 level (Figs. 4.31B and 6.6). It

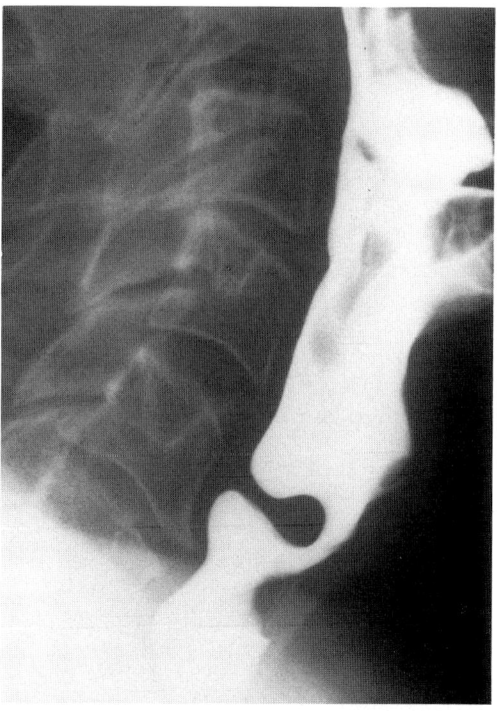

FIGURE 6.6. Cricopharyngeal impression on the hypopharynx. Defect in the posterior aspect of barium column in the hypopharynx.

results in contraction of the inferior pharyngeal sphincter at the moment when it should be relaxed. Delayed relaxation of the muscle may be a dysfunction related to achalasia of the lower esophageal segment (LES, the vestibule). While the pharynx and the esophagus participate synchronously in distal transport of the bolus and in retrograde transport, regurgitation, and vomiting, normal contraction of the inferior pharyngeal constrictor prevents reflux into the pharynx and aspiration.

Spasm of the LES, gastroesophageal reflux, hiatus hernia of the stomach, or a ring of Schatzki may result in hypertonia of the inferior pharyngeal constrictor. Patients with altered esophageal motility may have an excessively wide hypopharyngeal lumen and transient lateral pharyngeal diverticula (Fig. 6.1). Impression by an inferior pharyngeal constrictor is also seen in patients with posterior pharyngeal diverticulum (Fig. 6.7) and foreign bodies in the pharynx. Neurologic diseases may also cause a cricopharyngeal impression.

PHARYNGEAL WEBS

Pharyngeal webs are mucosal duplications that project into the lumen. They are either solitary or multiple. The majority of pharyngeal webs are located at the pharyngoesophageal junction (Fig. 6.8). Unlike a cricopharyngeal impression, which is seen on the posterior wall, they originate from the anterior pharyngeal wall, and affect a shorter segment of the hypopharynx.

Plummer–Vinson syndrome affects the middle-aged female population. It is featured by

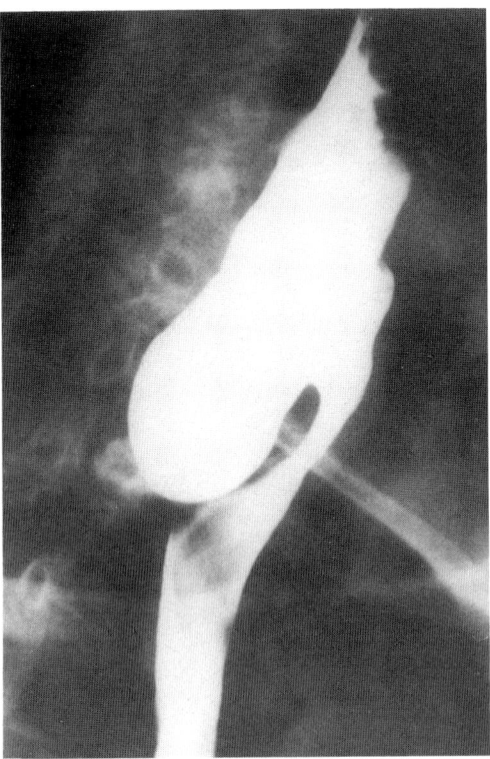

FIGURE 6.7. Large Zenker's diverticulum with cricopharyngeal impression.

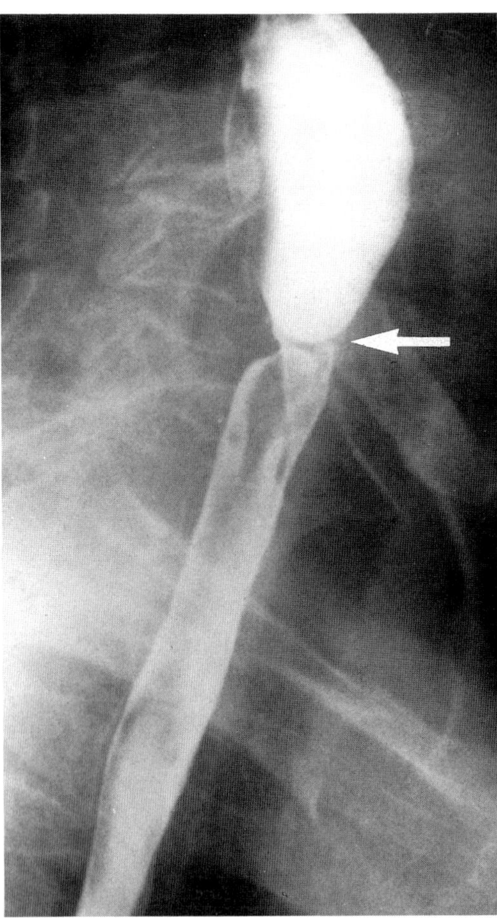

FIGURE 6.8. Web at the transition from pharynx to esophagus (arrow).

the formation of webs on the anterior pharyngeal wall, just above the transition to the esophagus. This may be associated with dysphagia, angular stomatitis, glossitis, and sideropenic anemia. However, both etiology and pathogenesis of this entity are obscure.

Esophageal webs should not be confused with the small venous plexus, a normal anatomical structure, which slightly impresses the barium column originating from the anterior aspect of esophageal wall (Fig. 6.9).

RELATIONS BETWEEN THE HYPOPHARYNX AND ADJACENT ORGANS

Pathologically altered organs adjacent to the pharynx may impress and/or infiltrate the pharyngeal wall. Large osteophytes of the cervical spine sometimes impinge on the posterior pharyngeal wall (Fig. 6.10). An enlarged thyroid gland occasionally narrows the pharyngeal lumen (Fig. 6.11).

PHARYNGEAL DIVERTICULA

Pharyngeal diverticula are either congenital or acquired. The location of diverticula is generally posterior and lateral.

Posterior diverticula (Zenker's or paraesophageal diverticula) occur in the midsagittal plane between the oblique and transverse muscle bundles of the inferior pharyngeal constrictor (Lannier's triangle). These diverticula are mucosal prolapses through muscle fibers, and are called *pulsion* diverticula. They may cause dysphagia and regurgitation, as well as aspiration. Dimensions vary from a few millimeters to sev-al centimeters in diameter (Figs. 6.7, and 6.11

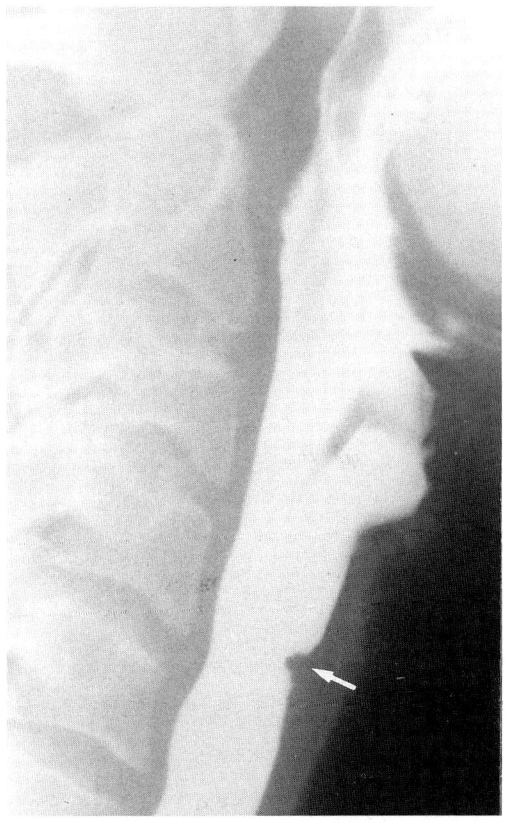

FIGURE 6.9. Defect of the anterior pharyngeal wall caused by a small venous plexus (arrow).

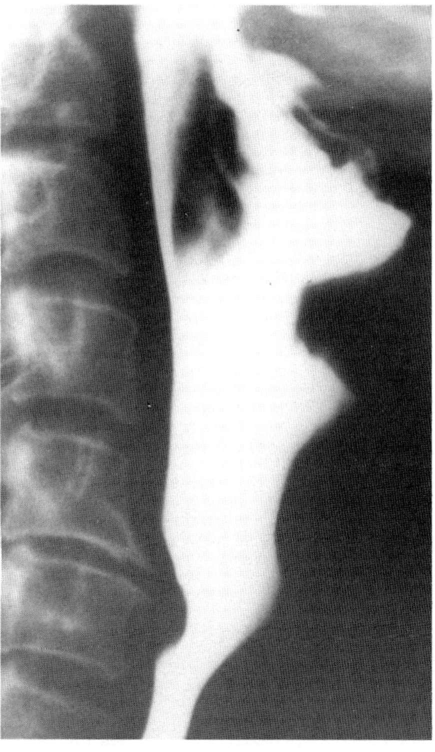

FIGURE 6.10. Impingement on the posterior pharyngeal wall by osteophytes of the cervical spine.

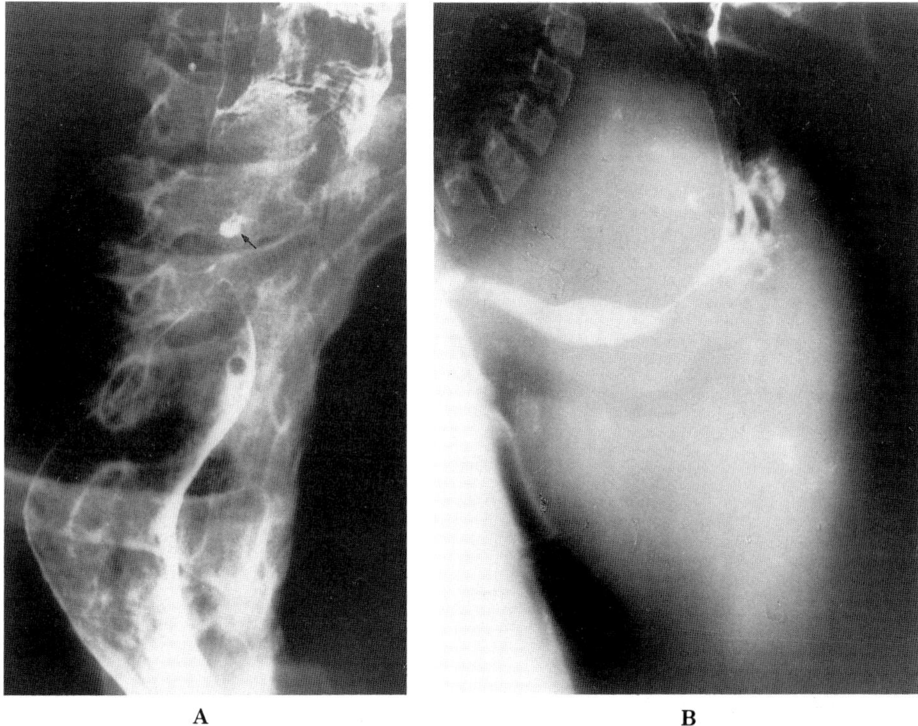

Figure 6.11. (A) Deviation of the hypopharynx and cervical esophagus with an enlarged thyroid gland. Small Zenker's diverticulum (arrow). (B) Anterior displacement of the hypopharynx, cervical esophagus, and trachea by a gigantic thyroid goiter with numerous calcifications.

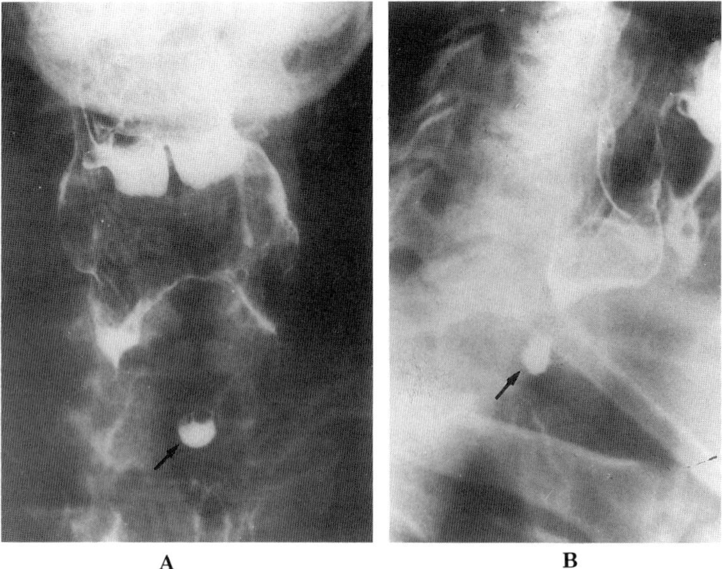

Figure 6.12. Small Zenker's diverticulum (arrows) seen in (A) AP and (B) lateral projections..

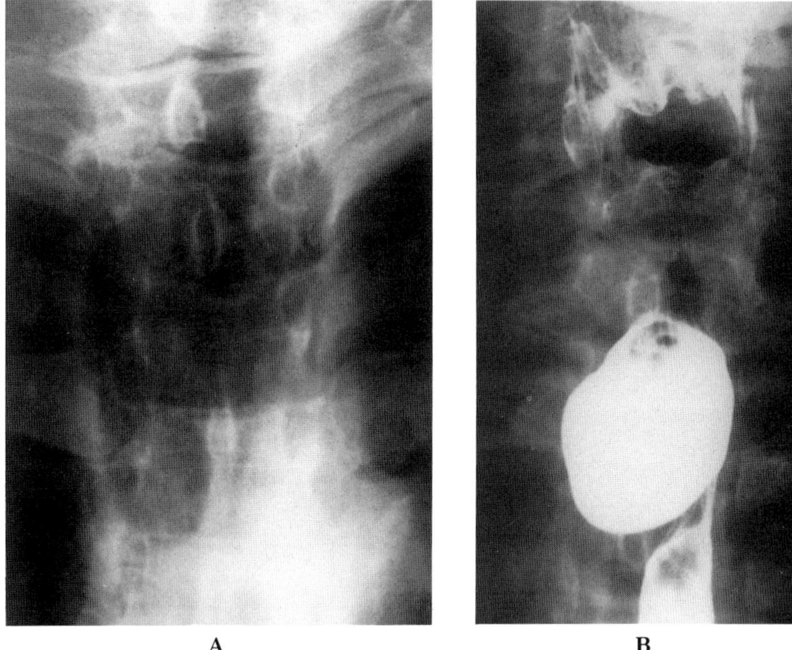

FIGURE 6.13. Giant Zenker's diverticulum, as seen on (A) plain film and (B) barium swallow.

to 6.13). Giant diverticula may extend through the upper mediastinum (Fig. 6.13). Small diverticula empty quite well. Large ones often have broad necks and contain food residues which appear as radiolucencies with barium contrast media. Radiographic examination should also detect any alterations in the passage of a barium bolus through the esophagus.

Four phases are recognizable in the development of posterior diverticula. The first is characterized by a small thorn-like diverticulum, the second with a club-shaped one; the third and the fourth phases are characterized by saccular diverticula, which in the fourth phase have a wide neck. In initial stages mucosal prolapse may be reversible.

Lateral pharyngeal diverticula are related to embryonic branchial clefts and are extremely rare (Fig. 6.14).

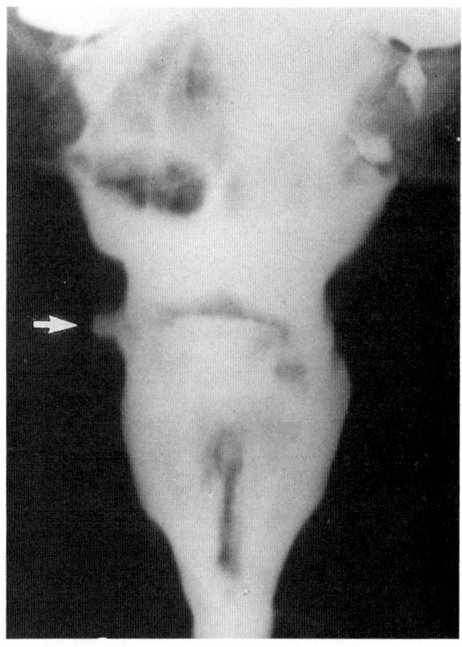

FIGURE 6.14. Lateral pharyngeal diverticulum (arrow).

RETROPHARYNGEAL ABSCESS

Widening of the retropharyngeal space characterizes a retropharyngeal abscess. It may develop from propagation of tonsillitis, presence

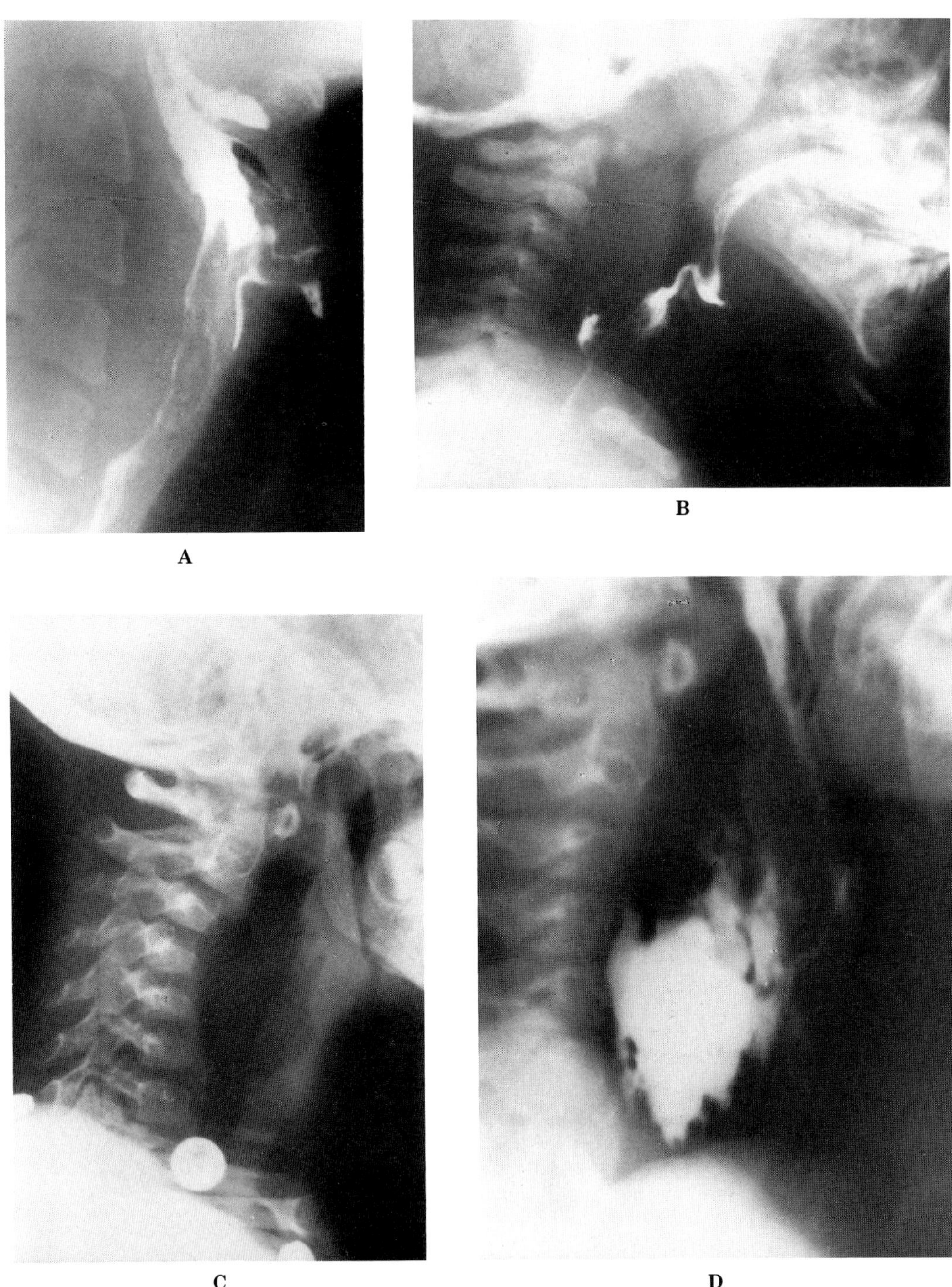

FIGURE 6.15. Retropharyngeal abscess. (A) Widened retropharyngeal space. (B) Retropharyngeal abscess in a child. The pharynx and trachea are displaced anteriorly. Barium enters an abscess cavity. (C) Gas in the abscess cavity. (D) Abscess cavity communicates with the pharynx and fills with barium.

of a foreign body in the pharyngeal wall, or the spread of inflammation from adjacent structures, as for example with tuberculous spondylitis. The distance between air in the hypopharynx and the anterior faces of the vertebral bodies is increased (Fig. 6.15A and B). The cavity of an abscess, particularly when filled with gas, appears as a radiographic transparency. An abscess may, but need not, communicate with the pharyngeal lumen; when it does communicate, it may fill with barium during a contrast examination (Fig. 6.15C and D).

NEOPLASMS

The most common pharyngeal neoplasms are *carcinomas*. They cause dysphagia in more than 60% of patients. Sometimes, when protruding into the pharyngeal lumen which is filled with air, tumors may be visible on lateral plain films. The most appropriate radiographic method to demonstrate pharyngeal neoplasms is contrast pharyngography. Neoplasms are demonstrated as radiolucent, negative, protruding defects within the pharyngeal lumen filled with barium (Fig. 6.16). Details of tumor morphology are particularly well visualized on double-contrast studies. These neoplasms frequently have irregular surfaces that thicken pharyngeal walls (Figs. 6.3, 6.17, and 6.18). Carcinomas are mainly exophytic and rarely ulcerated. Circumferential carcinomas have not been reported in the pharynx.

Various other entities may produce symptoms similar to neoplasms of the hypopharynx (Table 6.1). Unlike laryngeal carcinomas, which share biological features with cutaneous carcinomas, pharyngeal carcinomas have properties of visceral carcinomas; the prognosis is poor,

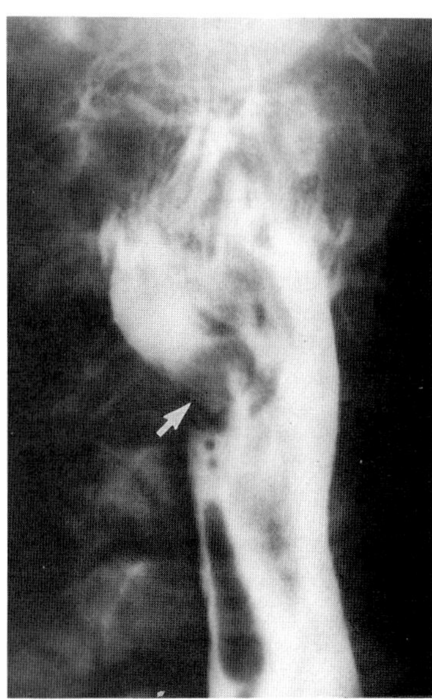

Figure 6.16. Carcinoma of the hypopharynx (arrow).

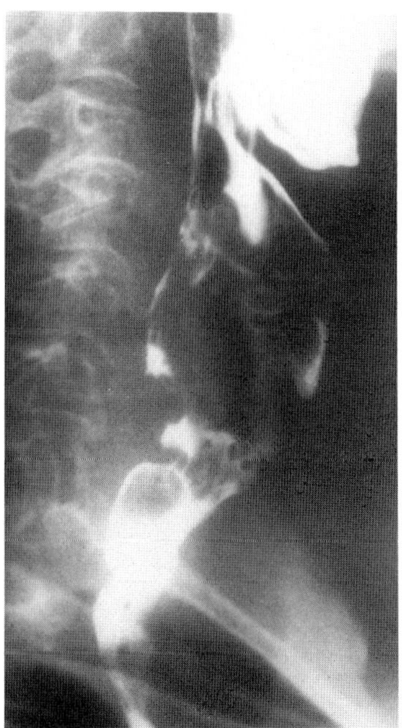

Figure 6.17. Ulcerated carcinoma involving the posterior wall of hypopharynx and esophagus.

Table 6.1. Disorders with Symptoms of Hypopharyngeal Neoplasia

Malignant pharyngeal neoplasms
Disorders of the pharyngeal phase of swallowing
Pharyngeal paresis and paralysis
Impression on the pharynx by adjacent structures
Invasion by adjacent neoplasms

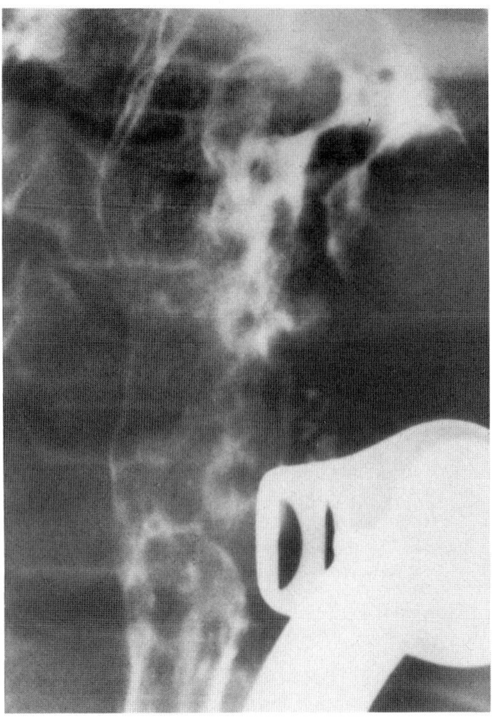

FIGURE 6.18. Carcinoma of the hypopharynx. A tracheostomy tube is in position.

and pharyngeal carcinoma is frequently fatal. Therapeutic irradiation can be followed by fibrosis of the pharyngeal wall and subsequent stenosis with decreased compliance (Fig. 6.19). Kaposi's sarcoma of the pharynx resembles carcinoma and occasionally arises in AIDS patients (Fig. 4.51).

During single-contrast pharyngography, discrete negative defects can be observed in the epiglottic valleculae. These formations mimic minute expansive growths on double-contrast studies. However, they result from irregularities at the root of the tongue, particularly when the lingual tonsil is enlarged.

FOREIGN BODIES OF THE PHARYNX

Impacted foreign bodies often lodge in the hypopharynx and cervical section of the esophagus. The position of the foreign body as well as possible perforation are examined radiologically. Foreign bodies may provoke retropharyngeal abscesses.

Radiopaque foreign bodies such as lodged bones or metallic foreign bodies are visible on plain films (Figs. 1.3 and 6.20). Foreign bodies

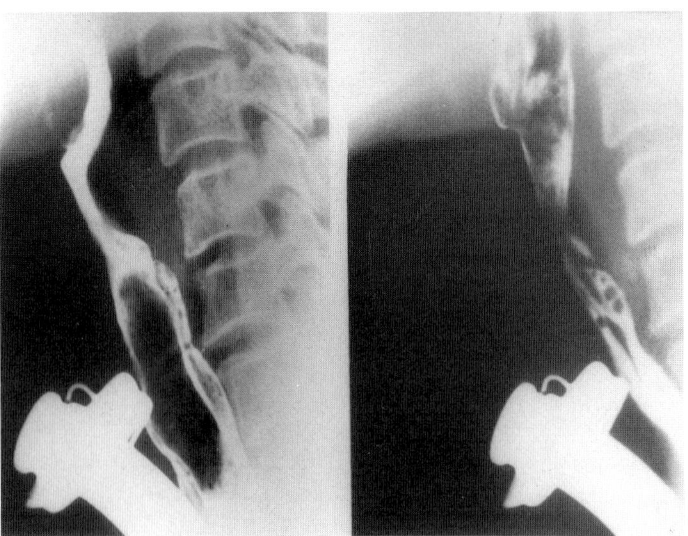

FIGURE 6.19. Laryngectomy and therapeutic radiation. Narrowing with loss of compliance of the pharyngeal wall.

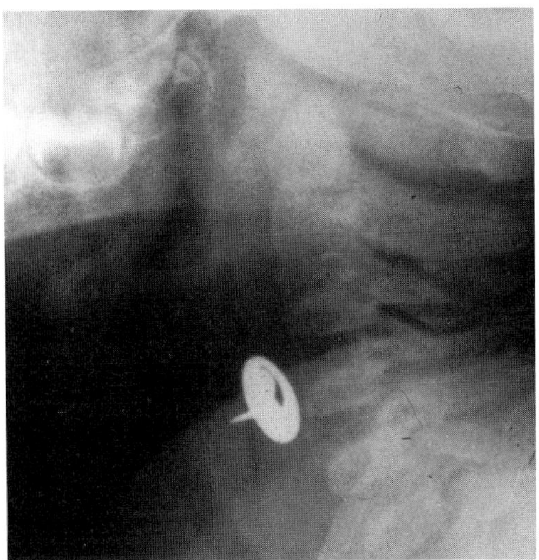

Figure 6.20. Foreign body of the hypopharynx—pushpin.

may be removed either by a balloon catheter, or by basket or forcep extraction.

Radiologic Examination and Signs in Dysphagia

The etiology of dysphagia, difficult swallowing, and odynophagia, painful swallowing, are controversial. Both entities reflect altered oral, pharyngeal, or esophageal phases of swallowing. Dysphagia may also be due to more difficult transport of the bolus into distal sections of the upper gastrointestinal tract. Difficult entry of the bolus into the stomach is the most common cause of dysphagia. Functional disorders of pharyngeal and esophageal motility are the most common causes of difficult and painful swallowing. The next most common causes are organic stenoses of the upper gastrointestinal tract, including the duodenum. These include hiatal herniation of the stomach, benign esophageal stenoses, esophagitis, achalasia, neoplasms, and scleroderma.

Dysphagia, as a consequence of esophageal stenosis, is not manifested until the lumen is reduced to approximately one-half of normal, or even less. In most cases the patient cannot locate the site of obstruction accurately. Alterations of pharyngeal and esophageal motility that cause dysphagia and odynophagia may result from organic or functional disorders. Gastric carcinoma which causes a loss of compliance of the wall and does not involve the cardia may provoke dysphagia. If esophageal motility is normal and brain metastases are excluded, dysphagia should be regarded as a nonspecific regional response to functional obstruction of the stomach. There can be increased excitability of the LES in patients with carcinoma of the gastric fornix that does not compromise transit through the cardia. "Secondary achalasia" results from damage of myenteric and submucosal plexuses by intramural growth of a neoplasm. Therefore, in patients with dysphagia the entire upper gastrointestinal tract should be examined, starting with an analysis of the oral phase of swallowing.

The technique of choice in searching for the cause of dysphagia is multiphasic examination, which includes single-contrast, double-contrast, and mucosal relief presentation of the upper gastrointestinal tract. This modality is more accurate than endoscopy in detection of altered motility, and less expensive and less uncomfortable for the patient. Videotape recording allows excellent frame-by-frame analysis.

Functional dysphagia due to primary disorders of pharyngeal and esophageal motility is a subject of the esophageal function tests discussed in chapter 4.

Bibliography

Arendt J, Wolf A. Vallecular sign; its diagnosis and clinical significance. AJR. 1947;57:435.

Akerlund A, Welin S. Roentgen diagnosis of malignant tumors within the boundary region between the pharynx and the esophagus. Acta Radiol. 1944;25:883.

Blendis LM, Sahay BM, Kreel L. The etiology of "sideropenic" web. Br J Radiol. 1965;38:112.

Borushok KF, Jeffrey RB Jr, Laing FC, Townsend RR. Sonographic diagnosis of perforation in patients with acute appendicitis. AJR. 1990;154:275.

Bucholz DW, Bosma JF, Donner MW. Adaptation, compensation and decompensation of the pharyngeal swallow. Gastrointest Radiol. 1985;10:235.

Buckstein J, Reich S. Lateral pharyngeal diverticula as a cause of dysphagia. JAMA. 1950;144:1154.

Crishlow TVL. The cricopharyngeus in radiography and cineradiography. Br J Radiol. 1956;29:546.

Curtis DJ, Crusess DF, Berg T. The cricopharyngeal muscle – a videorecording review. AJR. 1984;142: 497.

Donner MW, Silbiger ML. Cinefluorographic analysis of pharyngeal swallowing in neuromuscular disorders. Am J Med Sci. 1966;251:134.

Donner MW, Bosma JF, Robertson DL. Anatomy and physiology of the pharynx. Gastrointest Radiol. 1985;10:196.

Dunhill TF. Pharyngeal diverticulum. Br J Surg. 1940;37:404.

Ekberg O, Nylander G. Lateral diverticula from the pharyngoesophageal junction area. Radiology. 1983;146:117.

Ekberg O, Wahlgren L. Pharyngeal dysfunctions and their interrelationship in patients with dysphagia. Acta Radiol Diagn. 1985;26:695.

Halpert RD, Spickler E, Feczko PJ. Dysphagia in patients with gastric cancer and normal esophagogram. Radiology. 1985;154:589.

Halpert RD, Feczko PJ, Spickler EM, Ackerman LV. Radiologic assessment of dysphagia with endoscopic correlation. Radiology. 1985;157:599.

Hilding DA, Tachdjian MO. Dysphagia and hypertrophic spurring of the cervical spine. N Engl J Med. 1960;263:11.

Holmgren BS. Sideropenic dysphagia or cancer of the hypopharynx? Acta Radiol. 1943;24:455.

Hoover WB: The syndrome of anemia, glossitis and dysphagia. N Engl J Med. 1935;213:394.

Jones B, Ravich WJ, Donner MW, Kramer SS. Pharyngoesophageal interrelationships: observations and concepts. Gastrointest Radiol. 1985;10: 225.

Margulis AR, Koehler RE. Radiologic diagnosis of disordered esophageal motility. Radiol Clin North Am. 1976;14:429.

Pfakler GE. The roentgen diagnosis of treatment of carcinoma of the larynx and pharynx. Radiology. 1939;33:42.

Phillips MM, Hendrix TR. Dysphagia. Postgrad Med. 1971;50:81.

Shaffer HA Jr, Alford BA, de Lange EE, Meyer GA, McIlnenny J. Basket extraction of esophageal foreign bodies. AJR. 1986;147:1010.

Torres WE, Clements L Jr, Austin GE, Knight K. Cricopharyngeal muscle hypertrophy: radiologic – anatomic correlation. AJR. 1984;141:927.

Welin S. Deglutition anomaly simulating hypopharyngeal cancer. Acta Radiol. 1939;20:452.

Chapter 7

Radiology of the Esophagus

Although ingested food or contrast media do not change in character while passing from the pharynx to the stomach, the esophagus is not a simple elastic tube. It transports contents from a region of low pressure in the thorax, into a region of much higher but also variable pressure in the abdomen. A complex peristaltic process transports swallowed contents of the esophagus in all body postures, and, by a still insufficiently explained mechanism, prevents the reflux of gastric contents (except in vomiting, when gastric and duodenal contents empty via the esophagus). Complex coordination of striated and smooth muscles by the central nervous system is necessary for all esophageal motoric functions. On account of its close contacts with adjacent anatomical structures, the esophagus is essential as an indicator of pathologic events in the mediastinum.

Introduction of multiphasic examination of the esophagus has improved diagnosis of esophageal diseases and adjacent pathology. Hypotonic esophagography using glucagon or Buscopan can provide additional data. Abnormalities were found in the esophagus of 15% of the patients who underwent multiphasic upper gastrointestinal tract examination.

The anterior contour of the esophagus is indented by normal anatomical structures. These are, from the cephalad direction, the aortic arch, left primary bronchus or left pulmonary artery, and left inferior pulmonary veins. When the patient is not swallowing, the esophagus remains collapsed.

The similar subjective symptoms of various esophageal diseases make their mutual differentiation difficult. Dysphagia (difficulty in swallowing) and less commonly odynophagia (pain on swallowing) are the most important manifestations of esophageal diseases and functional disorders.

FUNCTIONAL DISORDERS

Motor functions of the esophagus are well-balanced and develop in a rapid sequence. In view of this, and because of good visualization by radiologic procedures, motility is better studied in the esophagus than in any other alimentary canal organ. Consequently, motility dysfunctions seem to be more common in the esophagus. Esophageal motility can be studied by upper gastrointestinal series with films and video-recording or rapid-sequence radiography, as well as by radionuclide or manometric studies. Esophageal peristalsis is studied by observation of the tail of the barium column.

Disorders of motility can be primary or secondary. In the former the main affected organ is the esophagus and in the latter the esophagus is one of several diseased organs. *Primary motility disorders* are manifested by disturbed peristalsis, dysfunction of the gastroesophageal vestibule, or a combination of both of these. Primary dysfunctions of esophageal motility are achalasia, symptomatic idiopathic diffuse esophageal spasm, and nonspecific motoric disturbances, such as increased frequency of tertiary esophageal contractions and focal esophageal contractions, breaking of the primary peristaltic wave, or lack of peristalsis.

Secondary disorders include scleroderma

and other collagenoses. Gastric neoplasms can affect esophageal motility without infiltrating the cardia (Fig. 7.1). However, narrowing of the cardia results in proximal dilatation. Pseudo-achalasia results from malignancies of distant organs. Secondary achalasia is the consequence of infiltration of the vestibule (LES) with a malignant growth (Fig. 7.1B).

The width of the esophageal lumen depends on muscle tone in the main esophageal muscular layer. There is an inversely proportional relationship between tone and the threshold for provocation of peristalsis. The destruction of the intramural neuronal network by infiltrative processes leads to dilatation of the esophagus. The esophagus should be considered hypotonic when the lumen is wider than 3 cm and when a bolus initiates only a faint wave of primary peristalsis or fails to initiate peristalsis altogether. While assessment of the rate of distal propagation and amplitude of peristaltic waves is being made, the patient is to lie flat on a horizontal fluoroscopic table, in order to minimize the influence of gravity on the bolus transportation.

Both primary and secondary esophageal peristaltic waves transport a bolus into the stomach. Tertiary waves do not have propulsive properties (see chapter 2 describing the act of swallowing). When peristalsis and esophageal contractions are fluoroscopically studied, compliance of the esophageal wall can be estimated.

In patients with scleroderma and achalasia, primary peristaltic waves are of low amplitude. They do not transport the bolus adequately, and can even be missing.

A secondary peristaltic wave propagates bi-

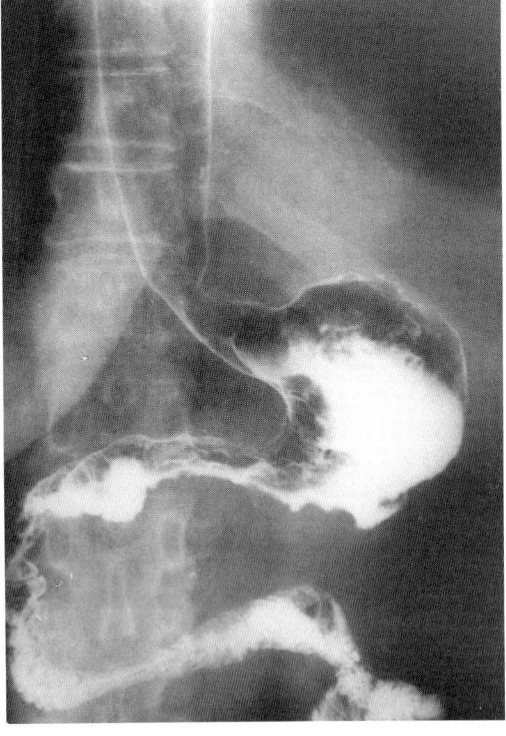

A

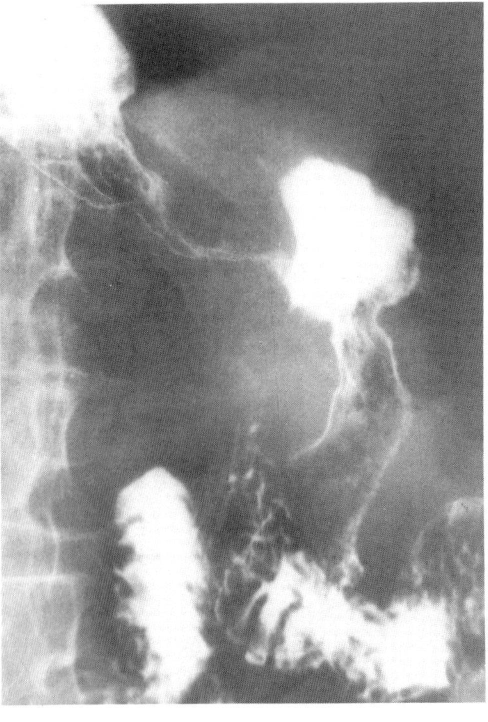

B

Figure 7.1. Distension of the esophagus resulting from carcinoma affecting the body and antrum of the stomach. Cardia and vestibule (lower esophageal segment) are not involved. (B) Distension of the esophagus results from carcinoma narrowing the vestibule and infiltrating the entire gastric stump.

directionally from the place of origin. However, the proximal wave extends only a few centimeters leaving a predominantly distal wave. Secondary peristalsis is the normal phenomenon by which food remnants are cleared from the esophagus to the stomach.

Tertiary contractions of the esophagus (Fig. 7.2) are a series of local ring-shaped muscular contractions. They are not peristaltic and do not propel esophageal contents into the stomach. When associated with a significant increase in intraluminal pressure they can be the cause of dysphagia and odynophagia. In normal middle-aged subjects tertiary contractions can represent 20% of esophageal motility. With aging, this ratio increases. In very old individuals, tertiary contractions can provide a majority of esophageal motility.

Functional disorders of the esophagus result in slowed transport of the bolus into the stomach. The rate of transportation of a bolus through the esophagus can be estimated by tests of esophageal function. These tests are not valid in the presence of organic lesions. However, they are useful when dealing with "pure," that is, isolated, functional disorders. Abnormal esophageal motility recorded during barium examination indicates the necessity of a multiphasic examination to reveal underlying lesions. Not infrequently, discrete inflammatory lesions, gastroesophageal reflux, or small neoplasms can be detected.

Several months after myocardial infarction, functional disorders of the esophagus may be found in one-third of the patients. These disorders can be confirmed by barium swallow, ma-

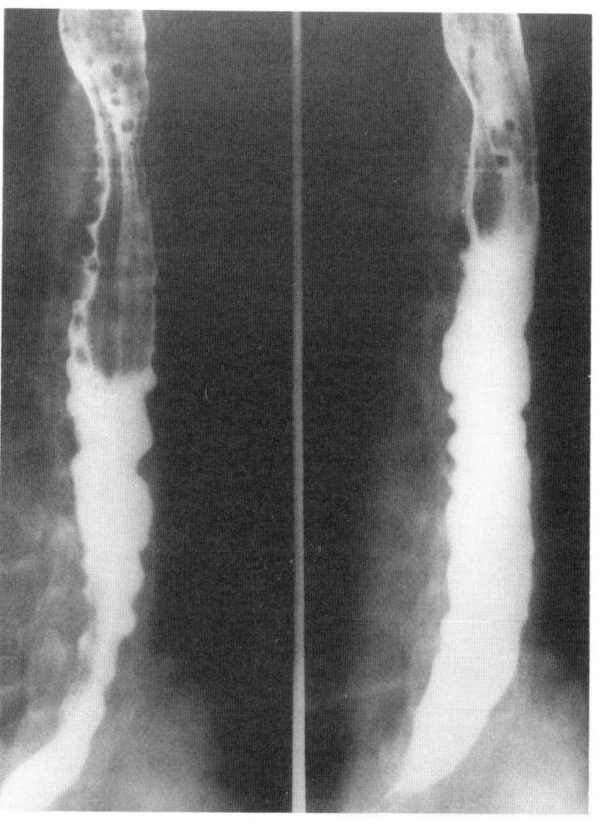

A

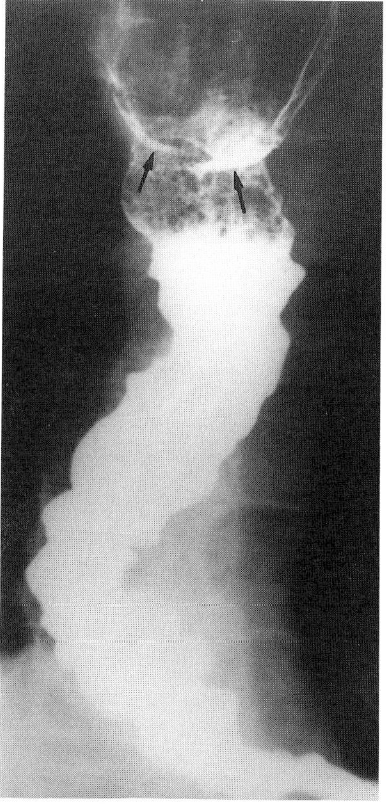

B

Figure 7.2. (A) Tertiary contractions of the esophagus manifest as a series of ring-like narrowings. (B) Tertiary esophageal contractions in achalasia. Large diverticulum of the proximal esophagus (arrows).

nometry, or by pH measurement, referring to dysfunction of the gastroesophageal vestibule.

The muscular tone of the gastroesophageal vestibule is increased by gastrin and acetylcholine. In contrast, glucagon, secretin, cholecystokinin, and some of the prostaglandins lower the tone of the vestibule.

SYMPTOMATIC IDIOPATHIC DIFFUSE ESOPHAGEAL SPASM

Symptomatic diffuse esophageal spasm is characterized by intense, relatively short-lasting chest pain, dysphagia, and odynophagia. Fluoroscopic examination during an attack reveals deep tertiary contractions accompanied by manometrically established increase in intraluminal pressure. The principal muscles and muscularis mucosae are often hypertrophic. Degenerative changes in the fibers of the vagus nerve exist. Hot beverages, emotional stress, and gastroesophageal reflux are provocative factors.

THE "NUTCRACKER ESOPHAGUS"

The main complaints of nutcracker esophagus, also called esophageal contractions of high amplitude, are odynophagia and dysphagia. Manometrically and fluoroscopically normal primary peristalsis is demonstrated in the proximal two-thirds of the esophagus. However, contractions of very high amplitude appear distally. Radiologic findings are normal or demonstrate nonspecific changes. In addition to normal primary peristalsis, in one-half of patients, tertiary contractions can appear during swallowing. Opinions of various authors disagree on whether nutcracker esophagus transforms into symptomatic diffuse esophageal spasm. There are indications that these disorders are related. The major role of the radiologic examination is to rule out organic lesions such as inflammation, ulcer, and neoplasia.

ACHALASIA

Achalasia is absence of smooth muscle relaxation within the alimentary canal. This results in muscle hypertrophy and proximal dilatation. Achalasia is most common in the lower esophagus where the peristaltic wave does not cause relaxation of the LES, the gastroesophageal vestibule.

The disease is not hereditary, and can be found, with the same frequency in both sexes, in 1/100,000 of the general population. A very rare form of familial achalasia was found in 5% of affected patients and begins in childhood. The exact mechanism of esophageal achalasia is not completely understood, since spasm of the lower esophageal segment has not been demonstrated.

In patients with achalasia, cells of the myenteric plexus are missing, particularly in the region of the esophagogastric junction. Fibrosis of the muscles gives rise to loss of intermuscular connections. In a similar manner as retrograde degeneration of axons and perikaryons of ganglion cells that occurs in the brain, there is comparable data about degeneration and destruction of myenteric plexus cells.

In achalasia, function of the upper esophageal segment is preserved. However, the lower esophageal segment is particularly sensitive to nervous stimulation and gastrin. In patients with achalasia, inhibitory impulses which maintain the resting tone are missing. In the course of deglutition the relaxation of the lower esophageal segment is incomplete. Consequently, proximal dilatation of the esophagus gradually develops.

It is not completely understood why proximal dilatation of the esophagus is less pronounced in patients with long-standing distal stenoses of the esophagus as a result of corrosive lesions or reflux esophagitis than in patients with achalasia. A neuromuscular abnormality most probably affects the entire esophagus. In patients with achalasia, slowly evolving changes are one of the factors leading to massive dilatation of the esophagus.

Chest films may reveal widening of the mediastinum and, at times, an air-fluid level in the distended esophagus. The air bubble in the stomach is reduced or missing (Fig. 7.3). A sip of barium will demonstrate the widened esophageal lumen. The lower esophageal segment appears narrowed with a regular contour resembling a "rat's tail" (Fig. 7.4). Peristalsis is lacking in the thoracic segment of the esophagus and superficial tertiary contractions may be seen. In the earlier stages of the disease, deep indentations of the barium column caused

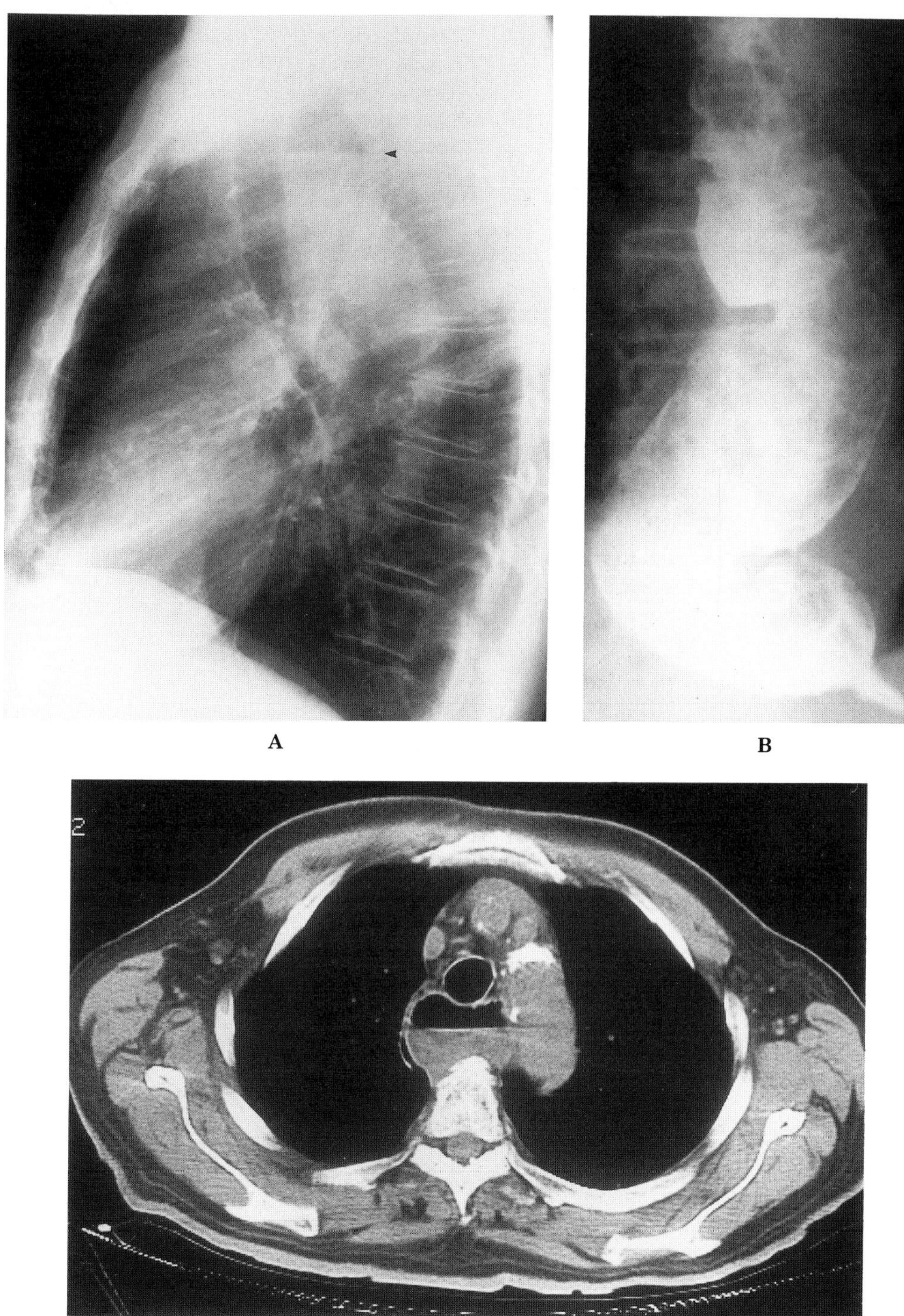

FIGURE 7.3. Advanced achalasia. (A) Air-fluid level in a widened esophagus (arrowhead) with displacement of the trachea anteriorly. (B) Barium study. (C) CT examination.

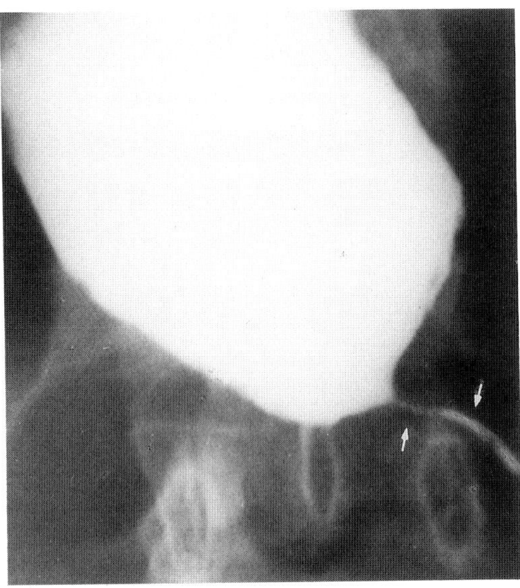

FIGURE 7.4. "Rat's-tail" appearance of the lower esophageal segment (arrows) with significant dilatation of the tubular segment in achalasia.

by tertiary contractions with vigorous achalasia may occur (Fig. 7.5); later there may be a transformation into the hypotonic or atonic form of the disease (Fig. 7.6). Esophageal contents stagnate in the widened lumen and present as negative defects (Fig. 7.3B and C). The LES allows passage of the esophageal contents into the stomach when the hydrostatic pressure is high enough to overcome the resistance caused by the resting tone of the sphincter. Mecholyl provokes painful contractions of denervated esophagus, and therefore can be used in diagnosing achalasia. Muscles of the proximal esophagus react inadequately to ganglionic cell stimulators, and confirm the data which support lack of ganglionic cells in this region. Inhibitory β-adrenergic receptors function normally.

Disorders with symptoms similar to those of achalasia are presented in Table 7.1. Of utmost importance is distinguishing achalasia from infiltrating carcinoma of the lower esophageal segment. Stenosis caused by malignant growth has irregular contours, and pliability of

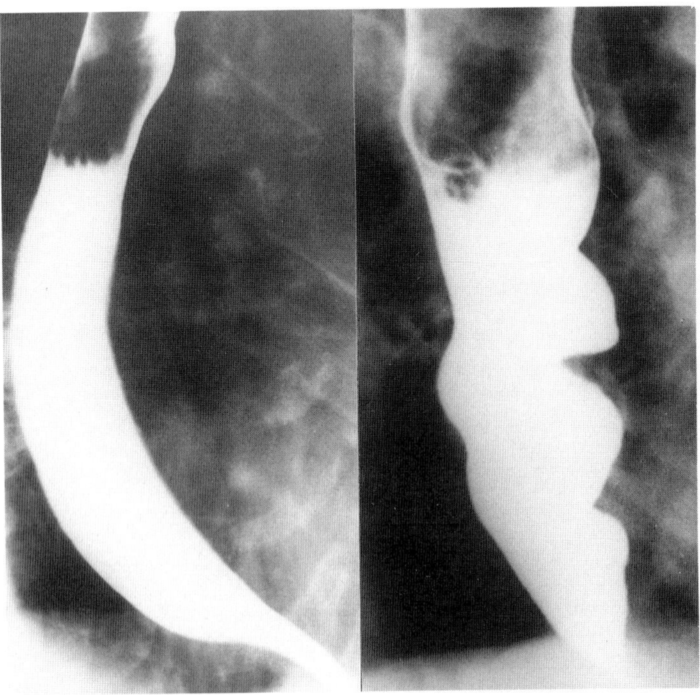

FIGURE 7.5. Moderate achalasia (left). Vigorous achalasia with deep tertiary contractions (right).

Table 7.1. Disorders with Symptoms of Achalasia

Idiopathic (primary) achalasia
Primary malignancy of the distal esophagus
Gastric carcinoma affecting the distal esophagus
Neoplasms of the tubular esophagus affecting the distal esophagus
"Pseudoachalasia" due to neoplasms in distant organs

the wall is completely lacking. However, sometimes only a sloping of the esophageal contour can be seen. Patients with newly discovered achalasia must be examined endoscopically and biopsy should be performed.

Synchronous carcinoma of the lower esophageal segment can develop in patients with achalasia (Fig. 7.7). Such tumors are difficult to discover by radiologic examination, especially when they are small. Proximally situated carcinomas are discovered more readily.

Invasive carcinoma affecting the lower esophageal segment is usually adenocarcinoma of the stomach (Fig. 7.8); this may be difficult to distinguish from achalasia. By infiltrating the esophageal wall this tumor destroys the myenteric plexus. When adenocarcinoma of the stomach infiltrates the lower esophageal segment, the narrowed portion is often longer than in achalasia. The presence of even slightly prominent sloping or "shoulders" at the transition between normal and tumor tissue indicates the malignant nature of the lesion.

Chagas' disease is caused by *Trypanosoma cruzi*. The esophageal appearance mimics achalasia with a *megaesophagus* pattern. However, the alimentary canal may also be affected distal to the stomach. Megaesophagus is a common finding in patients with Riley-Day's syndrome (familial dysautonomia).

Radiologic, endoscopic, and manometric signs closely resembling achalasia may appear in patients with extragastrointestinal malignancies. These are carcinomas of the bronchus, prostate, pancreas, and liver as well as lymphomas. They do not directly affect the esophagus or other segments of the alimentary canal. In patients with primary idiopathic achalasia, the onset of dysphagia is sudden, despite the more gradual evolution of other symptoms. The real causes for this phenomenon are not well understood. Infiltration of the cerebral stem by metastatic growth or destruction of periesophageal nervous plexuses by secondary tumors may be the cause. The "pseudoachalasia" may be part of a paraneoplastic syndrome. Withdrawal of

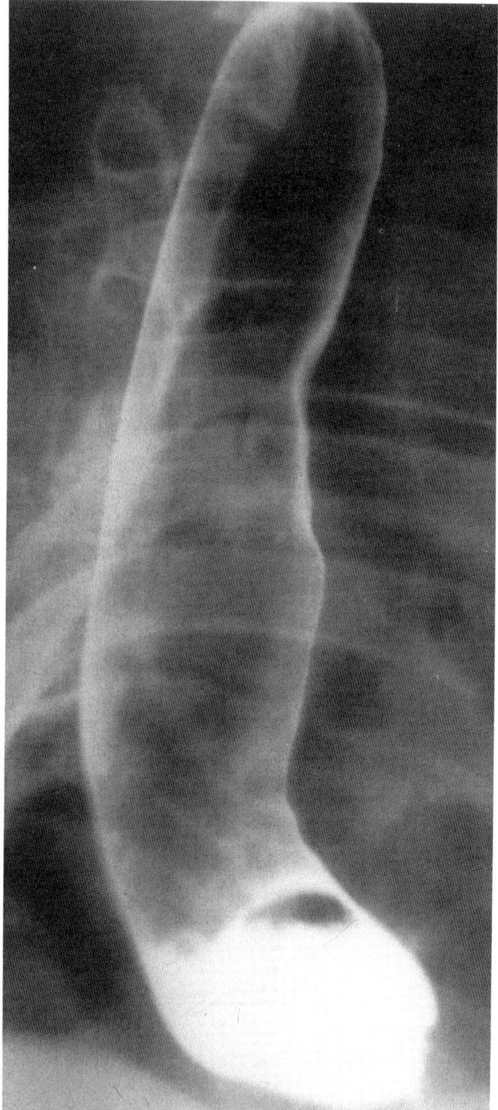

Figure 7.6. Advanced achalasia with significant dilatation of the esophagus.

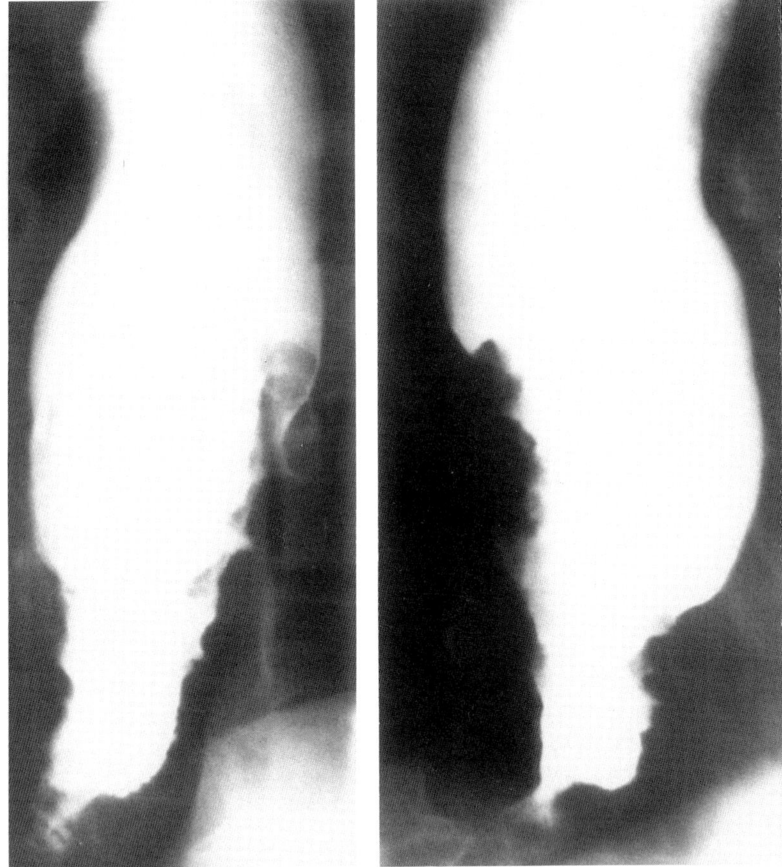

FIGURE 7.7. Esophageal carcinoma in achalasia.

the symptoms has been reported with treatment and resolution of the tumor.

CHALASIA

Chalasia denotes relaxation of sphincters that should be contracted. Chalasia of the gastric cardia is relaxation of the lower esophageal sphincter, resulting in gastroesophageal reflux. Radiologically, there is displacement of gastric contents into the esophagus (Fig. 7.9).

In the majority of newborns, the sphincteric function of the LES is not established until the third week of life. However, chalasia should not be considered a pathologic state even in the first six months after birth. It is commonly seen in prematures, and has even been evident in newborns and children with lesions of the central nervous system. Peptic esophagitis secondary to gastroesophageal reflux in newborns can result in stenosis and shortening of the esophagus.

Idiopathic chalasia in adults is the result of decreased tone of the LES.

MISCELLANEOUS MOTILITY DISORDERS

A series of diseases may affect motility of the esophagus. These are:

1. Diseases of the central nervous system:
   - Parkinson's syndrome
   - Vascular disorders
   - Amyotrophic lateral sclerosis

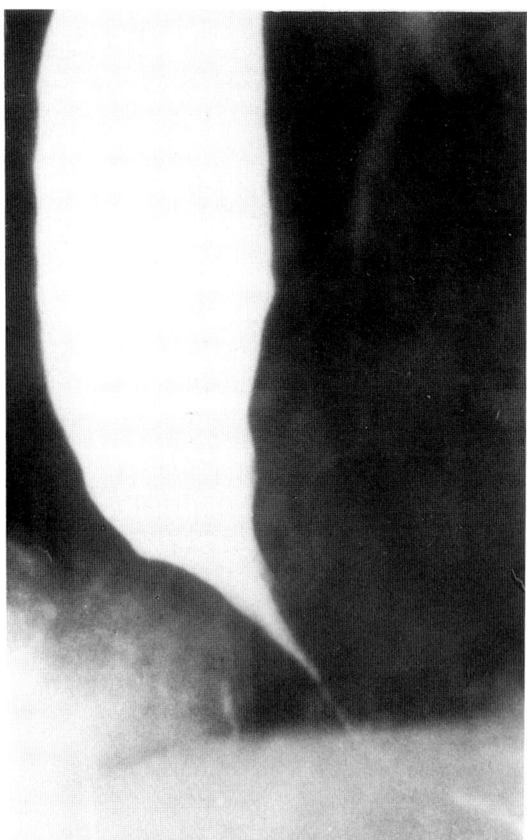

FIGURE 7.8. Gastric adenocarcinoma affecting the distal esophagus. Narrowed section is longer than the lower esophageal segment (vestibule). Sloping of the right contour results from carcinomatous infiltration.

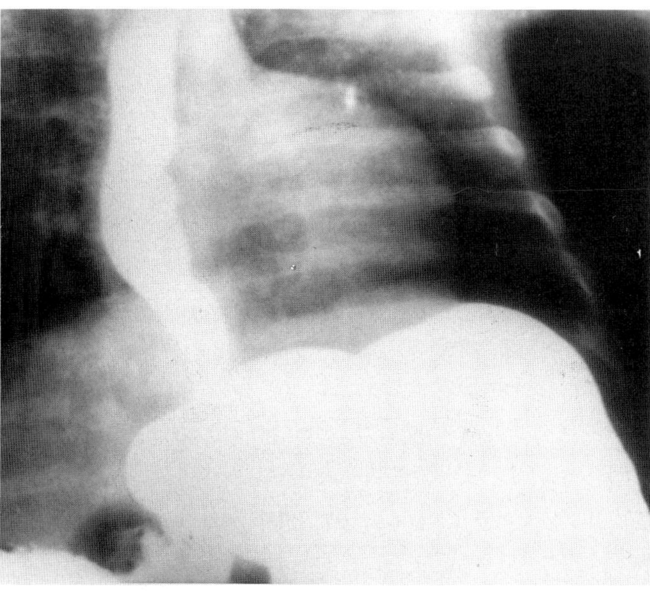

FIGURE 7.9. Free gastroesophageal reflux in the supine position.

2. Peripheral neuropathies:
   Diabetes
   Alcoholic damage
3. Changes of local ganglionic systems:
   Decreasing number of ganglionic cells:
      Achalasia
      Neoplastic diseases
4. Irritation of ganglia:
   Gastroesophageal reflux
   Esophagitis
   Caustic lesions
   Stress
5. Myoneural junction disorders:
   Myasthenia gravis

PRESBYESOPHAGUS

Presbyesophagus is characterized by slowed transport of esophageal contents, tertiary contractions, dilatation of the lumen, and gastroesophageal reflux. Primary and secondary peristaltic waves are infrequent and superficial. Function of the lower esophageal segment is often abnormal and sphincteric action may be diminished or may resemble the early phase of achalasia. Since this disorder occurs primarily in elderly patients a degenerative process is suspected. Dysphagia is a common symptom.

TABLE 7.2. STENOSES AND IMPRESSIONS ON THE ESOPHAGUS

CAUSED BY EXTERNAL COMPRESSION
Struma of the thyroid gland
Fibrosis of apical and mediastinal pleura
Spondylophytes
Anomalous and aberrant vessels
Enlarged left cardiac atrium
Widened and tortuous aorta
Mediastinal neoplasms
CAUSED BY ESOPHAGEAL WALL LESIONS
Benign
Reflux esophagitis
Corrosive strictures
Postinflammatory strictures
Neoplasms
Malignant
Primary esophageal neoplasms
Secondary esophageal neoplasms

ABNORMAL POSITION OF THE ESOPHAGUS

Numerous conditions alter the course and/or lumen of the esophagus (Table 7.2). Pronounced *spondylosis* or *osteochondrosis* of the cervical spine can impinge on the posterior aspect of the pharynx or esophagus (Fig. 6.10). Similar effects can be produced by deformities and spurring, resulting from trauma or degenerative process, of the cervical or thoracic segments of the vertebral column (Fig. 7.10). *Pleuritic* changes and *fibrosis* of pulmonary api-

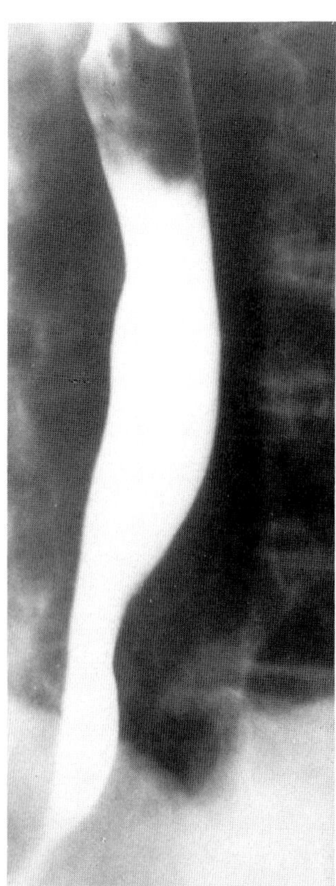

FIGURE 7.10. Impingement of large thoracic spine spondylophytes on the posterior aspect of the esophagus.

ces may cause deviation of the esophagus and trachea (Fig. 7.11). An enlarged *thyroid* gland may displace the cervical segment of the esophagus (Figs. 7.12 and 7.13).

An elongated and tortuous aorta may push the esophagus anteriorly and leftward. This is particularly pronounced when there is aneurysmal enlargement (Fig. 7.14).

An enlarged *left atrium* (Fig. 7.15) displaces the esophagus posteriorly and to the right. Impingement is below the bifurcation of the trachea and is one of the earliest radiographic signs of left atrium enlargement. When pronounced, the impression mimics an esophageal tumor on films taken in the supine position (Fig. 7.15B). *Neoplasms of the posterior mediastinum*, for example, lymphoma, neurogenic tumors, and metastases in mediastinal lymph nodes, can indent the esophagus or infiltrate its wall (Fig. 7.16).

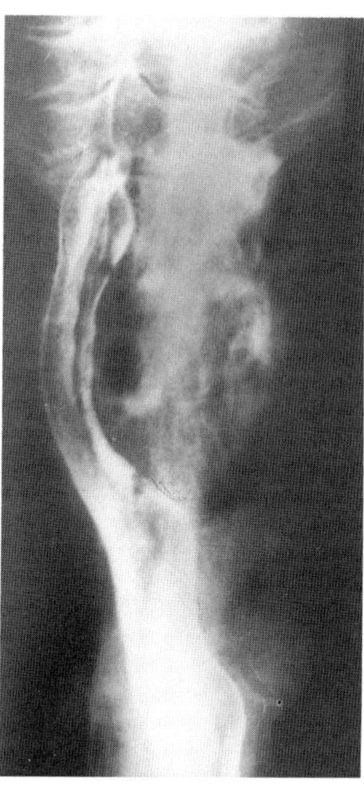

Figure 7.12. Deviation of the esophagus by a thyroid goiter with calcifications.

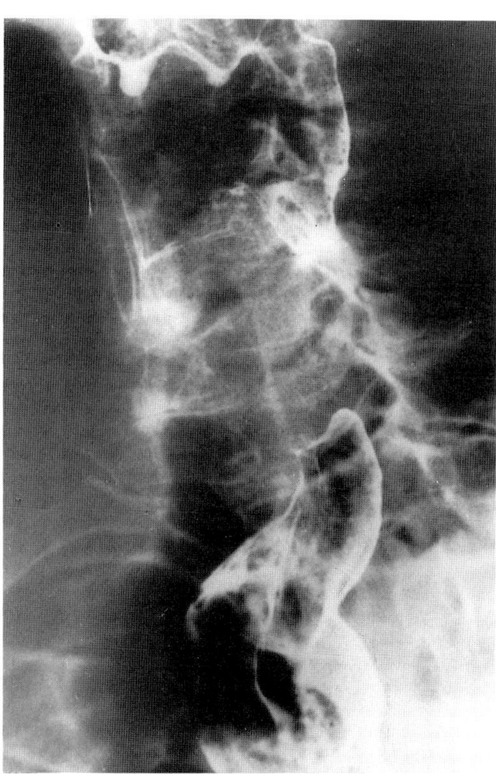

Figure 7.11. Deviation of the distal cervical and proximal thoracic esophagus by pleural fibrosis.

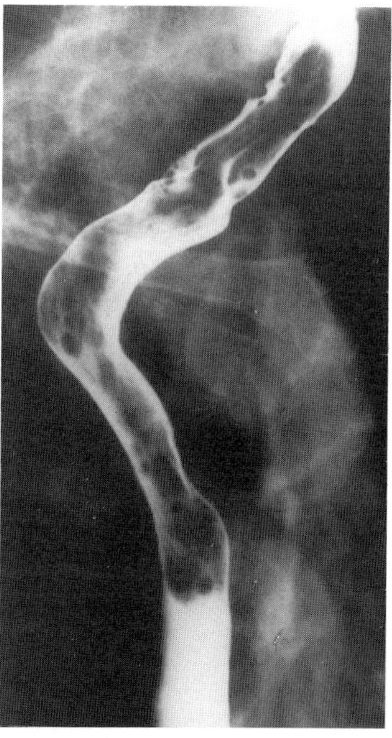

Figure 7.13. Displacement of the esophagus by a substernal goiter.

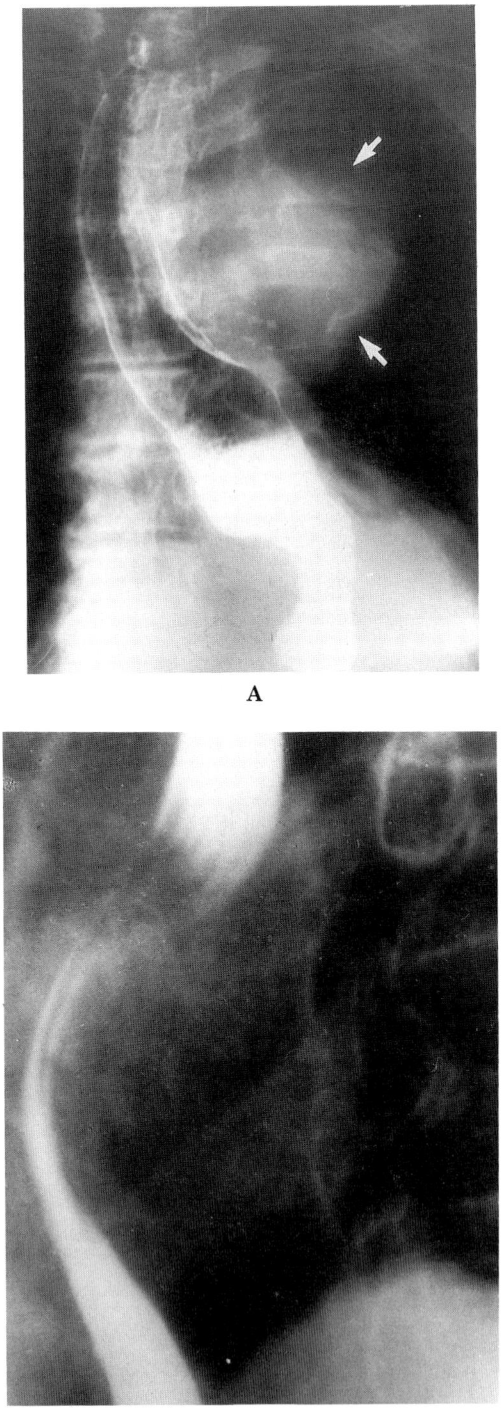

A

B

FIGURE 7.14. Aortic aneurysm. (A) Calcification (arrows) and dislocation of the esophagus. (B) Anterior dislocation of the distal esophagus.

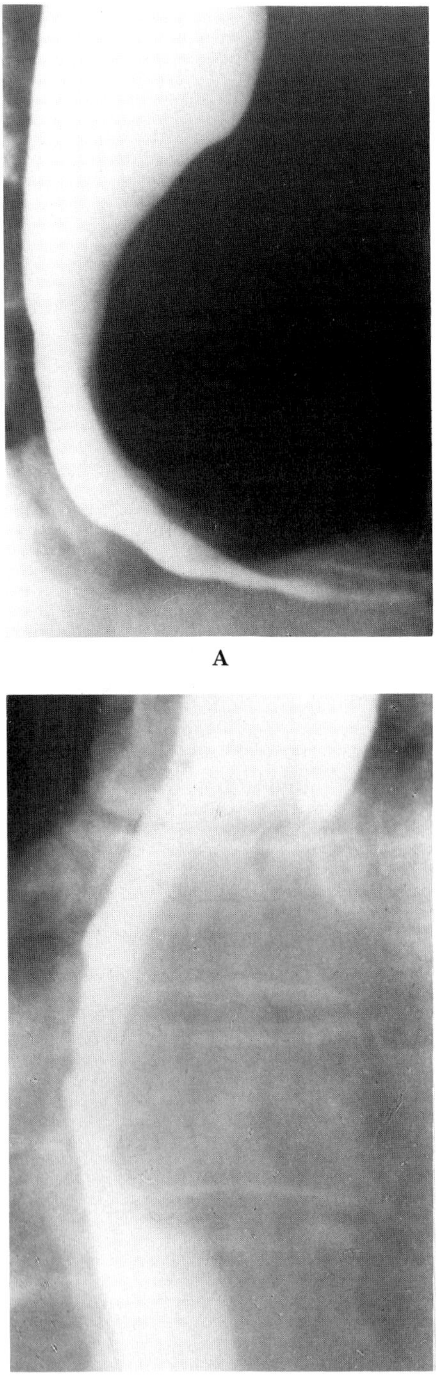

A

B

FIGURE 7.15. Impression on the esophagus by an enlarged left cardiac atrium. (A) Profile projection. (B) Supine position. The finding resembles an esophageal neoplasm.

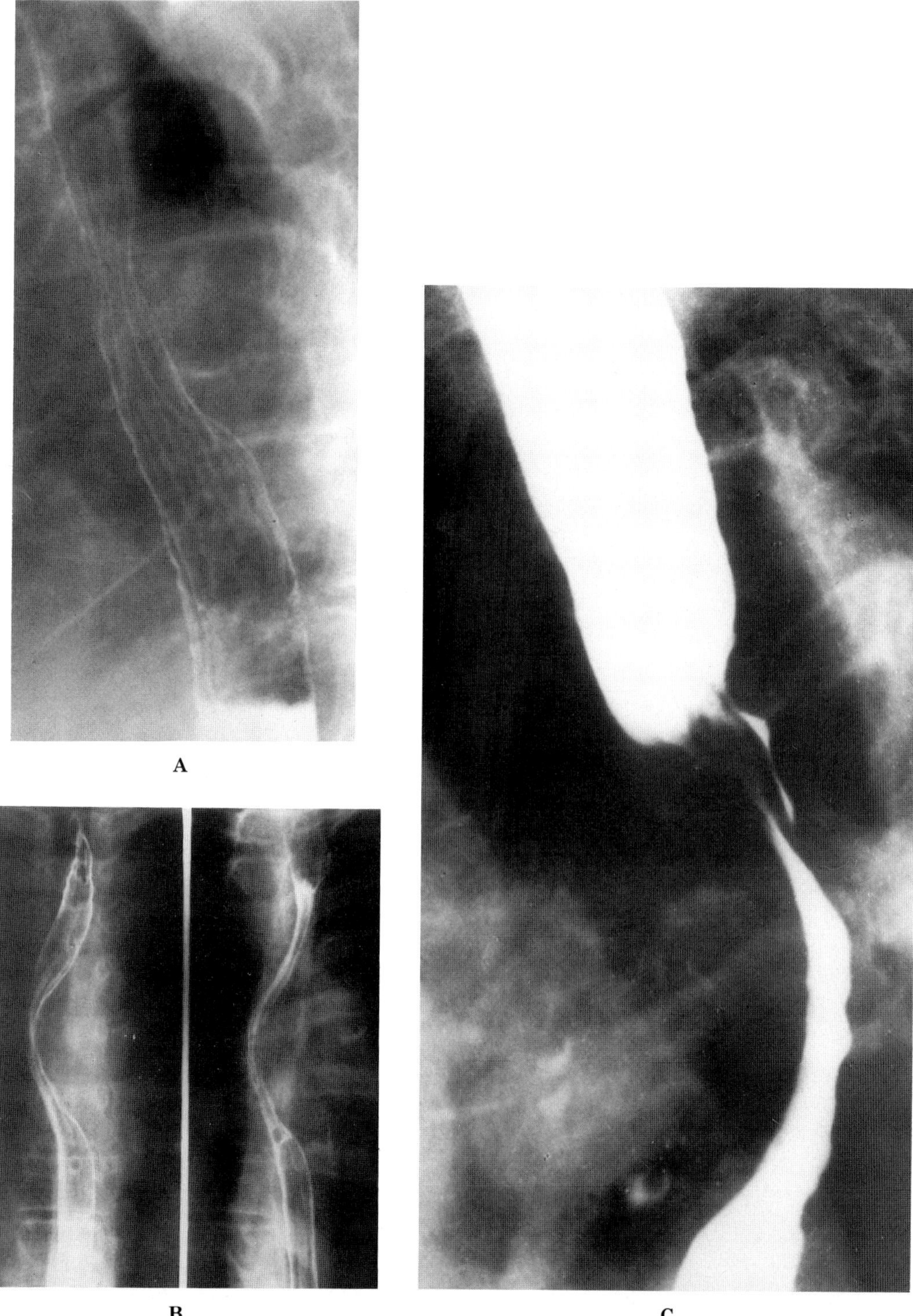

Figure 7.16. (A) and (B) Displacement of the esophagus by enlarged mediastinal lymph nodes. (C) Infiltration of the esophagus by lung carcinoma.

CONGENITAL MALFORMATIONS

Children with esophageal *atresia* cannot feed or handle secretions. If the lower segment does not communicate with the airway the alimentary canal is devoid of gas. Atresia can be proved by chest radiography following introduction of a radiopaque catheter into the blind pouch. Routine use of contrast media is usually contraindicated. If utilized, less than 1 mL of water-soluble, isotonic, nonionic solution should be injected through a flexible, soft tube with careful fluoroscopic guidance. After the proximal pouch has been demonstrated (Fig. 7.17), contrast medium should be removed. In fact, in all children with symptoms of upper alimentary tract obstruction, contrast medium should be introduced through a thin tube and immediately evacuated after the examination.

The morphology of various types of esophageal atresia is presented in Diagram 7.1. In more than 90% of patients with atresia com-

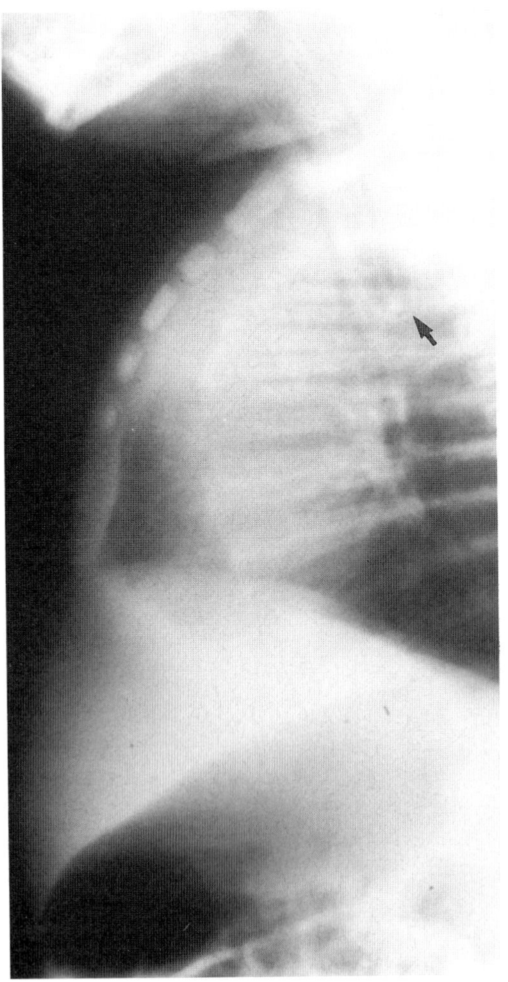

A

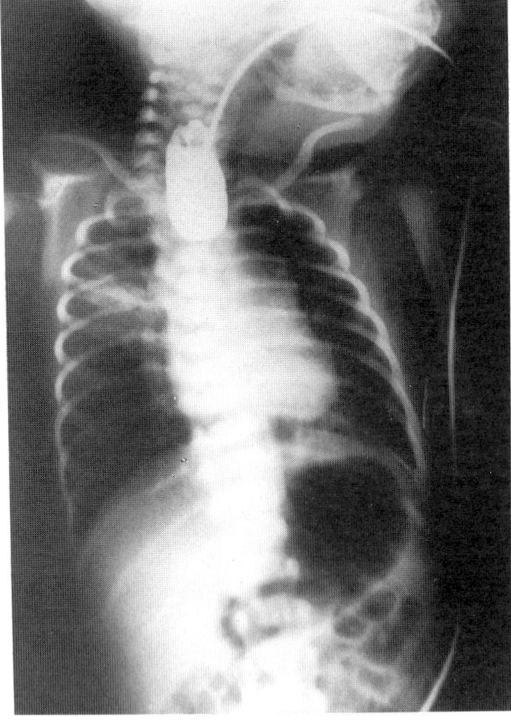

B

Figure 7.17. Esophageal atresia with distal tracheo-esophageal communication. Air is present in the stomach and gut. Demonstration of the blind pouch by (A) catheter coiling (arrow). (B) Administration of water-soluble, isotonic, nonionic contrast medium through a thin, soft catheter. Contrast medium should be removed immediately after examination. Air in the stomach and bowel indicates distal fistula. Right-sided pneumonia is probably related to previous aspiration. Contrast medium is unnecessary to establish the diagnosis. The figure is used only for purpose of illustration.

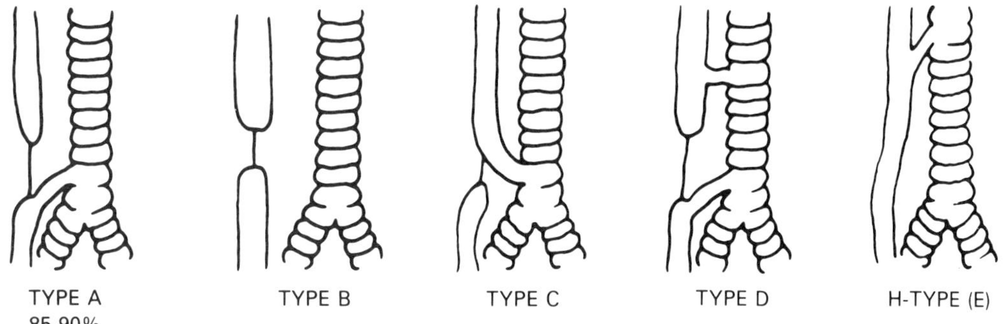

DIAGRAM 7.1. Types of esophageal atresia.

munication with the trachea is present. It is not always possible to determine the type of atresia by conventional radiologic examination.

Esophageal atresia appears with a prevalence of 1 in 2000 live births. There is no sex predilection. It is commonly associated with other congenital anomalies, but a hereditary basis has not been proved.

Esophagotracheal fistula can be present without esophageal atresia. It is most likely to be discovered when the child begins to eat solid food. Presence of a fistula is manifested by recurrent, sometimes chronic pneumonia, particularly in the right lung. The fistulous canal is often very narrow and may not be shown by initial barium examination (Fig. 7.18).

Esophageal *duplications* are very infrequent. They rarely communicate with the main lumen (Fig. 7.19) or fill with contrast medium. However, when they do not communicate, they only impress the esophageal wall.

There are several types of esophageal *steno-*

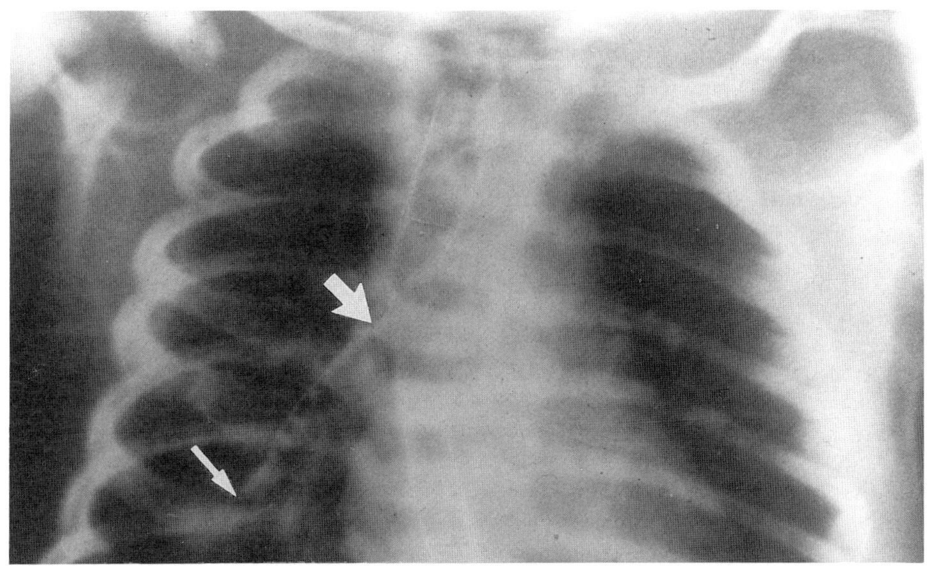

FIGURE 7.18. Tracheosophageal fistula (upper arrow). Contrast medium in the bronchus (lower arrow).

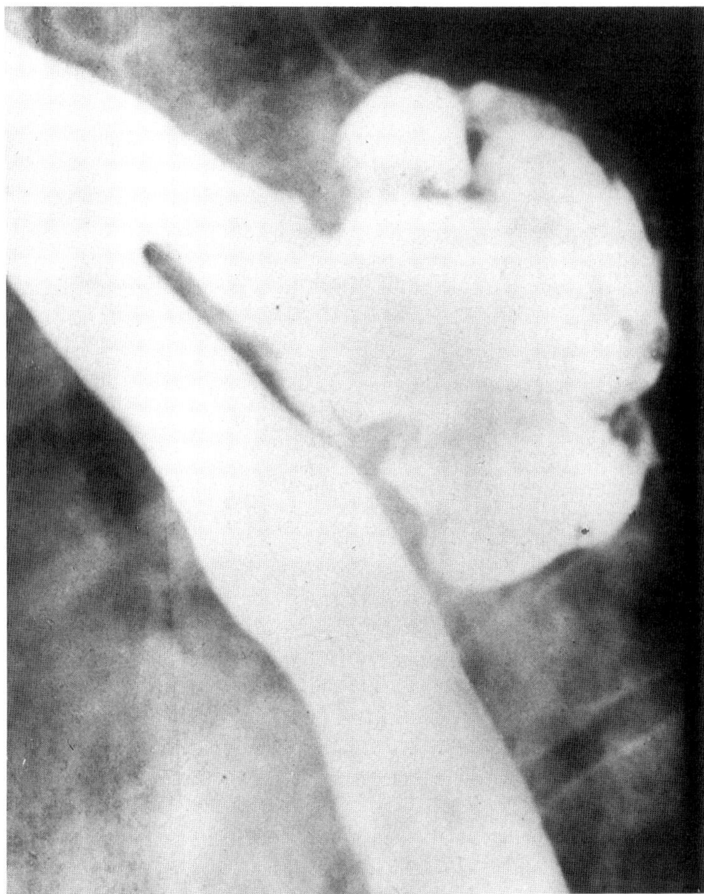

FIGURE 7.19. Communicating duplication of the esophagus.

ses. In *tubular* stenoses, the narrowed esophageal segment is usually 1–3 cm long (Fig. 7.20). However, congenital stenoses may be longer (Fig. 7.20B). The majority of congenital tubular stenoses are located at the transition between the middle and distal portions of the esophagus, and are more common in the lower than in the upper portion. The etiology of congenital esophageal stenoses is unknown. Failure of fusion in epithelial vacuoles, intrauterine vascular insufficiency, and peptic esophagitis have been mentioned as possible causative factors. However, congenital stenoses might be the consequence of failed differentiation of the respiratory system. Congenital tubular stenoses possess benign features. Transition to the normal wall is gradual and mucosal surface is preserved. In contrast, stenoses due to malignant processes have an abrupt transitional zone and destroy mucosal relief in the region occupied by the tumor. The esophagus can be narrowed by compression caused by adjacent anatomical structures (Table 7.2). A double aortic arch narrows the esophagus by bilateral impression, with one side higher than the other (Fig. 7.21). *Valvular stenoses*, also known as *webs* (Fig. 7.22), may resemble a ring or a sail. Multiple congenital stenoses have also been described. Symptoms of dysphagia manifest later if food is insufficiently masticated, and a larger bolus results. In 20% of patients with dysphagia, webs can be found in the cervical portion of the esophagus. As large webs are not common, the usual discrete webs often escape detection on conventional barium examination. Diagnosis is facilitated by video-recording of the bar-

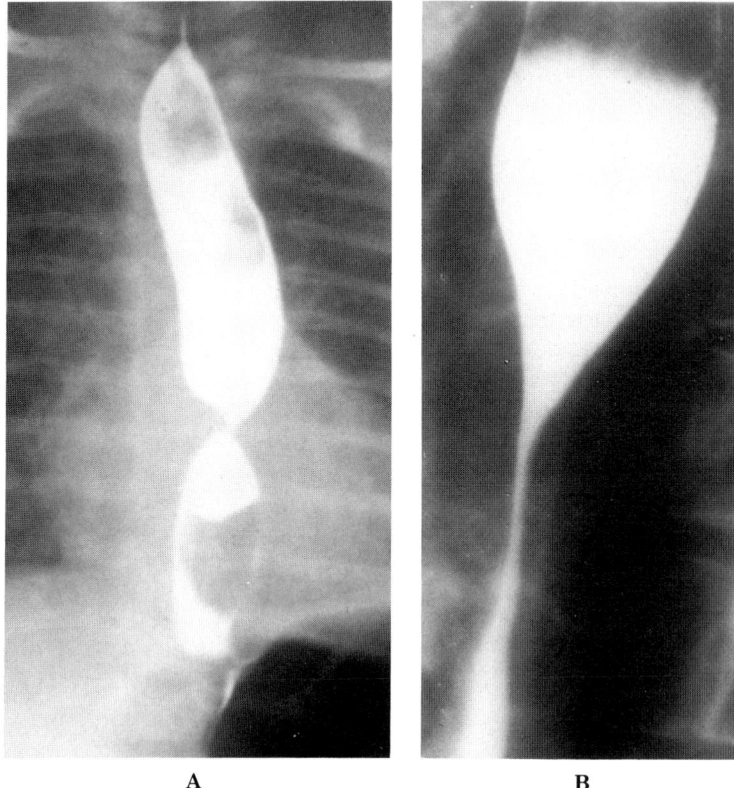

FIGURE 7.20. Congenital esophageal tubular stenoses. (A) Short esophageal stenosis at the junction of the middle and distal third of the esophagus with proximal dilatation. (B) Long stenosis with significant proximal dilatation.

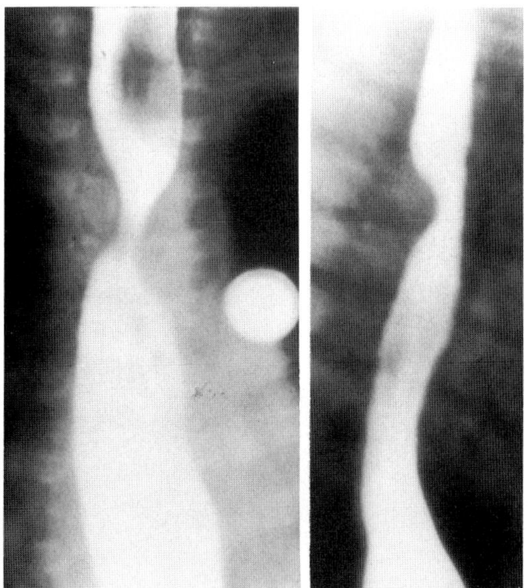

FIGURE 7.21. Double aortic arch causing bilateral impingement on the esophagus, and tracheal narrowing.

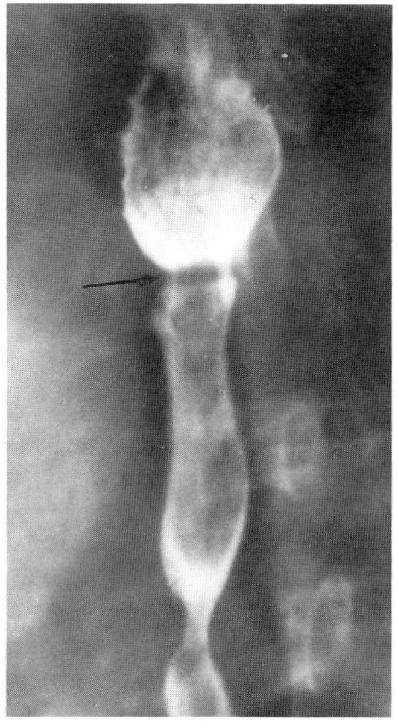

A

B

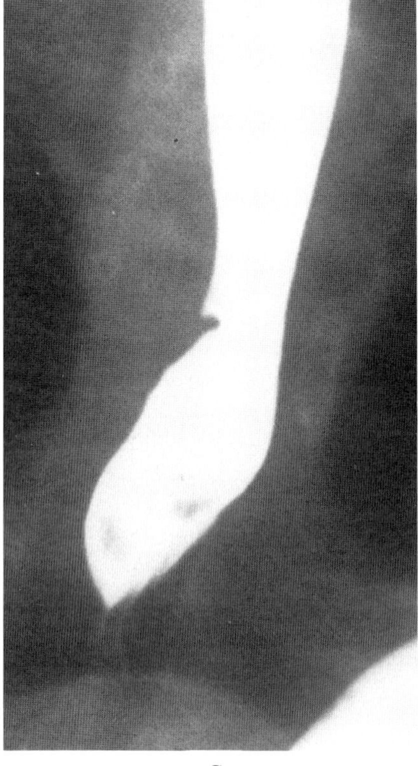

C

FIGURE 7.22. Congenital esophageal webs. (A) Web of the proximal esophagus (arrow). (B) Small anterior wall web of the proximal esophagus (arrow). (C) Web of the anterior wall of distal esophagus.

ium swallow. Webs can be easily differentiated from other pathologic states of the esophagus. They typically have the appearance of thin radiolucent defects protruding from the anterior wall into the esophageal lumen.

The *aorta* physiologically impresses the esophagus from the left anterior direction. A left-sided aortic arch descending to the right of the esophagus indents its posterior and left aspects. A right-sided aortic arch which descends ipsilaterally is associated with imprints on the posterior right aspect of the esophagus (Fig. 7.23).

An *aberrant right subclavian* artery, *arteria lusoria*, arises from the aortic arch distal to the left subclavian artery. Traversing upward to the other side, it passes between the esophagus and the spine causing a band-like horizontal or slightly oblique regular defect on the posterior esophageal wall (Fig. 7.24). A comparable defect can originate from a right aortic arch and extend in a similar manner to the left. This finding is usually incidental but associated symptoms have been referred to as dysphagia lusoria.

CONGENITALLY SHORT ESOPHAGUS

Congenitally short esophagus, *brachyesophagus*, is a very rare congenital anomaly. Since the stomach never appears under the diaphragm, this condition should not be consid-

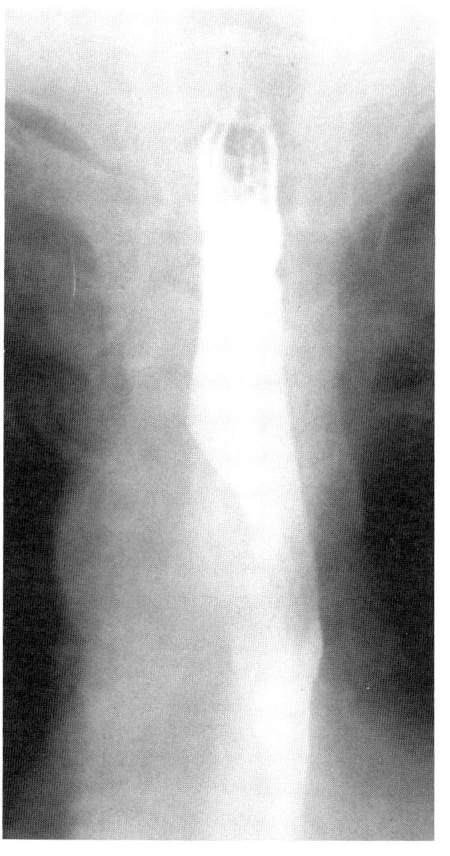

A

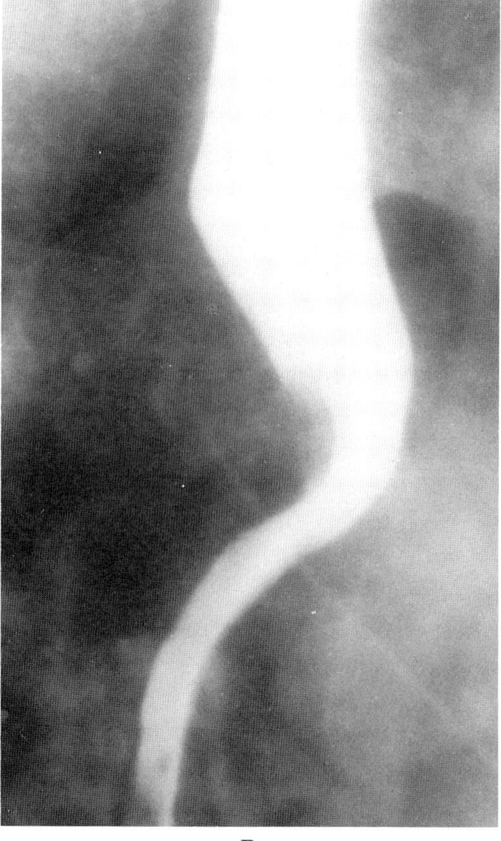

B

FIGURE 7.23. Right-sided aortic arch. (A) P-A projection demonstrates impingement on the esophagus from the right side. (B) Profile projection.

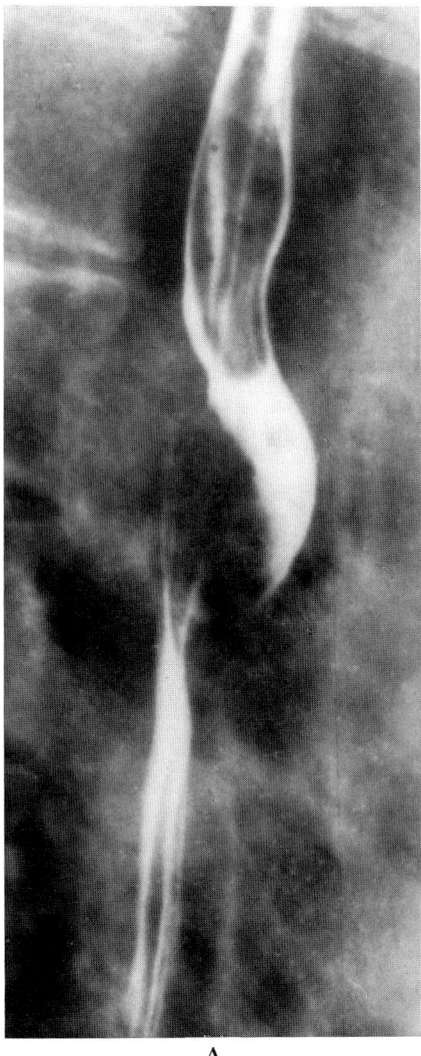

A

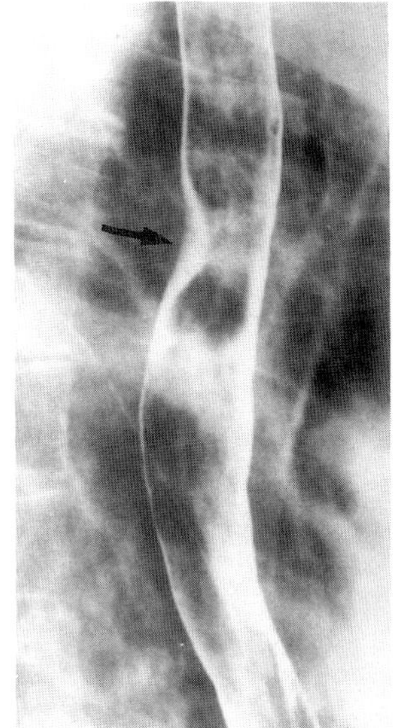

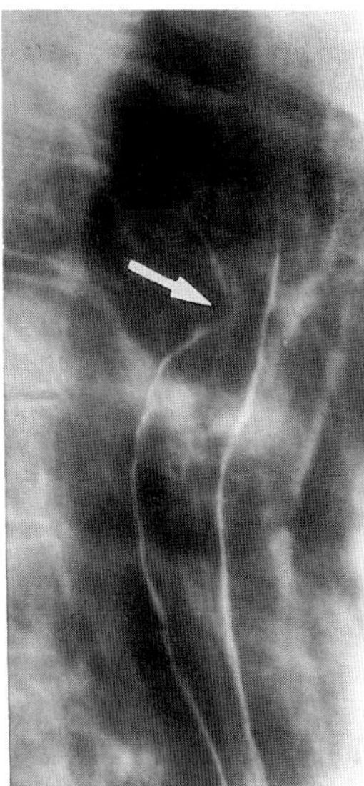

B

Figure 7.24. Aberrant right subclavian artery producing a negative linear defect on the posterior esophageal aspect. (A) Pronounced impression on single-contrast study. (B) Double-contrast study (arrow).

ered a hiatus hernia. Peptic esophagitis may result when gastroesophageal reflux is present. Differential diagnostic considerations should include hiatal hernia and a phrenic ampulla.

Congenitally Narrow Esophagus

This is an extremely rare phenomenon. The entire esophageal lumen is narrow (Fig. 7.25). Patients are without symptoms and therefore it is an incidental finding. Esophageal functions are well preserved.

ESOPHAGEAL DIVERTICULA

True diverticula of the esophagus are protrusions of all layers of the wall. In contrast, false diverticula are prolapses of mucosa and submucosa between the bundles of the main muscular layer. Distinction between the two is not possible on radiologic grounds alone. Radiologic examination should document the capability of the diverticulum to empty its contents. Prolonged stagnation of material in the lumen of the diverticulum is considered an indication

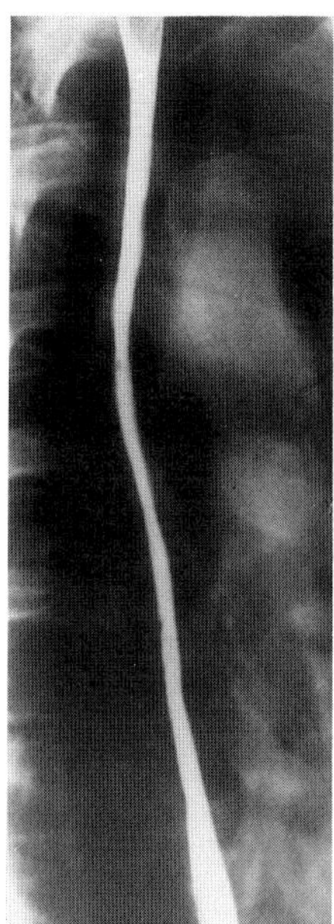

FIGURE 7.25. Congenitally narrowed esophagus.

for therapy. Diverticula of the esophagus are demonstrated in at least 3% of correctly performed examinations of the esophagus. Pulsion diverticula (Figs. 7.26 and 7.27) can be either

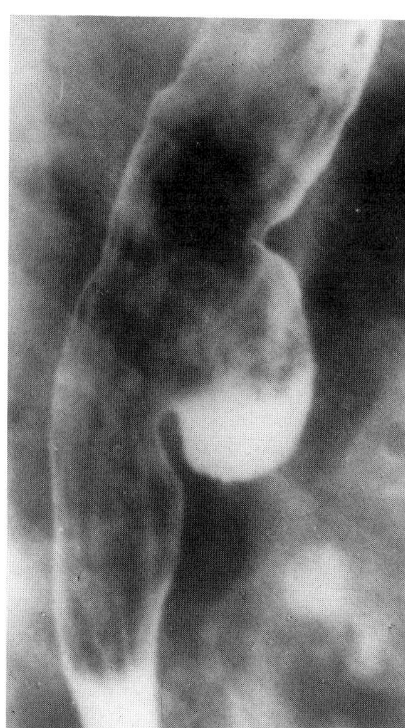

FIGURE 7.26. Pulsion diverticulum of the esophagus.

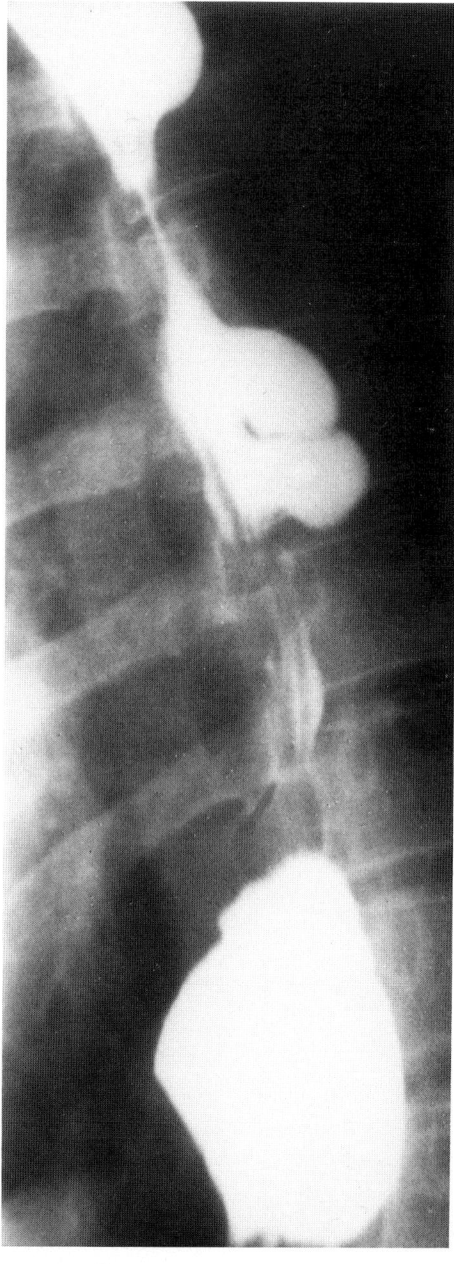

FIGURE 7.27. Multiple esophageal pulsion diverticula. Gastric hiatus hernia.

congenital or acquired. They are of round shape and directed caudally. They communicate with the esophageal lumen via the neck, which may be of various widths.

Traction diverticula resemble a tilted tent and have a wide neck (Fig. 7.28). They result from adhesions to inflammatory lymph nodes. Traction-pulsion diverticula possess combined features (Fig. 7.29). About 70% of esophageal diverticula are situated in the middle third of the esophagus. The anterior wall diverticula are the commonest. All types of diverticula are best shown when the esophageal wall is contracted (Fig. 4.3). In contrast to esophageal ulcers, diverticula change their dimensions during the course of examination.

Only epiphrenic diverticula may cause differential diagnostic problems (Figs. 7.30 and 7.31). They should be differentiated from phrenic ampullae, hiatal hernias, and large esophageal ulcers (Table 7.3).

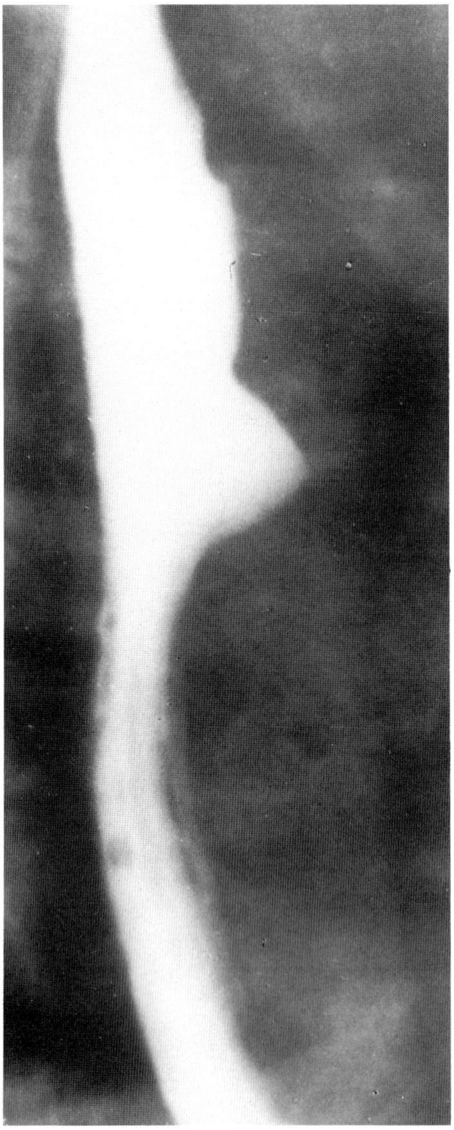

FIGURE 7.28. Traction diverticulum of the esophagus.

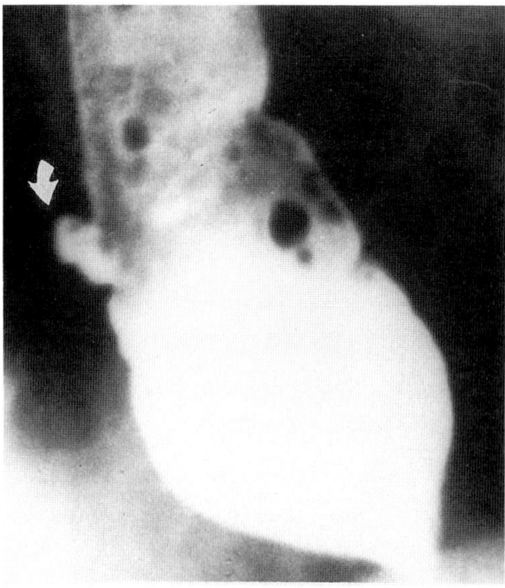

FIGURE 7.29. Epiphrenic traction-pulsion diverticulum of the lower esophageal segment (arrow) with hiatus hernia of the stomach. Several air bubbles are in the esophageal lumen.

TABLE 7.3. DIFFERENTIAL DIAGNOSIS OF AN EPIPHRENIC DIVERTICULUM

Phrenic ampulla
Hiatus hernia
Paraesophageal hernia
Large esophageal peptic ulceration
Ulcerated esophageal neoplasm

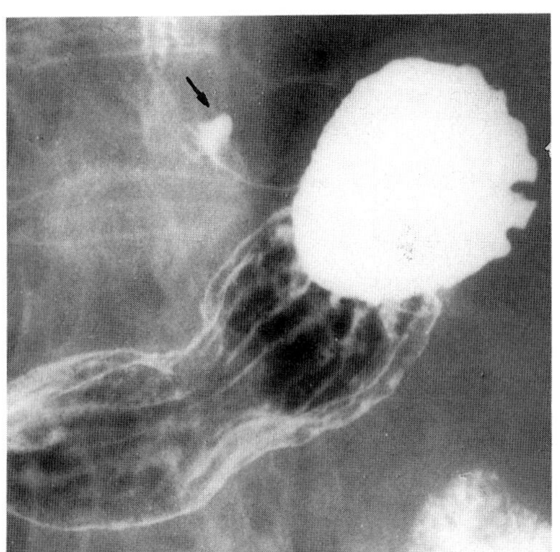

FIGURE 7.30. Epiphrenic diverticulum of the esophagus.

Esophageal duplication, a very rare congenital anomaly, may be manifested by symptoms similar to those of diverticula. Intramural pseudodiverticula are a separate pathologic entity.

Complications of the diverticula include inflammations which may, in some instances, be the result of prolonged stasis of esophageal contents. Bleeding is not a common complication. Free perforations of esophageal diverticula may result in acute mediastinitis.

INTRALUMINAL DIVERTICULA

Patients can develop intraluminal diverticula, from various causes, such as increased intraluminal esophageal pressure, acquired weakness of the wall, and traumatic or inflammatory discontinuity of the mucosal integrity. The structure resembles a membrane. When filled with contrast medium, the diverticulum resembles a sack filled with barium lying in the lumen of the esophagus. A thin transparent line, the wall of the diverticulum, is seen between the contrast in the esophageal lumen and that within the lumen of the diverticulum (Fig. 7.32). An identical finding could be made in the presence of a flexible partial membrane of the esophagus (see chapter 9, on intraluminal duodenal diverticulum). In addition, congenital partial duplication of the esophagus may cause a similar radiologic finding. Inconstancy of findings on repeated examinations suggests the presence of transient intramural diverticula.

TRANSIENT INTRALUMINAL DIVERTICULA

Rarely, an oval or spherical accumulation of barium sulfate surrounded by a thin radiolucent rim may be seen while swallowing a barium suspension; it closely resembles an intraluminal esophageal diverticulum. However, the find-

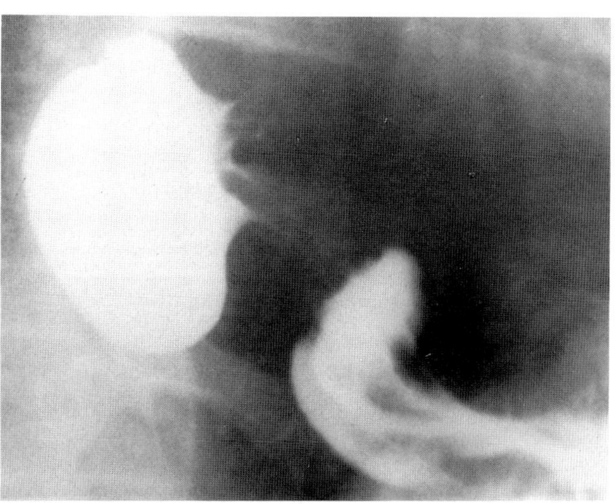

FIGURE 7.31. Very large epiphrenic diverticulum of the esophagus. Such a finding may mimic gastric hiatus hernia.

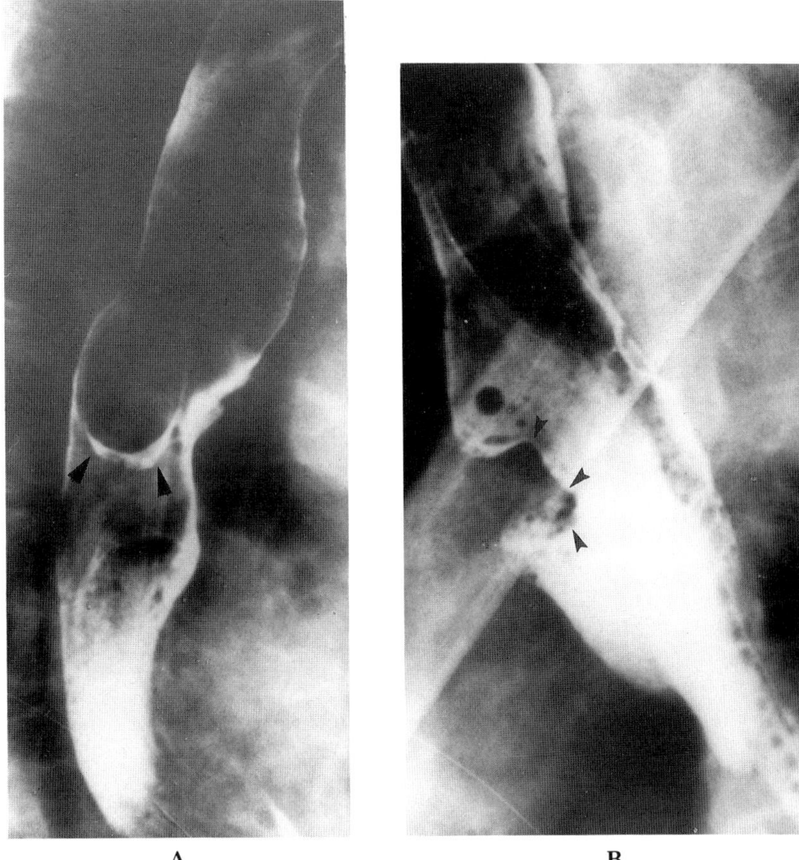

Figure 7.32. (A) and (B) Intraluminal esophageal diverticulum (arrowheads).

ings are irreproducible and cannot be corroborated endoscopically. These formations are transient; seemingly the phenomena are caused by primary or secondary dysmotility of the esophagus, with tertiary contractions and retention of air in the lumen. Inadequate mixing of the contrast suspension with air may cause this phenomenon.

Intramural Pseudodiverticula

The frequency of esophageal intramural pseudodiverticula is less than 0.1% in patients undergoing single- or double-contrast examinations of the esophagus. This entity is characterized by multiple saccular narrow-necked protrusions out of the column of contrast medium. They resemble tiny diverticula 1–4 mm long (Fig. 7.33). When diluted barium suspension is utilized, they are better visualized by single-contrast rather than by double-contrast examinations. The openings by which intramural pseudodiverticula communicate with the esophageal lumen are very narrow and therefore hardly seen at endoscopy. Pseudodiverticula may be distributed diffusely or segmentally. They are most commonly encountered in the distal portion of the esophagus.

Intramural pseudodiverticula are the dilated excretory canals of the deep esophageal mucosal glands. Dilatations result from intrinsic obstruction of excretory canals by plugs of viscous mucus and desquamated cells, or by extrinsic compression of the canals by periductal

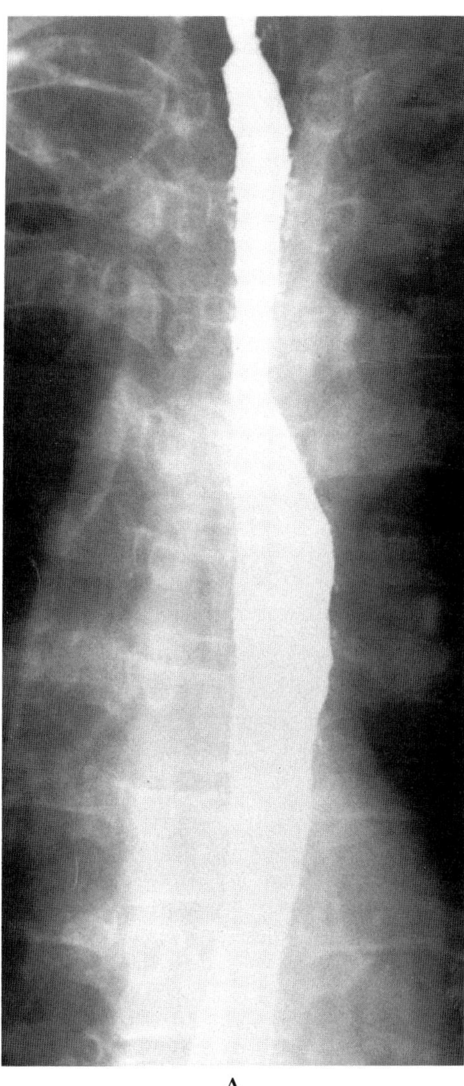

A

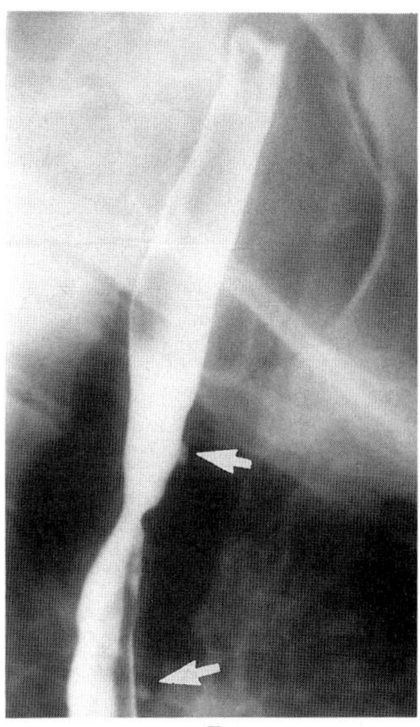

B

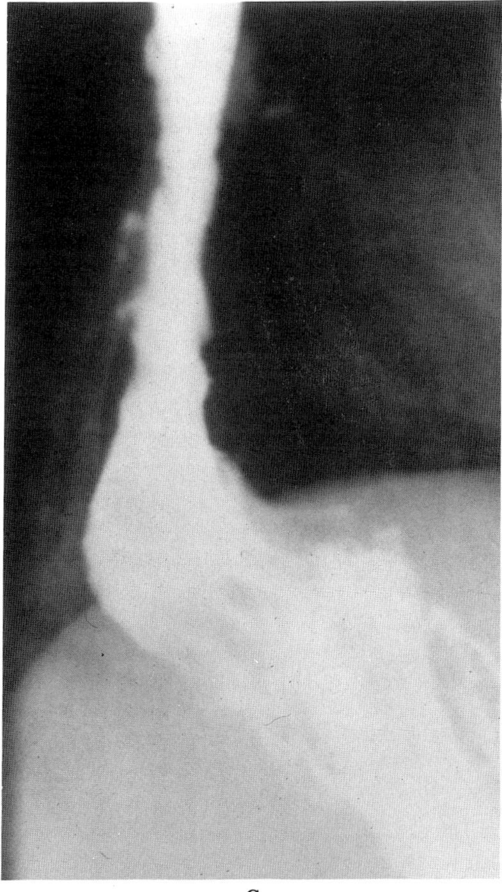

C

Figure 7.33. Intramural pseudodiverticula of the esophagus. (A) Multiple pseudodiverticula. (B) Two intramural pseudodiverticula (arrows). (C) Intramural pseudodiverticula and gastric hiatus hernia. (Courtesy R.F. Thoeni, M.D., University of California, San Francisco.)

inflammatory infiltrates and fibrotic tissue. Indeed, inflammatory changes seem to have an essential role in the development of intramural diverticula. In some 90% of patients, esophageal intramural pseudodiverticula are accompanied by chronic reflux esophagitis with strictures. Moniliasis or herpes simplex esophagitis may be an associated finding. Intramural pseudodiverticula may be seen in patients with Barrett's esophagus, varices, or squamous cell carcinoma of the esophagus. However, it remains unclear why the intramural pseudodi-

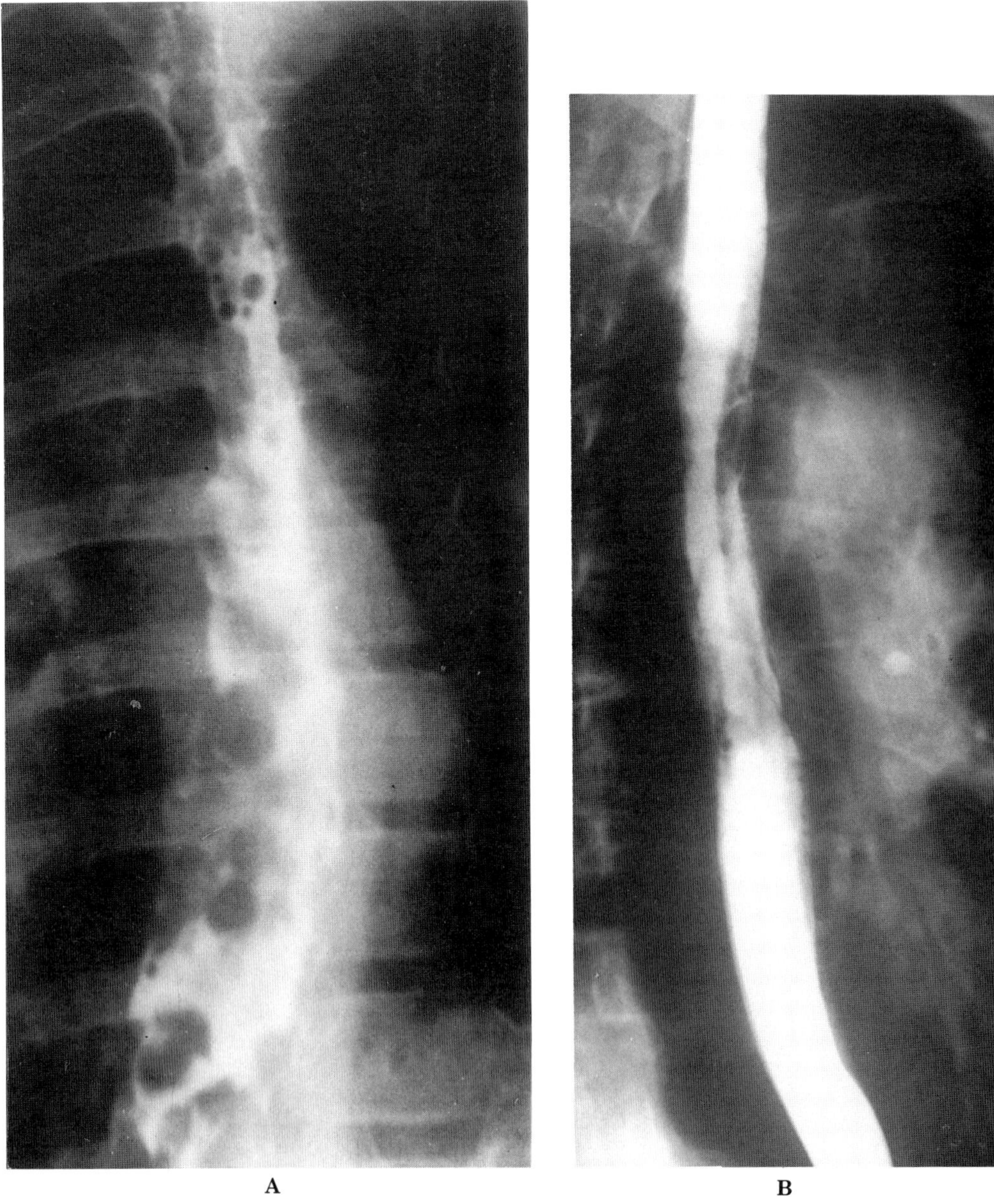

FIGURE 7.34. Esophageal varices. (A) The entire esophagus is affected. (B) Downhill varices secondary to superior vena cava obstruction.

verticula develop in only a small number of patients with reflux esophagitis.

ESOPHAGEAL VARICES

In patients with portal hypertension, submucosal varices are common in the distal two-thirds of the esophagus (below the level of confluence of the azygos vein into the superior vena cava). Obstruction of normal blood flow results in a change in direction of the portal circulation. Blood is drained via the left gastric vein and submucosal venous plexuses of the esophagus into the paraesophageal veins, and through them into the azygos and hemiazygos veins.

Varices of the proximal two-thirds of the esophagus, downhill varices, are the consequence of obstruction of the superior vena cava resulting from chronic mediastinitis or infiltration by bronchogenic carcinoma (Fig. 7.34). Downhill varices are much less common than the varices found in patients with portal hypertension. After the injection of contrast medium into the left jugular vein, barium swallow and CT may reveal varices. They possess the radiologic properties of varices in other parts of the esophagus.

If varices of the esophagus are not adequately filled with blood during conventional radiologic examination, enhancement can be accomplished by specific procedures (see examination of the esophagus, page 84) as well as by deep inspiration, forced expiration, and coughing.

Early esophageal varices cause esophageal folds to be slightly widened (Fig. 7.35A) and the lumen dilated. Peristaltic waves are of low

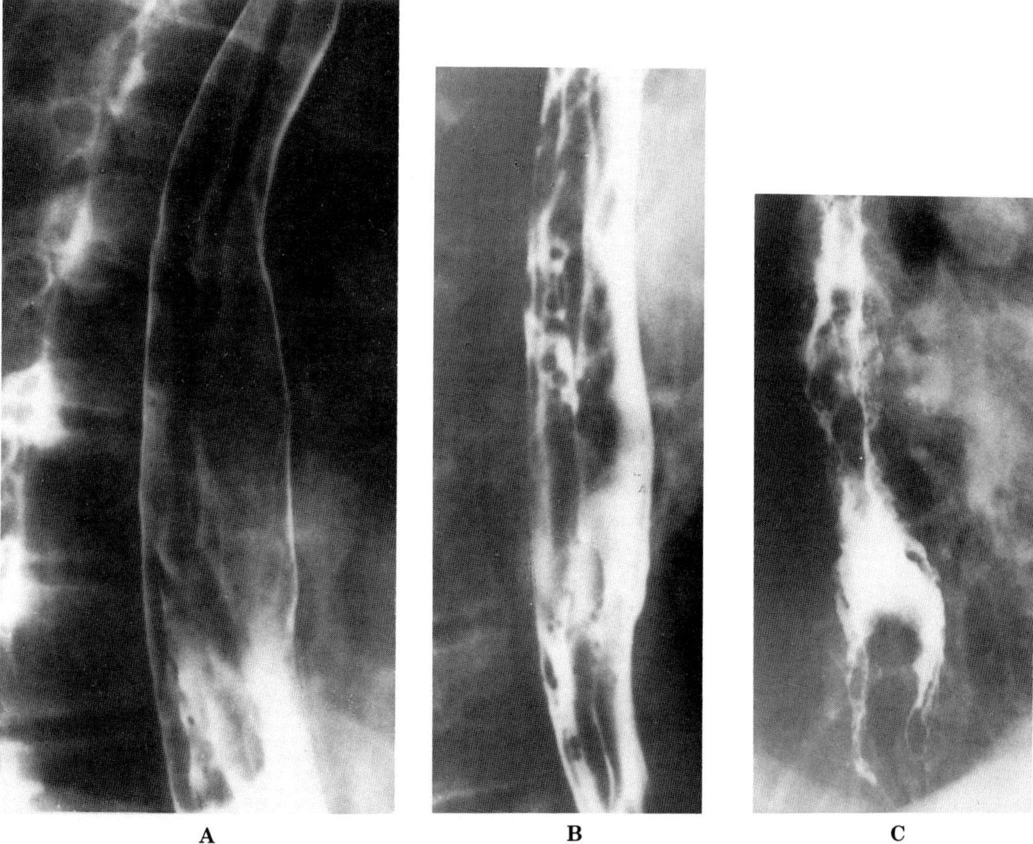

A B C

FIGURE 7.35. Esophageal varices. (A) Serpiginous. (B) Advanced. (C) Large caliber.

amplitude and the motility may be uncoordinated with tertiary contractions. Advanced varices are demonstrated by wide, regular, well circumscribed, sometimes serpiginous formations protruding into the lumen (Fig. 7.35B and C). They are best visualized by double-contrast examination. However, significant dilatation of the esophagus may cause flattening of less pronounced varices making them imperceivable. The variation in findings depending on body posture, phase of respiration, and contraction of esophageal wall is characteristic (Fig. 7.36). Radiologic diagnosis is equally accurate or even superior to esophagoscopic examination.

Varices should be differentiated from tertiary contractions, air bubbles (Fig. 7.37), esophagitis (Fig. 7.38), and superficial tumor infiltration.

ESOPHAGITIS

Esophagitis is commonly associated with other diseases. It can be caused by pathogenic microorganisms, gastroesophageal reflux, corrosive and thermal injuries, ionizing radiation, and drugs (Table 7.4) (Figs. 7.39 and 7.40).

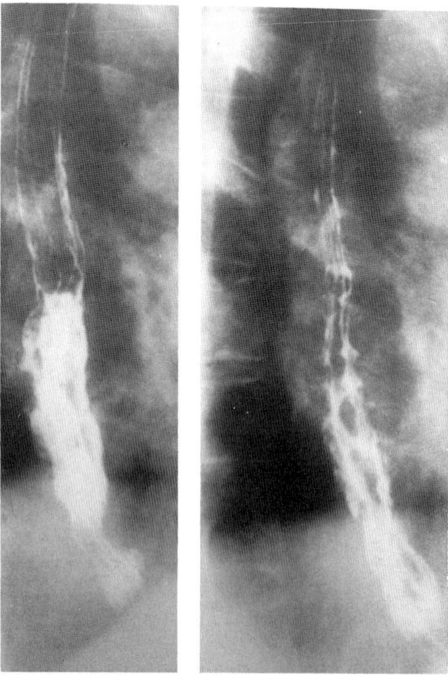

Figure 7.36. Esophageal varices change morphology with breathing, swallowing, or changes of body position.

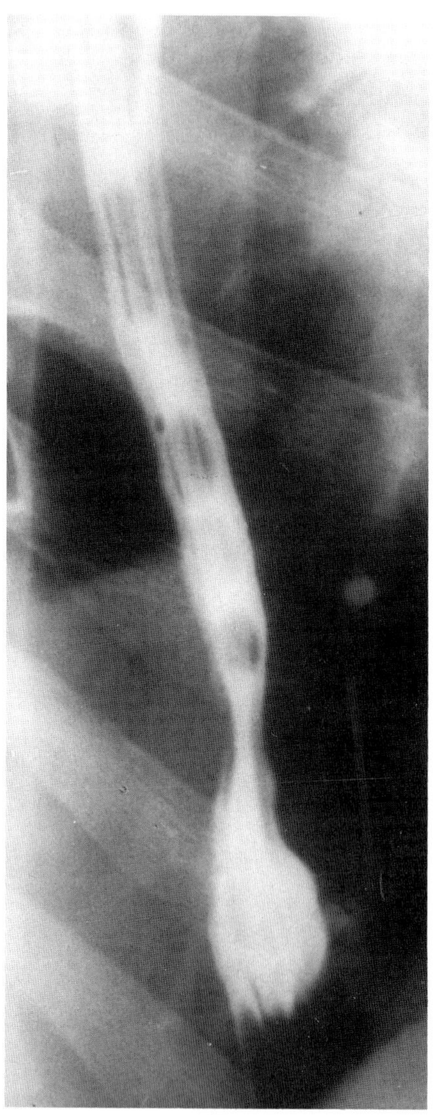

Figure 7.37. Air bubbles in the esophagus.

Reflux esophagitis is described with hiatal hernia and gastroesophageal reflux.

Moniliasis

Moniliasis or candidiasis is an infectious esophagitis caused by the fungus *Candida albicans*. It occurs primarily in immunologically

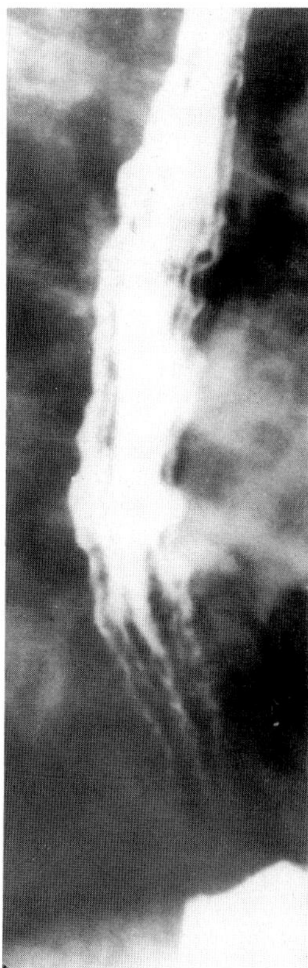

FIGURE 7.38. Reflux esophagitis may mimic esophageal varices. These findings are constant regardless of changes in intrathoracic or intra-abdominal pressure.

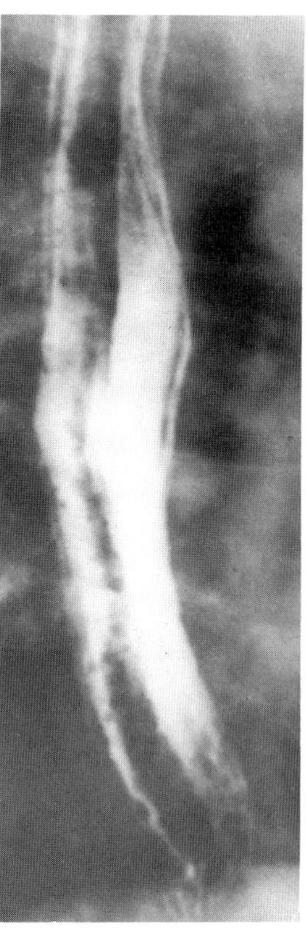

FIGURE 7.39. Esophagitis. Widened esophageal folds with granularity of the mucosa and erosions.

TABLE 7.4. CAUSES OF ESOPHAGEAL INFLAMMATION

Reflux esophagitis
Moniliasis
Herpes simplex esophagitis
Zollinger-Ellison syndrome
Chemical injuries
Crohn's disease

impaired patients, and has been seen more often since cytostatic and immunosuppressive drugs are in use for the treatment of malignant tumors and management of transplanted organs. Candidiasis appears also in patients with AIDS. Therapy with corticosteroids, chemotherapy, radiotherapy, and the uncritical use of antibiotics are favorable to the development of moniliasis. The main local predisposing factor may be stasis of esophageal contents in patients with abnormalities of motility, such as those that occur in achalasia, strictures, and scleroderma. Delayed emptying of the esophagus allows colonization with fungi. Clinically, odynophagia and dysphagia are the main symptoms.

Single-contrast examination reveals abnormalities in motility, thickening of esophageal folds, and ulcers. In advanced moniliasis the contours of the esophagus may resemble cobblestones or appear shaggy (Fig. 7.41) due to multiple mucosal plaques and ulcers. Moniliasis is successfully diagnosed in only 50% of patients undergoing single-contrast examination, which is particularly insensitive in detecting the earliest radiologic signs of esophagitis.

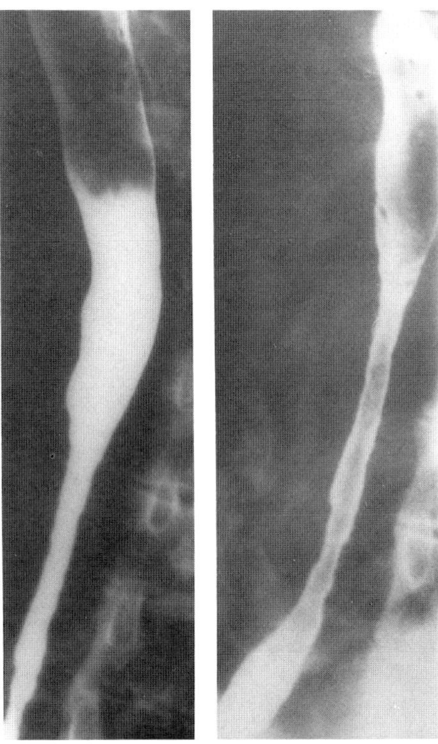

FIGURE 7.40. Postesophagitic stricture.

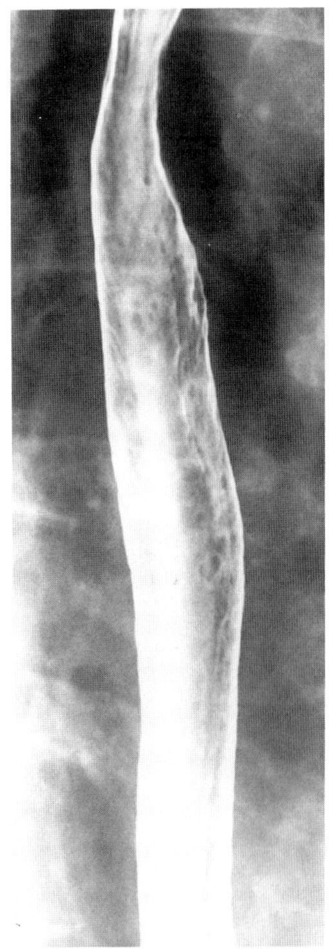

A

FIGURE 7.41. Esophageal moniliasis. (A) In the early phase, the plaques are lined along the longitudinal esophageal axis.

However, double-contrast examination may reveal early signs such as mucosal plaques and granular surface of the mucosa. The plaques consist of necrotic epithelial cells and colonies of fungi presenting as irregular, well-demarcated layers on the mucosal surface. They are aligned along the longitudinal axis of the esophagus (Fig. 7.41A). The earliest esophageal strictures may be seen one year after the onset of the disease. The sensitivity of double-contrast esophagography in detection of candidiasis exceeds 80%.

Advanced monilial esophagitis may radiographically resemble esophageal varices. Esophagitis resulting from *herpes simplex* infection may mimic candidiasis except that shallow ulcers on the otherwise unchanged mucosa are present, and mucosal plaques are not a common finding. Edema and inflammation are the most constant findings in patients with reflux esophagitis. Mucosal lesions are predominantly nodular rather than plaque-like. Glycogenic acanthosis is a benign degenerative disease in which hyperplastic columnar cells accumulate glycogen. Plaques seen in this disorder are of uniform dimensions measuring 1–4 mm in diameter.

HERPES ESOPHAGITIS

Immunosuppressed patients have a greater risk of developing herpes simplex type 1 esophagitis than immunocompetent patients. Odynophagia and dysphagia are dominant clinical

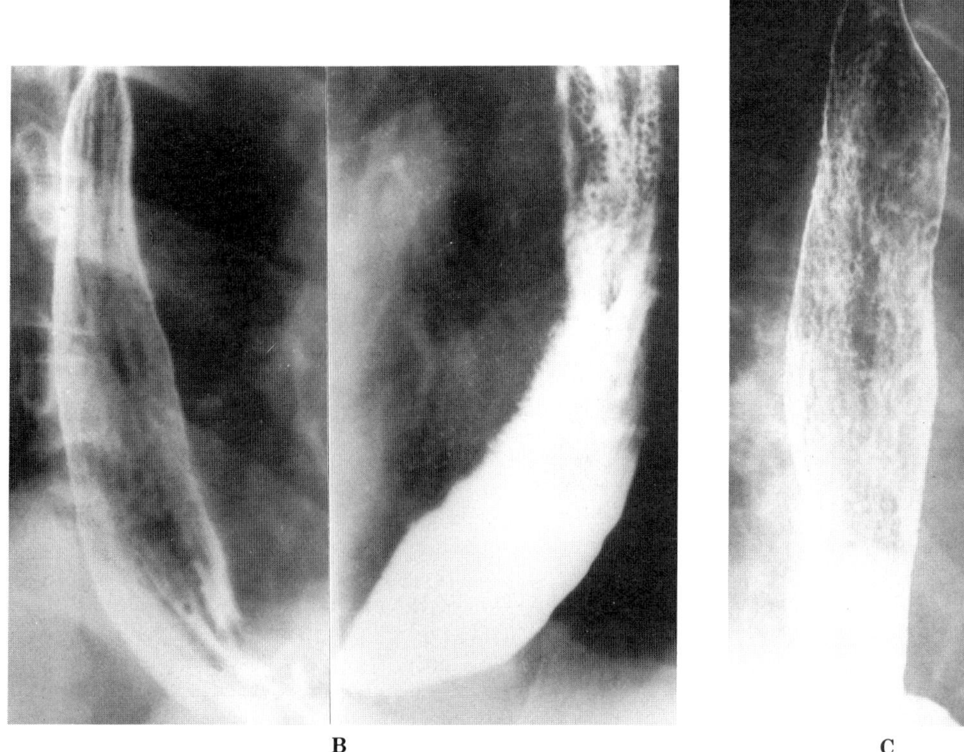

FIGURE 7.41. *continued.* (B) More advanced stage. (C) Advanced stage.

symptoms. Radiologic examination reveals multiple, shallow, tiny ulcers and, less frequently, plaques which are not ulcerated. Ulcers are found on the mucosa without other pathologic changes (Fig. 7.42). Inflammatory changes are most common in the middle and less common in the distal esophagus.

The differential diagnosis includes moniliasis, reflux and drug-induced esophagitis, Crohn's disease, and Behcet's syndrome.

Crohn's disease seldom affects the esophagus. Even then simultaneous changes are present in the small and large intestine. Electron microscopic research has revealed that Crohn's disease affects the entire alimentary canal, with macroscopic manifestations in only a few portions. It is characterized as a segmental, granulomatous, ulcerative, transmural process. Early lesions, aphthoid ulcers, are only detected when seen *en face* on double-contrast roentgenograms. They are less likely to be seen when filmed in profile (Fig. 7.43). Owing to their tiny dimensions and slight protuberance into the lumen, they are not likely to be observed at esophagoscopy. Aphthoid ulcers resemble the erosions of reflux esophagitis, herpetic and mycotic esophagitis, and lesions caused by medication. In advanced Crohn's disease longitudinal and transverse ulcers result in a cobblestone appearance of the mucosa. Strictures and fistulae with adjacent organs are late manifestations of Crohn's disease.

In patients with allogenic bone marrow transplant, radiologic examination of swallowing disorders, which result from chronic *graft-versus-host* disease, may reveal webs and stenoses of the upper esophageal segment. However, small bowel lesions are still more

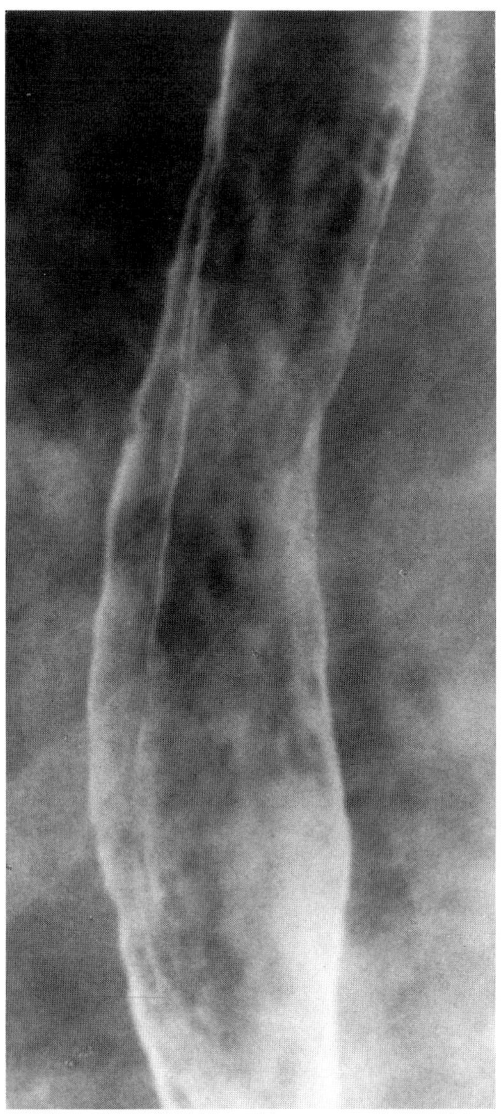

Figure 7.42. Esophagitis resulting from herpes simplex virus.

common in transplant patients than are esophageal stenoses.

HIATUS HERNIA

Hiatus hernia is a protrusion of a portion of the stomach through the esophageal hiatus into the thoracic cavity.

Hiatal insufficiency denotes permanent presence of the lower esophageal segment above the diaphragm without herniation of the stomach. Namely, in the course of swallowing, the abdominal portion of the esophagus temporarily enters the chest but readily returns to the abdominal cavity (see the discussions on lower esophageal segment, page 6, and act of swallowing, page 25).

It is to be realized that symptoms caused by hiatus hernia may mimic those of coronary artery disease. In addition, hiatal hernia can result in gastroesophageal reflux with subsequent reflux esophagitis. Since Barrett's esophagus may result, esophageal adenocarcinoma must also be anticipated. However, patients may be without symptoms.

The radiologic diagnosis of hiatus hernia requires one or more of the following signs:

1. Gastric folds of the stomach are seen passing through the esophageal hiatus into the thoracic cavity (Fig. 7.44).
2. Areae gastricae are present in that portion of the alimentary canal within the chest (Fig. 7.45). This is the most reliable sign of hiatal herniation of the stomach but it is not often demonstrated.
3. Three ring-shaped narrowings are demonstrated in the LES and on the proximal portion of the stomach. These are, in the caudo-cranial direction, indentation of the stomach by diaphragmatic crura in the region of the hiatus, cardia, and the tubulovestibular junction (Figs. 1.7 and 7.44).
4. That portion of the alimentary canal above the diaphragm is significantly wider than the LES (Fig. 7.27).
5. The transverse mucosal fold at the transition between gastric and esophageal mucosa (B ring) is above the diaphragm (Fig. 1.7).
6. The lateral imprint in the region of the cardia resulting from contraction of sling fibers of the stomach lies above the diaphragm (Fig. 1.8).
7. The esophagogastric (Hiss's) angle is significantly increased.
8. The width of the infradiaphragmatic segment of the "vestibule" is equal to or even exceeds the length.
9. The portion of the alimentary tube just above the diaphragm is aperistaltic, and is

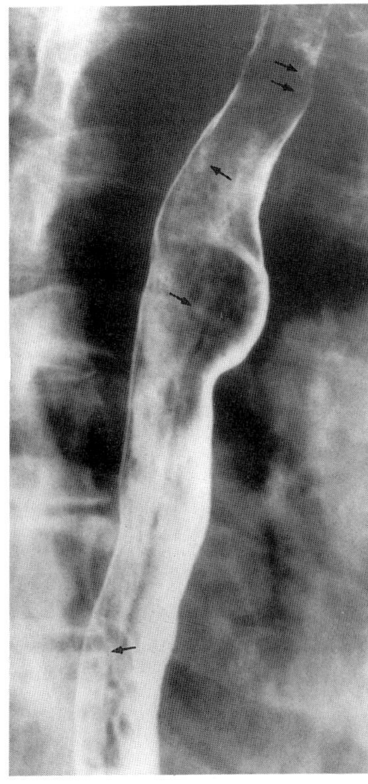

A

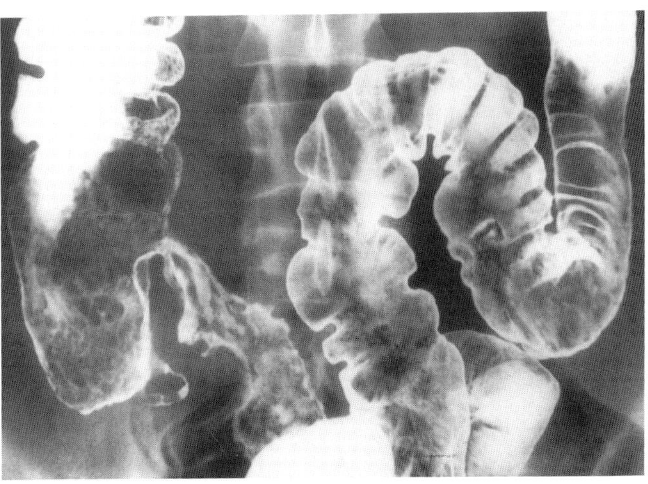

B

Figure 7.43. Crohn's disease. (A) Aphthoid ulcers in the esophagus (arrows). (B) Affection of terminal ileum and colon in the same patient.

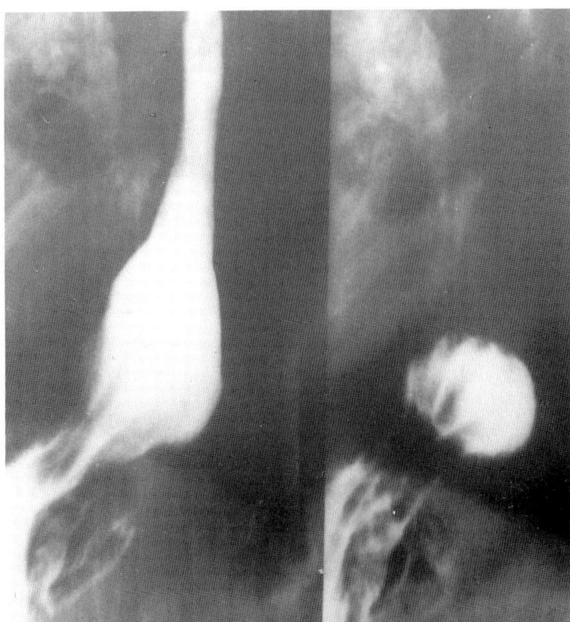

Figure 7.44. Hiatus hernia. Gastric folds are seen above the diaphragm.

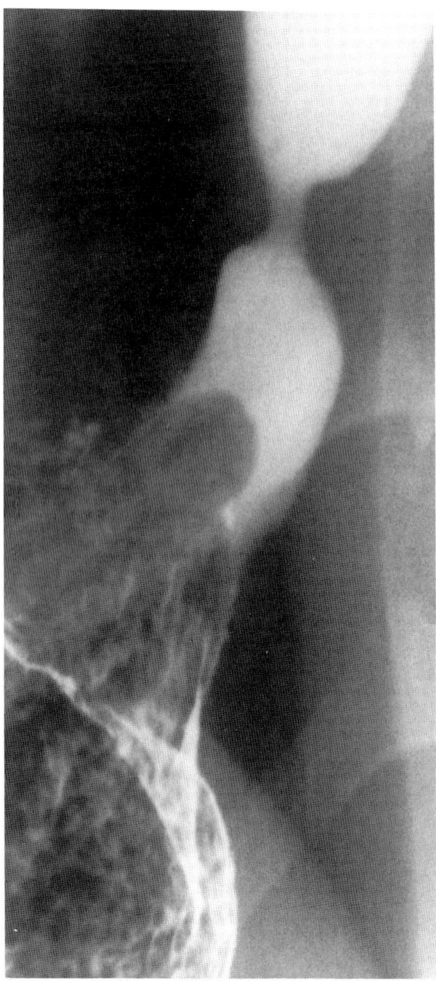

FIGURE 7.45. Hiatus hernia. Area gastricae are seen above the diaphragm.

often eccentric or parallel with the longitudinal axis of the esophagus (Fig. 7.46).

10. In the upright position gastric folds above the diaphragm are seen to converge, while those below the diaphragm diverge (Fig. 7.44). In normal circumstances, folds below the diaphragm also converge.

Paraesophageal hernia is most commonly the result of a defect in the phrenoesophageal membrane (see discussion on LES, page 8). Part, or all, of the gastric fundus herniates through the hiatus into the chest with the esophagus alongside (Fig. 7.47). The cardia may be situated above or below the hiatus. If the cardia is below the hiatus, gastroesophageal reflux is not likely to occur, and vice versa.

Hiatal hernias over 5 cm in diameter are considered to be large. While large hernias may be easy to diagnose, small hiatal hernias cause considerable diagnostic problems. If the cardia is displaced 1 cm above the esophageal hiatus the possibility of hiatal hernia should be considered. In elderly patients, this displacement should not be considered pathologic unless gastroesophageal reflux can be demonstrated. Small hiatal hernias are difficult to diagnose by radiologic means. When performing provocation maneuvers, hiatus hernia could be demonstrated in 50% of asymptomatic patients.

Hiatus hernia can produce opacity at the base of the left lung. While incarceration of hiatal hernias is rare, paraesophageal hernias are more frequently incarcerated. The fixation of herniated portions is evaluated by raising the patient from the horizontal to the vertical position. In most patients with hiatus hernia the LES and the cardia are situated in the chest, resulting in gastroesophageal reflux. Indeed, hiatus hernia is the commonest cause of reflux esophagitis.

Hiatus hernia should be distinguished from a dilated thoracic portion of the LES (phrenic ampulla). This is easily accomplished during the course of fluoroscopy but may be difficult when only films are examined. The phrenic ampulla dilates on inspiration and the abdominal portion of the esophagus is collapsed. The herniated portion of the stomach is devoid of peristalsis, while the LES shows lively motility. The possible existence of a very rare, congenitally short esophagus should be considered when making a differential diagnosis. On CT scans hiatal hernia can resemble a tumor of the esophagogastric junction.

The diagnosis of paraesophageal hernias does not cause difficulties. A large epiphrenic diverticulum can mimic this type of hernia.

COMPLICATIONS

Incarceration of hiatus hernia is characterized by gas-fluid level in the herniated portion of the stomach (Fig. 4.26). While changing posture, the herniated part does not change position.

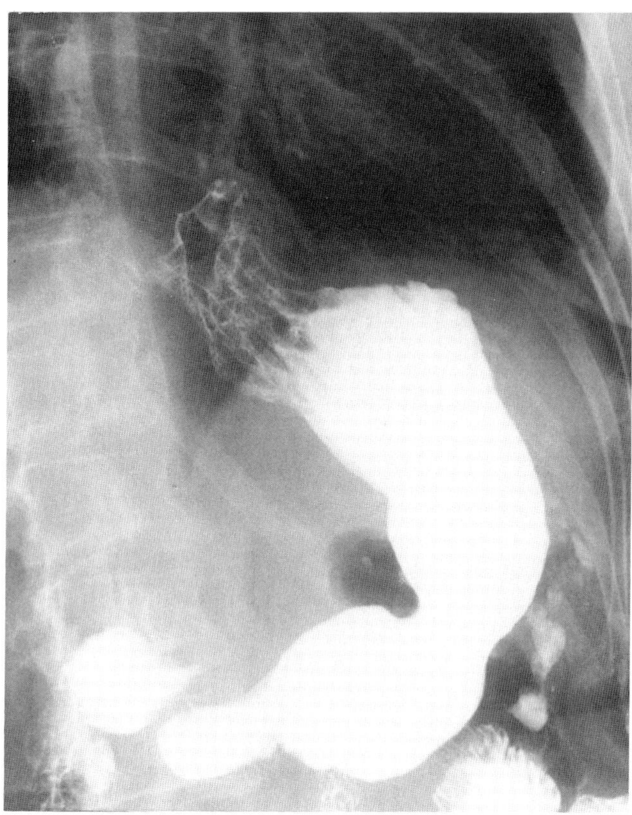

FIGURE 7.46. Hiatus hernia of the stomach.

Gastroesophageal reflux is a common consequence of hiatus hernia and may result in *reflux esophagitis* with ulcers, strictures, and shortening of the esophagus. When Barrett's esophagus occurs, adenocarcinoma of the esophagus may result.

Esophagogastric and gastroesophageal intussusceptions of herniated stomach are transitory phenomena. The former resembles a ring and the latter a mushroom. Portions of the herniated stomach can undergo intussusception (Fig. 7.48) which disappears spontaneously.

Lesions, such as ulcers and neoplasms, can be more difficult to detect in the herniated stomach (Fig. 7.49).

GASTROESOPHAGEAL REFLUX

Gastroesophageal reflux is a passive and involuntary flow of gastric juice into the esophagus. It appears without vomiting or eructation.

Examination for gastroesophageal reflux is described in the section on examination of the esophagus (see page 89). After the stomach is filled with 250 mL or more of barium suspension, saliva should be swallowed several times before starting provocation of the reflux. This will help evacuate remnants of contrast medium from the esophagus.

Normally, the abdominal portion of the esophagus is under the same pressure as the stomach. An increase in intra-abdominal pressure does not cause a gradient between the stomach and the esophagus. However, in patients with hiatal insufficiency and hernia, the situation is different.

Deep inspiration of air gives rise to differences in pressure between the chest and the abdomen in the order of 10 kPa (75 mm Hg), sufficient to enhance reflux. Compression of the abdomen or a change of posture can make this gradient even higher, further stimulating reflux.

Gastroesophageal reflux is prevented by the

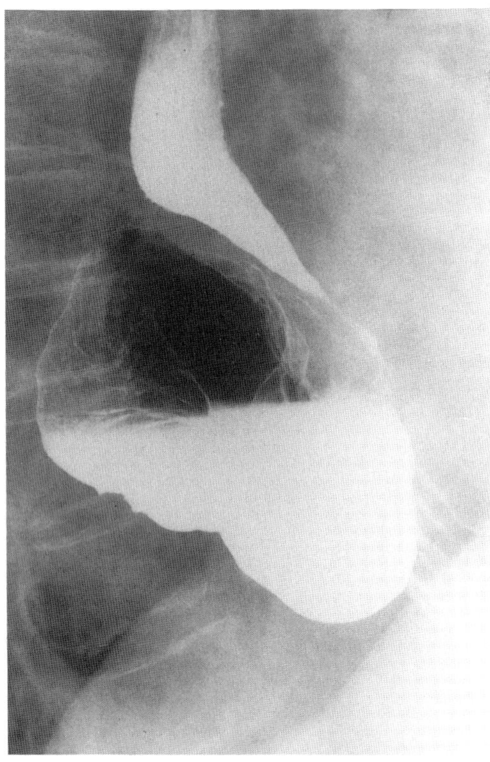

A

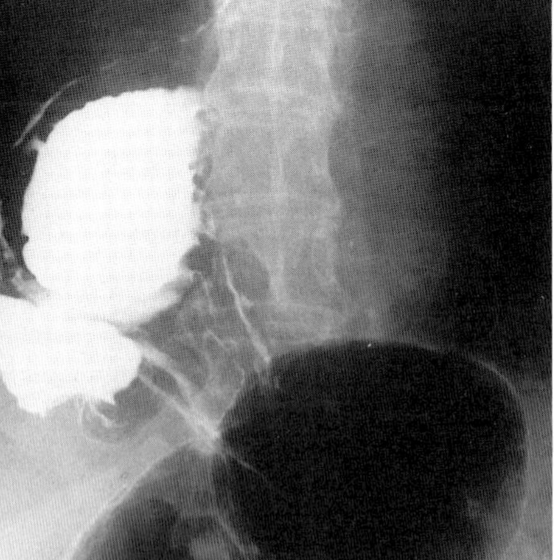

B

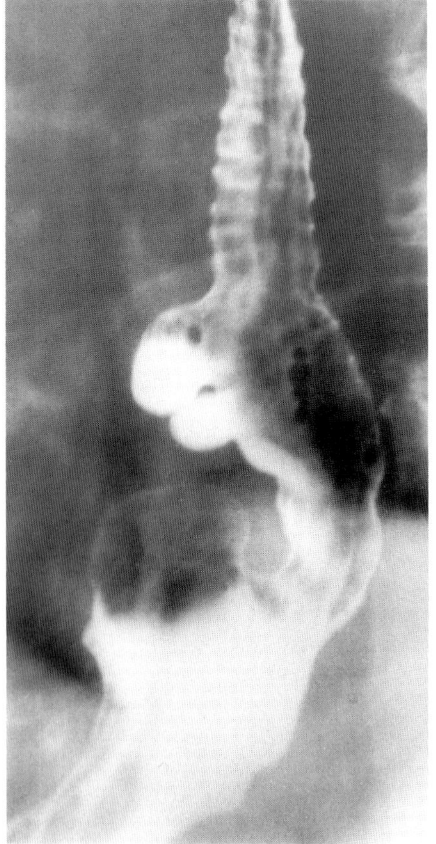

C

Figure 7.47. Paraesophageal hernia. (A) Discrete irregularities of the esophagus by reflux esophagitis. (B) Large hernia. (C) Two large epiphrenic diverticula of the esophagus with transverse striations of reflux esophagitis.

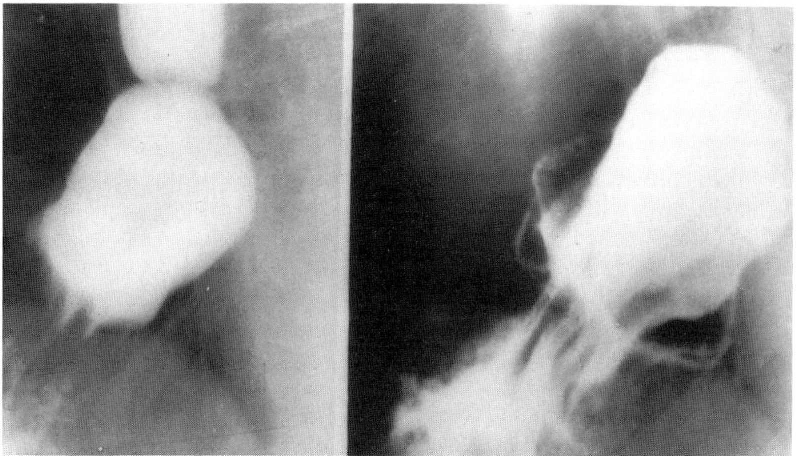

Figure 7.48. Hiatus hernia with transient gastro-gastric intussusception (right).

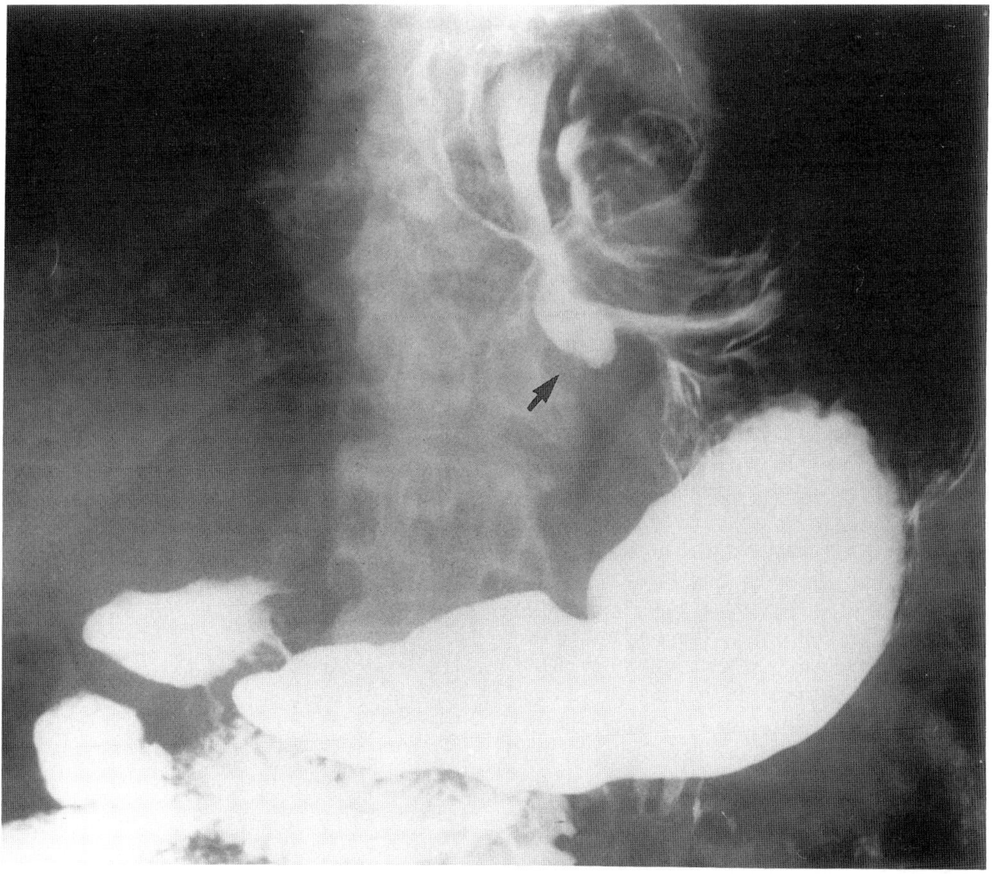

Figure 7.49. Large peptic ulcer in a herniated stomach (arrow).

sphincteric function of the lower esophageal segment, the esophageal hiatus and esophagogastric angle of Hiss, that is, the angle between the abdominal portion of the esophagus and the gastric fundus. With a more acute Hiss's angle, greater force is required for retrograde opening of the esophagogastric junction. In patients with a hiatus hernia little force is required for reflux to be provoked.

Since systemic progressive sclerosis lessens the sphincteric function of the LES, gastroesophageal reflux also readily occurs in this condition. In addition, mucosal folds in the region of cardia can result from contraction of the muscular coat of the mucosa. While these are presumed to prevent gastroesophageal reflux, mechanical valves have not been demonstrated in this region.

An antireflux role for a normally functioning esophageal hiatus seems to be definitely established and to have an importance equal to that of the LES, since repositioning of herniated portions of the stomach with surgical narrowing of the hiatus, but without change in the LES, can still prevent gastroesophageal reflux.

Gastroesophageal reflux in adults is most frequently the consequence of hiatus herniation of the gastric cardia into the thoracic cavity (Table 7.5). Reflux is also the most important consequence in idiopathic chalasia.

Passive reflux occurs when contrast medium passes, under gravitational influence, from the infradiaphragmatic segment of the stomach into the herniated portion of the stomach and then into the esophagus (Fig. 7.50). This occurs when the patient is supine, recumbent on the right side, or prone. Patients with passive reflux have subjective symptoms such as heartburn.

Induced reflux may result from abdominal compression, from swallowing of water or contrast suspension in the horizontal position, or as a result of assuming the Trendelenburg position. However, the latter maneuver is believed to be nonphysiologic and should be avoided when searching for hernia and reflux.

Gastroesophageal reflux causes reflux esophagitis. In addition to esophageal lesions, radiologic examination for reflux esophagitis should demonstrate the presence of hiatal herniation and reflux as well as evaluate the propulsive ability of esophageal peristalsis to displace esophageal contents such as contrast medium.

Gastroesophageal reflux may be classified into three stages. In stage I, refluxed material reaches midway between the diaphragm and the aortic arch. In stage II, it reaches the aor-

TABLE 7.5. ETIOLOGIC FACTORS IN GASTROESOPHAGEAL REFLUX

Chalasia in newborns and adults
Hiatal insufficiency and hiatal hernia
Damage to diaphragmatic crura
Scleroderma
Failed antireflux surgery

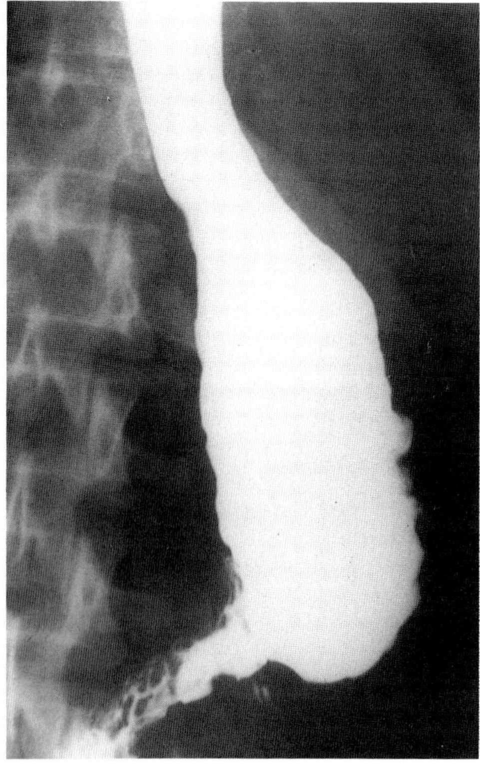

FIGURE 7.50. Passive, free gastroesophageal reflux in the supine position after Billroth I surgery.

tic arch, and in stage III, it reaches the proximal one-third of the esophagus.

In infants and small children gastroesophageal reflux is classified into five stages:

1. Reflux into the LES
2. Reflux to the height of the tracheal bifurcation
3. Reflux into the cervical part of the esophagus
4. "Chalasia"
5. Reflux with aspiration into the trachea.

Prominent gastroesophageal reflux with entrance of barium into the tympanic cavity through the auditory tubes has even been described.

Results obtained by barium upper gastrointestinal series and acid reflux measurements are of equal validity in diagnosing gastroesophageal reflux. This conclusion was reached after comparing results with clinical symptomatology, as well as endoscopic and biopsy findings. Food-stimulated radiologic examination of the upper gastrointestinal tract has been proposed as the first procedure in the algorithm of examinations for diagnosing gastroesophageal reflux.

However, use of these highly accurate tests in the evaluation of gastroesophageal reflux in children shows minimal correlation between demonstrated reflux and clinical symptoms. Abnormal esophageal pH does not always correlate with the results of upper gastrointestinal series. Both examinations need to be evaluated in association with clinical symptomatology.

Periodic regurgitation is frequent in infants and is not the cause or the consequence of pathologic events. It may disappear spontaneously in most instances. However, it is not always easily differentiated from significant gastroesophageal reflux. An important criterion in estimating whether reflux is significant is the age of the child. Gastroesophageal reflux which occurs three times over the course of an upper gastrointestinal examination lasting five minutes can be considered pathologic in children over six weeks of age.

With appropriate concern for technique and standardization of the results, high sensitivity can be achieved, but a high false-positive rate decreases the specificity for diagnosis of gastroesophageal reflux by upper gastrointestinal series. In half the normal infants examined, regurgitation of esophageal contents and gastroesophageal reflux occur without reflux esophagitis. The use of an upper gastrointestinal series in revealing clinically significant reflux may achieve 85% sensitivity and 25% specificity. The predictive value of a positive test is 54% and the negative predictive value is 65%. Reflux could be proved in 76% of children with clinical symptoms, but reflux was also demonstrated in 37% of asymptomatic examinees. Pathologic conditions develop in 2% of infants with reflux, and this is still a significant number.

Fluoroscopic assessment may be less reliable than scintigraphy, manometry, measurement of pH in the esophagus, and esophagoscopy in revealing gastroesophageal reflux. However, roentgenologic examination also allows accurate and simple evaluation of anatomical changes of obstruction of the gastric outlet and of esophageal stenosis, both of which may cause similar symptoms. It can demonstrate signs of reflux esophagitis and hiatal herniation. In fact, reflux esophagitis seems to be as common as peptic ulceration in the upper gastrointestinal tract.

REFLUX ESOPHAGITIS

Reflux or peptic esophagitis is the sequela of esophageal mucosal damage by acid gastric contents. The most common cause of gastroesophageal reflux is hiatus hernia. In addition, reflux esophagitis is often associated with peptic ulceration of the duodenum.

Reflux esophagitis may be divided into several pathologic stages. Mild esophagitis is characterized by erythema of the mucosa, surface irregularity, and exudation. Erosions and ulcers can be found in patients with moderately developed esophagitis. Severe forms are denoted by deep ulcers and strictures. A comparison of radiologic and endoscopic findings reveals that a multiphasic barium examination, consisting of single-contrast examination in the prone position, mucosal relief studies, and double-contrast examinations in the upright position, is best for demonstration of abnormalities caused by reflux esophagitis. The specificity of the multiphasic radiologic procedure equals 98%. Sensitivity for all the stages of reflux esophagitis equals 65%. However, the sensitivity of a multiphasic examination in advanced forms of esophagitis is 90%. A routine upper gastrointestinal series has low sensitivity in detecting mild forms of esophagitis.

Discrete transverse folds seen on double-contrast esophagograms may well be the earliest radiologic sign of reflux esophagitis (Fig. 7.51) and can result from transversely oriented esophageal ulcers or early longitudinal scarring. However, the majority of ulcers in reflux esophagitis are longitudinally directed (Figs. 7.52A and 7.53). Tertiary contractions can mimic this phenomenon on roentgenograms. Both phenomena resemble the transverse folds occasionally seen in normal cases, the so-called feline appearance of the esophagus (Fig. 2.1). The nature of the latter variant is unexplained, but most probably results from contraction of lamina muscularis mucosae. However, longitudinal ulcers are most common in reflux esophagitis. An esophageal lumen diameter exceeding 25 mm on single-contrast esophagograms also suggests the diagnosis of reflux esophagitis. In patients with reflux esophagitis mucosal folds in the distal portion of the esophagus are widened, their width exceeding 3 mm. The mucosal surface is granulated. In later phases erosions appear (Fig. 7.52). The contour of the barium-filled esophagus is often serrated. Mucosal ulcers and submucosal plaques, with resultant decreased compliance of the esophageal wall and

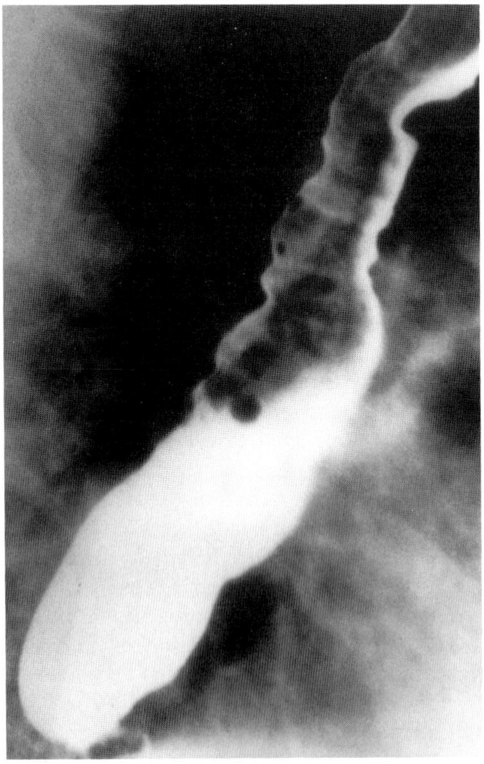

Figure 7.51. Reflux esophagitis. Discrete transverse striations.

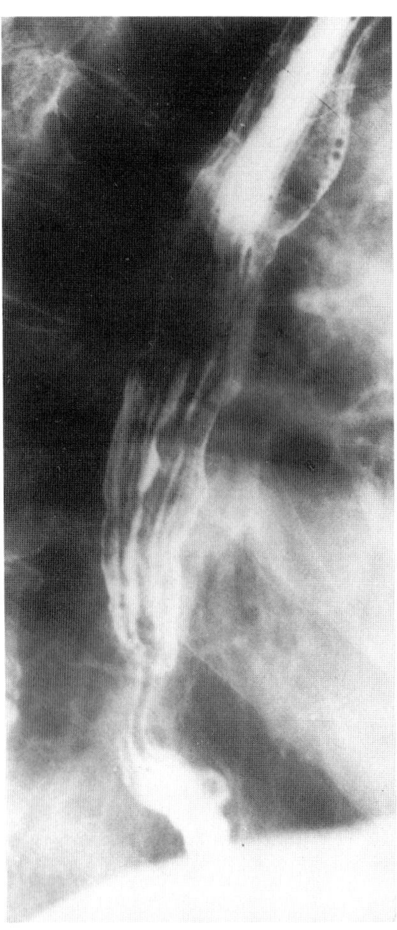

Figure 7.52. Marked reflux esophagitis. (A) Widened, nodular folds, erosions, and peptic ulcer of the anterior esophageal aspect.

hypotonia or hypertonia of the esophageal muscular coat, may develop in the subsequent phase of the disease (Fig. 7.53). Fibrous changes and strictures affecting the LES develop in deeper layers of the wall. Consequently, the sphincteric function of the lower esophageal segment weakens, increasing the likelihood of gastroesophageal reflux.

Reflux esophagitis strictures are smoothly contoured. Mucosal relief may be preserved

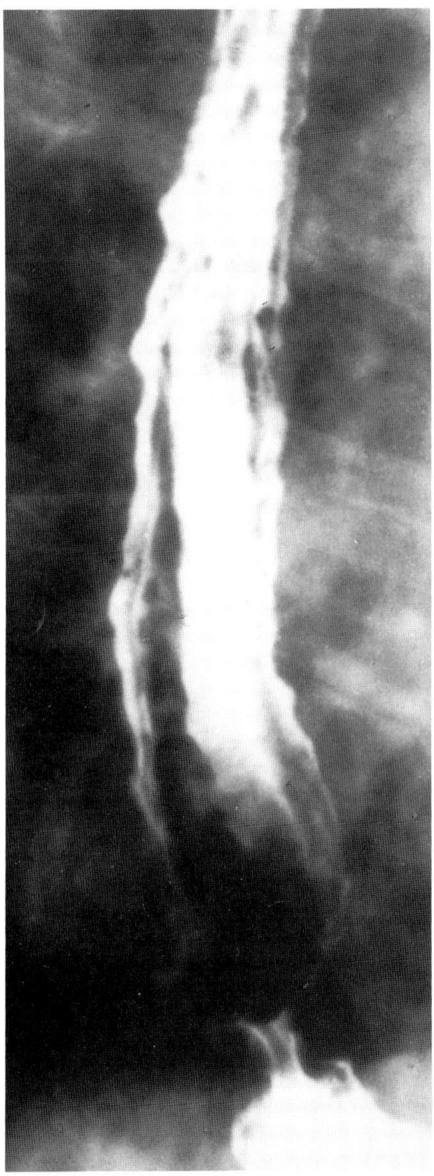

FIGURE 7.52. *continued.* (B) Thickened esophageal folds, erosions, ulcers, and tertiary contractions. Hiatus hernia of the stomach.

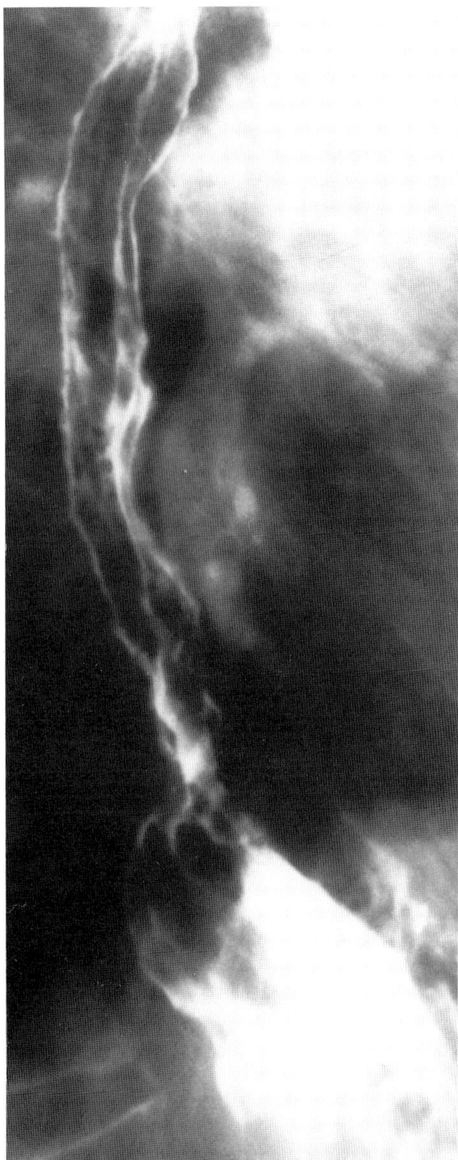

FIGURE 7.53. Marked reflux esophagitis with longitudinal ulcerations. Large gastric hiatus hernia is evident.

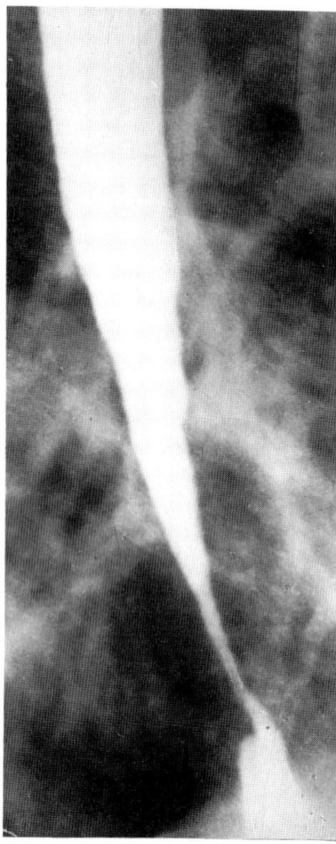

Figure 7.54. Stricture of the distal esophagus with reflux esophagitis.

and the transition between the normal and stenosed portions is gradual (Fig. 7.54). Proximal dilatation is frequently moderate. Acute inflammatory changes are common proximal to the stricture.

Gastroesophageal reflux in children may also result in reflux esophagitis, formation of strictures, and aspiration pneumonia. Development of reflux esophagitis is influenced by the frequency and degree of reflux and the capability of secondary peristalsis to remove remnants of esophageal contents.

BARRETT'S ESOPHAGUS

Barrett's esophagus (BE) is characterized by metaplasia of stratified squamous to simple columnar epithelium. In contrast to islets of ectopic gastric mucosa, the columnar epithelium of BE is continuous with the epithelium of gastric mucosa, but does not secrete HCl. There are no parietal cells, which are normal constituents of gastric mucosa. However, goblet cells are present and the situation is similar to villous (intestinal) metaplasia of gastric mucosa in patients with chronic atrophic gastritis. Since intestinal metaplasia of gastric mucosa increases the risk of cancer, the high malignant potential of BE makes early detection of critical importance to patient management.

Barrett's esophagus is present in 10% of patients with advanced chronic reflux esophagitis. Men and women are equally affected with maximal prevalence in middle age. Thickening and irregularity of esophageal folds are found in 95% of patients. Hiatal hernia of the stomach with resultant gastroesophageal reflux and peptic esophagitis is often present. Gastroesophageal reflux with or without hiatal hernia is verified in 90% of patients with BE.

More than three-quarters of affected patients have esophageal strictures (Fig. 7.55). Approximately 60% of these strictures affect the middle third of the esophagus, while the remainder are located in the distal portion of the esophagus. Radiologic signs of reflux esophagitis are visible, mostly proximal to the stenoses. There are opinions that strictures are located at the transition of stratified squamous epithelium to columnar epithelium. However, this has not been definitely proved.

Peptic ulcer of the esophagus, a common finding in reflux esophagitis, is present in 30% of patients with BE. It is the most specific sign of BE but is of relatively little importance because of the low prevalence.

On double-contrast roentgenographs, that portion of the esophagus covered with columnar epithelium is wider than 25 mm in 65–90% of cases. Decreased tone of the distal part of the esophagus, one of the signs of hiatal herniation, reflux esophagitis and BE, may be confirmed by manometry (Fig. 7.55). Scintigraphic data demonstrate the inherent dysmotility of the esophagus in patients with BE.

Diffuse granularity and a fine reticular pattern of the esophageal mucosa may be found with reflux esophagitis and BE. Granular, spheroid extrusions of the mucosa are rarely larger than 2–3 mm in diameter (Figs. 7.55A and B). Reticularity of the mucosa is a consequence

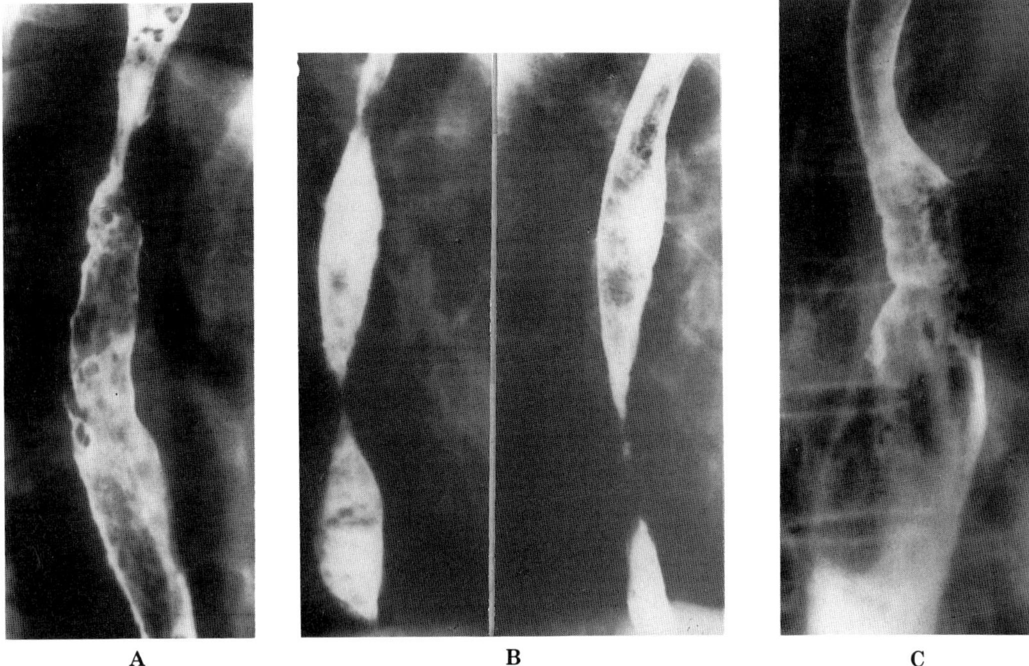

FIGURE 7.55. Barrett's esophagus. (A, B, C) Sign of reflux esophagitis, stricture, and flaccidity of distal segment.

of residual barium in shallow grooves and impressions of the mucosa. Both these patterns of the mucosa are present distal to strictures. Granular bulges are visible on double-contrast roentgenographs in half of the patients with BE. These result from villous metaplasia of the epithelium. The granular mucosal pattern may indicate a higher cancer risk. A granular and reticular mucosa may also be found in moniliasis, herpetic esophagitis, leukoplakia, superficially spreading carcinoma, and glycogenic acanthosis of the esophagus.

There are no specific radiologic signs of BE. All the signs are, at the same time, characteristic of advanced reflux esophagitis, and reflect a common pathophysiologic basis for these two entities. As a matter of fact, BE is a result of long-lasting severe reflux esophagitis.

Progressive systemic sclerosis also affects the esophagus in 50–80% of diseased patients. Because of lowered tone of the LES, gastroesophageal reflux and reflux esophagitis often develop, thus increasing the risk of BE. Whatever is the cause of gastroesophageal reflux, long-lasting reflux esophagitis creates the danger of columnar metaplasia of the esophageal epithelium. In areas of columnar metaplasia, redness of the mucosa is visible endoscopically. This change in color is more important as an indicator of BE than the change in relief of the mucosa.

Some authorities do not even favor double-contrast and mucosal relief studies in diagnosing BE and early Barrett's carcinoma. Radiologic properties of BE are not specific and the sensitivity of the radiologic examinations is relatively low. Although a more "aggressive" examination increases sensitivity, specificity decreases at the same time because of a higher number of false-positive results. Thus, a large number of patients will be unnecessarily examined endoscopically.

Compared with control subjects, the probability of developing esophageal cancer is 40 times higher in patients with BE (see text concerning esophageal cancer, page 227).

PEPTIC ULCERS

Peptic ulcers are of similar morphology throughout the alimentary canal. They arise in the presence of HCl and heal by forming a scar. After prompt therapy of an acute ulcer the scar may be so minute that only microscopic analysis will detect residual pathology.

Esophageal peptic ulcerations resulting from gastroesophageal reflux are most commonly situated in the distal portion of the esophagus, especially in the region of the cardia. Affected patients commonly harbor duodenal or gastric ulcers.

Peptic ulcers of the esophagus create a crater in the wall (Fig. 7.56) with folds converging toward the crater of a healing or chronic ulcer. These ulcers may alter normal esophageal motility. Strictures are the sequelae of chronic ulcers (Fig. 7.56D). Ulcer walls, in contrast to diverticula, are without mucosal folds. Unlike malignant ulcers, peptic ulcers may have mucosal relief preserved along the edges. More accurate differentiation is possible by esophagoscopy with biopsy.

Peptic ulceration on ectopic gastric mucosa (also referred to as Barrett's ulcer and unrelated to Barrett's esophagus) can develop in

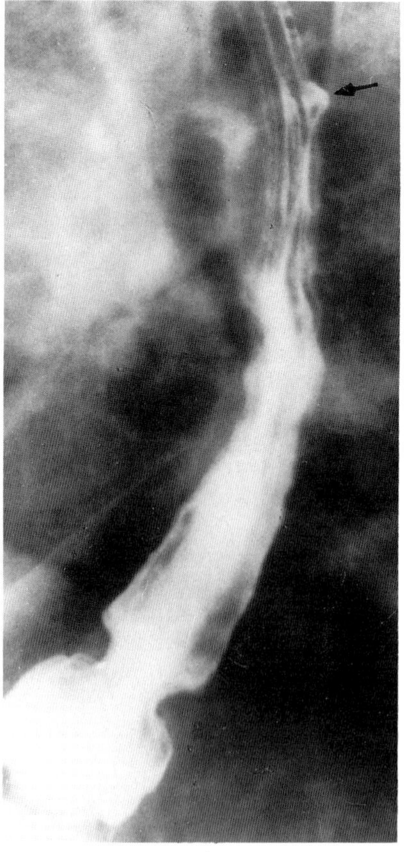

A

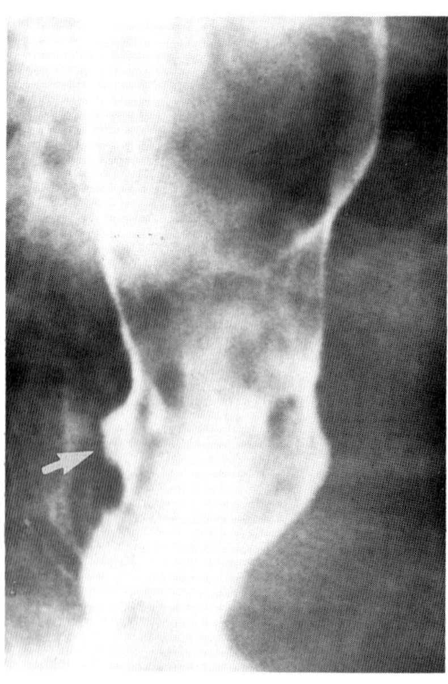

B

Figure 7.56. Peptic ulcer of the esophagus. (A) Proximal segment ulcer with signs of reflux esophagitis and hiatus hernia. (B) Distal segment ulcer.

any portion of the esophagus and is not the result of reflux. Stenoses caused by peptic ulceration should be distinguished from malignant stenoses and achalasia. Criteria for distinguishing benign from malignant stenoses are described in chapter 3 (see page 52).

During embryonic development, the esophagus is lined with stratified columnar epithelium which is replaced by ciliated epithelium, and then with stratified squamous epithelium. Changes start in the mid portion of the esophagus and progress in both proximal and distal directions. Columnar epithelium of the cervical segment of the esophagus is the last to undergo change. Any remaining columnar epithelium contains parietal and chief cells; this is not the case with Barrett's esophagus. Islets of columnar epithelium manifest as webs or ring-like protruding lesions.

ZOLLINGER-ELLISON SYNDROME

Autopsy results suggest esophageal involvement in 33% of patients with Zollinger–Ellison syndrome. Esophagitis is common, with ulcers of various depth, and with stenoses (Fig. 7.57) resulting from gastroesophageal reflux in association with excessive secretion of HCl in the stomach. Barrett's esophagus may result. However, the high gastrin levels associated with Zollinger–Ellison syndrome provoke increased LES tone, making gastroesophageal reflux uncommon.

THE RING OF SCHATZKI

The lower esophageal or Schatzki ring is a web at the junction of esophageal and gastric mucosa (Fig. 7.58); it is a membranous struc-

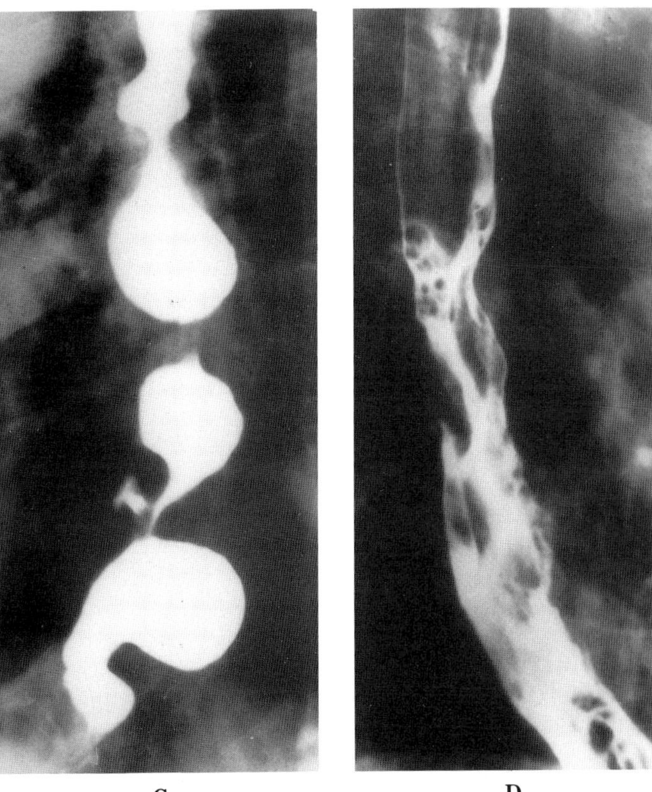

FIGURE 7.56. *continued.* (C) In distal segment with deep tertiary contraction. (D) Mild mid-esophageal stricture after healed peptic ulcer with thickened folds.

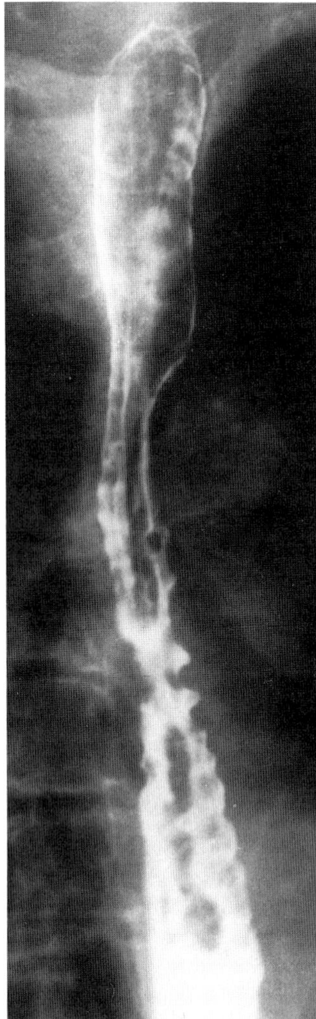

Figure 7.57. Esophagitis in Zollinger-Ellison syndrome.

ture in the region of the B-ring (sphincter of the cardia), resulting from esophagitis. Dysphagia in patients with a lower esophageal ring depends on its diameter. Some data indicate that the lower esophageal ring commonly causes dysphagia of solid food in adults; whether dysphagia occurs is dependent on the diameter of this esophageal ring.

Since there is great distensibility of the LES, the ring may protrude up to 6 mm into the esophageal lumen without causing subjec-

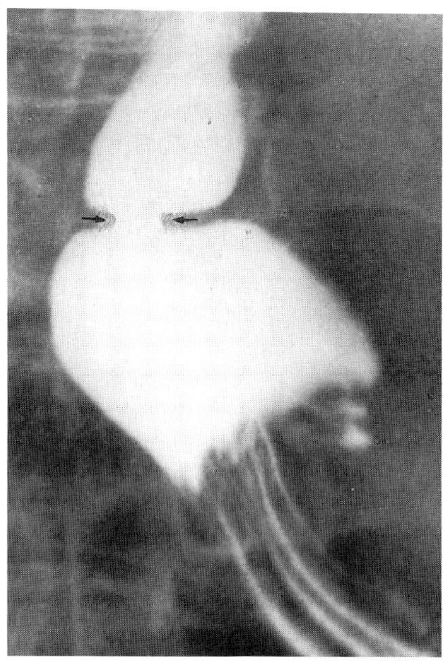

A

B

Figure 7.58. Lower esophageal ring—ring of Schatzki. (A) Projection of the ring (arrows) demonstrating the residual esophageal lumen. Also evident is a large hiatus hernia. (B) Typical ring.

tive symptoms. However, it can also cause significant dysphagia. The ring is only evident when there is hiatal gastric herniation with the cardia above the diaphragm. In this case the esophagus may be shortened by esophagitis. The ring is optimally shown when both proximal and distal segments of the esophagus are filled with barium suspension. It may also be demonstrated using double-contrast technique, when the lower esophageal segment is dilated. Spot films should be taken after swallowing of the contrast medium has been followed by a deep inspiration.

Single-contrast examination of the esophagus in the prone position reveals 95% of lower esophageal rings. However, the detection rate for double-contrast examination does not exceed 46%. The sensitivity of endoscopy in defining lower esophageal rings equals 58% and is dependent on the diameters of the ring and the endoscope. Discrete rings can easily be overlooked, particularly when small-caliber endoscopes are used. The radiologic examination is more accurate, and is the method of choice in patients whose dysphagia is suspected to be related to narrowing of the lower esophageal segment. A lower esophageal ring may narrow the esophageal lumen significantly, but stasis of the contrast medium and proximal dilatation are infrequent (Fig. 7.59).

A lower esophageal ring should be distinguished from a functional "contraction" ring, which represents an abnormally contracted tubulovestibular sphincter in the presence of hi-

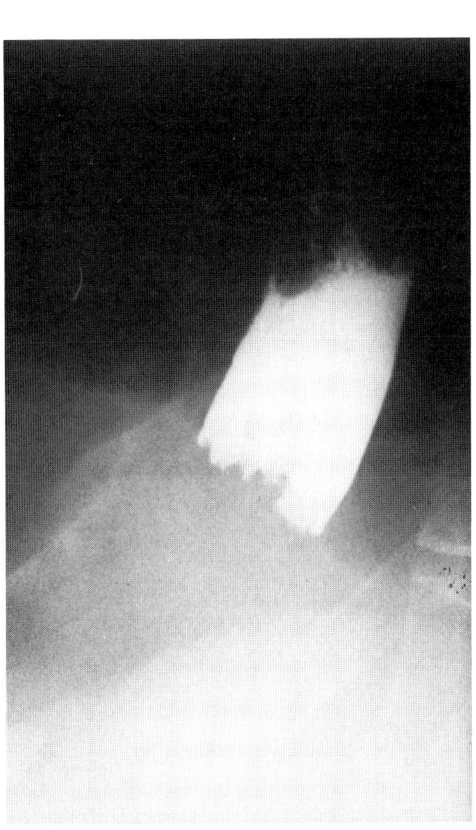

A

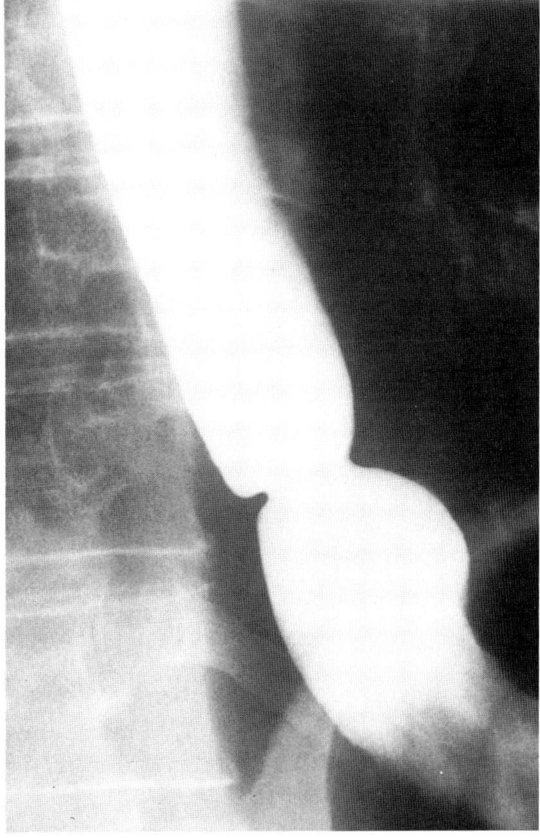

B

FIGURE 7.59. (A) Bolus of food lodged in the distal esophagus. (B) Ring of Schatzki impaction.

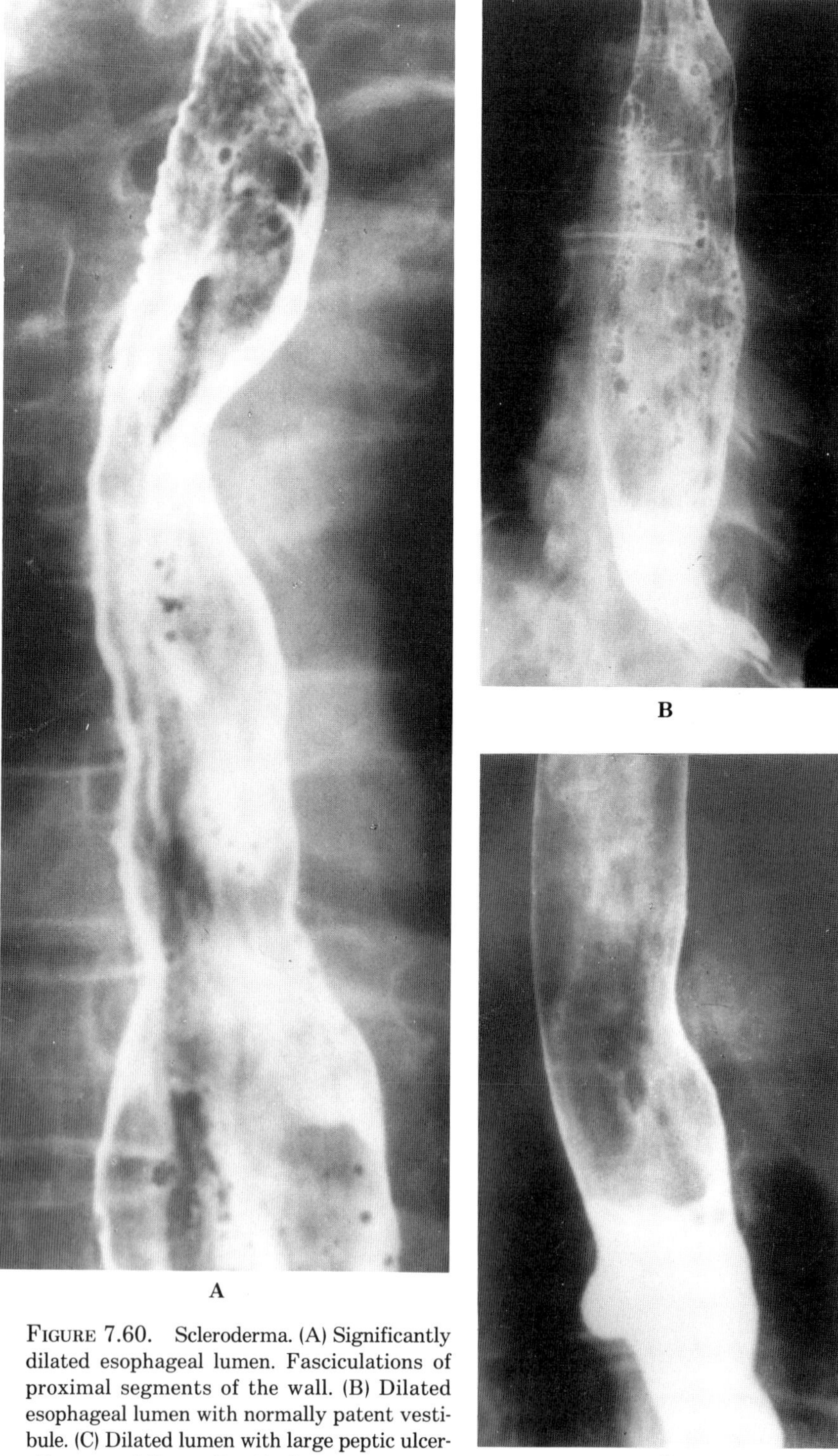

FIGURE 7.60. Scleroderma. (A) Significantly dilated esophageal lumen. Fasciculations of proximal segments of the wall. (B) Dilated esophageal lumen with normally patent vestibule. (C) Dilated lumen with large peptic ulceration resembling a diverticulum.

atal herniation. Differentiation from ring-like narrowings in portions of the stomach affected by hiatal herniation is necessary. Membranous formations may be detected up to 6 cm proximal to the esophagogastric junction in 0.14% of upper gastrointestinal examinations. Like webs in the cervical segment of the esophagus, they are the consequence of chronic irritation. Gastroesophageal reflux may cause these webs to be formed in the distal segments of the esophagus, as a rare and unusual response of the esophageal mucosa. They can be mistaken for the B-ring (mucosal ring in the region of the cardia) or the ring of Schatzki.

Various examination techniques may be used in the detection of hernias, strictures, and rings of the LES. These are single-contrast examination while the patient is in the prone position, demonstration of the mucosal relief, and double-contrast examination. A sensitivity of almost 100% is achieved by use of single-contrast examination. Demonstration of mucosal relief during a single-contrast examination reveals these lesions in 52% of the cases when they occur. Since they are performed mainly while the patient assumes a standing posture, double-contrast studies are successful in only 34%.

SCLERODERMA – PROGRESSIVE SYSTEMIC SCLEROSIS

The esophagus is affected in more than half the patients with scleroderma. Other collagenoses cause similar esophageal changes. Scleroderma results in atrophy of the smooth muscles of the esophagus with deposition of collagen in the submucosa. Striated muscles of the esophagus are not affected. The thoracic portion of the esophagus is hypotonic, with a widened lumen; peristaltic waves appear rarely, look shallow, or are even missing (Fig. 7.60). In advanced stages a bolus of highly concentrated barium "falls" as if traversing a rigid tube. The inner esophageal surface is smooth as a result of changes in the lamina muscularis mucosa. Peristalsis is uncoordinated, and shallow tertiary contractions or fasciculations may be noticed (Fig. 7.60A).

The threshold for eliciting peristalsis is increased. With the progression of disease, a decrease in the amplitude of primary peristaltic waves is accompanied by the disappearance of resting tone in the lower esophageal segment and symptoms of dysphagia. These changes are most pronounced when the patient is supine. Video-radiography demonstrates impaired motility of the esophagus. The specificity of the examination in revealing a lack of peristalsis reaches almost 100%. However, it decreases to 70% in individuals sixty or more years of age. Weakened and deficient peristalsis can be detected with a sensitivity of 70%. Hypotonia of the lower esophageal segment results in gastroesophageal reflux with resultant reflux esophagitis, ulceration, and shortening of the esophagus (Fig. 7.60C).

GRANULOMATOUS DISEASES

Involvement of the esophagus with Crohn's disease is rare, although any segment of the alimentary canal, as well as organs not belonging to the gastrointestinal tract, may be affected. Esophageal involvement with Crohn's disease is described in the section on esophagitis (see page 205).

NEOPLASMS

BENIGN NEOPLASMS

Benign esophageal neoplasms grow slowly. Like malignant tumors, they can cause dysphagia, but not before the tumor mass occupies approximately one-half of the esophageal lumen. Benign tumors do not interfere significantly with peristalsis.

Mesenchymal benign tumors – leiomyomas, lipomas, and fibromas – are more common than those that are epithelial. Submucosal tumors are mesenchymal in most instances. They cause regular radiolucent negative defects, transparencies, in an esophagus filled with contrast medium, and cause the overlying mucosa to bulge into the lumen. The mucosal folds are preserved, but shifted aside. They may even be formed in the manner of an arch. *Epithelial* tumors include adenomas and papillomas. These tumors originate from the mucosa and protrude into the lumen. They are most often spherical or oblong with contours that are sharply demarcated. They may have a stalk.

Leiomyomas are the most common benign esophageal tumors. They are most frequently found in the distal two-thirds of the esophagus. Growth may be limited to the submucosa (Fig. 7.61) but these tumors can develop a stalk and become movable. When they assume large dimensions they cause symptoms of intermittent obstruction. The mucosa overlying an esophageal myoma is infrequently ulcerated. This is not the case with alimentary tube myomas in other locations.

Radiologic examination should be used to differentiate benign tumors from extrinsic compression of the esophageal wall by adjacent structures, air bubbles, varices, or foreign bodies. It is most important to distinguish benign from malignant tumors. The latter cause destruction of mucosal surface and rigidity of the esophageal wall. Air bubbles are mobile. Submucosal varices affect longer segments of the esophagus and their morphologic appearance varies with the degree to which they are filled with blood.

MALIGNANT NEOPLASMS

Malignant esophageal tumors are more common than benign. They primarily affect the older male population. Unfortunately, subjective symptoms start only when the disease is advanced. About 90% of esophageal malignancies are carcinomas, and the remainder are sarcomas such as leiomyosarcoma (Fig. 7.62) or liposarcoma (Fig. 7.63), and lymphomas.

Carcinoma. Although it represents only about 5% of all alimentary canal carcinomas, esophageal carcinoma is the most significant esophageal disease because of its high mortality rate.

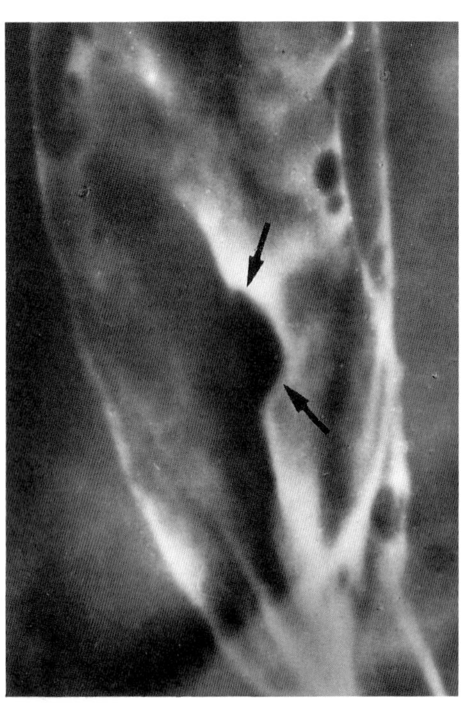

A

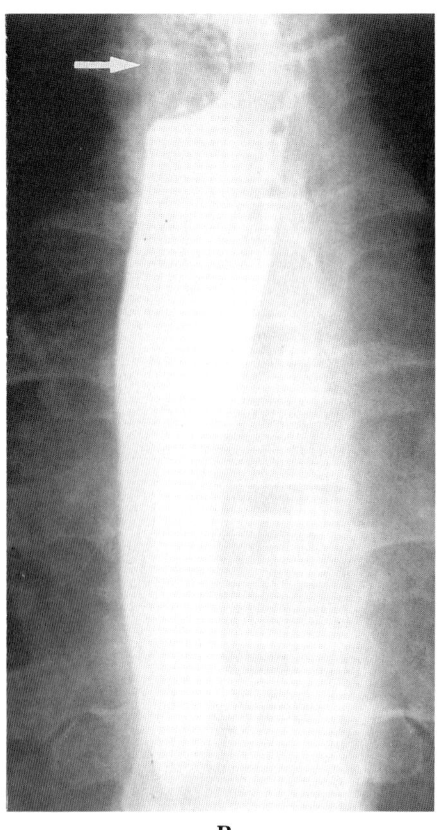

B

FIGURE 7.61. (A) Small esophageal leiomyoma (arrows). (B) Large esophageal leiomyoma (arrow).

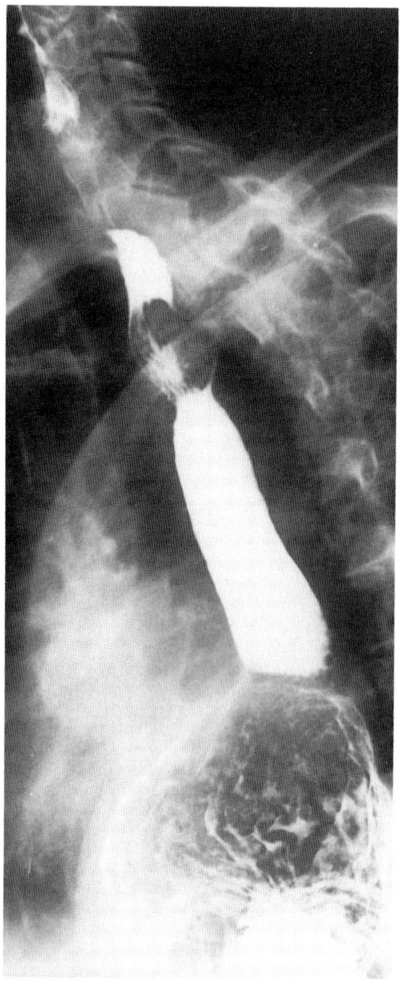

FIGURE 7.62. Ulcerated leiomyosarcoma of the esophagus. Hiatus hernia of the stomach.

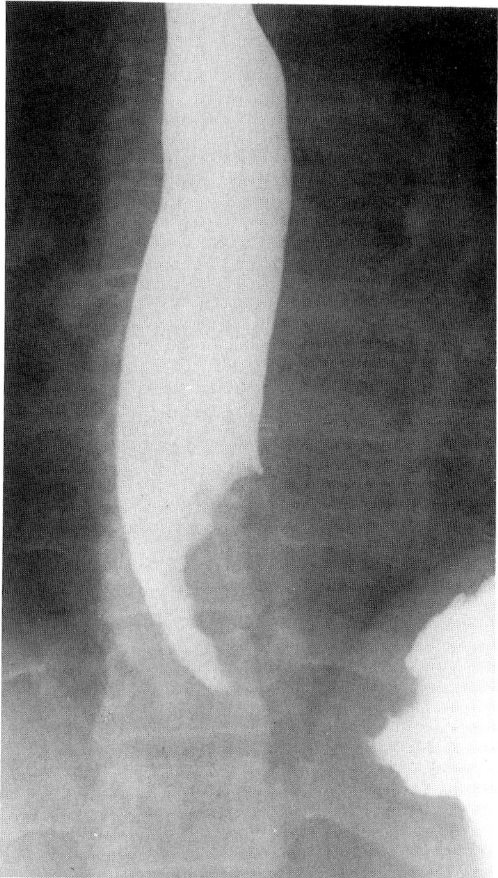

FIGURE 7.63. Liposarcoma of the distal esophageal segment.

The five-year survival rate is low, being only about 5% in patients who undergo therapy. Heavy drinking of alcohol and smoking significantly increase the risk of developing the disease. Patients with tylosis have a 100% chance of developing carcinoma of the esophagus. Carcinoma is more common in distal segments of the esophagus, where it has a better prognosis since it lacks close contact with vital structures.

The more distal the occurence of the stenosis in the esophagus, the more pronounced is the proximal dilatation. As a result of rapid growth, malignant tumors cause less pronounced proximal dilatation than benign stenoses. *Early esophageal carcinoma* does not penetrate deeper than the submucosa and is without metastases. It has a much better prognosis than advanced carcinoma, the five-year survival rate being almost 90%. The diagnosis of early carcinoma is rarely made on the basis of clinical symptoms. Indeed, dysphagia is the result of tumors which affect lymph nodes and other mediastinal structures.

To determine the relationship between progression of carcinoma and survival rate, several types of carcinoma have been defined. *Early carcinoma* is a superficial carcinoma without metastases. *Superficial carcinoma* of the esophagus may penetrate up to but does not involve the main muscular layer of the wall. Regional lymph nodes may be infiltrated with tumor cells. *Small carcinoma* is a tumor less than 35 mm in diameter. The sensitivity in diagnosing small carcinoma by upper gastrointestinal series is less than 73%, 6% of lesions being missed and 21% being mistaken for benign disease.

Superficial and small carcinomas may be early carcinomas. However, both superficial and small carcinoma with regional lymph node metastases have practically the same prognosis as advanced carcinoma. All these carcinomas may be of various microscopic types – squamous cell, adenocarcinoma, or small cell carcinoma.

The morphology of superficial and small carcinomas is that of a flat lesion with or without central ulceration. However, these carcinomas may be sessile polyps with smooth or lobulated surfaces. The macroscopic appearance of esophageal carcinoma does not vary with microscopic structure.

The radiologic appearance of early esophageal carcinoma may be similar to that of advanced carcinoma. Differentiation is established by microscopic analysis of the tumor, surrounding tissue, and lymph nodes. With deeper infiltration of the esophageal wall, lymph node involvement is more likely. Less than 1% of patients whose carcinoma affects only the mucosa have regional lymph node metastases. The prognosis depends on the depth of infiltration of the esophageal wall and involvement of lymph nodes. While these parameters are practically impossible to estimate by radiographic analysis, CT can determine both.

Carcinomas originating from the mucosal surface are often smoothly nodular and sharply demarcated from the adjacent wall, but they may have a reticular or granular surface. Carcinomas originating from deep mucous glands are mound-like.

Esophageal carcinomas can present with several macroscopic appearances. *Stenotic carcinoma* causes destruction of the mucosa, abrupt discontinuity of normal wall contour, interrupted mucosal folds, and "shouldering." The stenosed area may vary in length (Fig. 7.64A

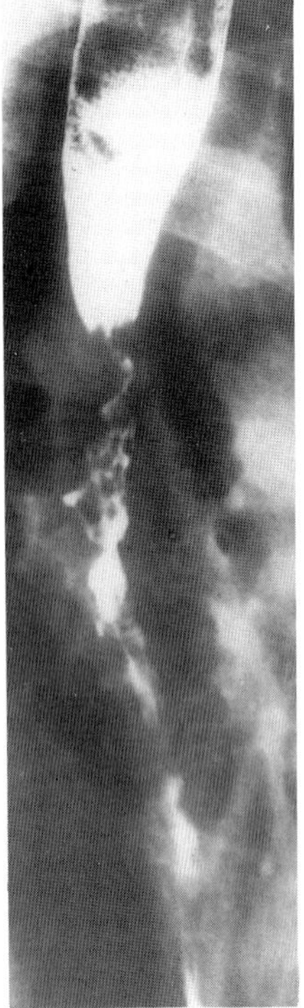

A

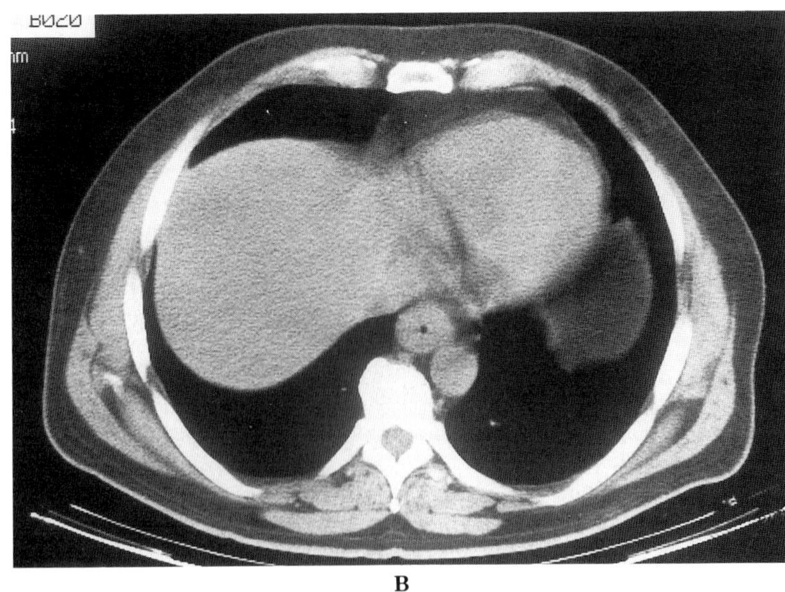

B

FIGURE 7.64. Esophageal carcinoma: Stenotic, annular esophageal carcinoma. (A) Barium studies. (B) CT examination. (*Figure continued on the following three pages.*)

and B). In exceptional cases, when the tumor is mainly confined to the wall, espohageal folds can be temporarily preserved. Esophageal segments proximal to the stenosis will be dilated.

Advanced *polypoid carcinoma* affects a major portion of the esophageal circumference and protrudes into the lumen (Fig. 7.64C–E). At times it may resemble esophageal varices and is then called varicoid carcinoma (Fig. 7.65C and D).

An *ulcerated, volcano-like carcinoma* frequently results from necrosis of a polypoid tumor, but may originate as a mucosal defect with irregular margins. An ulcerated carcinoma produces rigidity of the wall, but causes less severe obstructive symptoms than annular or polypoid forms (Fig. 7.64F and G). Differential diagnosis of esophageal carcinoma is presented in Table 7.6. Radiologic examinations should demonstrate the morphology, dimensions, and extension of a carcinoma into the mediastinum (lymph node metastases, communication with the respiratory system), and other complications, such as free perforation.

The majority of esophageal *adenocarcinomas* possess common radiologic properties. They arise from:

1. Gastric adenocarcinoma affecting the esophagus.
2. Submucosal and deep esophageal glands.
3. Elements of ectopic gastric mucosa in the esophagus.
4. Columnar epithelium lining Barrett's esophagus (Barrett's carcinoma).

A decrease in the incidence of squamous cell carcinoma and an increase in esophageal adenocarcinoma has been noted, with 19% of esophageal carcinoma being adenocarcinoma. Most adenocarcinomas originate in the distal segment, the majority being carcinoma of the cardia which affects the esophagus (Fig. 7.65A). They are primarily stenosing neoplasms and

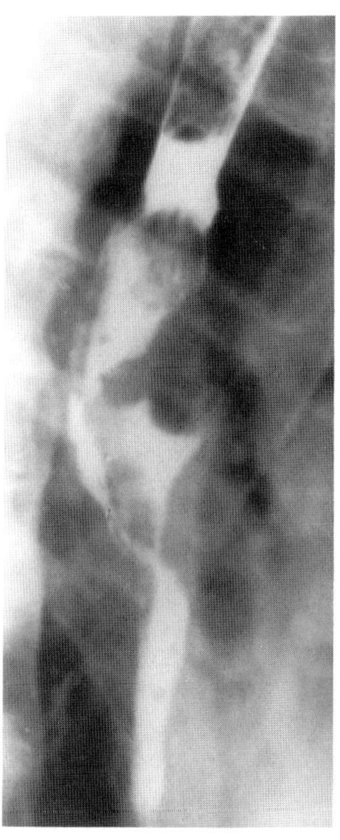

C

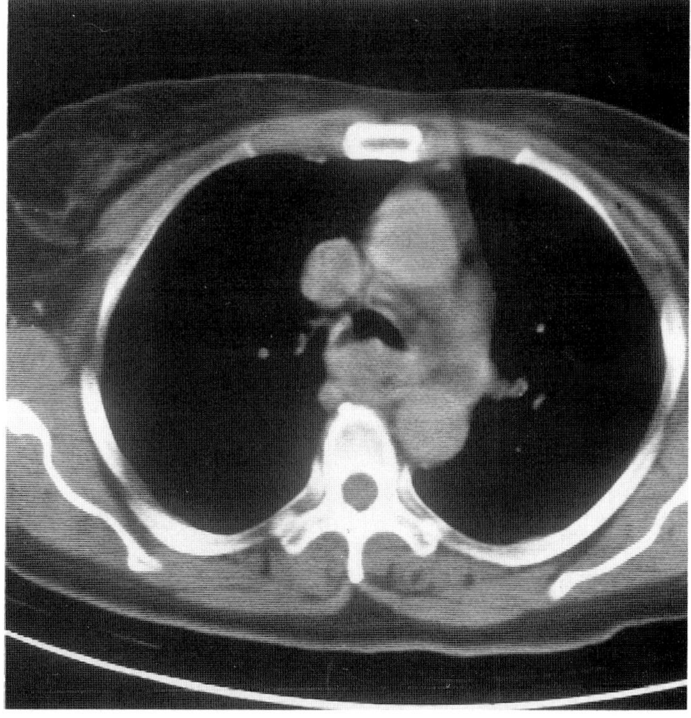

D

FIGURE 7.64 *continued.* Esophageal carcinoma: Polypoid. (C) Barium studies. (D) CT examination.

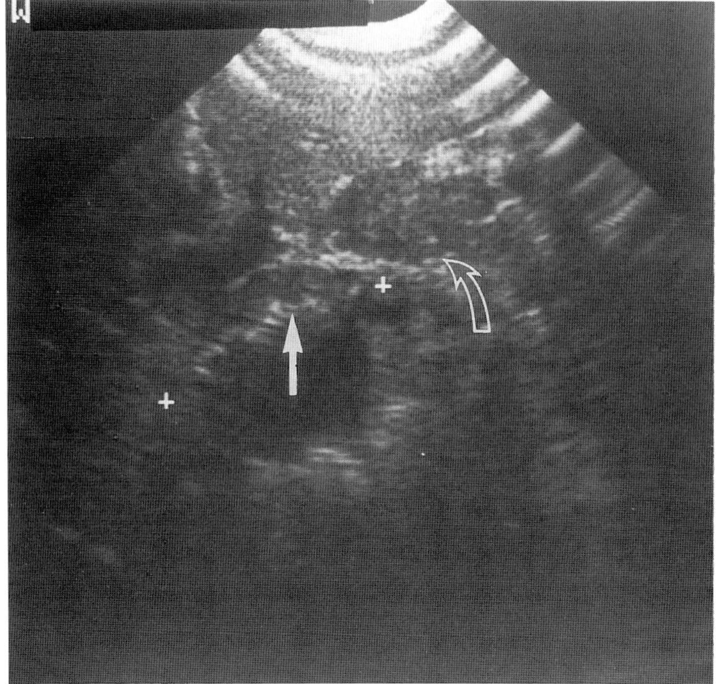

E

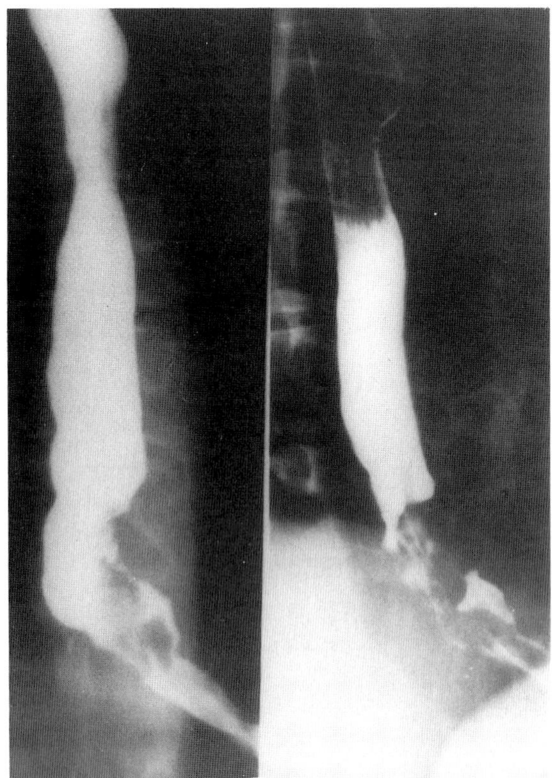

F

Figure 7.64 *continued.* Esophageal carcinoma: Polypoid. (E) Ultrasound examination showing thickened distal esophagus (closed arrow) with enlarged lesser omental nodes (open arrow). Courtesy of W.L. Wells, M.D., Louisiana State University, New Orleans. Esophageal carcinoma: Ulcerated. (F) Barium studies.

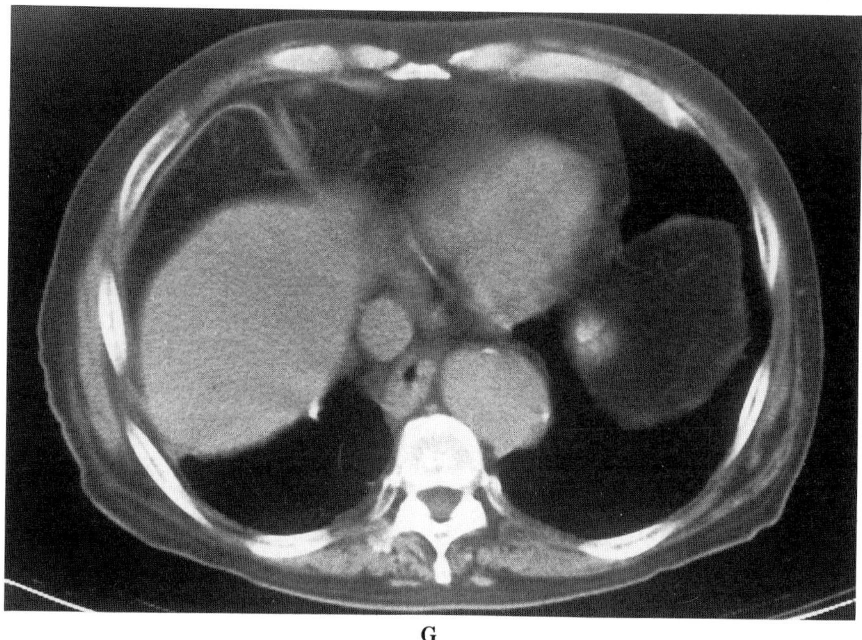

G

Figure 7.64 *continued.* Esophageal carcinoma: Ulcerated. (G) CT examination showing thickened esophageal wall.

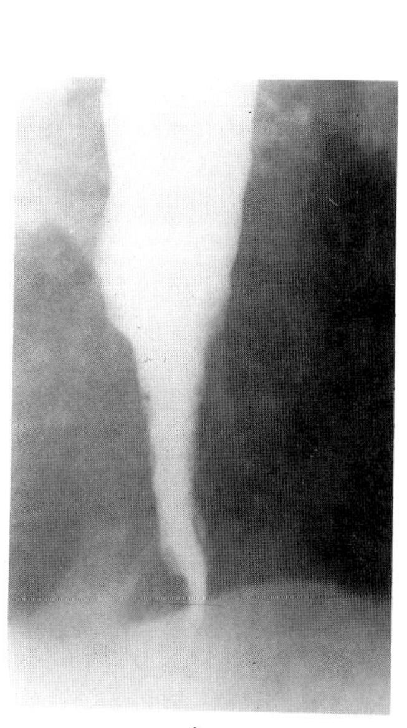

A

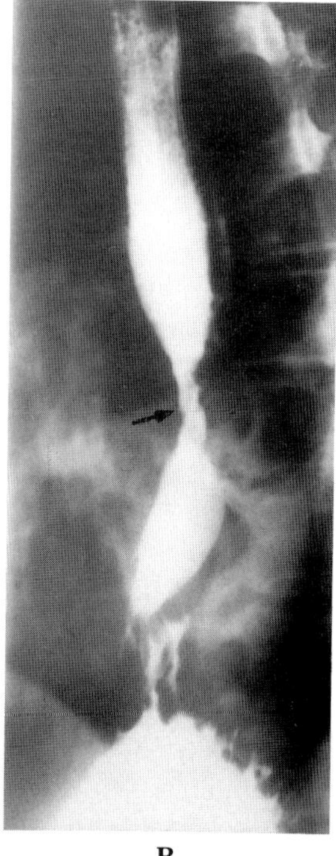

B

Figure 7.65. Adenocarcinoma of the esophagus. (A) Adenocarcinoma of the cardia infiltrating the distal portion of the esophagus, which is much longer than the lower esophageal segment. (B) Barrett's carcinoma in the region of a peptic stricture (arrow). (*Figure continued on overleaf*)

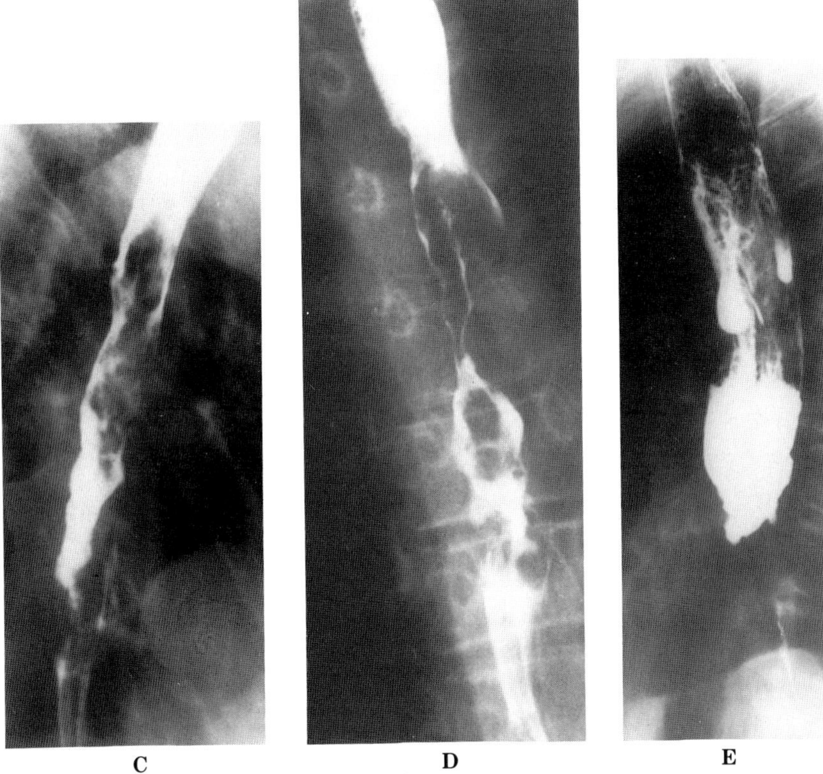

FIGURE 7.65 *continued.* Adenocarcinoma of the esophagus. (C, D) Varicoid Barrett's carcinoma. (E) Barrett's carcinoma affecting the distal segment of the esophagus. Pulsion diverticulum on the anterior wall.

TABLE 7.6. DIFFERENTIAL DIAGNOSIS OF ESOPHAGEAL NEOPLASIA

Varices
Benign stricture
Foreign body
Neoplasm of adjacent organs
Esophageal impression

may, in the early stage, resemble achalasia, except that the narrowed segment is longer than the vestibule, and shouldering may be present. Adenocarcinomas originating from esophageal glands and islets of heterotopic gastric mucosa in the esophagus are very rare.

Some 10% of patients with Barrett's esophagus develop esophageal adenocarcinoma. These tumors represent only 4% of all esophageal carcinoma and 20% of adenocarcinomas of the esophagus. The male-to-female ratio is 4:1, and the average age is 53 years. Subjective symptoms may be present for eight years and are related to reflux esophagitis and Barrett's esophagus. Exacerbation of dysphagia and weight loss frequently last for months before the diagnosis is established. Two-thirds of Barrett's carcinomas are situated in the lower third of the esophagus and one-third in the middle portion. However, one-third of patients have simultaneous involvement of the middle and distal thirds of the esophagus. Barrett's carcinoma arises near strictures and ulcers (Fig. 7.65B). These tumors are circumferential or varicoid and may spread along the submucosa and resemble benign strictures or varices (Fig. 7.65C and D). In two-thirds of patients, Barrett's carcinoma tends to affect long sections of the esophagus causing irregular stenosis whose average length is 8 cm (Fig. 7.65E). Barrett's carcinoma should be suspected when there are long strictures or varicoid defects of the distal segment of the esophagus. A history of chronic reflux esophagitis, hiatal hernia, and gastroesophageal reflux is important.

The most significant factors for estimating survival of patients with esophageal carcinoma are tracheal, aortic, and pericardial invasion. Patients with esophageal carcinoma can be categorized by CT into groups:

1. Those without evidence of invasion or metastases.
2. Those with mediastinal invasion and metastases, and
3. Those with inconclusive evidence of invasion requiring follow-up CT studies.

Mediastinal and subdiaphragmatic adenopathy can be revealed by CT. The main indicator of metastases is the enlargement of lymph nodes. In patients with esophageal carcinoma, upper abdominal lymph nodes, particularly those above the celiac axis and in the gastrohepatic ligament, are frequently involved; consequently, CT of the upper abdomen should not be omitted. It is not possible to determine accurately the depth of esophageal wall infiltration by CT. Carcinoma of superior and middle segments of the esophagus directly invades the trachea and bronchi. These organs are not always separated by fat planes, so indentation or displacement of the tracheal wall can be signs of invasion. The aorta is infrequently invaded directly, therefore absence of a fat plane between the esophagus and the aorta should not be considered abnormal. Preservation of a fat plane indicates the absence of pericardial invasion, but its absence should not be considered abnormal.

There are many controversies regarding CT staging of esophageal carcinoma. It is unreliable in patients with carcinoma of the cervical esophagus, carcinoma of the LES, and nonsquamous cell primary carcinoma. Sensitivity for detecting mediastinal lymphadenopathy is only 48% and, for abdominal lymph nodes, 61%. However, specificity exceeds 90% for mediastinal and abdominal lymph nodes. Progression of a carcinoma can be estimated according to the TNM classification in only 37% of patients with esophageal carcinoma.

Leiomyosarcoma is the most common malignant mesenchymal neoplasm of the esophagus. These polypoid, submucosal, oval masses of solid consistency are larger than myomas, and arise from the main muscular layer, and exceptionally, from the *lamina muscularis mucosae*. Ulcerations are not seen as often as in leiomyosarcoma from other locations in the alimentary canal (Fig. 7.62). Pedunculated leiomyosarcomas are uncommon.

Also referred to as *lymphosarcoma, lymphoma* affects the esophagus in 1% of patients with generalized lymphoma. Irregular narrowing of the distal segment of the esophagus is a most common radiographic finding and may mimic a polypoid carcinoma. Diffuse submucosal infiltrates may assume various dimensions and resemble varices (Fig. 7.66). Nodular lymphoma of the esophagus is characterized by multiple nodes protruding into the lumen and resembling moniliasis. Indeed, both conditions are, in addition, characterized by immunological impairment. Superficially spreading carcinoma,

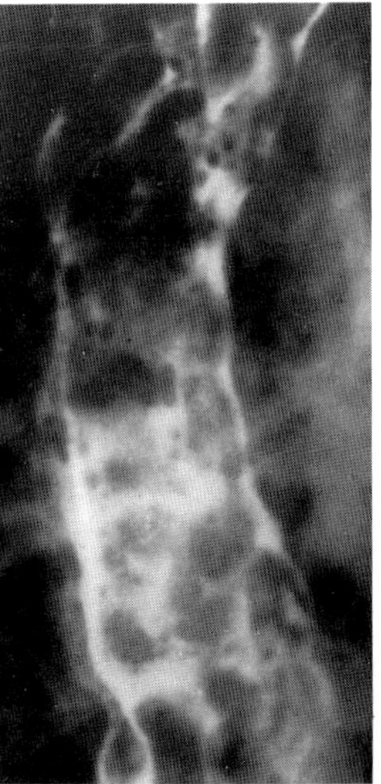

Figure 7.66. Nodular lymphoma of the esophagus. Findings resemble esophageal varices or oat cell esophageal carcinoma.

glycogenic acanthosis, and viral esophagitis should also be of consideration in differential diagnosis.

Carcinosarcoma of the esophagus (spindle cell variant of squamous cell carcinoma) develops silently. This very rare tumor originates in the middle third of the esophagus and represents not more than 0.1–1.5% of all esophageal neoplasms. It is a large bulky mass with a lobulated surface and local expansion causing little obstruction. The lobulated structure results in a dome-like configuration of the proximal portion of the tumor (Fig. 7.67). Occasionally, carcinosarcomas have been detected with a stalk. A carcinosarcoma consists of two components – squamous epithelial carcinoma cells and sarcoma spindle cells. Both components can metastasize.

Differential diagnosis of large polypoid esophageal lesions, such as carcinosarcoma, should include lesions such as myofibroma, lipoma, fibrovascular polyp and myoma, which are benign. However, sarcoma and adenocarcinoma can give rise to similar radiographic findings. For definitive diagnosis, microscopic examination is inevitable.

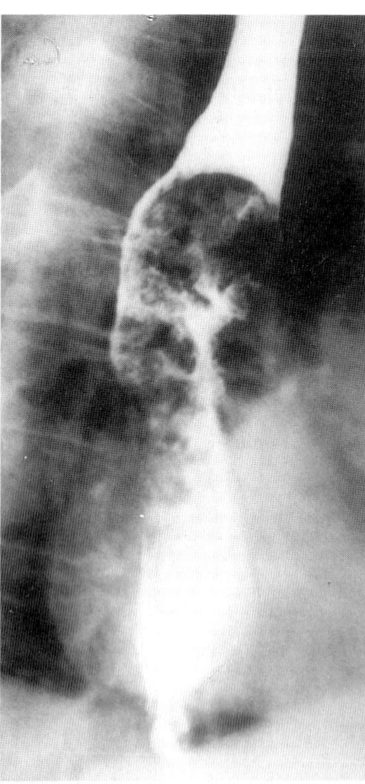

FIGURE 7.67. Carcinosarcoma of the esophagus. A characteristic finding.

Malignant esophageal tumors should be differentiated from benign tumors, esophagitis, peptic ulcer, achalasia, corrosive esophagitis and varices. Oat cell esophageal carcinoma may cause a macroscopic appearance similar to that of varicoid carcinoma and may be impossible to differentiate from esophageal nodular lymphoma.

Tumors of the lower esophageal segment should be differentiated from retrograde prolapse of gastric mucosa into the esophagus. Signs of such a prolapse are a mushroom-like defect in the lower esophageal segment, slow entering of barium suspension into the stomach, and gastroesophageal reflux.

The esophagus may be the site of *secondary tumors*, particularly bronchogenic and breast carcinoma. Metastatic tumors can cause obstructive symptoms, and their morphology may resemble benign esophageal strictures. However, they cannot always be differentiated from primary esophageal malignancies. Metastatic tumors may result in fistula formation (Fig. 7.68).

FOREIGN BODIES IN THE ESOPHAGUS

Foreign bodies impact more commonly in the pharynx than in the esophagus. When they lodge in the esophagus, they do so at sites of physiologic narrowings (Fig. 7.69).

Esophageal stenoses, regardless of etiology, predispose to impaction of solid contents, which then become a foreign body. The position of a foreign body is established and controlled fluoroscopically. When perforation is not suspected, plain roentgenography and fluoroscopy may be followed by a barium swallow.

Esophageal foreign bodies may be removed by proteolytic enzymes like papain, treatment with glucagon or Buscopan, or swallowing of effervescent agents, as well as by the use of an endoscope or by retrograde balloon extraction. Carbonated beverages may empty esophageal contents in patients with achalasia and stenosing carcinoma of the distal esophagus.

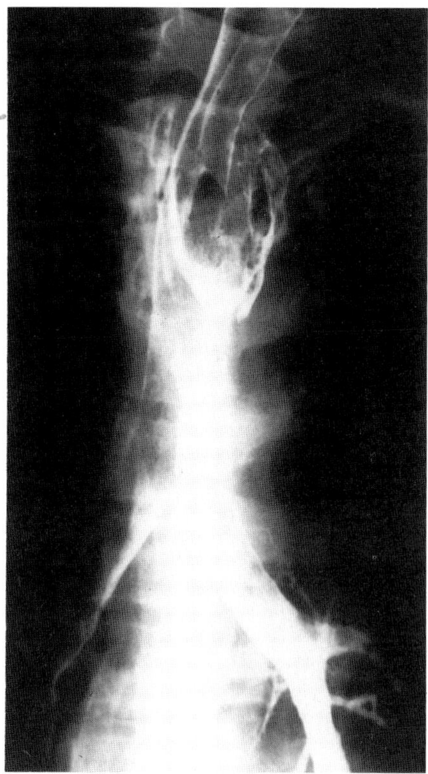

FIGURE 7.68. Esophagotracheal fistula in Hodgkin's disease.

INJURIES

Trauma to the esophagus may result from foreign bodies, particularly during their extraction (Figs. 7.70 and 7.71). Esophageal peptic ulcers, and less commonly carcinomas, may result in perforation.

An abnormal chest X-ray, showing pneumomediastinum and air in soft tissues of the neck, is seen in 90% of patients with a perforated thoracic esophagus. Esophageal perforation is life threatening. The abdominal segment of the esophagus, which is least frequently involved, perforates into the retroperitoneal space. Iatrogenic instrumental procedures are a causative factor in 70% of perforations, but spontaneous rupture may also occur.

Rupture of the esophagus may result from compression of the chest or from swallowing a sharp foreign body. Rupture of a single esophageal layer is found in Mallory-Weiss's syndrome. As a result of vigorous vomiting, Boerhaave's syndrome is characterized by ruptures of all layers of the distal esophagus. Sudden increase of pressure in the esophageal lumen is a common pathophysiologic factor. Perforation or rupture of the distal esophagus results in left-sided hydropneumothorax, while perforation of the middle portion results in

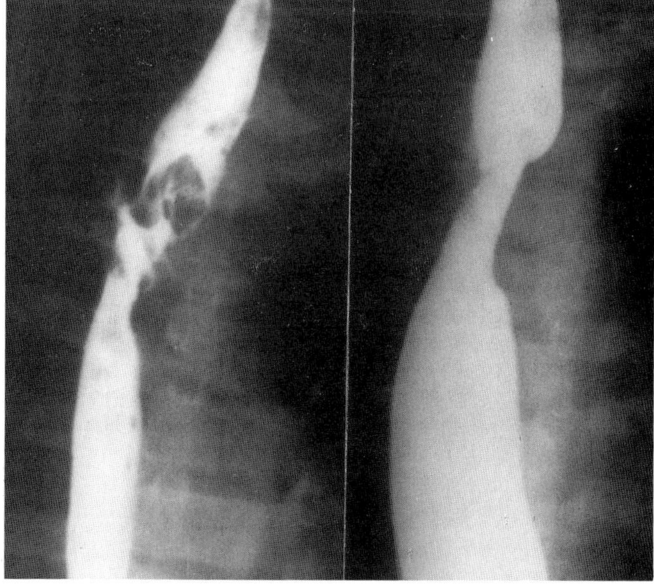

FIGURE 7.69. Foreign body in the esophagus. A button that the patient swallowed three weeks earlier has lodged in the esophagus with surrounding tissue reaction (left figure). Esophageal stenosis is seen two weeks after endoscopic extraction. Previous stenosis caused foreign body impaction, or stenosis resulted from tissue reaction to the foreign body.

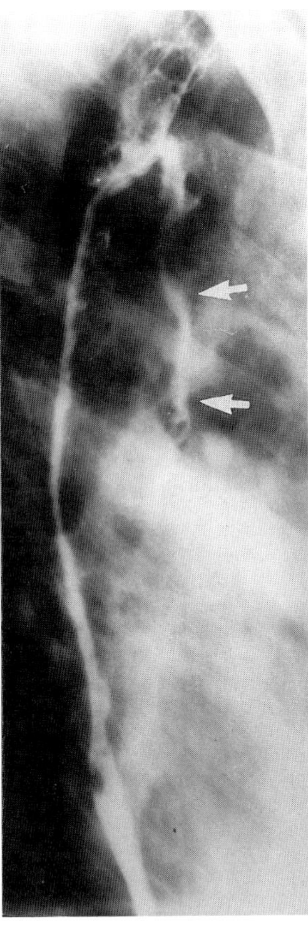

Figure 7.70. Perforation of the esophagus by a rigid endoscope. Water-soluble contrast medium is seen leaking into the mediastinum (arrows).

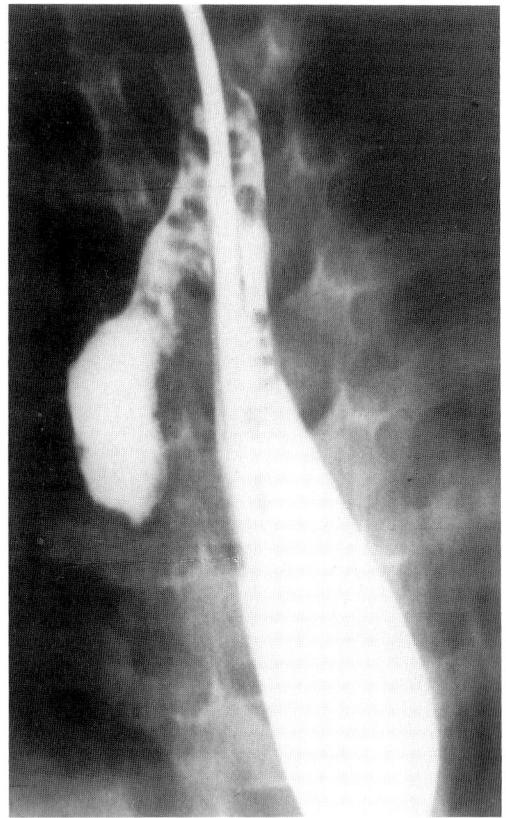

Figure 7.71. Perforation of the esophagus. Water-soluble contrast medium is administered via a catheter.

right-sided hydropneumothorax. The chest roentgenogram may be negative in 12% of patients with a perforated esophagus. In the case of esophageal trauma, evaluation by water-soluble contrast medium should be used. If an endoscopic procedure caused traumatization, it should not be repeated. *Hematoma* of the esophageal wall clinically and radiologically mimics esophageal tumors.

Radiation injuries to the esophagus result in the thickening of esophageal folds and in mucosal ulcers. Stenoses appear in chronic phases (Fig. 7.72). Intracavitary irradiation of esophageal carcinoma can result in pronounced stricturing after 12 to 20 months. The length of the stricture depends on the length of the esophageal segment affected by both tumor and radiation.

CORROSIVE LESIONS

Ingestion of caustic substances such as alkali and acids results in corrosive injuries of the esophagus. The former causes more severe injury. The degree of injury depends on the concentration, viscosity, and length of contact with the mucosa. Initially, an examination should be performed with water-soluble iso-osmolar contrast medium.

Edema of the mucosa and submucosa, accompanied by ulcers, bleeding, and the disappearance of mucosal relief, characterizes the

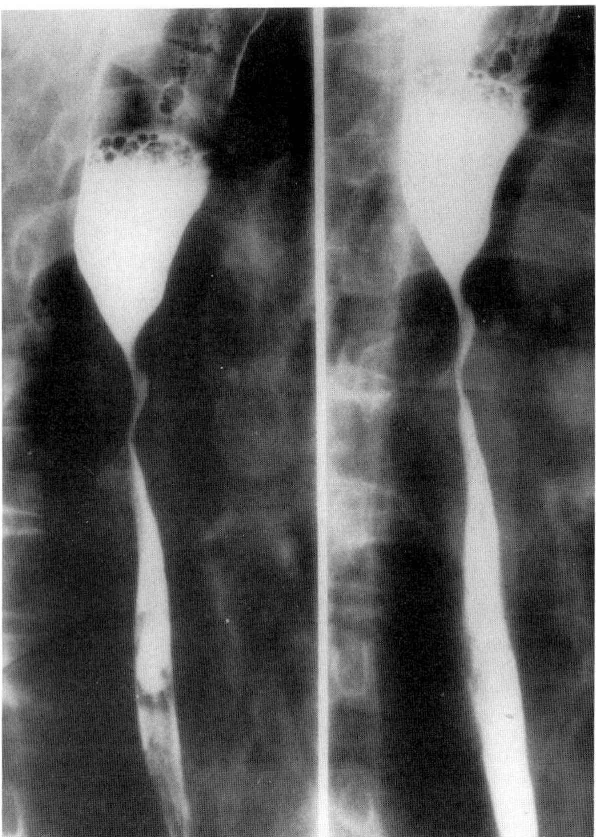

FIGURE 7.72. Radiation injury to the esophagus. Note rigidity of the wall.

acute phase (Fig. 7.73A). The esophagus may be either atonic or hypertonic during the first several hours subsequent to injury. The acute phase lasts 10 days, and the subacute approximately 20 days, after injury. Chronic changes occur four weeks following ingestion of a corrosive agent and may result in stricturing (Fig. 7.73B). The most common sites for the stricture to develop are the lower and middle portions of the esophagus, accompanied by prestenotic dilatation. These strictures have a typically benign radiographic appearance. When situated in the lower esophageal segment, corrosive strictures may mimic early achalasia, a traumatic lesion, or stenosis resulting from chronic reflux esophagitis. History is helpful in establishing a diagnosis. In addition to the esophagus, the stomach may also be injured by a corrosive agent. The lesser curvature will be shortened and the antrum stenosed.

Esophageal injuries by *drugs* are infrequent. Causative agents are tetracyclines, slowly releasing KCl tablets, quinidine, doxicycline, ferric sulfate, clindamycin, and ascorbic acid. A proximal segment of the esophagus, particularly at the level of aortic arch, is most commonly injured. This results in edema of the mucosa, erosions, and shallow ulcers. Esophageal injury induced by tetracycline may mimic a malignant tumor.

THE POSTOPERATIVE ESOPHAGUS

The outer surface of the esophagus, unlike other organs of the alimentary tube, is covered

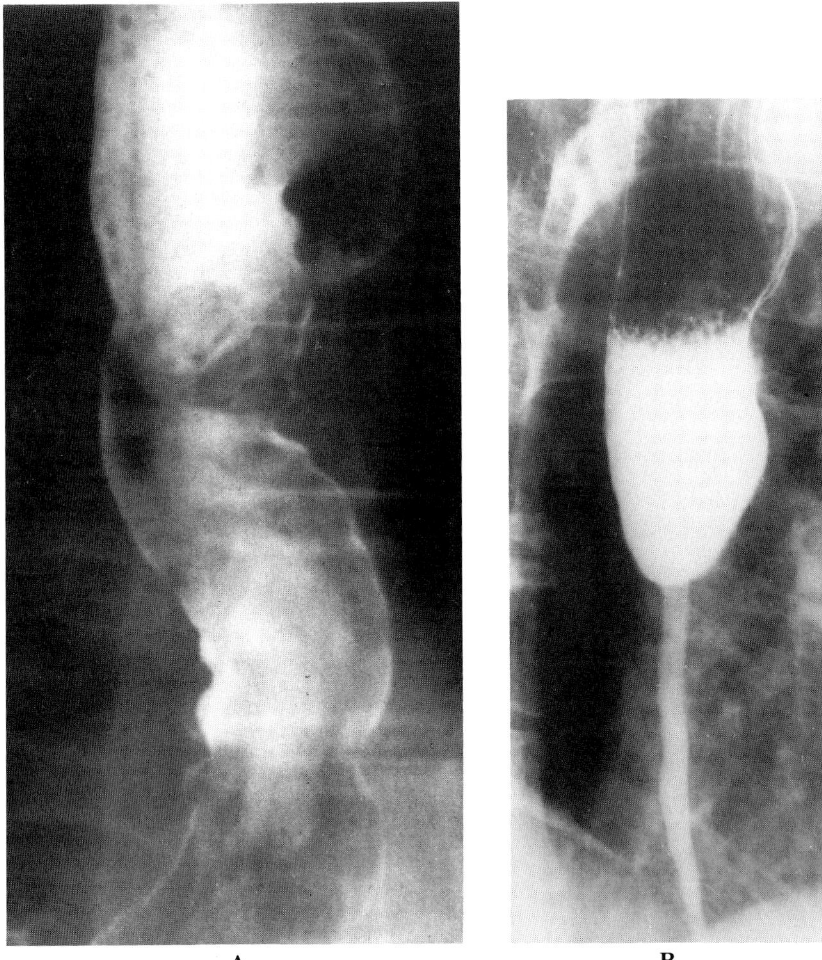

Figure 7.73. Corrosive injury of the esophagus. (A) Acute phase two hours after alkali ingestion. Hypotonia with shallow tertiary contractions. (B) Chronic phase. Stricture of the distal half of the esophagus with proximal dilatation.

by adventitia and not by serosa. This results in slow postoperative healing, with possible leakage of minute amounts of liquid esophageal contents. However, healing commonly occurs spontaneously. If dehiscence of sutures with subsequent leakage of esophageal contents is suspected, water-soluble contrast medium should be used for radiologic examination.

After endoscopic injection sclerotherapy of esophageal varices, two types of changes can be recorded. In the *early* period, lasting up to one month following sclerotherapy, mucosal ulcers, stenoses, fistulae, dissections, and perforations of the esophageal wall may occur. In the *late* period, one month or more after sclerotherapy, irregularities of esophageal contour, strictures, wall defects, dysmotility, and sometimes obstructive symptoms can be found. A careful history can eliminate problems in differential diagnosis.

Congenital stenoses, and some acquired stenoses, including malignant neoplasms, can be *dilated* with a balloon catheter (Fig. 7.74).

Gastric interposition is performed without

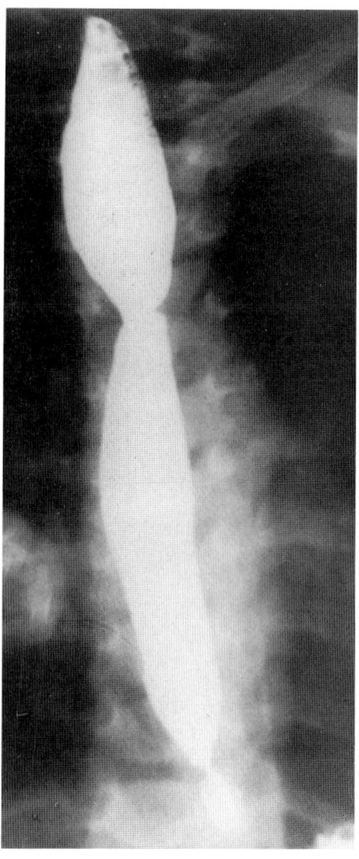

Figure 7.74. Esophagogram taken after dilatation of a congenital esophageal stenosis.

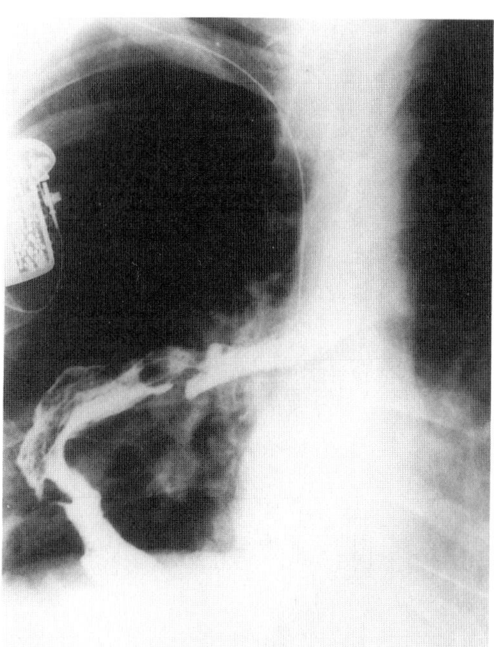

Figure 7.75. "Pull-through" surgery. Stomach is moved into the chest to replace a segment of resected esophagus.

thoracotomy following transhiatal esophagectomy. After cervical esophagogastrostomy, interposition of the stomach into the posterior mediastinum can be performed. This operation may be palliative or, in lucky persons, a definitive procedure (Fig. 7.75). Complications encountered in the *early period* are anastomotic leaks, cricopharyngeal incoordination with aspirations, and gastric perforation. *Late complications* are strictures in the region of the anastomosis, pyloric stenosis, tumor recurrence, and transhiatal herniation of abdominal organs.

Excised portions of the esophagus can be replaced by jejunal autotransplant (Fig. 7.76). *Free jejunal autotransplant* is suitable for reconstruction of the cervical segment of the

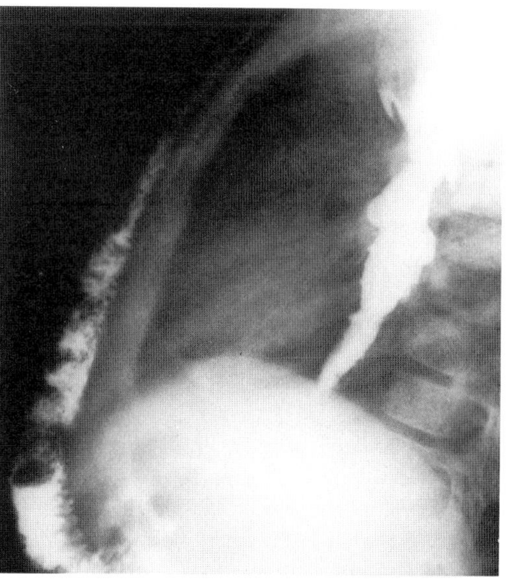

Figure 7.76. Subcutaneous interposition of bowel between the pharynx and abdominal segments of the alimentary canal in a patient with esophageal carcinoma.

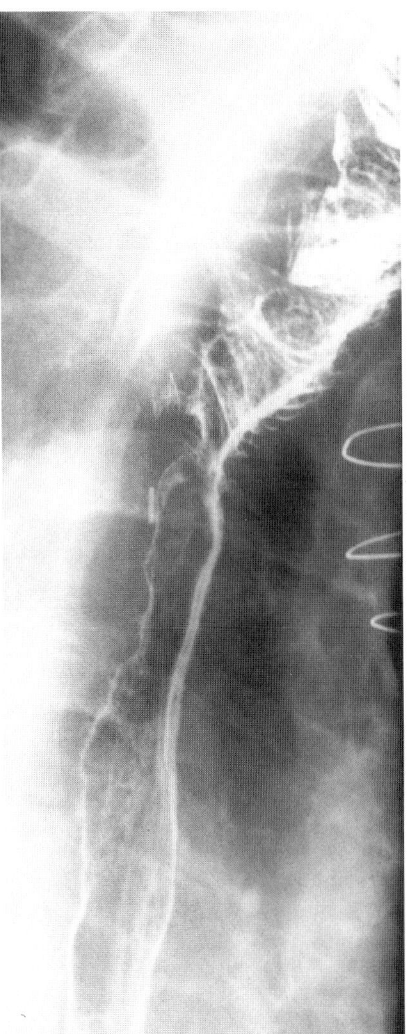

Figure 7.77. Free jejunal autotransplant interposed in place of resected cervical esophagus for carcinoma.

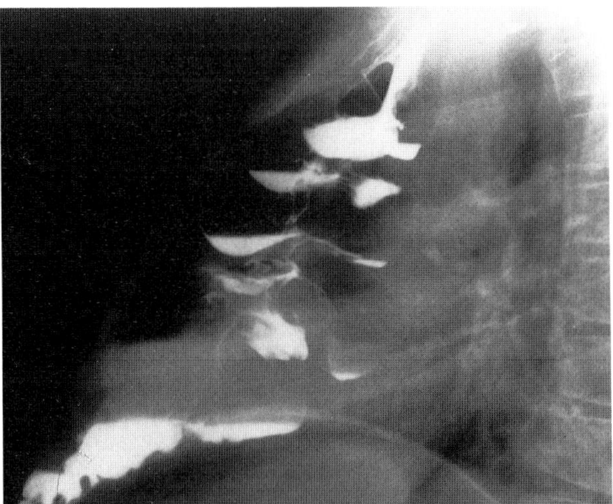

Figure 7.78. Colon autotransplant replacing an esophagus resected for carcinoma.

esophagus (Fig. 7.77). Barium swallow is the method of choice for estimating success of the operation and finding later complications.

Following an interposition of the colon as a transplant in place of a resected segment of the esophagus, an examination during the first 10 days should be performed using water-soluble contrast medium (Fig. 7.78). Ischemia of the interpositioned portion of the colon, character-

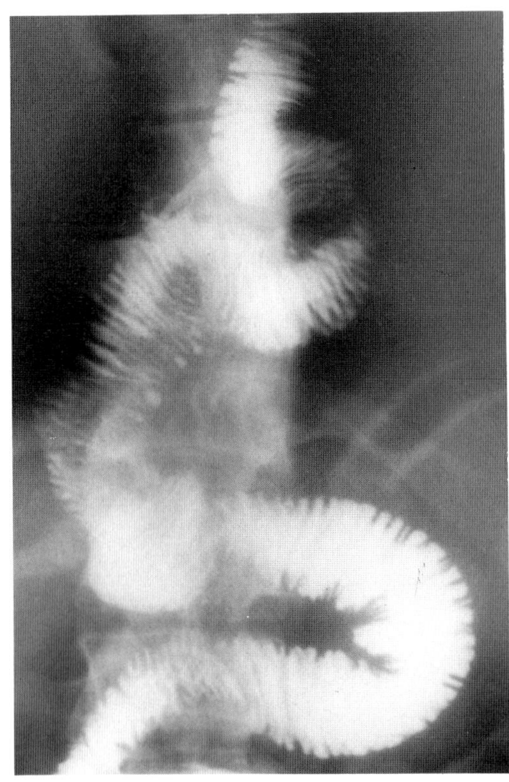

Figure 7.79. Interposition of jejunum for resected esophagus and stomach.

ized by mucosal edema, spasms, ulcers, loss of haustral markings, and leakage of contrast medium into the mediastinum, along with incoordination of swallowing, are frequent findings. Late complications are stenoses, reflux, and stasis of esophageal contents.

A prosthesis made of artificial materials may be used in patients with gastroesophageal reflux.

Esophagogastrectomy is performed in patients with carcinoma of the tubular portion of the esophagus, lower esophageal segment, and cardia. Barium is the agent of choice for examining interpositioned small intestine in these patients (Fig. 7.79). Alternatives are water-soluble contrast medium or CT.

Bibliography

Abrams L, Heath D. Lower esophagus lined with intestinal and gastric epithelia. Thorax. 1965;20:66.

Adler RH. What is the cardia? JAMA. 1962;182: 1045.

Agha FP, Orringer MB. Colonic interposition—radiographic evaluation. AJR. 1984;142:703.

Agha FP. The esophagus after endoscopic injection sclerotherapy: acute and chronic changes. Radiology. 1984;153:37.

Agha FP. Esophageal involvement in Zollinger-Ellison syndrome. AJR. 1985;144:721.

Agha FP. Transient intraluminal diverticulum of the esophagus: a significant flow artifact. Gastrointest Radiol. 1984;9:99.

Agha FP, Orringer MB, Amendola MA. Gastric interposition following transhiatal esophagectomy: radiographic evaluation. Gastrointest Radiol. 1985:10:17.

Agha FP, Dabich L. Barrett's esophagus complicating scleroderma. Gastrointest Radiol. 1985;10: 325.

Agha FP. Barrett carcinoma of the esophagus: clinical and radiographic analysis of 34 cases. AJR. 1985;145:41.

Agha FP, Keren DF. Spindle-cell squamous carcinoma of the esophagus: a tumor with biphasic morphology. AJR. 1985;145:541.

Agha FP, Wilson JAP, Nostrand T. Medication-induced esophagitis. Gastrointest Radiol. 1986;11:7.

Anderson MF, Harell GS. Secondary esophageal tumors. AJR. 1980;135:1243.

Andren L, Theander G. Roentgenographic appearances of esophageal moniliasis. Acta Radiol. 1956; 46:571.

Appleton DS, Sandrasagra FA, Flower CDR. Perforated esophagus: review of twenty eight consecutive cases. Clin Radiol. 1979;30:493.

Bane AE. Bleeding from lacerations of the cardia: the Mallory Weiss syndrome. JAMA. 1963;184:325.

Barret NR. Benign stricture of the lower esophagus. Proc Roy Soc Med. 1960;53:402.

Barsony T. Funktionelle Speiserohrendivertikl. Wien Klin Wschr. 1926;39:1963.

Berenberg W, Nenhauser EBD. Cardioesophageal relaxation (chalasia) as a cause of vomiting in infants. Pediatrics. 1950;5:414.

Blane, CE, Klein MD, Drongowski RA, Sarahan TM. Gastroesophageal reflux in children: is there a place for the upper gastrointestinal study? Gastrointest Radiol. 1986;11:346.

Bleshman MH, Banner MP, Johnson RC, De Ford J. The inflammatory esophagogastric polyp and fold. Radiology. 1978;128:589.

Blum DS, Weis A, Weiselberg HM, Siegel WB. Retrograde prolapse of gastric mucosa into the esophagus. Gastroenterology. 1961;41:408.

Botha GMS. Mucosal folds at the cardia as a component of the gastroesophageal closing mechanism. Br J Surg. 1958;45:569.

Bremer JL. Diverticula and duplication of intestinal tract. Arch Path. 1944;38:132.

Burhenne LJW, Frathin LB, Flak B, Burhenne HJ. Radiology of the angelohic prosthesis for gastroesophageal reflux. AJR. 1984;142:507.

Butler ML. Radiologic diagnosis of Mallory-Weiss syndrome. Br J Radiol. 1973;46:553.

Chen YM, Gelfand DW, Ott DJ, Wu WC. Barrett esophagus as an extension of severe esophagitis: analysis of radiologic signs in 29 cases. AJR. 1985;145:278.

Chen YM, Ott DJ, Gelfand DW, Munitz HA. Multiphasic examination of the esophagogastric region for strictures, rings and hiatal hernia: evaluation of the individual techniques. Gastrointest Radiol. 1985;10:311.

Chen YM, Ott DJ, Hewerson EG, Richter JE, Wu WC, Gelfand DW, Castell DO. Diffuse esophageal spasm: radiographic and manometric correlation. Radiology. 1989;170:807.

Chermin MM, Amberg JR, Kogan FJ, Morgan TR, Sampliner RE. Efficacy of radiologic studies in the detection of Barrett's esophagus. AJR. 1986; 147:257.

Christiensen T, Thommesen P. Food stimulated gastroesophageal reflux demonstrated by barium examination. Acta Radiol Diagn. 1986;27:45.

Cleveland RH, Kushner DC, Schwartz AN. Gastroesophageal reflux in children: results of standardized fluoroscopic approach. AJR. 1983;141:53.

Cohen, S, Lipshutz W. Lower esophageal dysfunction in achalasia. Gastroenterology. 1971;61:814.

Cohen S, Lipshutz W, Hughes W. Role of gastrin supersensitivity in pathogenesis of lower esophageal sphincter hypertension in achalasia. J Clin Invest. 1971:150:1241.

Cohen S, Harris LD. The lower esophageal sphincter. Gastroenterology. 1972;63:1066.

Cohen S. Motor disorders of the esophagus. N Engl J Med. 1979;301:184.

Conway-Hughes JHL. Esophageal reflux. An analysis of 453 consecutive barium meal examinations. Br J Radiol. 1956;29:321.

Cynn WS, Chon H, Gureghian PA, Levin BL. Crohn's disease of the esophagus. AJR. 1975;125:359.

Davis JA, Kantrowitz PA, Chandler HL, Schatzki SC. Reversible achalasia due to reticulum-cell sarcoma. N Engl J Med. 1975;293:130.

De Gaeta L, Levine MS, Guglielmi GE, Raffensperger EC, Laufer I. Herpes esophagitis in an otherwise healthy patient. AJR. 1985;144:1205.

Degryse HRM, De Schepper MAP. Aphthoid esophageal ulcers in Crohn's disease of ileum and colon. Gastrointest Radiol. 1984;9:197.

Dreyfuss JR, Wilkos RG. The elevator esophagus. A fluoroscopic clue to possible organic disease. Radiology. 1960;75:914.

Edwards DAW. Concepts of esophageal disorders. J Roy Soc Med. 1980;73:402.

Ekberg O. Cervical esophageal webs in patients with dysphagia. Clin Radiol. 1981;32:633.

Feczko PJ, Halpert RD. Achalasia secondary to non-gastrointestinal malignancies. Gastrointest Radiol. 1985;10:273.

Felson B, Lessure AD. "Downhill" varices of the esophagus. Dis Chest. 1964;46:740.

Frager DH, Frager JD, Brandt LJ, Wolf EL, Rand LG, Klein RS, Beneventano TC. Gastrointestinal complications of AIDS: radiologic features. Radiology. 1986;158:597.

Fransson SG, Sokjer H, Johansson KE, Tibbing L. Radiologic diagnosis of gastroesophageal reflux. Acta Radiol. 1989;30:187.

Friedland GW. Historical review of the changing concepts of lower esophageal anatomy: 430 B.C–1977. AJR. 1978;131:373.

Fuhrman M, Dragutsky D, Rooh G, Drossman A. Congenital atresia of the esophagus. Radiology. 1942;38:326.

Gedgaudas-McClees RK, Maglinte DDT. Lymphomatous esophageal nodules: the difficulty in radiological differential diagnosis. Am J Gastroenterology. 1985;80:529.

Gefter WB, Laufer I, Edell S, Goehel VK. Candidiasis in the obstructed esophagus. Radiology. 1981;138:25.

Gelfand MD, Krone CL. Dysphagia and esophageal ulceration in Crohn's disease. Gastroenterology. 1968;55:510.

Ghahremani GG, Gore, RM, Breuer RI, Larson RH. Esophageal manifestations of Crohn's disease. Gastrointest Radiol. 1982;7:199.

Goldin NR, Burns TW, Ferrante WA. Secondary achalasia: association with adenocarcinoma of the lung and reversal with radiation therapy. Am J Gastroenterol. 1983;78:203.

Goldman A, Masters H. Leiomyoma of the esophagus. Arch Surg. 1950;60:559.

Gore RM, Margulis AR, Moss AA, Thoeni RF, Mahony BS. Diverging gastroesophageal folds: a useful sign for detecting hiatal hernias in the erect position. Europ J Radiol. 1985;5:27.

Graziani L, Nigris ED, Pasaresi A, Baldelli S, Dini L, Montesi A. Reflux esophagitis: radiologic-endoscopic correlation in 39 symptomatic cases. Gastrointest Radiol. 1983:8:1.

Halvorson RA, Magruderhabib K, Foster WL, Roberts L. Esophageal cancer staging by CT—long term follow-up study. Radiology. 1986;161:147.

Halvorsen RA, Thompson WT. CT of esophageal neoplasm. Radiol Clin North Am. 1989;27:667.

Han SY, Tishler JM. Perforation of the abdominal segment of the esophagus. AJR. 1984;143:751.

Han SY, McElvein RB, Aldrete JS, Tishler JM. Perforation of the esophagus: correlation of site and cause with plain film findings. AJR. 1985;145:537.

Harris LD, Kelly JE, Kramer P. Relation of the lower esophageal ring to the esophagogastric junction. N Engl J Med. 1960;263:1232.

Heiken JP, Balfe DM, Roper CL. CT evaluation after esophagogastrectomy. AJR. 1984;143:555.

Hirose J, Takashima T, Suzuki M, Matsui O. "Downhill" esophageal varices demonstrated by dynamic computed tomography. J Comput Assist Tomogr. 1984;8:1007.

Hishikawa Y, Kamikonya N, Tanaka S, Miura T. Esophageal stricture following high-dose rate intracavitary irradiation for esophageal cancer. Radiology. 1986;159:715.

Ingelfinger FJ, Kramer P. Dysphagia produced by contractile ring in the lower esophagus. Gastroenterology. 1953;23:419.

Ingelfinger FJ, Kramer P, Sanchez GC. The gastroesophageal vestibule—its normal function and its role in cardiospasm and gastroesophageal reflux. Am J Med Sci. 1954;228:417.

Itai Y, Kogure T, Okuyama Y, Akiyama H. Superficial esophageal carcinoma. Radiology. 1978;126:597.

Jackson C. Peptic ulcer of the esophagus. JAMA. 1929;92:369.

Karvelis KC, Drane WE, Johnson DA, Silverman ED. Barrett's esophagus: decreased esophageal clearance shown by radionuclide esophageal scintigraphy. Radiology. 1987;162:97.

Katsura S, Ischikawa F, Okayama G. Transplantation of partially resected middle esophagus with jejunal graft. Ann Surg. 1958;147:146.

Kelling G. Osophagusplastik mit Hilfe des Quercolon. Zbl Chir. 1911;38:1209.

Koeberle F, Penha PD. Chagas megaesophagus. Z Tropenmed Parasit. 1959;10:291.

Koehler RE, Moss AA, Margulis AR. Early radiographic manifestations of carcinoma of the esophagus. Radiology. 1976;119:1.

Koehler RE, Weyman PJ, Oakley HP. Single- and double-contrast techniques in esophagitis. AJR. 1980;135:15.

Laufer I. Radiology of esophagitis. Radiol Clin North Am. 1982;20:687.

Leonidas JC. Gastroesophageal reflux in infants: role of the upper gastrointestinal series. AJR. 1984;143:1350.

Lepke RA, Libshitz HI, Dory MA. Radiation-induced injury of the esophagus. Radiology. 1983;148:375.

Levine MS, Kressel HY, Caroline D, Laufer I, Herlinger H, Thompson JJ. Barrett esophagus: reticular pattern of the mucosa. Radiology. 1983;147:663.

Levine MS, Goldstein HM. Fixed transverse folds in the esophagus – a sign of reflux esophagitis. AJR. 1984;143:275.

Levine MS, Caroline D, Thompson JJ, Kressel HY, Laufer I, Herlinger H. Adenocarcinoma of the esophagus – relationship to Barrett mucosa. Radiology. 1984;150:305.

Levine MS, Macones AJ, Laufer I. Candida esophagitis: accuracy of radiographic diagnosis. Radiology. 1985;154:581.

Levine MS, Sunshine AG, Reymonds JC, Saul SH. Diffuse nodularity in esophageal lymphoma. AJR. 1985;145:1218.

Levine MS, Dillon EC, Saul SH, Laufer I. Early esophageal cancer. AJR. 1986;146:507.

Levine MS, Moolten DN, Herlinger H, Laufer I. Esophageal intramural pseudodiverticulosis: a reevaluation. AJR. 1986;147:1165.

Levine MS, Gilchrist AM. Esophageal deviation: pushed or pulled. AJR. 1987;149:513.

Lindel D, Sandmark S. Hiatal incompetence and gastro-esophageal reflux. Acta Radiol Diagn. 1979;20:626.

Lipa FH, Thal AP. Experimental reflux esophagitis. Arch Surg. 1966;93:148.

Lipschultz BM, Fisher S. Leiomyosarcoma of the esophagus. Gastroenterology. 1964;27:661.

Maglinte DDT, Schultheis TE, Krol KL, Caudill LD, Chernish SM, McCune WM. Survey of the esophagus during the upper gastrointestinal examination in 500 patients. Radiology. 1983;147:65.

Mangala JC. Barrett's esophagus: an old entity rediscovered. Gastroenterology. 1981;3:347.

Margulies SI, Brunt PW, Donner MW, Silbiger ML. Familial dysautonomia. Radiology. 1968;90:107.

Margulis AR, Koehler RE. Radiologic diagnosis of disordered esophageal motility. A unified physiologic approach. Radiol Clin North Am. 1976;14:429.

Margulis AR, Shapiro HA. Barrett esophagus. Radiology. 1984;150:602.

McCanley RKG, Darling DB, Leonidas JC, Schwartz AM. Gastroesophageal reflux in infants and children: a useful classification and reliable physiologic technique for its demonstration. AJR. 1978;130:47.

McDonald GB, Sullivan KM, Plumley TF. Radiographic features of esophageal involvement in chronic graft-vs-host disease. AJR. 1984;142:501.

McNally EF, Katz J. The roentgen diagnosis of diffuse esophageal spasm. AJR. 1967;99:218.

Mellow MM. Symptomatic diffuse esophageal spasm. Manometric follow-up and response to cholinergic stimulation and cholinesterase inhibition. Gastroenterology. 1977;73:237.

Miller JDR, Lewis RB. Esophageal webs in man. Radiology. 1963;81:489.

Mohammed SH, Hegediis V. Dislodgement of impacted esophageal foreign bodies with carbonated beverages. Clin Radiol. 1986;37:589.

Morson BC. Carcinoma arising from areas of intestinal metaplasia in the gastric mucosa. Br J Cancer. 1955;9:377.

Moss AA, Koehler RE, Margulis AR. Initial accuracy of esophagograms in detection of small esophageal carcinoma. AJR. 1976;127:909.

Muhletaler CA, Gerlock AJ Jr, de Soto L, Halter SA. Acid corrosive esophagitis: radiographic findings. AJR. 1980;134:1137.

Muhletaler CA, Gerlock AJ, de Soto L, Halter SA. Gastroduodenal lesions of ingested acid: radiographic findings. AJR. 1980;135:1247.

Ott DJ, Gelfand DW, Wu WC. Reflux esophagitis: radiographic and endoscopic correlation. Radiology. 1979;130:583.

Ott DJ, Dodds WJ, Wu WC, Gelfand DW, Hogan WJ, Stewart ET. Current status of radiology in evaluating for gastroesophageal reflux disease. Clin Gastroenterol. 1982;4:365.

Ott DJ, Chen YM, Wu WC, Gelfand DW, Munitz HA. Radiographic and endoscopic sensitivity in detecting lower esophageal mucosal ring. AJR. 1986;147:261.

Ott DJ, Chen YM, Gelfand DW, Munitz HA. Analysis of multiphasic radiographic examination for detecting reflux esophagitis. Gastrointest Radiol. 1986;11:1.

Ott DJ, Richter JE, Wu WC, Chen YM, Gelfand DW, Castell DO: Radiologic and manometric correlation in "nutcracker esophagus." AJR. 1986;147: 692.

Pinckney LE, Currarino G. Reflux of barium into the middle ear during upper gastrointestinal series. Radiology. 1980;135:653.

Pupols A, Ruzicka FF. Hiatal hernia causing a cardia pseudomass on computed tomography. J Comput Assist Tomogr. 1984;8:699.

Quint LE, Glaser GM, Orringer MB, Gross BH. Esophageal carcinoma: CT findings. Radiology. 1985;155:171.

Rice BT, Spiegel PK, Dombrowski PJ. Acute esophageal food impaction treated by gas-forming agents. Radiology. 1983;146:299.

Robins AH, Vincent ME, Saini M, Schimmel EM. Revised radiological concepts of the Barrett esophagus. Gastrointest Radiol. 1978;3:377.

Sabanathan S, Salama FD, Morgan WE. Esophageal intramural pseudodiverticulosis. Thorax. 1985;40: 849.

Sato T, Sakai Y, Kajita A, Fujino Y, Taniguchi K, Kabuto T, Ishiguro S. Radiographic microstructures of early esophageal carcinoma: correlation of specimen radiography with pathologic findings and clinical radiography. Gastrointest Radiol. 1986;11:12.

Schatzki R, Gary JE. Dysphagia due to a diaphragm-like localized narrowing in the lower esophagus ("lower esophageal ring"). AJR. 1953;70:911.

Schatzki R. Esophagus progress and problems. AJR. 1965;94:523.

Schreiber MH, Davis M. Intraluminal diverticulum of the esophagus. AJR. 1977;129:595.

Siebert JJ, Byrne WJ, Euler AR, Letture T, Leach M, Campbell M. Gastroesophageal reflux—the acid test; scintigraphy or the pH probe. AJR. 1983;140:1087.

Swamy N. Esophageal spasm: clinical and manometric response to nitroglycerin and long-acting nitrates. Gastroenterology. 1967;42:435.

Tishler JMA, Helman CA. Crohn's disease of the esophagus. J Can Assoc Radiol. 1984;35:28.

Treacy WL, Baggenstoss AH, Slocumb CH, Code CF. Scleroderma of the esophagus. Ann Intern Med. 1963;59:351.

Ulmas J, Sakhuja R. The pathology of esophageal intramural pseudodiverticulosis. Am J Clin Pathol. 1976;65:314.

Uzunov G. Familial achalasia of the esophagus in infancy. Radiol Diagn. 1982;23:31.

Vogt EC. Congenital esophageal atresia. AJR. 1929; 22:463.

Waldmann HK, Turnball A. Esophageal webs. AJR. 1957;78:567.

Weaver JW, Kaude JV, Hamlin DJ. Webs of the lower esophagus. A complication of gastroesophageal reflux. AJR. 1984;142:289.

Williams SM, Harned RK, Kaplan PH, Cinsigny PM. Work in progress: transverse striations of the esophagus: association with gastroesophageal reflux. Radiology. 1983;146:25.

Williams SM, May C, Krause DW, Harned RK. Symptomatic congenital ectopic gastric mucosa in the upper esophagus. AJR. 1987;148:147.

Williford ME, Rice RP, Kelvin FM, Fisher SR, Meyers WC, Thompson WM. Revascularized jejunal graft replacing the cervical esophagus: radiographic evaluation. AJR. 1985;145:533.

Wolf BS. The inferior esophageal sphincter. Anatomic, roentgenologic and manometric correlation, contradictions and terminology. AJR. 1970;11: 260.

Chapter 8

Radiology of the Stomach

The stomach unselectively accepts esophageal contents regardless of their osmolarity, corrosive properties, or substantial difference in temperature. Conversely, the stomach permits passage of contents into the duodenum in minute divided portions, this material being mostly liquid in consistency. In the fasting state the stomach contains about 50 mL of secretions.

Radiographic contrast medium should enter the stomach in one stream. Separation of the contrast bolus most frequently results from a tumor of the cardia. Analysis of the dynamics of gastric evacuation provides useful data. Spasm of the pylorus can be an indirect sign of a peptic ulcer in the pyloric canal or the duodenal bulb. Structural stenoses and spasms can be differentiated by the use of a spasmolytic and by gaseous distension.

Analysis of the form and dimension of gastric folds is essential in each segment of the stomach. Fundic rugae resemble a mosaic pattern which becomes more regular in the region of the gastric body, where the folds become parallel. The contour of the greater curvature may normally be serrated, but the lesser curvature is always smoothly contoured in normal individuals. In the pyloric portion of the stomach, the folds are parallel and regular, while the folds of the duodenal bulb are similar to those in the antrum, being almost parallel, slightly spiral in shape, and smaller in caliber than gastric folds. The dimensions of the gastric folds depend on the blood supply to the submucosa and on gastric distension. With remarkable distension, folds may be effaced. During contraction of the gastric wall, folds become flatter or seemingly disappear. In double-contrast studies of a properly distended stomach, gastric folds are effaced or only faintly noticeable (Fig. 8.1). However, significantly widened rugae cannot be effaced by gaseous distension.

DISORDERS OF TONE AND MOTILITY

Functional disturbances of gastric motility are not easy to quantify because of the wide range of normal motility. Changes of motility are not pathologic phenomena but may be symptoms of pathologic events. Gastric motility can be studied using barium sulfate suspensions, radionuclide studies, or by monitoring myoelectric phenomena.

Tone and Peristalsis

Changes in tone of the principal muscular layer affect the shape of the stomach and the threshold for provocation of peristalsis. An *orthotonic* stomach has the shape of a fishhook. The angular notch is clearly discernible. The diameter of the gastric body immediately below the cardia and at the angular notch are approximately equal. A *hypertonic* stomach is hori-

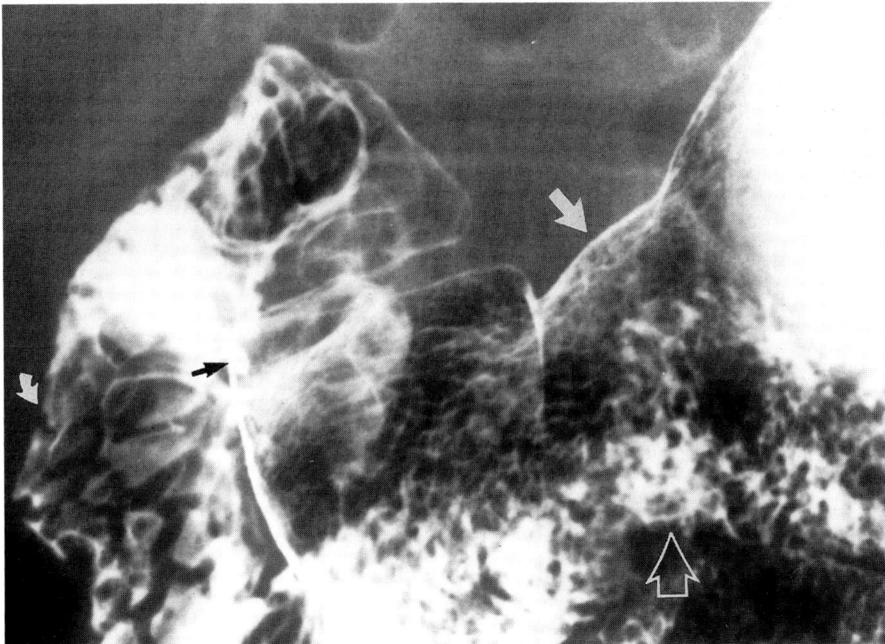

FIGURE 8.1. Relief of the stomach, duodenum, and proximal small bowel. Areae gastricae (white arrow), discrete transverse folds of the antrum (black arrow), relief of the second portion of the duodenum (white curved arrow), small bowel relief (open arrow).

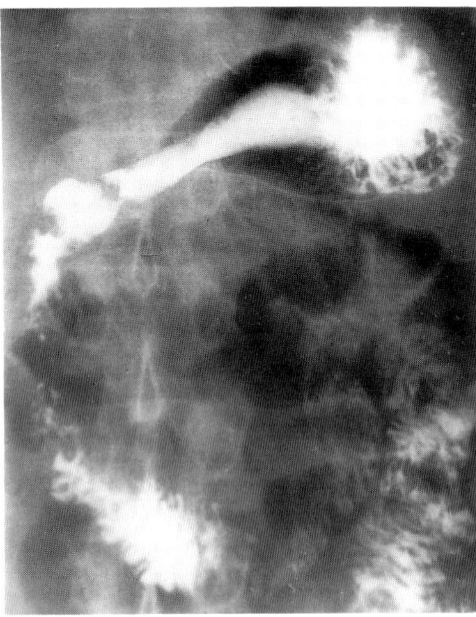

FIGURE 8.2. Hypertonia of the stomach. Duodenal sweep appears widened.

zontally situated (Fig. 8.2) with the subcardiac diameter of the body longer than the region of the angular notch. These relations are quite opposite in a *hypotonic* stomach where the angulus is below the crest of the iliac bone.

Sympathetic stimulation in acute emotional stress, as in the reaction of "fight or flight," lowers the tone of gastric muscles. Chronic emotional stress, on the contrary, increases muscular tone by stimulating the parasympathetic system.

The intensity of muscle tone is inversely proportional to the threshold for peristalsis. A *peristaltic wave* appears every 15–35 seconds, and three to four peristaltic waves are usually seen simultaneously. In the supine or upright position they appear in the region of the angular notch, but originate more proximally in the prone position. Emptying of the stomach also causes peristalsis to originate proximally. Hypertonia is associated with an increase in the number and amplitude of peristaltic waves. Increased tone in the circular muscular coat may result in a serrated appearance of the greater curvature.

Deep peristaltic waves are found when pyloric and duodenal stenoses are well compensated. This type of peristalsis most probably results from absence of an inhibitory enterogastric reflex.

Peristalsis is altered by inflammatory, fibrotic, and neoplastic processes. A peristaltic wave does not propagate along a rigid wall but will continue along the opposite wall, if that wall is not affected with the pathologic process. Distal to the lesion, a peristaltic contraction is visible along the entire circumference of the gastric wall. *Localized hypertonia*, spasm, may be seen on the gastric wall opposite a peptic ulcer. Quite opposite phenomena characterize hypotonia.

Gastric emptying into the duodenum is dependent on the tone of the muscular layer (i.e., the number and intensity of peristaltic waves) and on opening of the pylorus. The analysis of barium evacuation from the stomach is qualitative, since the residual volume of barium suspension cannot be measured practically. Barium examination results are not easily extrapolated to the emptying of food. Radionuclide studies offer quantitative data on gastric emptying. During fasting, periods of standstill alternate with motor activity.

Emptying of the stomach depends on the volume, consistency, and chemical properties of the contents. Solid contents are displaced by strong antral contractions, and liquids are evacuated by contractions of more proximal portions of the stomach which cause intraluminal pressure to increase. Fatty substances and hyperosmolar and hypo-osmolar contents are evacuated more slowly than iso-osmolar contents. Emptying is also influenced by body posture, being enhanced by the right lateral decubitus position.

The quantity of barium suspension required for an upper gastrointestinal series is normally eliminated in less than four hours, with an average evacuation time of two hours. A retention time longer than six hours needs to be explained, and retention longer than eight hours should be considered definitely abnormal even in children.

The stomach empties rapidly in patients with peptic ulcer, Zollinger–Ellison syndrome, and malabsorption syndromes. Delayed emptying may result from functional or organic changes in distal portions of the stomach and/or proximal duodenum. Chronic retention of gastric contents results from paresis of the alimentary canal secondary to hyperglycemia or low intracellular concentrations of potassium, as well as from gastroesophageal reflux, duodenal peptic ulceration, anorexia nervosa, and idiopathic intestinal obstruction. Secretions can fill the stomach at a rate of approximately 1.5 L per day.

Gastric atonia, a rare event, appears as part of the paralytic ileus syndrome and may accompany vascular shock and diabetic coma. It is often encountered in the postoperative period. Causative factors for acute gastric paresis also include infectious diseases and the effects of medication. The stomach appears significantly dilated by gas (Fig. 8.3). Atonia should be differentiated from the dilatation which results from obstruction, such as pylorospasm, or stenoses of the gastric outlet or proximal duodenum. Chronic gastroparesis appears in patients with myotonic dystrophy, progressive muscular dystrophy, and long-lasting diabetes mellitus. Vagotomy and pyloroplasty may cause chronic gastroparesis (Table 8.1).

TABLE 8.1. ETIOLOGY OF GASTRIC DISTENSION

Mechanical Obstruction
Pylorostenosis
Benign-postulcerative
Malignant-pyloric carcinoma
Stenoses or compression of the proximal duodenum
Paralytic Illeus (acute dilatation)
Peritonitis
Trauma
Coma (diabetic, uremic)
Shock
Medication
Aerophagia

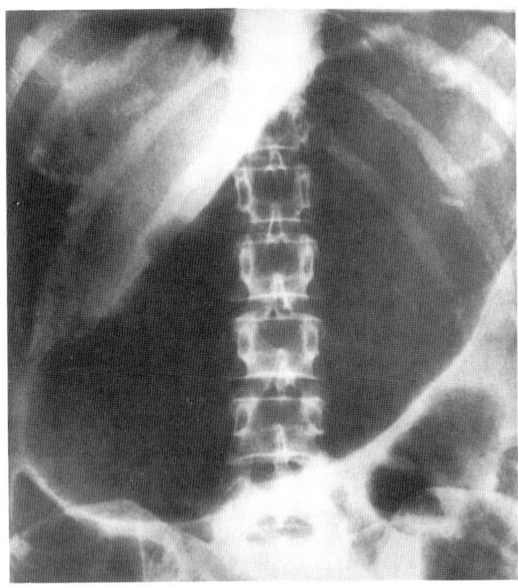

A

Figure 8.3. Acute gastric atonia. The stomach is greatly distended by gas. (A) Plain abdominal film. (B) CT examination.

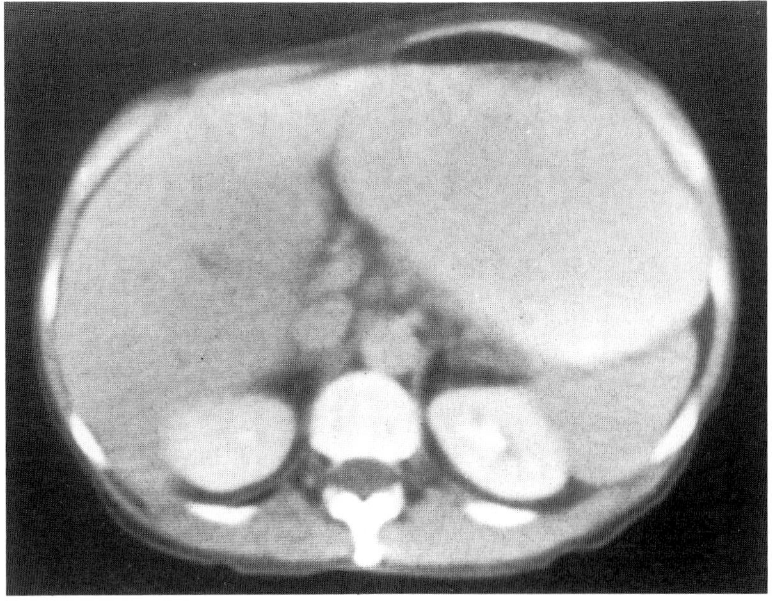

B

ACQUIRED CHANGES OF GASTRIC POSITION

The stomach is "J" shaped in a majority of normal healthy adults. In children and in adults in the supine position, the longitudinal gastric axis is almost perpendicular to the longitudinal body axis. Even though the stomach is bound by numerous duplications of the peritoneum, it may be displaced or impinged upon by adjacent anatomical structures (Diagram 8.1). Either the entire stomach or portions of it may be

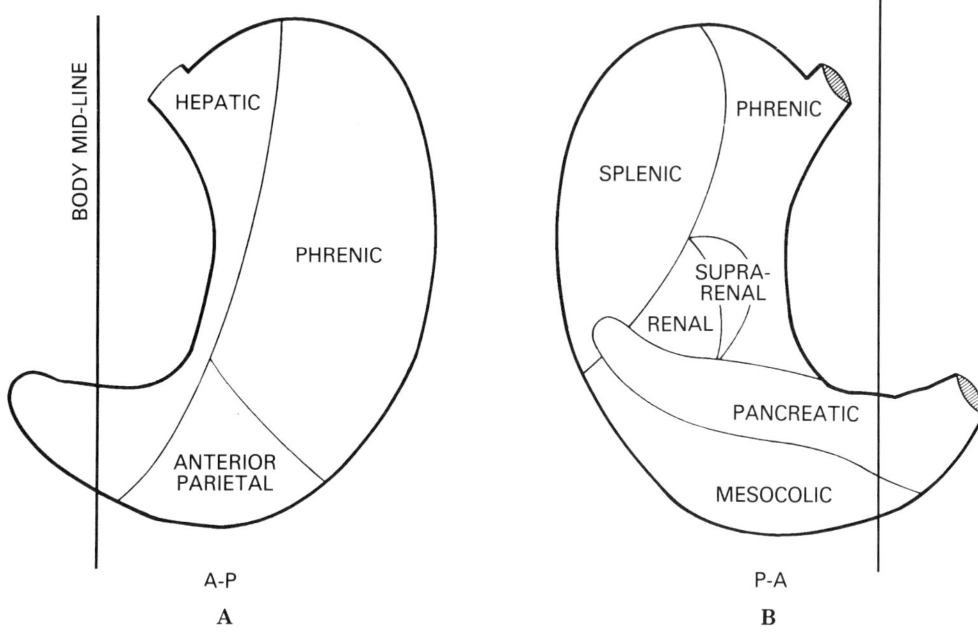

Diagram 8.1. Portions of the stomach surface in contact with adjacent anatomical structures. (A) Anterior surface. (B) Posterior surface.

displaced (Fig. 8.4). An analysis of dislocation or imprint on the stomach is possible with full-column or double-contrast studies.

An enlarged pancreas, particularly an enlarged body and tail, will displace the stomach *anteriorly* (Fig. 8.5). The normal retrogastric space should not exceed the width of a lumbar vertebral body. However, in obese individuals, or in patients with gastric hypertonia, the distance between the posterior wall of the stomach and the anterior surfaces of vertebral bodies may be several times greater without pathologic significance.

The distance between the gas in an air-filled (or distended) gastric fundus and the air in the lungs is usually 0.5–2 cm and should be considered outside the normal range when it exceeds 2 cm after gaseous distension of the fundus. Thickening of the gastric wall such as that caused by varices, neoplasms, or pathologic processes of the peritoneum and/or pleura can increase this distance.

Abdominal and pelvic masses may displace the stomach *cranially*. Pregnancy, as well as omental, small intestinal, and retroperitoneal processes, such as enlargement of the head of the pancreas, may also displace the stomach superiorly (Fig. 8.6).

Anterior and *inferior* displacement is caused by enlargement of the tail of the pancreas. An enlarged spleen dislocates the stomach to the *right* and indents the greater curvature, while an enlarged liver displaces the stomach to the *left* and posteriorly.

The gastric fundus may be indented by enlargement of the left ventricle, the spleen, or the left lobe of the liver. The body of the stomach is imprinted by an enlarged liver (Fig. 8.7), spleen, or pancreas. In contrast to an enlarged pancreas or left kidney, which would impress the stomach anteriorly, the liver impresses and displaces the stomach in a posterior direction. The pyloric portion may be impressed or dislocated by an enlarged pancreas (Diagram 8.1). When the left leaf of the diaphragm is paretic, paralyzed, or eventrated, the stomach is displaced cranially (Fig. 8.8). Displacement of the stomach can be shown by double-contrast examination but CT demonstrates any displacement in a superior fashion and allows differentiation

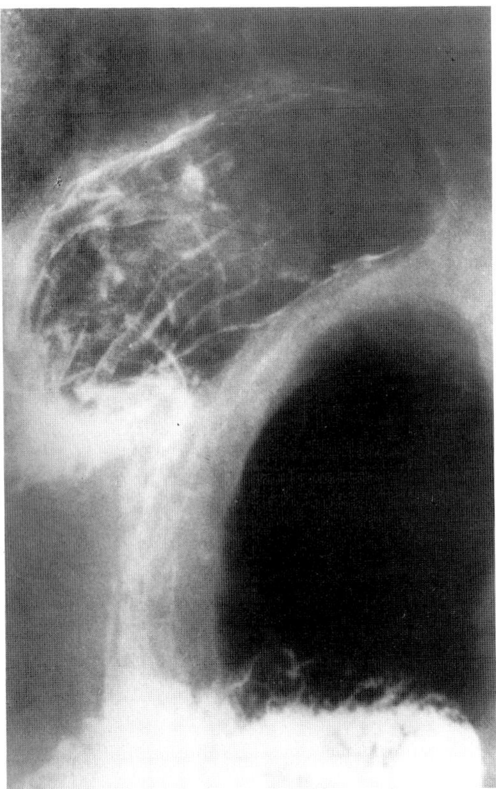

Figure 8.4. Gas-filled colon impinges on the stomach.

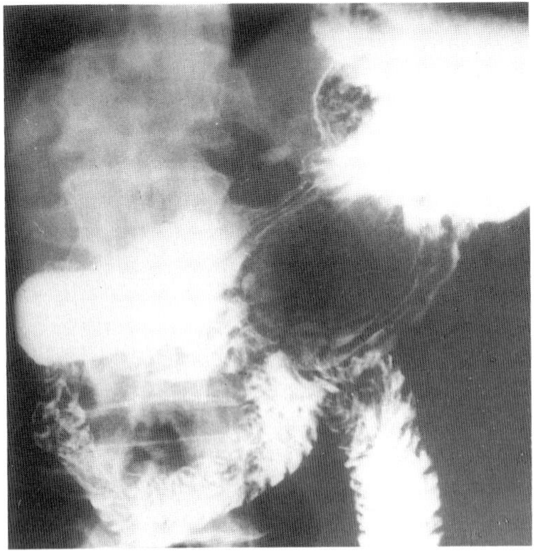

Figure 8.5. Pseudocyst of the pancreatic tail. An extrinsic mass displaces gastric rugae in an arcuate manner.

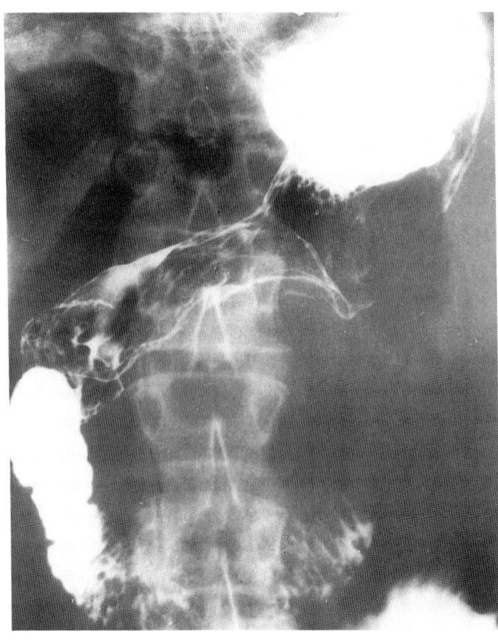

Figure 8.6. Pancreatitis. The gastric antrum is displaced cranially and the duodenal sweep is widened by an enlarged pancreas.

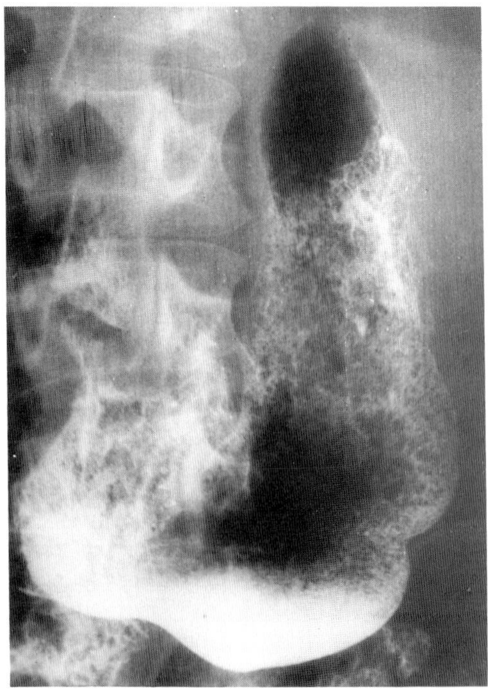

Figure 8.7. (A) Cone shaped gastric fundus.

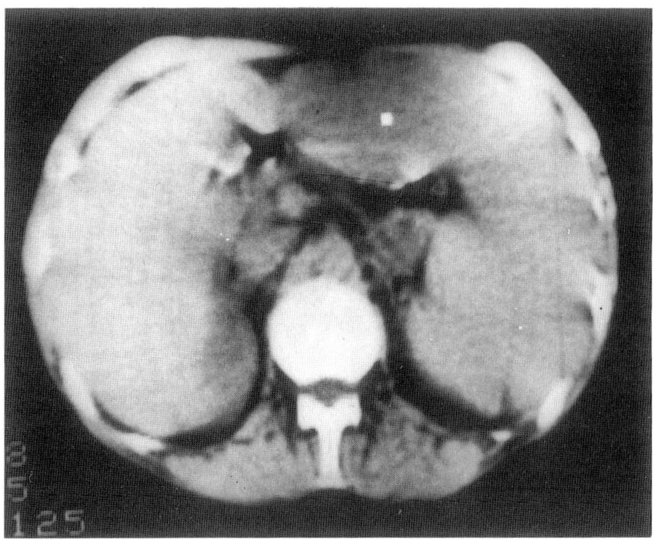

Figure 8.7. *continued.* (B) Liver duplication fills the entire upper and mid-abdomen compressing the stomach. (Used by permission, Ugarkovic B, Tezak S, Plavsic B, et al., A case of bizarre liver form variation. Clin Nucl Med. 1986;12:461.)

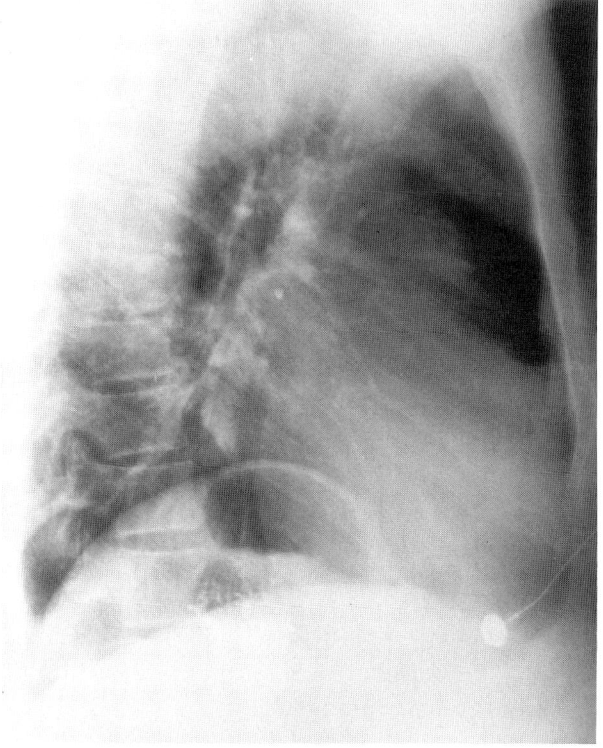

Figure 8.8. Relaxation of the left leaf of the diaphragm. (A) Lateral chest. (*Figure continued on overleaf.*)

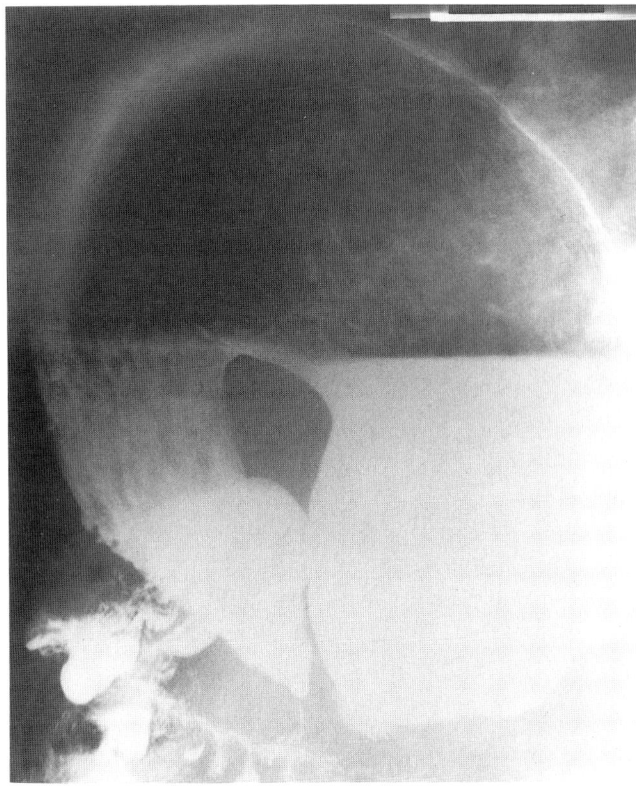

Figure 8.8. *continued.* Relaxation of the left leaf of the diaphragm. (B) Cranial displacement of the stomach.

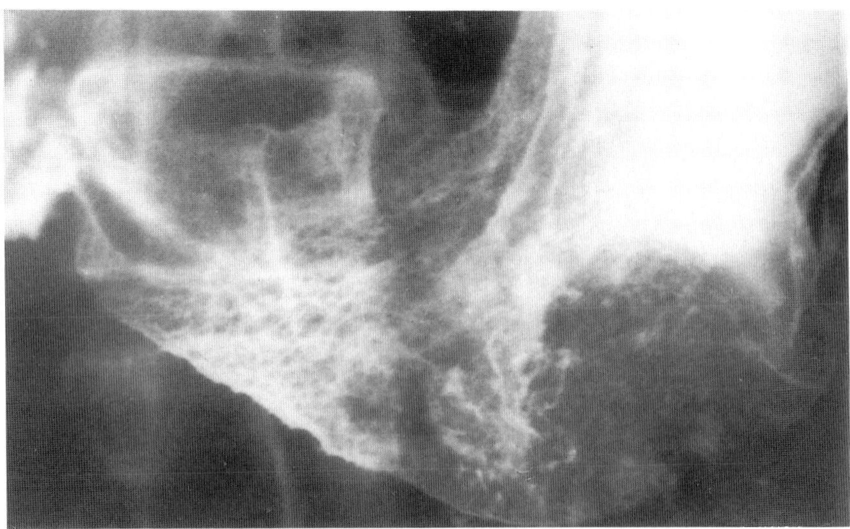

Figure 8.9. Submucosal gastric neoplasm: (A) Posterior wall leiomyosarcoma.

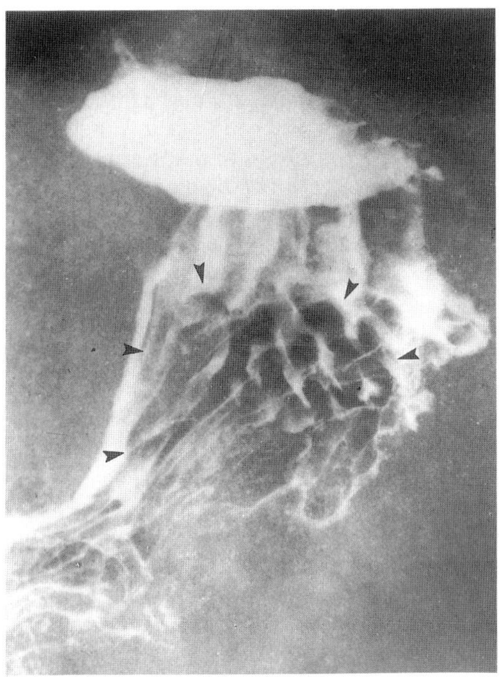

FIGURE 8.9. *continued.* Submucosal gastric neoplasm: (B) Large posterior wall lipoma.

between mural and extramural lesions. Barium studies sometimes distinguish extrinsic impressions from submucosal masses (Fig. 8.9).

ADHESIONS

Adhesions can cause deformity of any portion of the stomach. They can be congenital or acquired, the latter resulting from inflammation or mechanical injury such as penetrating wounds and, rarely, surgical procedures (Fig. 8.10). In the region of adhesions, the stomach is fixed and wall distensibility is decreased. Adhesions may sometimes resemble infiltrative carcinoma as well as corrosive, eosinophilic, granulomatous, or phlegmonous gastritis.

CASCADE OF THE STOMACH

A cascade stomach is an acquired, transitory, or permanent condition in which the longitudinal axis of the fundus does not continue along the body axis in a rectilinear manner, but forms an angle of less than 180 degrees that opens posteriorly. A cascade stomach may re-

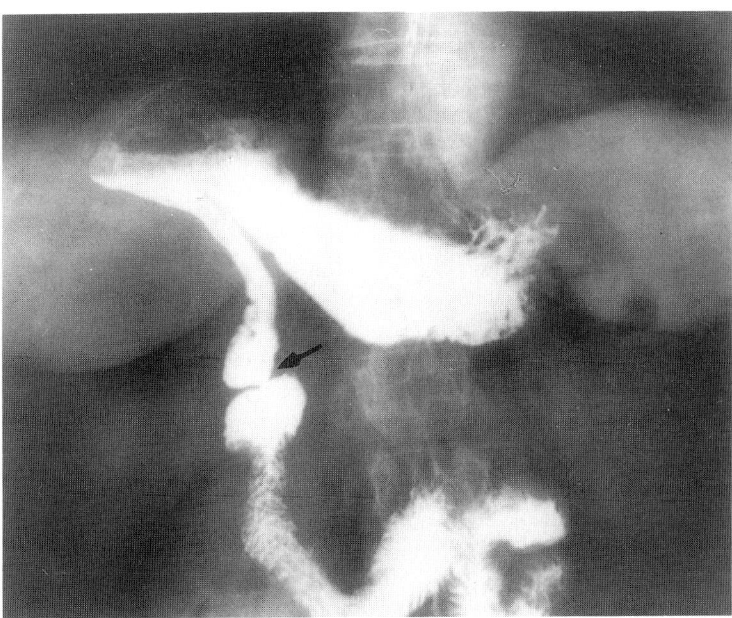

FIGURE 8.10. Gastric body displaced cephalad by adhesions after marsupialization of an echinococcal cyst. Pylorus (arrow).

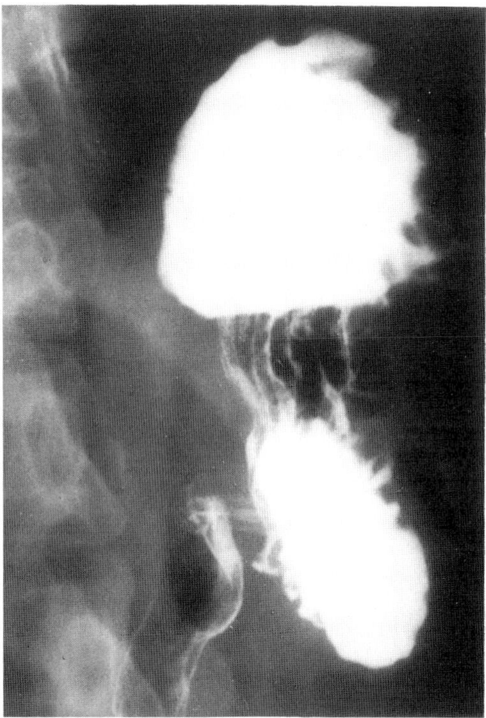

A

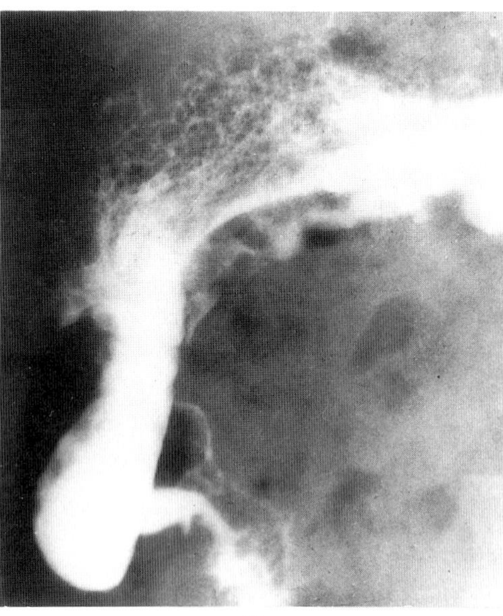

B

FIGURE 8.11. Gastric fundal cascade. (A) P-A projection. (B) Profile projection demonstrating posterior direction of the fundus.

sult from contraction of sling fibers, adhesions, compression of the stomach by dilated transverse colon or, most commonly, as an "idiopathic" cascade stomach. This cascade causes stagnation of gastric contents in the fundus, since the fundus of the cascade stomach lies significantly more dorsal than usual (Fig. 8.11). Examination of a patient with a cascade stomach is described in chapter 4, concerning special procedures during upper gastrointestinal series (see page 88).

VOLVULUS

Volvulus is a rotational torsion of the stomach around the longitudinal or transverse axis of 180 degrees or more. Volvulus around the longitudinal axis, organo-axial volvulus (Diagram 8.2 and Fig. 8.12), is four times as common as mesenteric-axial volvulus. In organo-axial volvulus, the greater curvature is situated cranially and the pylorus is directed caudally.

Volvulus of the stomach is associated with high morbidity and may be complete or partial, acute or intermittent. On an upright abdominal film, two gas-fluid levels may be seen in the epigastrium with the stomach elevated below the left hemidiaphragm. On a scout film, the gas-distended stomach should be differentiated from volvulus of the cecum. Partial volvulus

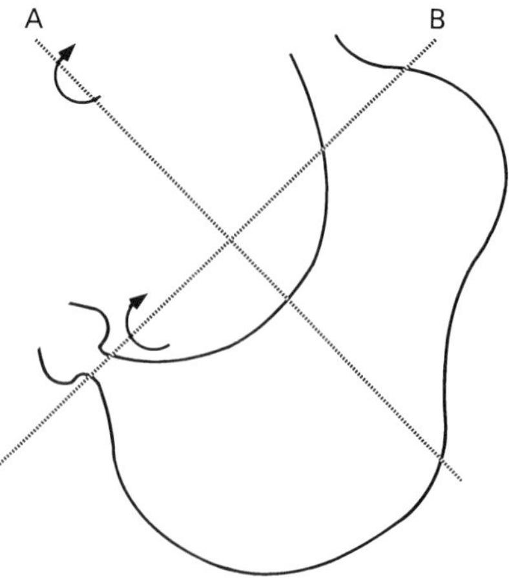

DIAGRAM 8.2. Volvulus of the stomach. (A) Organoaxial. (B) Mesenteroaxial.

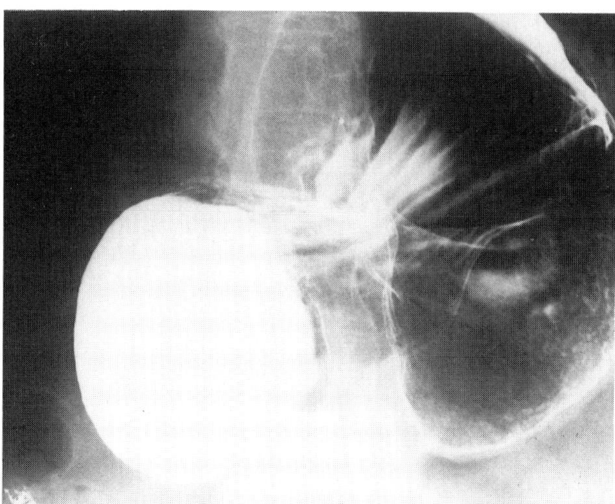

Figure 8.12. Organoaxial gastric volvulus with eventration of the left leaf of the diaphragm.

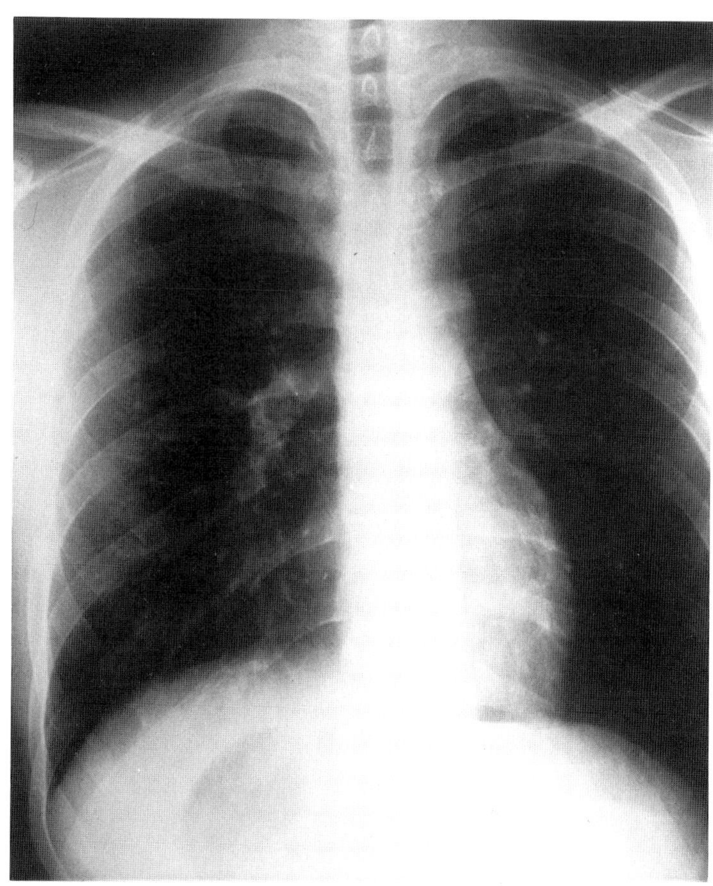

Figure 8.13. Visceral situs inversus. (A) P-A chest. Gastric air bubble in the right hypochondrium. (*Figure continued on the following two pages.*)

may resemble a cascade stomach. Obstruction is often present in the cardia and/or pylorus, making endoscopic examination impossible to perform.

CONGENITAL ANOMALIES

Congenital anomalies of the stomach are infrequent. *Transposition*, heterotaxia of the stomach, may be isolated or associated with *situs inversus* of all abdominal organs. It is usually asymptomatic. With *situs inversus* the stomach is in the right hypochondrium, behind the liver (Fig. 8.13). *Microgastria* is extremely rare. Congenital *membranes* (webs), mucosal duplications covered with epithelium, are situated in the prepyloric region, and originate from the greater curvature. Unless operatively relieved, complete membranes are incompatible with life. Incomplete membranes are more common (Fig. 8.14) and may sometimes interfere with gastric emptying. The degree of obstruction depends on the size of the membrane opening.

Diverticula

It is believed that a majority of gastric diverticula are congenital. They may be found in any portion of the stomach, but are most common near the cardia (Fig. 8.15). These are true diverticula containing all layers of the gastric wall. The width and the length of the neck of the diverticulum may vary considerably. Gas-

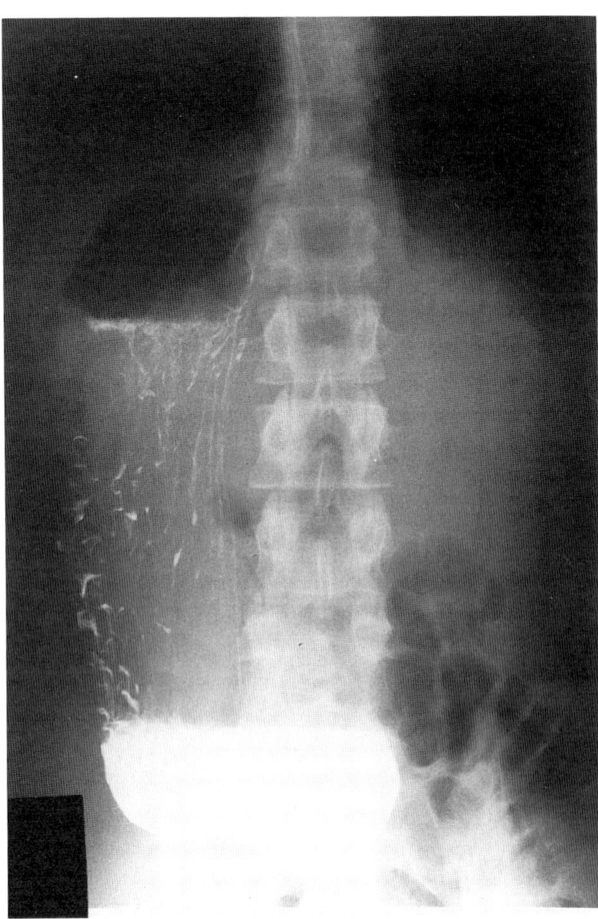

Figure 8.13 *continued.* Visceral situs inversus. (B) Barium studies.

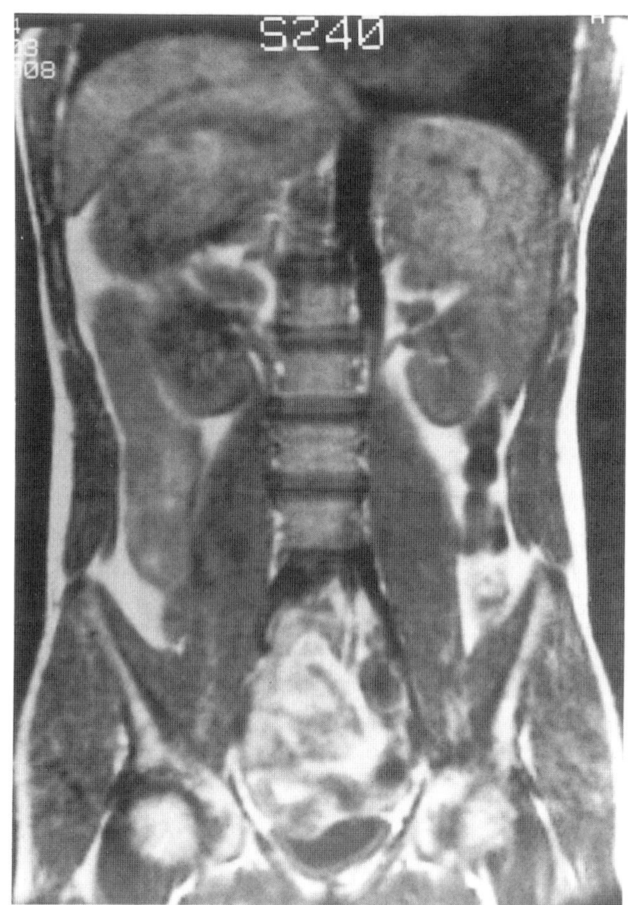

Figure 8.13 *continued.* Visceral situs inversus. (C) MRI, T1 weighted image demonstrates spleen on the right and liver on the left side.

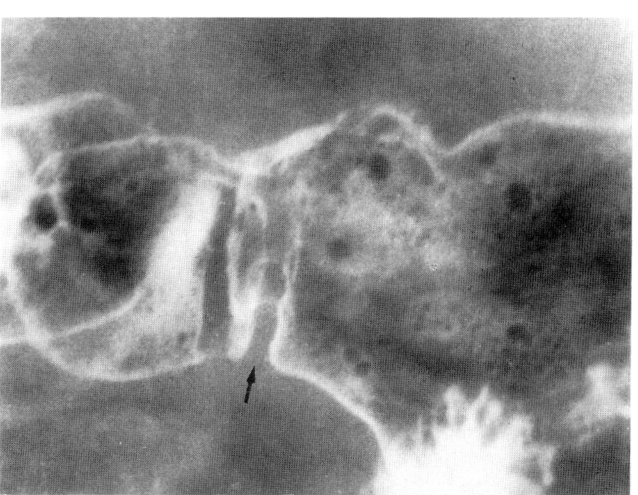

Figure 8.14. Partial antral membrane originates from the greater curvature of the stomach.

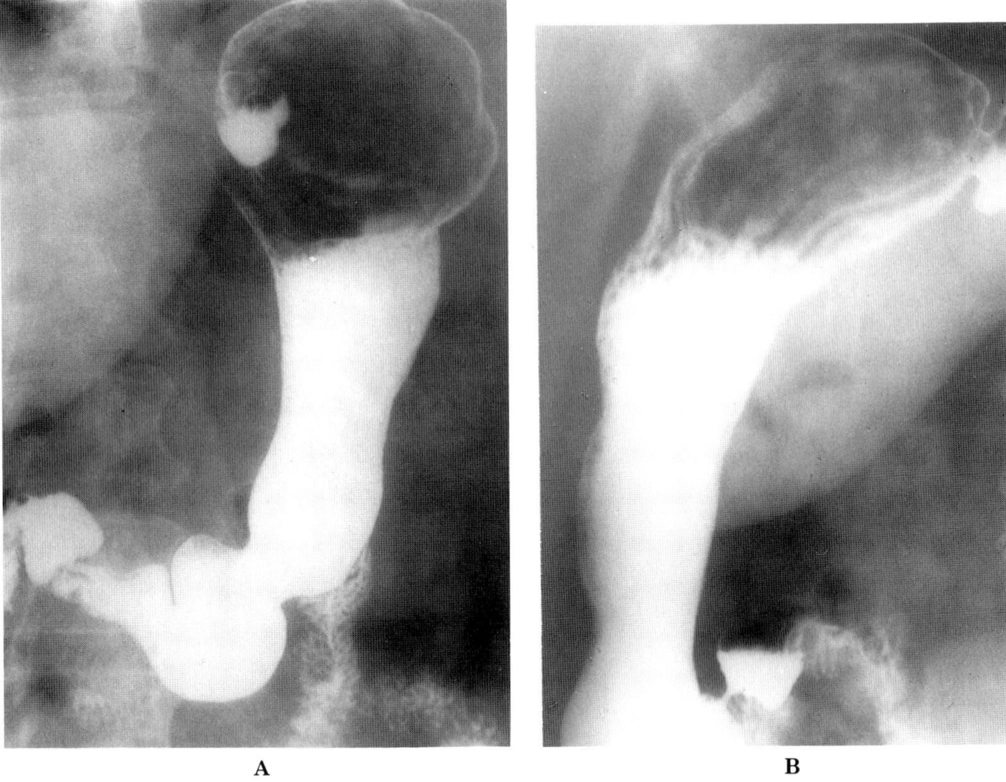

FIGURE 8.15. Typical gastric diverticulum just below the cardia: (A) *En face*. (B) In profile.

tric folds are often seen entering a diverticulum, while they do not enter an ulcer crater. In addition an ulceration does not change form and dimension during a radiologic examination. Radiologic examination may demonstrate retention of food in a diverticulum; this is manifested by irregular negative defects. Small diverticula may mimic barium collections between gastric rugae.

ACCESSORY PANCREATIC TISSUE

A rare occurrence, aberrant pancreatic tissue, is most common among heterotopic tissues in the gastric wall (Fig. 8.16). The choristoma, 1–2 cm in diameter, is a regular shaped, oval or spherical, submucosal protrusion with a central positive defect, representing the excretory canal. This resembles a peptic ulcer surrounded by edema or an ulcerated tumor.

PYLORIC HYPERTROPHY IN CHILDREN

Hypertrophic pyloric stenosis, 5 to 10 times more common in boys than in girls, is characterized by projectile bile-free vomiting. Onset of symptoms usually occurs in the sixth week of life; it rarely appears earlier, but may appear as late as five months after birth. A mother who had hypertrophic pyloric stenosis has a four times higher chance of having an affected offspring than does the father. Although the precise cause of hypertrophic pyloric stenosis remains unknown, etiologic factors may be hypergastrinemia and hyperacidity, together with a decreased number of ganglion cells and neurofibrils in the pyloric segment of the stomach. Propulsion of milk curds against the pylorus may cause spasm and edema of the mucosa and submucosa resulting in narrowing of the

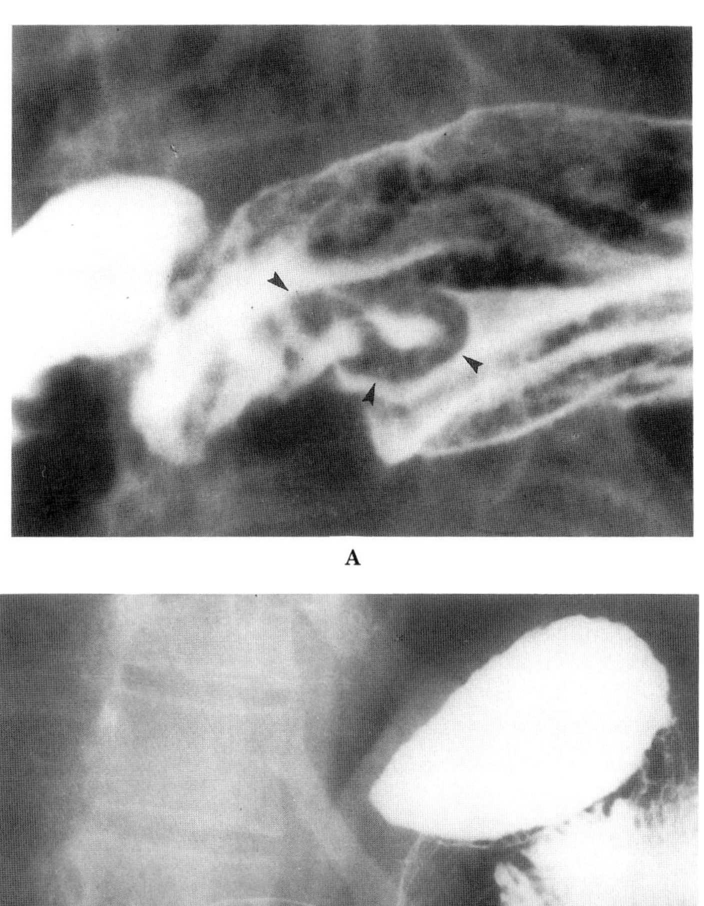

A

B

FIGURE 8.16. Heterotopic pancreatic tissue (choristoma) in the gastric antrum. (A) Spot film with controlled compression (arrowheads). (B) Double-contrast studies (arrows).

pyloric canal. Hypertrophy of the pyloric and gastric musculature results.

When an olive-shaped hypertrophic muscle mass is palpated in a child with typical clinical symptoms, further diagnostic procedures may not be necessary. However, when the diagnosis cannot be established by palpation, the next diagnostic choice is ultrasound. The thickened hypoechoic muscle tumor has a central collection of echoes that often forms a stellate pattern (Fig. 8.17A and B). The mural thickness is typically 4 mm or greater and the pyloric canal is at least 15 mm long. A negative ultrasound examination in a patient with clinical signs should be followed by a scout film and careful barium examination.

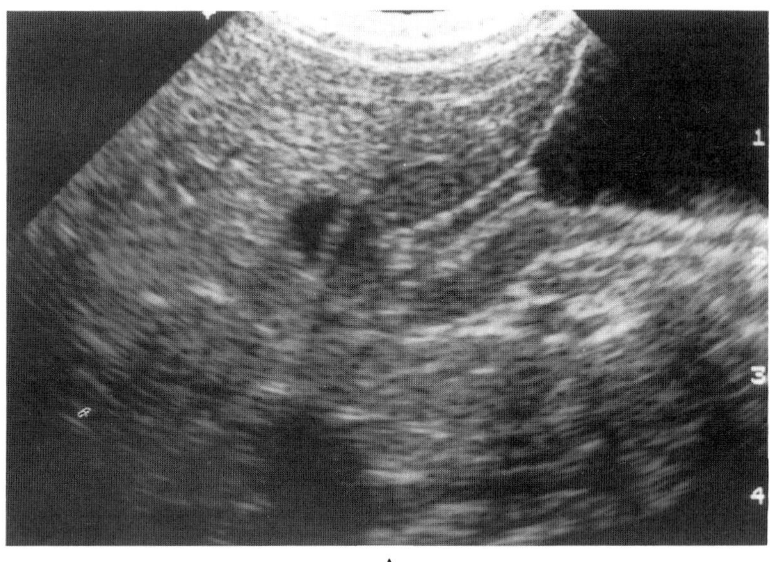

A

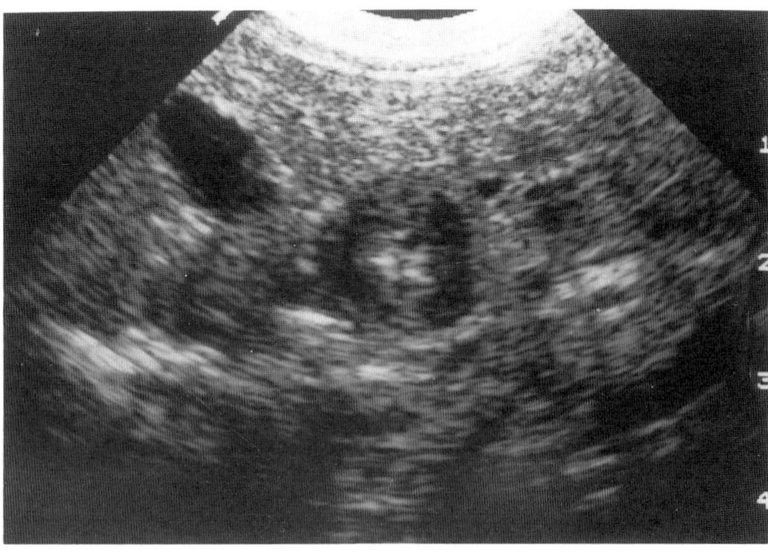

B

FIGURE 8.17. Hypertrophic pyloric stenosis in a child. (A) Ultrasound demonstrates a thickened pyloric muscle and elongated pyloric canal on a longitudinal section. (B) Transverse section. (Courtesy L.E. Swischuk, MD, University of Texas, Galveston.) (*Figure continued on the following two pages.*)

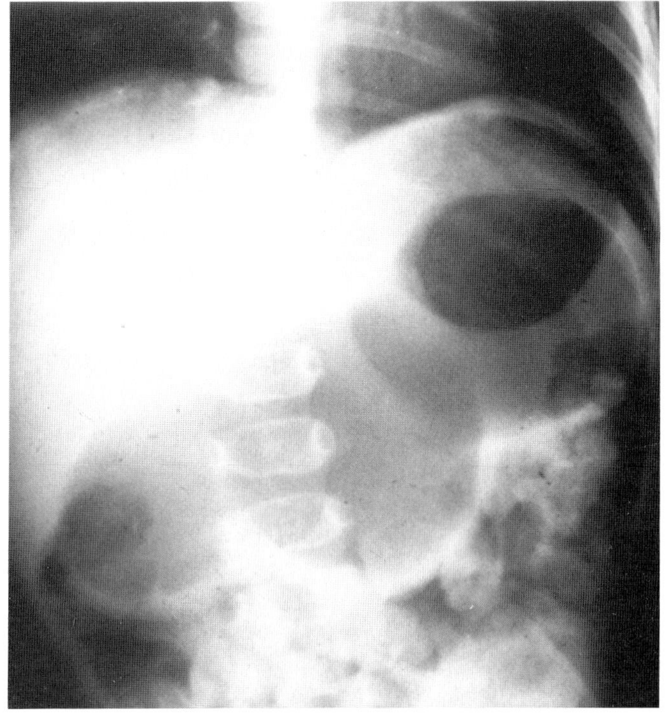

C

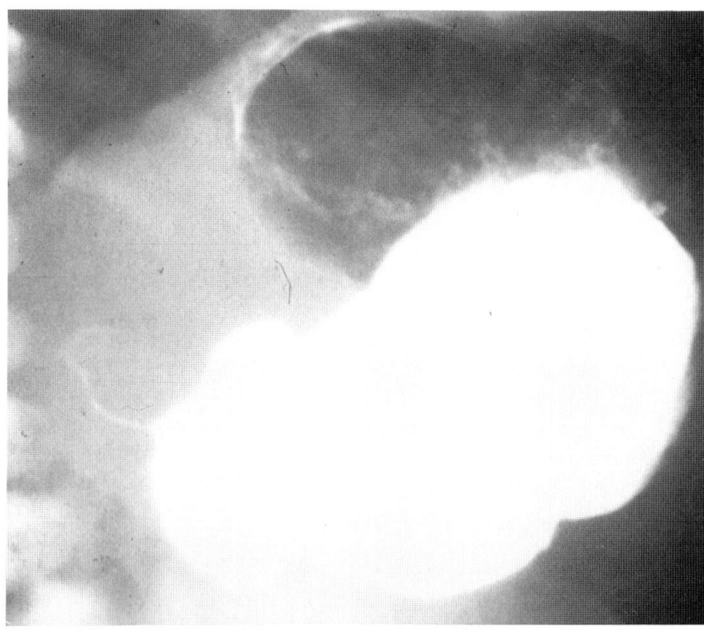

D

Figure 8.17 *continued.* Hypertrophic pyloric stenosis in a child. (C) Hyperperistaltic, gas-filled stomach on plain abdominal film. (D) Barium study. (See Diagram 8.3.)

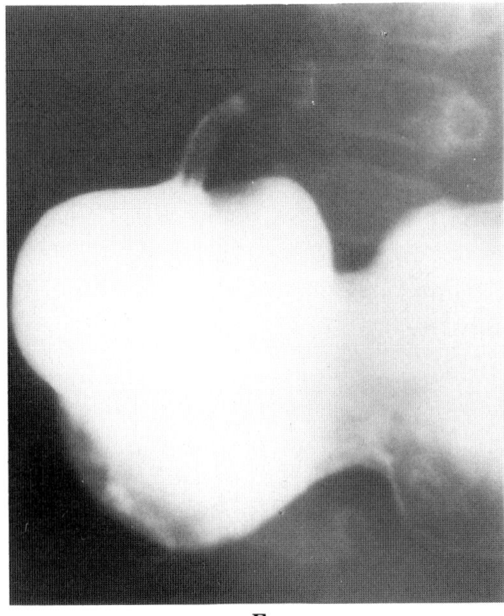

Figure 8.17 *continued.* Hypertrophic pyloric stenosis in a child. (E) Double-track sign.

A plain abdominal radiograph may demonstrate the following signs:

1. Gastric distension by air.
2. Food remnants in an air-filled stomach.
3. Sparse gas in both small and large bowel.
4. Gastric hypermotility (Fig. 8.17C).

Barium series can demonstrate all or some of the following signs (Fig. 8.17D):

1. Gastric dilatation.
2. Delayed and prolonged gastric emptying.
3. String sign, a streak of barium filling the pyloric canal.
4. Less commonly, a double-track sign of barium caught between folds of hypertrophic pyloric muscle (Fig. 8.17E).
5. Pyloric canal directed cranially.
6. Shoulder sign, resulting from hypertrophic muscle impinging on the barium column in the pyloric antrum.
7. Beak sign—barium entering the proximal segment of the pyloric canal.
8. Indentation of the base of the duodenal bulb by hypertrophic pyloric muscle (Diagram 8.3).

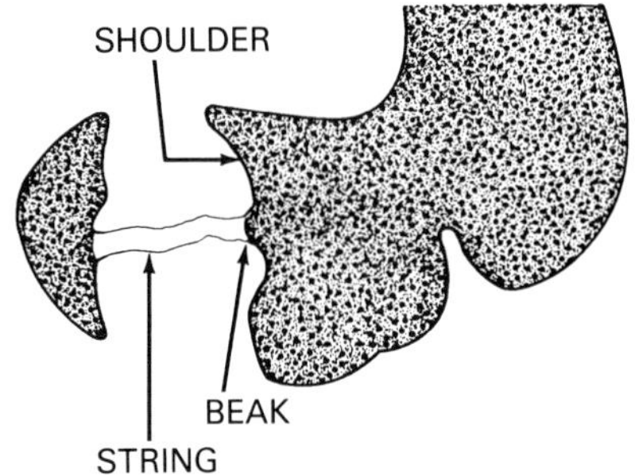

Diagram 8.3. Congenital pyloric stenosis.

The pyloric canal may be only several millimeters in diameter. Barium should be administered through an indwelling thin soft tube and removed at the end of the examination, since vomiting and aspiration with serious consequences may otherwise occur.

PYLORIC HYPERTROPHY IN ADULTS

Hypertrophic pyloric stenosis, characterized by pyloric muscle hypertrophy, may also result from healing of a pyloric canal peptic ulcer (Figs. 4.1 and 8.18). "Antral gastritis" may be seen in surgical specimens of patients with pyloric canal peptic ulcer. Inflammatory changes are present in the pyloric mucosa and submucosa, resulting in thickening of the pyloric sphincter. Sclerotic changes of the antrum, accompanied by motor dysfunction, are late sequelae. Endoscopy with biopsy is usually diagnostic.

Hypertrophic stenosis in adults may be a mild form of the same entity observed in children. In contrast to children, these adults are free of clinical symptoms. Response to spasmolytics is weak or negligible in the presence of any fibrosis. Focal muscular hypertrophy may affect the lesser curvature in the region of the torus only (see chapter 2 on physiology, page 29). Indeed, the pyloric muscle may be hypertrophied exclusively in the region of the greater curvature. The greater curvature then has a serrated appearance, while the lesser curvature has a smooth, concave configuration.

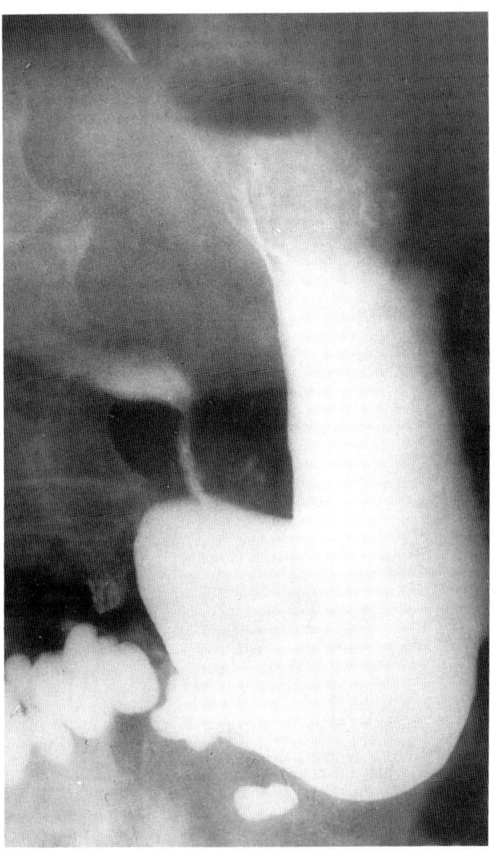

FIGURE 8.18. Hypertrophic pyloric stenosis in an adult.

GASTRIC VARICES

The configuration of the gastric mucosal surface pattern makes demonstration of gastric varices difficult, particularly in the early stages. Gastric varices are seen in less than 50% of patients with esophageal varices, but can arise in any portion of the stomach (Fig. 8.19). However, varices are not common in the fundus. They appear as serpiginous, regular protrusions or lobular submucosal masses, which may be filled with blood to a different degree during various stages of an examination and with different body postures, resulting in changing morphology.

Computed tomography after oral administration of radiographic contrast medium demonstrates nonspecific thickening of the gastric wall. However, IV administration of contrast medium is usually diagnostic, showing tubular or rounded structures that are enhanced to the same degree as adjacent vascular structures.

GIANT GASTRIC FOLDS

The lesser gastric curvature is perfectly smooth in normal individuals. However, indentation of the greater curvature, resulting from circular muscle contraction, is a normal finding. Some conditions, different from neoplasms, cause folds of certain portions, or of the entire stomach, to be significantly thickened (Fig. 8.20). When the number and activity of parietal cells are increased, hyperchlorhydria results with the formation of giant folds. Conversely, gastric atrophy (Fig. 8.21) is associated with hypochlorhydria or achlorhydria. Between these two extremes, moderately enlarged gastric folds are associated with hyperchlorhydria and duodenal peptic ulcer.

Hyperplasia of the gastric mucosa is characterized by enlarged gastric rugae which may have a polypoid appearance. Some degree of wall pliability may be preserved with hyperplasia, although this might be difficult to demonstrate. When the enlarged folds are due to lymphoma, pliability is completely lost.

Menetrier's disease, gigantic gastropathy, results from hyperplasia of superficial epithelium of the gastric mucosa. Gastric rugae are wider than 25 mm, and sometimes polypoid in appearance. While the diameter of normal folds does not exceed 5 mm, widening of folds may be seen in a number of neoplastic conditions. The fundus and greater curvature undergo the most significant changes in Menetrier's disease (Fig. 8.22), but the entire stomach may also be affected. Fundic glands are elongated with cystic dilatation in the gastric fundus and body, while lymphocytic infiltrates pervade the mucosa and submucosa. This form of hyperplasia is called *foveolar*.

Menetrier's disease is very rare, affecting mostly males. Only several hundred cases have been reported. Secretion of a large amount of mucus makes radiologic examination difficult to perform, since adherence of barium to the mucosal surface is poor. The excreted mucus is rich in proteins suggesting that this disease

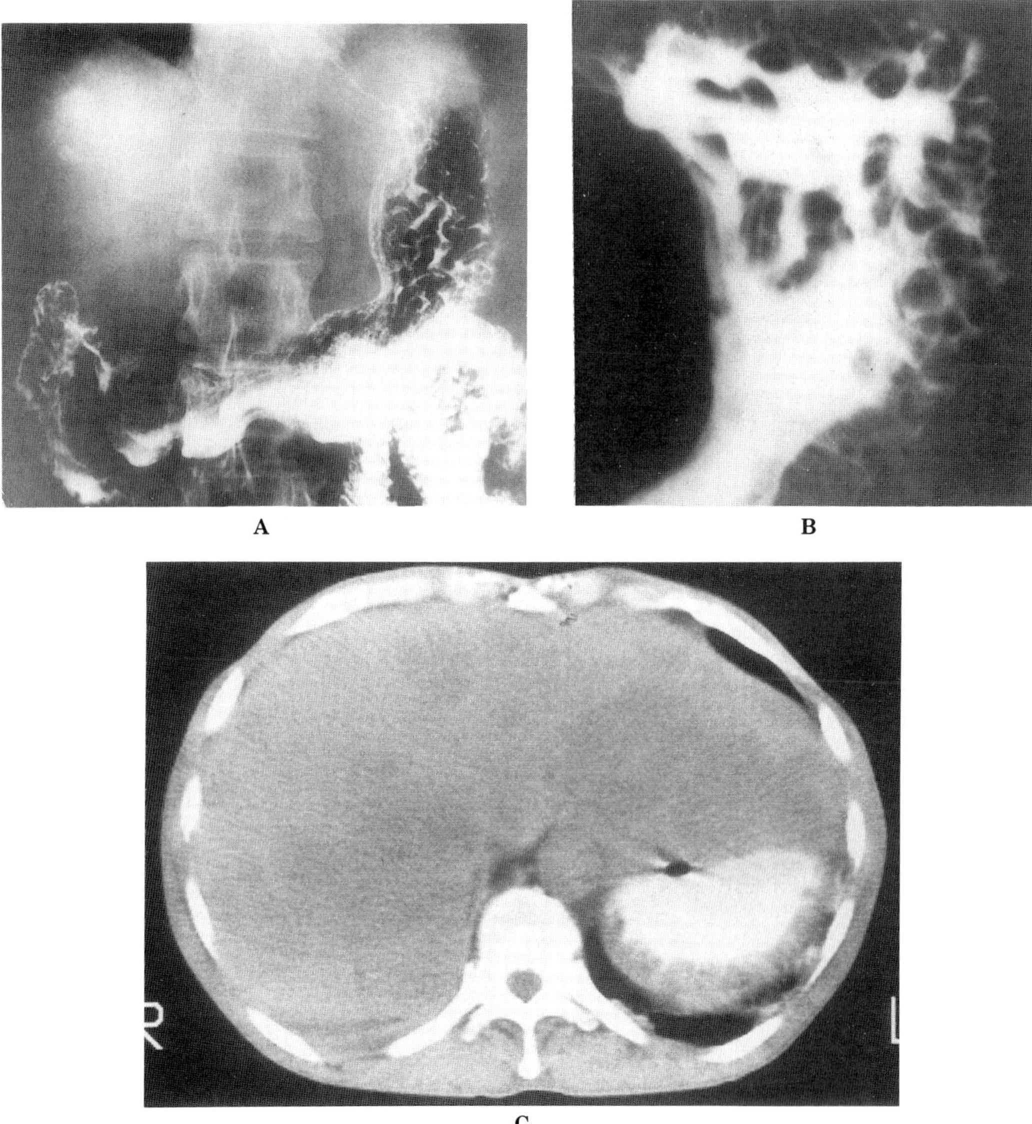

Figure 8.19. (A) Esophageal, gastric (fundic and antral), and duodenal varices. (B) Varices in the gastric fundus. (C) CT study.

process is related to protein-losing gastroenteropathies.

Radiologic distinction between Menetrier's disease and other benign diseases characterized by giant gastric rugae is not always accurate (Table 8.2). It is difficult to distinguish Menetrier's disease from lymphoma and diagnosis must be established by endoscopic biopsy. Localized foveolar gastric hyperplasia can be manifested by polypoid growth. Carcinoma, eosinophilic gastritis, and hypertrophic hypersecretory gastropathy should also be included in the differential diagnosis. Computed tomography does not always provide enough data for final confirmation of the diagnosis. Unlike barium series, CT gives insight into thickness of the

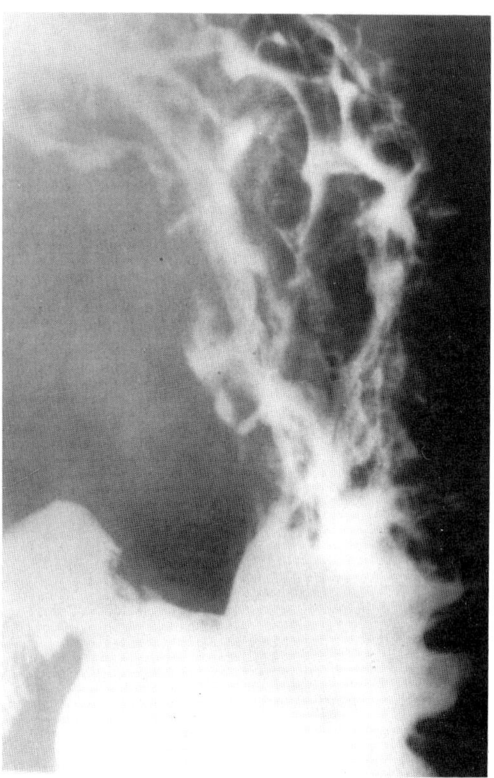

Figure 8.20. Giant gastric folds and peptic ulcerations in glandular gastric hyperplasia (confirmed by endoscopy).

gastric wall and into extramural extension of the process in patients with gastric neoplasia.

Glandular hyperplasia is characterized by thickened gastric folds, hyperchlorhydria, and peptic ulceration. In this form of hyperplasia, smaller amounts of mucus are secreted than in foveolar hyperplasia (Fig. 8.20).

In *foveolar-glandular* hyperplasia, another protein-losing gastroenteropathy, gastric rugae are thickened, excess mucus rich in proteins is secreted, and hyperchlorhydria is present.

Lymphoid hyperplasia is characterized by an increased number of normal lymphoid elements in the submucosa and mucosa of the stomach, resulting in giant gastric folds.

Table 8.2 Differential Diagnosis of Enlarged Gastric Folds

Carcinoma
Lymphoma
Pseudolymphoma
Varices
Zollinger–Ellison syndrome
Hyperplasia of gastric mucosa
Menetrier's disease
Corrosive gastritis

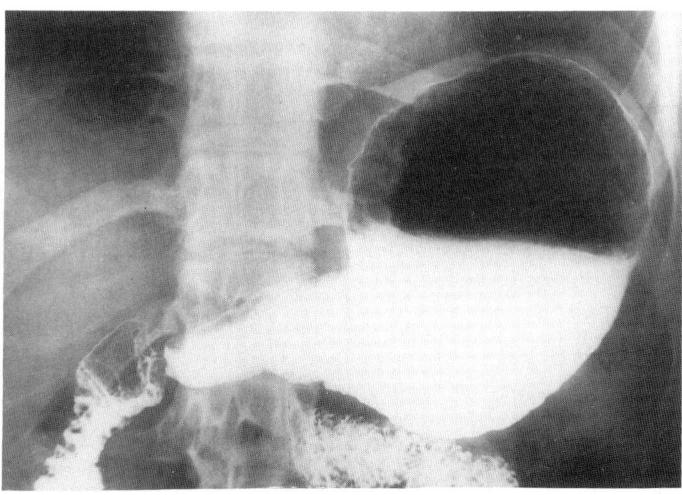

Figure 8.21. Atrophic gastritis of the gastric pouch after Billroth I surgery.

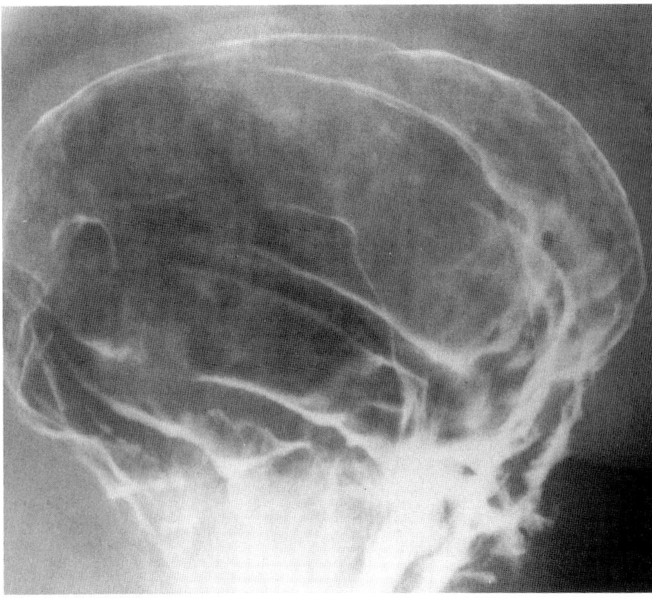

FIGURE 8.22. Menetrier's disease affecting the proximal stomach.

ZOLLINGER-ELLISON SYNDROME

Zollinger-Ellison syndrome comprises hyperacidity of gastric secretions, with thickened gastric rugae and multiple peptic ulcers in unusual locations. It results from malignant or benign gastrin-secreting, non-beta islet cell tumor(s) of the pancreas (Fig. 8.23). A gastrinoma sometimes occurs in sites other than the pancreas, such as the duodenum. Polyadenomatosis, including tumors of the pituitary gland, of the cortex of the adrenal glands, and of the parathyroid glands, is found in one-half of the patients. Gastric glandular hyperplasia results in hypersecretion of HCl and pepsin. Brunner's glands of the duodenum are hyperplastic, and plicae conniventes of the proximal jejunum are thickened. Signs of malabsorption may be present. Peptic ulcerations are found in the second and third portions of the duodenum and jejunum.

PROLAPSE OF GASTRIC MUCOSA

Prolapse of thickened antral mucosa into the duodenal bulb is a common finding which results from loose attachment of mucosa to the submucosa and the muscular layer. The prolapse has clinical significance only when there is bleeding or obstruction; otherwise, it is asymptomatic. Morphologically, three types of prolapse can be distinguished (Fig. 8.24):

1. Partial, reversible prolapse into the pyloric canal is represented by a negative defect on single-contrast examination, and shows as a mass protruding from the antrum on double-contrast studies.
2. Partial prolapse into the base of the duodenal bulb resembles a mushroom. However, it more often presents as a regular, umbrella-like defect indenting the base of the bulb.
3. Complete prolapse is seen as a lobulated mass protruding into the duodenal bulb; it may be either reversible or incarcerated.

The most common underlying cause for incarceration of a complete prolapse is the presence of a polyp(s) on the prolapsed mucosa. A polyp should be distinguished from thickened mucosa and enlarged Brunner's glands. Polypoid gastric folds can fill the entire duodenal bulb and cause obstruction.

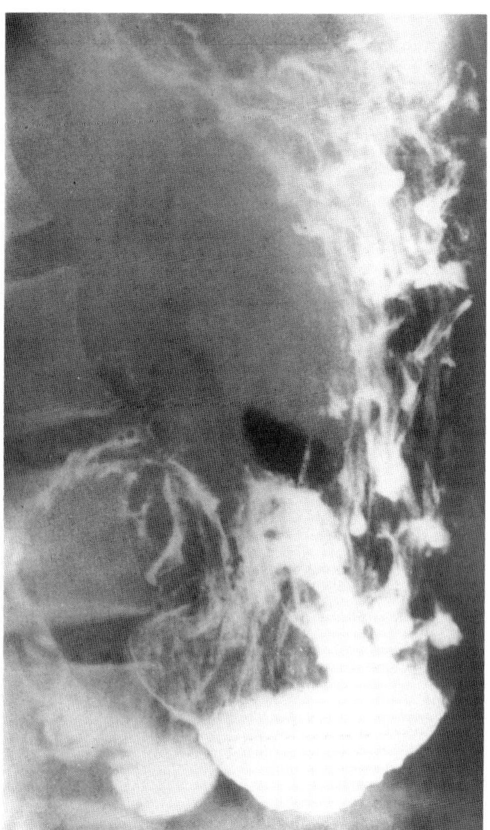

Figure 8.23. Zollinger-Ellison syndrome. Thickened gastric folds with multiple peptic ulcerations.

GASTRITIS

Acute Gastritis

The types of acute gastritis can be defined by clinical, endoscopic, pathologic, and radiologic criteria. The onset of symptoms may sometimes mimic an acute abdomen.

Erosive gastritis can result from chemical (including medicinal), thermal, or radiation damage. The role of infectious agents is not completely understood. However, *cytomegalovirus* may affect any portion of the stomach, resulting in an erosive gastritis appearance (Fig. 8.25A). In a majority of patients the causative factor remains unexplained. Erosive gastritis is also referred to as hemorrhagic gastritis, because melena and hematemesis can result in profuse bleeding. Erosions are depressed lesions no deeper than the muscular layer of the mucosa. The antrum and distal segments of the stomach, particularly near the lesser curvature, are the commonest sites of erosions. The diameter of typical erosions is 1-2 mm, and the depth about 1 mm. In contrast to peptic ulcers, erosions do not heal by forming a scar, but are subsequently covered by epithelium.

Erosions appear radiologically as accumulations of barium surrounded by a radiolucent brim of edema. Sometimes there are only elevated edematous nodules without central bar-

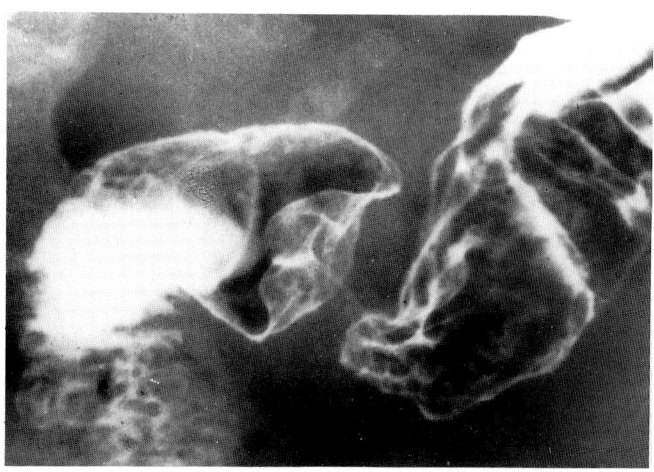

A

Figure 8.24. Prolapse of gastric mucosa into the duodenum. (A) Partial reversible prolapse into the duodenal bulb. (*Figure continued on overleaf.*)

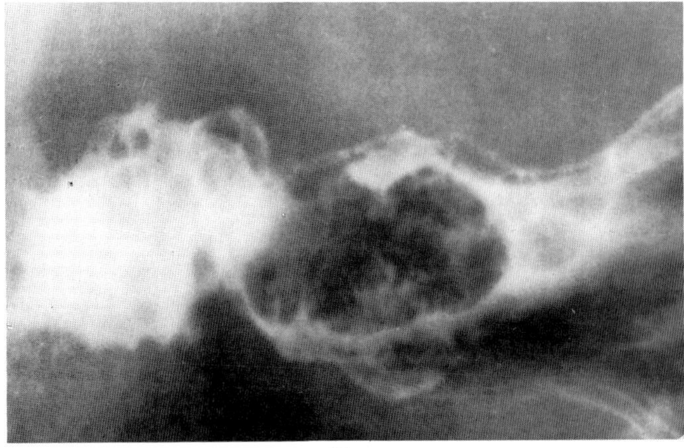

B

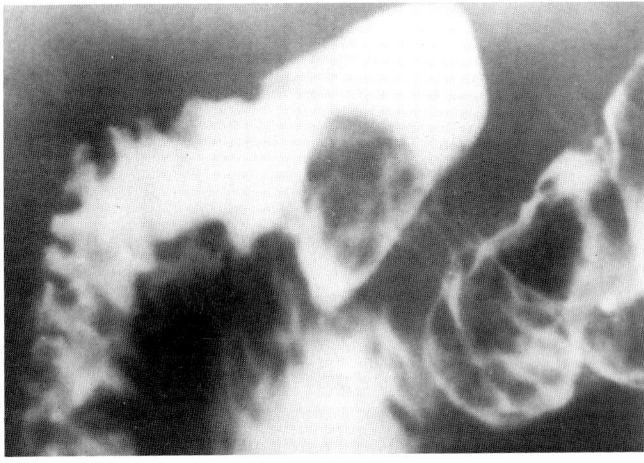

C

FIGURE 8.24. *continued.* Prolapse of gastric mucosa into the duodenum. (B) Polypoid mass in the gastric antrum. (C) Mass prolapses into the duodenal bulb.

ium collections. Endoscopically, erosions can be classified into three groups:

1. Complete erosions which are defects on nodules formed by edema (Fig. 8.25B).
2. Incomplete erosions in which there is no reaction of the wall (Fig. 8.25C).
3. Punctiform erosions which are the smallest.

The latter two types of erosions may be mistaken radiographically for flocculated barium (Fig. 8.26). Discrete, linear gastric erosions have also been described (Fig. 8.27).

Erosions may be demonstrated by double-contrast studies, or by controlled compression of the stomach during a single-contrast or multiphasic examination.

Corrosive gastritis results from ingestion of caustic substances such as acid, alkali, and salts of heavy metals. Findings depend on the degree of injury to the gastric wall and the interval after damage. Immediately after ingestion of a corrosive agent, the stomach is hypotonic, the rugae are edematous, and the sulci between them can disappear. Necrosis resulting in ulcerations may be seen in the acute phase, but perforations are rare, and, if suspected, water-soluble contrast medium instead of barium should be used. In the chronic phase,

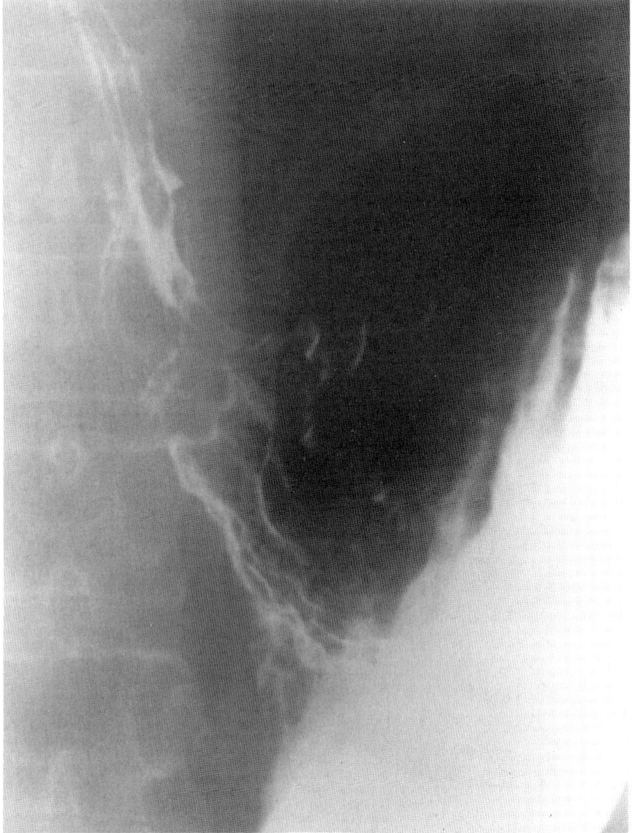

A

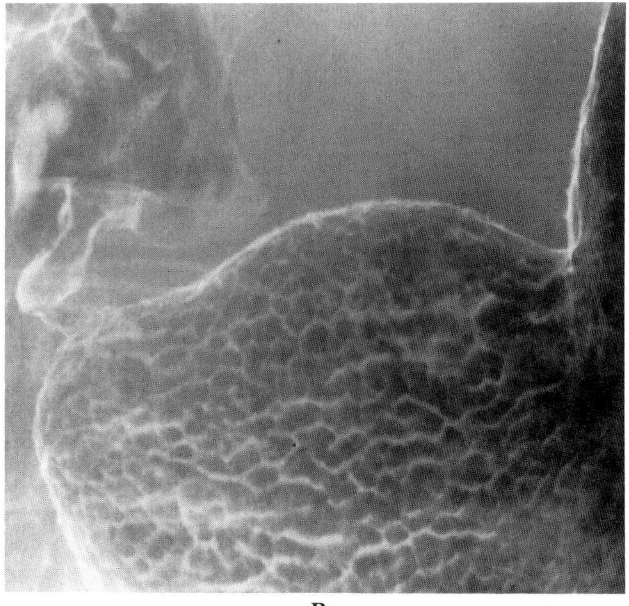

B

Figure 8.25. Gastric erosions. (A) Cytomegalovirus gastritis in a patient with AIDS. (B) Complete, with edema. (*Figure continued on overleaf.*)

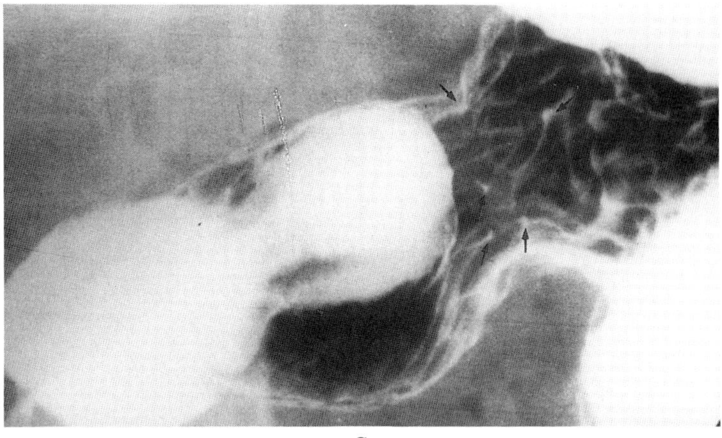

C

Figure 8.25 *continued.* Gastric erosions. (C) Incomplete (arrows).

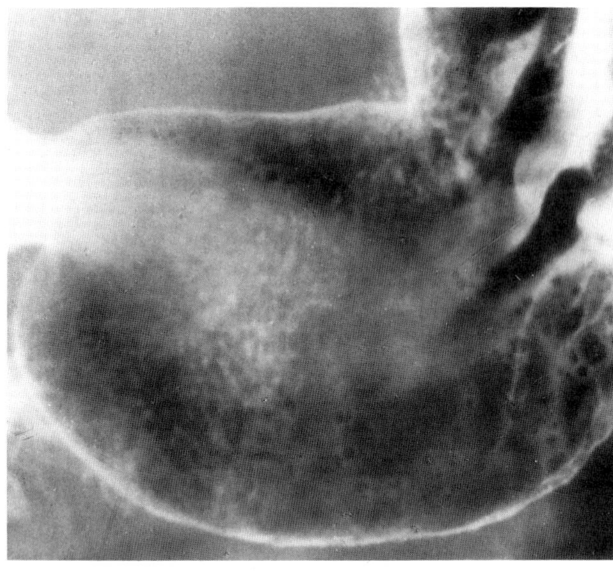

Figure 8.26. Flocculated barium may resemble incomplete erosions.

the lesser curvature is shortened and pyloric stenosis may result (Figs. 8.28 and 8.64). These findings may resemble scirrhous carcinoma.

Emphysematous gastritis (Fig. 8.29) is a rare but often fatal condition characterized by the presence of gas within the gastric wall. This may be seen on a plain roentgenogram. Emphysematous gastritis can be the sequel of dissection of the wall, resulting from vigorous vomiting, corrosive gastritis, infection by gas-producing microorganisms, or gastric infarction. Emphysema of the gastric wall may be mimicked by large amounts of food in the stomach. Computed tomography is diagnostic and can accurately locate gas within the gastric wall.

Granulomatous gastritis represents a rare group of diseases. Changes which are nonspecific in the early phases may later assume an appearance of hypertrophic gastritis with rigid-

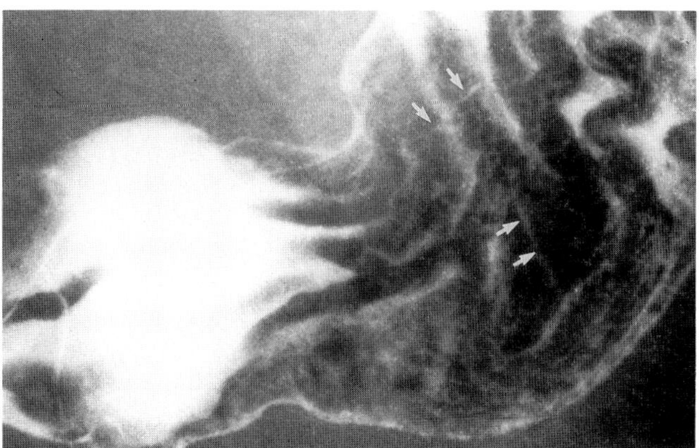

FIGURE 8.27. Linear gastric erosions (arrows).

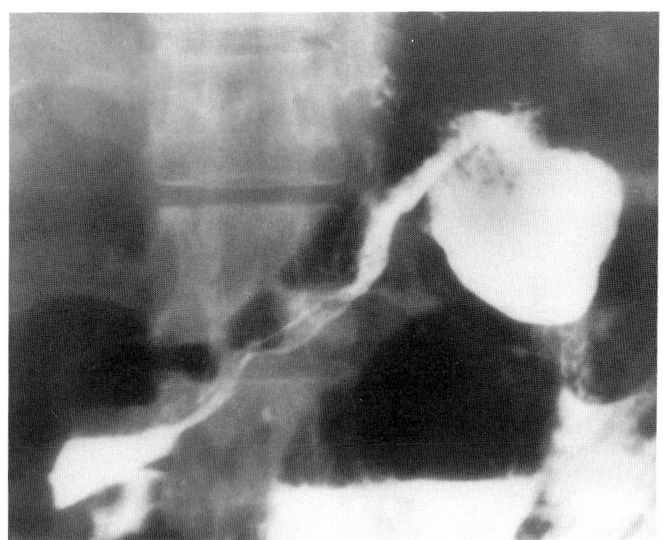

FIGURE 8.28. Chronic phase of corrosive gastritis.

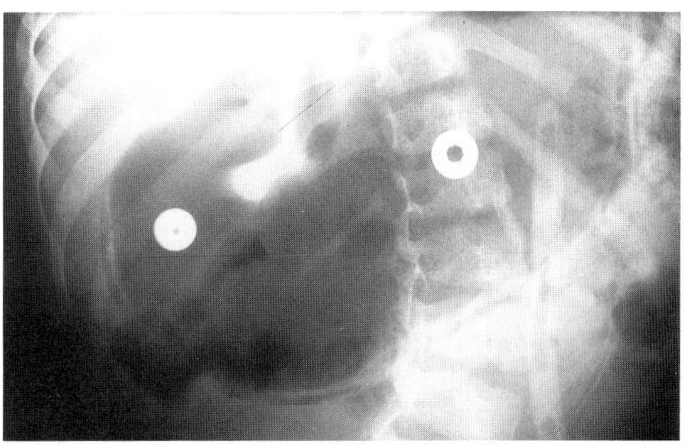

FIGURE 8.29. Emphysematous gastritis. Gas in the gastric wall.

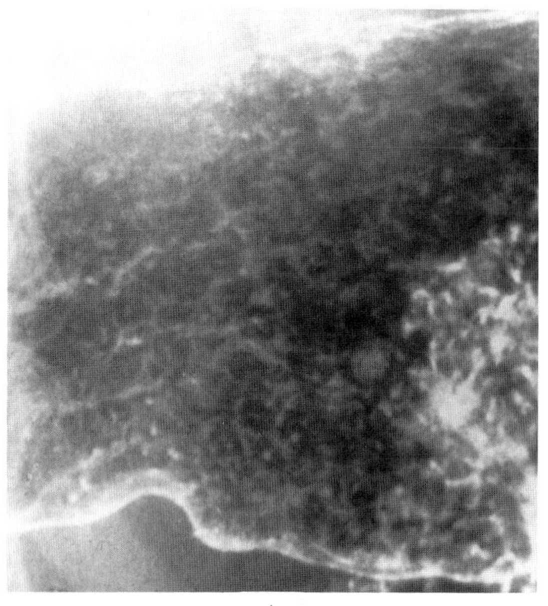

A

Figure 8.30. Aphthoid ulcers in Crohn's disease. (A) Gastric antrum. (B) Colon of the same patient.

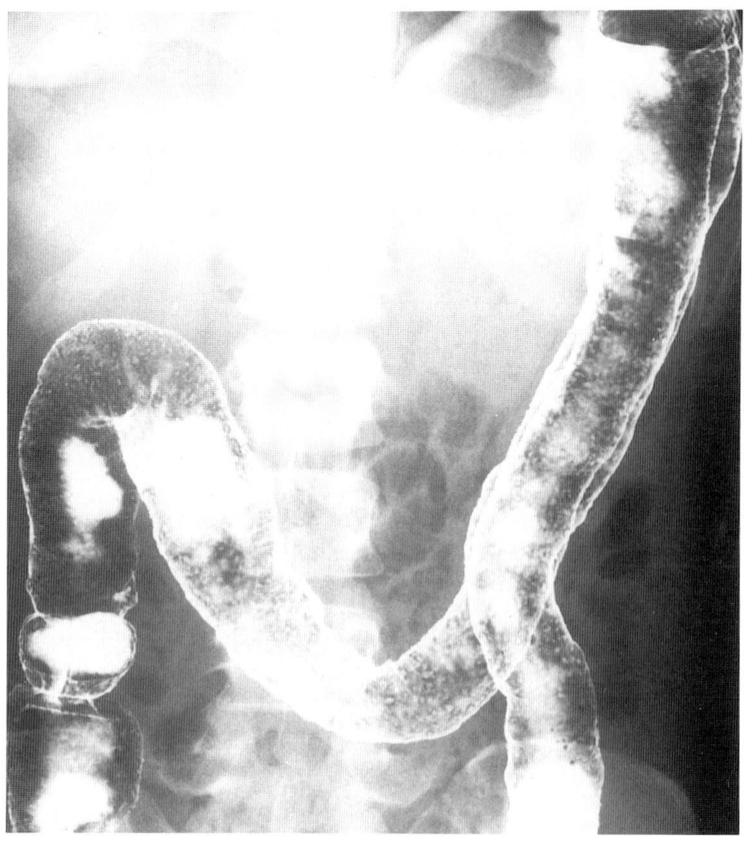

B

ity of the wall. Crohn's disease or granulomatous diseases of other etiologies can also affect the stomach. The prevalence of gastric affection in Crohn's disease is 0.5–4%, but some sources give a figure 10 times as high. Aphthoid ulcers, appearing alone or accompanied by thickening of gastric folds, are the earliest detectable sign of Crohn's disease (Figs. 8.30 and 11.20B). They cannot be differentiated from gastric erosions. Mucosa of distal portions of the stomach may assume a cobblestone appearance. However, a funnel-shaped stenosis of the antrum with narrowing of the proximal duodenum is rather characteristic for Crohn's disease affecting the stomach and duodenum (Fig. 8.31).

Candidiasis most commonly affects the stomach of immunosuppressed patients. Aphthoid ulcers, identical to those in Crohn's disease, are the earliest detectable lesions, and are often on thickened gastric rugae. In advanced candidiasis collections of fungi may resemble a bezoar.

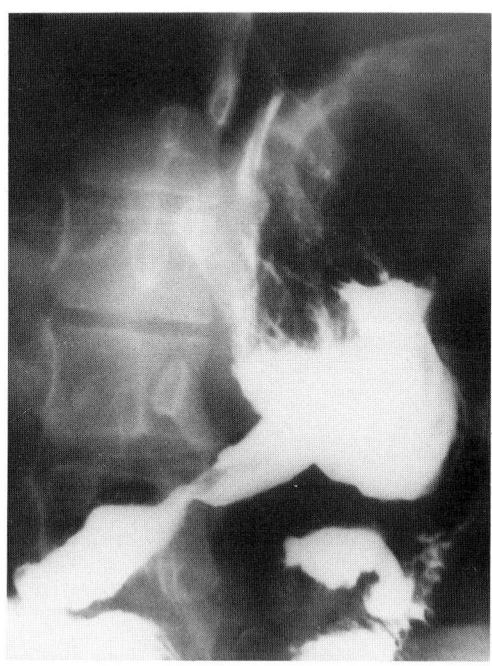

FIGURE 8.31. Advanced Crohn's disease affecting gastric antrum and proximal duodenum.

CHRONIC GASTRITIS

Clinical, endoscopic, macroscopic, and microscopic findings are seldom concordant in chronic gastritis. Even microscopic criteria for establishing the diagnosis are neither uniform nor accurate. Clinically healthy people may show vividly demonstrable accumulations of lymphocytes, plasma cells, eosinophils, mastocytes, and macrophages making it difficult to establish a demarcation between physiologic and abnormal events. However, it is likely that chronic gastritis represents an autoimmune disorder. The gastric antrum and regions adjacent to the lesser curvature are most commonly affected.

Three phases can be observed in the natural course of chronic gastritis:

1. *Superficial gastritis* confined to the mucosa.
2. Subsequent transformation to *atrophic gastritis* penetrating all layers of the wall. The mucosal epithelium acquires characteristics of intestinal epithelium through metaplasia, and parietal cells which secrete HCl and intrinsic factor are missing. Chief cells secreting pepsinogen are replaced by mucous cells similar to those in the small bowel. Such "intestinalized" mucosa has a high malignant potential (Fig. 8.32). Glandular atrophy also takes place and glands of the gastric body assume properties of pyloric glands by metaplasia.
3. Evolution of the inflammatory process leading to *gastric atrophy*. The mucosa of the entire stomach becomes extremely thin and fundic glands disappear irretrievably.

Thick, wide, and prominent gastric rugae do not indicate underlying chronic gastritis; however, rugae may be low or even disappear in patients with gastric atrophy. The stomach is tubular shaped and associated pernicious anemia is common.

Demonstration of areae gastricae is the only radiographic finding which corresponds to microscopic findings in patients with chronic gastritis. However, definition of normal areae gastricae is not always successful when increased gastric secretion interferes. In normal subjects, areae gastricae are regularly shaped,

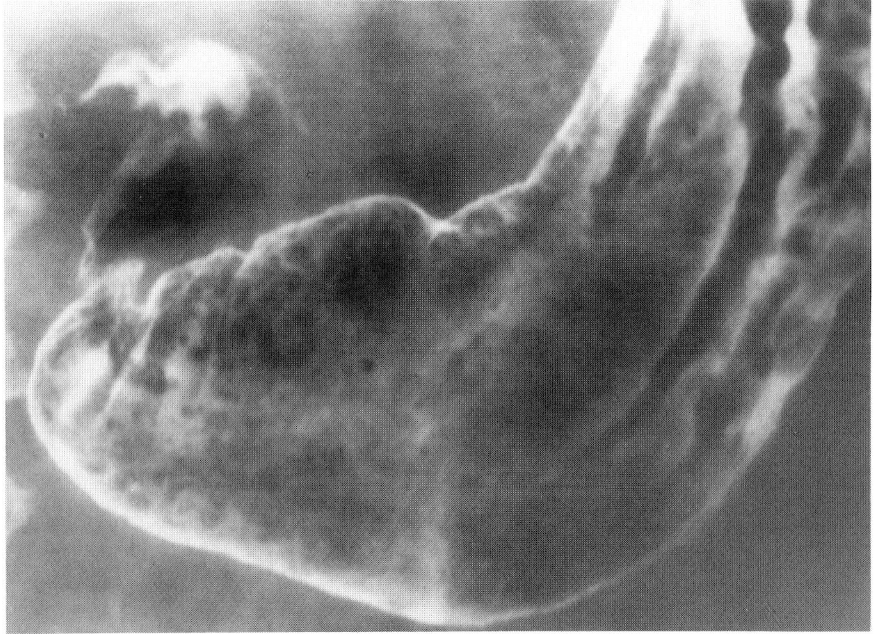

A

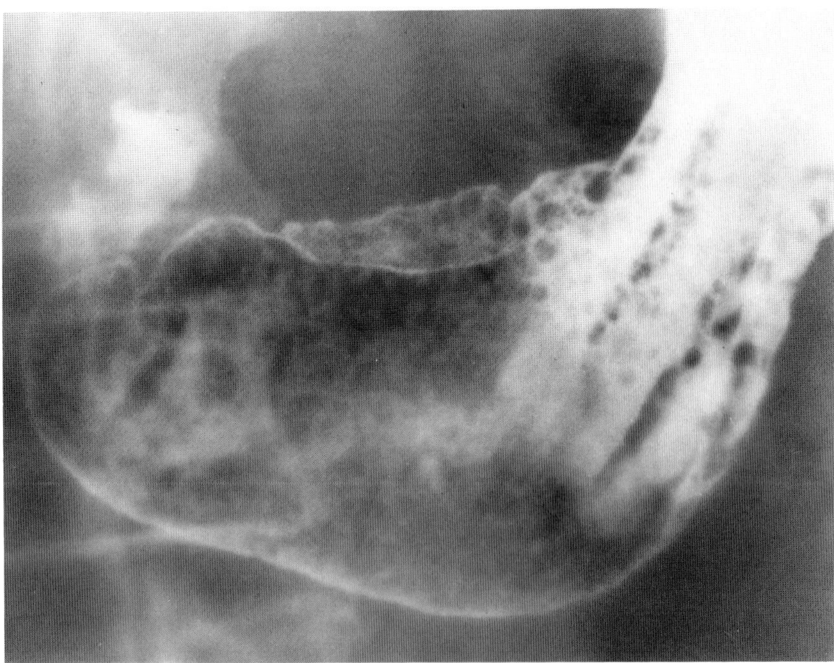

B

Figure 8.32. Atrophic gastritis. (A) Markedly reduced numbers of areae gastricae. Residual areae gastricae near the greater and lesser curvature are enlarged and irregular. (B) Two years later with carcinoma on the lesser curvature.

measuring 1–3 mm in diameter. Such normal findings rule out diffuse gastric atrophy. In early phases of atrophic gastritis, enlarged (3–5 mm) areae gastricae are polygonal or irregularly shaped, and a spasmolytic will not influence morphology. As the disease advances, areae gastricae become smaller and finally disappear (Fig. 8.32).

Hypertrophic Gastritis. Hypertrophic gastritis occurs infrequently but carries malignant potential. Enlargement of the rugae results from thickened mucosa and submucosa. Areae gastricae are enlarged up to a diameter of 5 mm, and are oblong or polygonal shaped (Fig. 8.33). Widened gastric rugae may bear erosions. Hypertrophic gastritis cannot be distinguished

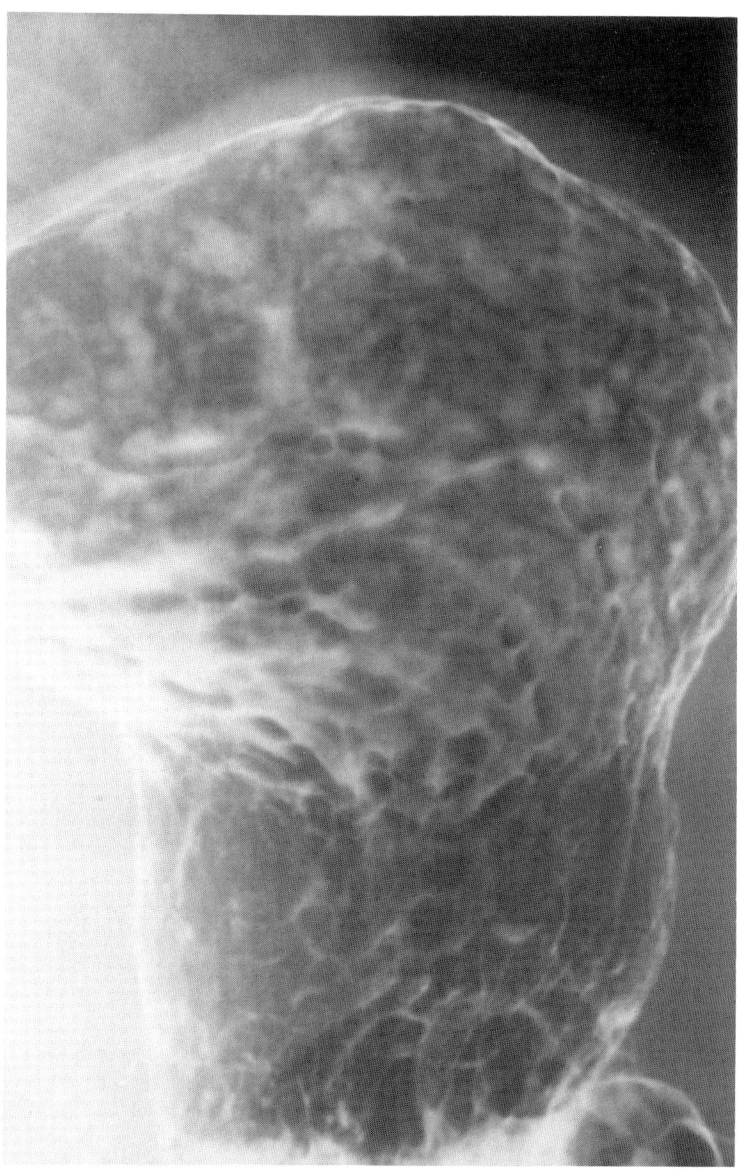

FIGURE 8.33. Hypertrophic gastritis.

radiographically from other conditions characterized by enlarged gastric rugae.

EOSINOPHILIC GASTROENTERITIS

A common radiographic finding in eosinophilic gastroenteritis is nodular mucosal thickening of a narrowed gastric antrum and of the valvulae conniventes, along with thickening of the entire wall of the small intestine (Fig. 8.34). Strictures may result in late phases. The esophagus and the large intestine are infrequently affected. Radiologic signs do not differ from those of other gastrointestinal inflammatory diseases.

The mucosal form of eosinophilic gastroenteritis is characterized by abdominal pain, loss of protein, and vomiting. Obstructive phenomena distinguish muscular forms of the disease, while the serosal form may result in ascites.

Eosinophilic infiltrates characterize the microscopic picture, and eosinophilia in peripheral blood is common. Eosinophilic gastroenteritis is more common in individuals with allergic diseases such as bronchial asthma.

BENIGN INFILTRATIVE DISEASES

The stomach may be affected by Crohn's disease (Figs. 8.30 and 8.31), tuberculosis, and lues. Mutual differentiation and distinction from a malignant infiltrative process such as scirrhous carcinoma, which narrows the gastric lumen and causes rigidity of the wall, is not always possible by radiologic means.

Sarcoidosis of the stomach is a rare extension of the disease, and is indistinguishable from other infiltrative lesions of the stomach.

CHRONIC GRANULOMATOUS DISEASE IN CHILDHOOD

This is a recessively inherited disorder transmitted by the X chromosome. Due to deficiency of NADPH oxidase, neutrophils do not produce hydrogen peroxide and do not destroy ingested bacteria. This results in recurrent infections with catalase-positive microorganisms. The sequelae of repeated infections are usually liver abscesses, osteomyelitis, and granulomas in the lungs, bones, and liver. Rugae of the body of the stomach are widened and the antrum is narrowed, with proximal portions of the stomach intact. Biopsy reveals edema and fibrosis in the submucosa with granulomatous infiltration of the muscular layer, while the epithelial layer of the mucosa is unchanged. Pathologic changes withdraw spontaneously in a majority of patients.

PEPTIC ULCER

Peptic ulceration is a defect of the alimentary canal wall caused by acid gastric secretions from normal or ectopic gastric mucosa. It develops from superficial erosion and extends deeper than the muscular layer of the mucosa. In contrast to simple erosions, peptic ulcers heal to form a scar, which may result in stenosis and deformity. Only with prompt and successful medical management can treated acute ulcers heal without macroscopic scarring.

A chronic peptic ulcer typically activates in the spring and late autumn. About 5–10% of the general population have peptic ulcers, males twice as often as females. Duodenal peptic ulcer is four times more common than gastric. Malignant transformation of a duodenal peptic ulcer has not been described. Multiple peptic ulcers of the stomach and proximal small bowel, especially when combined with significantly enlarged rugae, should arouse suspicion of Zollinger–Ellison syndrome. Simultaneous peptic ulcers of the stomach and duodenum are infrequent.

Microscopic analysis has revealed that peptic ulcers originate at junctions of mucosas of different properties, and are situated in the region of pyloric glands. More than 90% of gastric ulcers occur along the fundoantral junctional line. This junctional line may be situated at various locations in the stomach, resulting in gastric peptic ulcers at different sites. Intestinal metaplasia of gastric mucosa, and atrophic gastritis are common in patients with chronic ulcers.

The majority of peptic ulcers originate in regions where HCl is not secreted and where the mucosa is sensitive to the actions of acid gastric juice. Ulcers are most commonly found 1 cm proximal and distal to the mucosal junc-

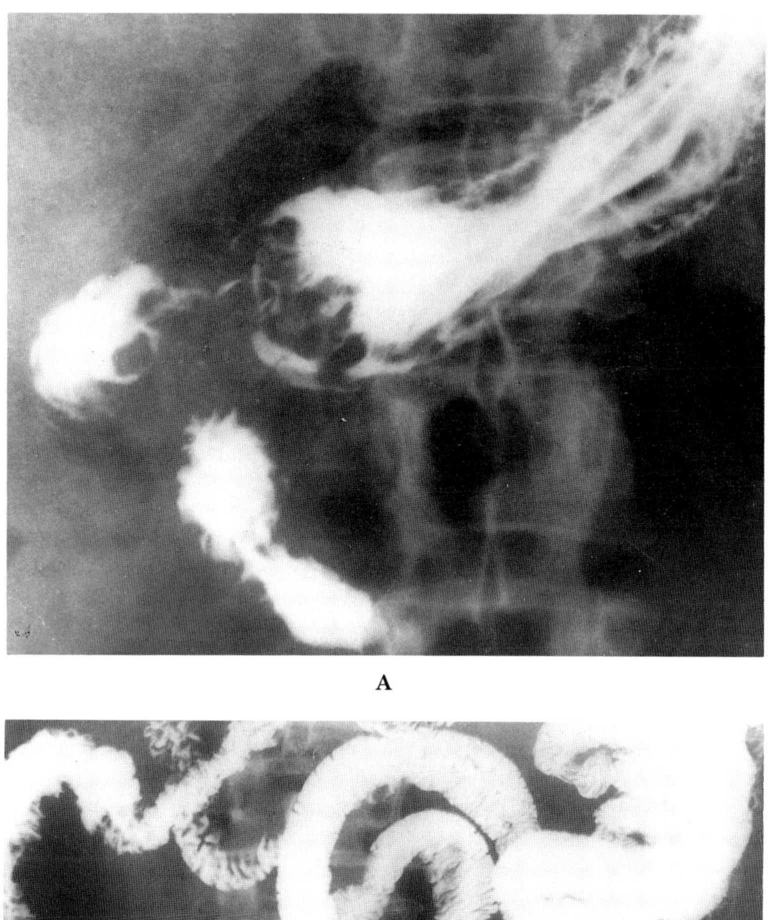

A

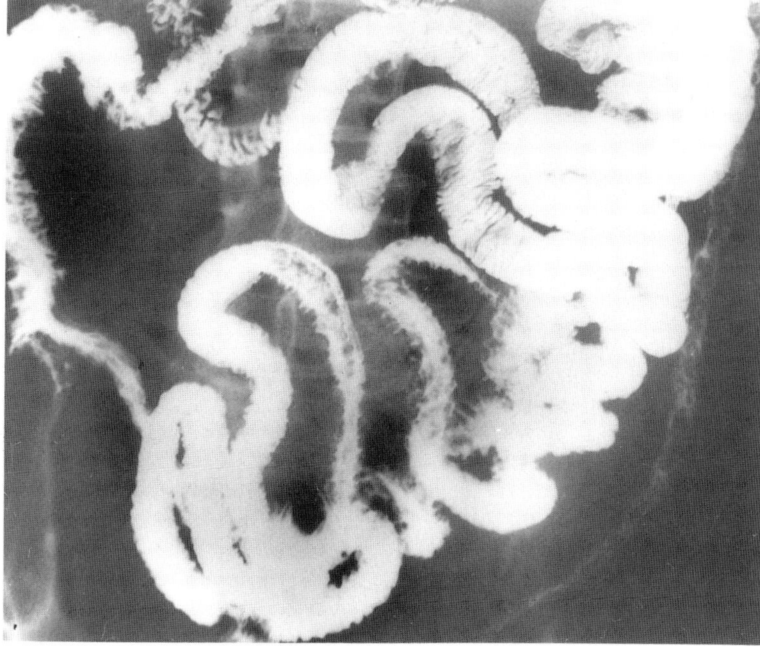

B

Figure 8.34. Eosinophilic gastroenteritis. (A) Nodularity of the gastric antrum. Controlled compression study. (B) Nodular lesions of small bowel circular folds.

tion of the corpus and the antrum. When this junction is more distal, ulcers appear in the pyloric canal. Peptic ulcers are more common along the lesser curvature. Ulcers of the anterior gastric wall represent only 1% of all gastric ulcers. They frequently cause minimal subjective symptoms, and may perforate into the peritoneal cavity. Ulcers of the gastric fundus should be considered malignant (Fig. 8.35).

Ulcers in the proximal portions of the stomach tend to be larger, and those in the distal portions smaller, than an average gastric peptic ulcer. Increased frequency of ulcers in the proximal portions of the stomach in elderly patients has not been demonstrated.

There is no site predilection for an *acute ulcer*. An acute, stress ulcer is a sequel to acute physical and/or psychologic trauma, including surgery, alcohol abuse, corticosteroid therapy, and severe infectious disease. In contrast, chronic stress contributes to the development of a duodenal ulcer.

Chronic ulcers are more common in the pyloric region and are, on average, smaller than an acute ulcer. Acute ulcers tend to occupy a larger area, but are shallow. However, acute ulcer perforation is more probable and the response to therapy is more satisfying. Single-contrast and double-contrast examinations are suitable for diagnosing gastric peptic ulcer. The main radiologic finding of an ulcer is a collection of contrast medium in the crater, the niche of an ulcer. Depending on the shape of the ulcer and projection, the niche may appear as a round or reniform collection of contrast medium (Fig. 8.36). When seen in profile, there is a protrusion of contrast medium outside the inner contour of the stomach (Figs. 8.37 and 8.38). The crater often has smooth edges and walls, but a thrombosed blood vessel, a blood clot, or necrotic masses may cause irregularities of the ulcer bottom. Mucosa surrounding the crater may be significantly thickened.

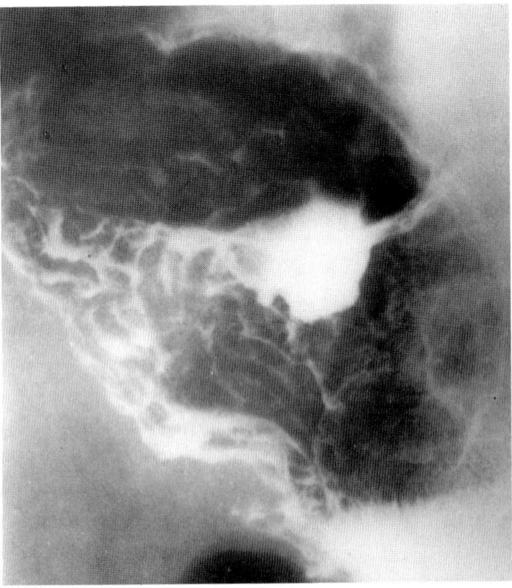

Figure 8.35. Ulcerating carcinoma of the gastric fundus.

Mucosal defects produced by shallow ulcers can only be demonstrated by means of double-contrast studies. Accumulation of barium in the ulceration is better presented *en face* than by profile projection. An ulcer on the dependent wall accumulates barium, while barium empties from an ulcer on the nondependent wall (Fig. 8.36A and B). Compression or changing the patient's position will not mobilize accumulated barium from the ulceration.

The crater of a *penetrating* ulcer is deeper than the expected thickness of the gastric wall (Fig. 8.39). Three layers separated by horizontal division lines may be seen in the crater, representing in the cranial-caudad direction, air, gastric secretions, and barium. The most common penetrations are into the pancreas. Shortening of the lesser curvature of the stomach results from penetration of an ulcer into the lesser omentum with the formation of fibrous tissue (Fig. 8.39C).

A chronic peptic ulcer is prone to recurrence. The surrounding gastric rugae appear as radiating folds and converge toward the crater, as a result of contraction of the wall by collagenous fibers; this results in wrinkling of the gastric wall (Fig. 8.39D). Scarring may result in prominent deformation, and an irregular fibrous rim can be seen surrounding an ulcer callus. Approximately 85% of gastric peptic ulcers can be diagnosed by a single-contrast examination; however, even higher sensitivity can be achieved with a double-contrast examination. If both single-contrast examination with compression and double-contrast examination fail to demonstrate signs suggesting a

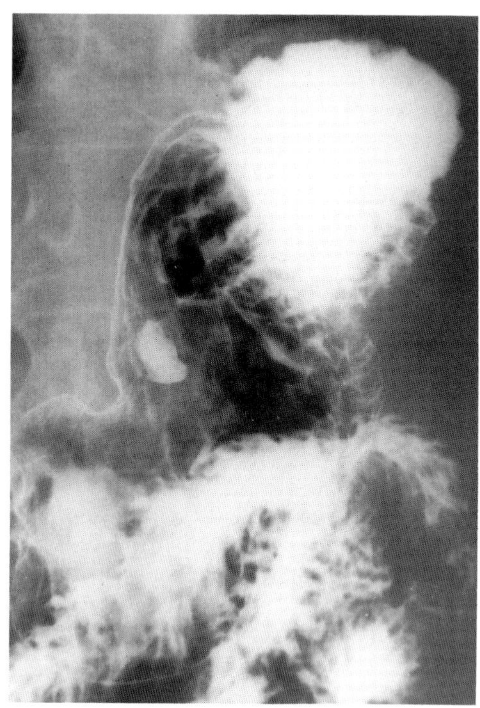

A

FIGURE 8.36. (A) and (B) Oval crater [arrow on (B)] of a posterior (dependent) gastric wall ulcer. (C) Intraspinal myelographic contrast medium mimics a peptic ulcer (arrow).

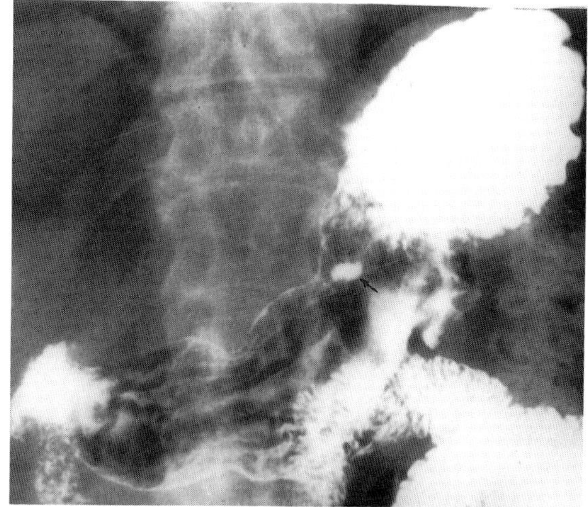

B

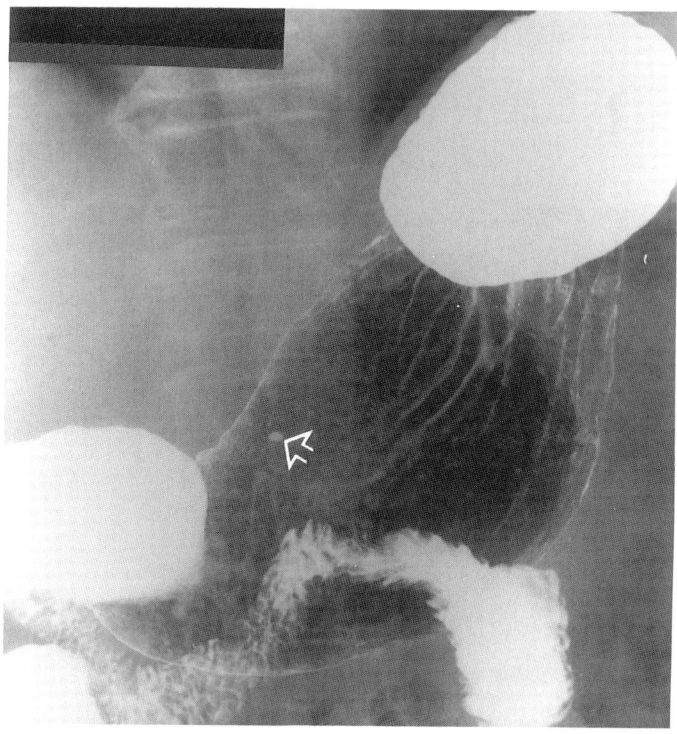

C

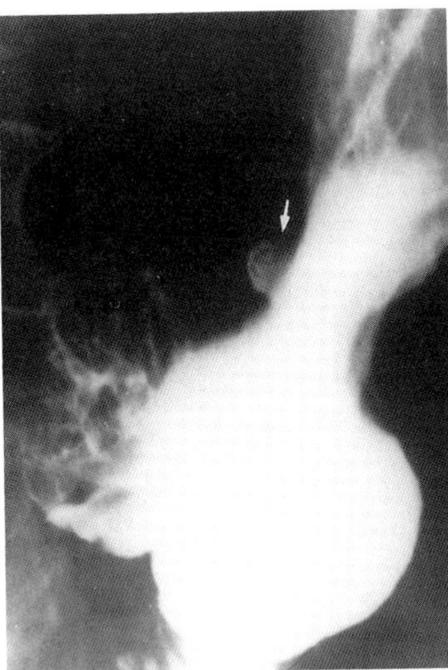

FIGURE 8.37. Peptic ulcer of the lesser gastric curvature exhibiting a Hampton line (arrow).

benign nature, or if the ulcer does not heal on therapy, gastroscopy is indicated. Such a protocol allows savings in time and cost of up to 30% in diagnostic procedures, and 80% in follow-up of patients, which is important considering the high prevalence of the disease. All ulcers diagnosed as benign by double-contrast examinations or multiphasic examinations were found to be benign at biopsy. Most suspicious ulcers are benign, but almost no benign-appearing ulcers are malignant. Indeed, a thorough radiologic and endoscopic follow-up study of 200 patients with benign-appearing ulcers confirmed the benign nature of the lesions. The fact that only 5% of gastric ulcers are malignant contributes to successful diagnosis of a benign peptic ulcer. Some benign ulcers may have indeterminate properties or properties which may suggest malignancy. In contrast, malignant ulcers almost never present with benign properties.

Benign ulcers seen *en face* present a round

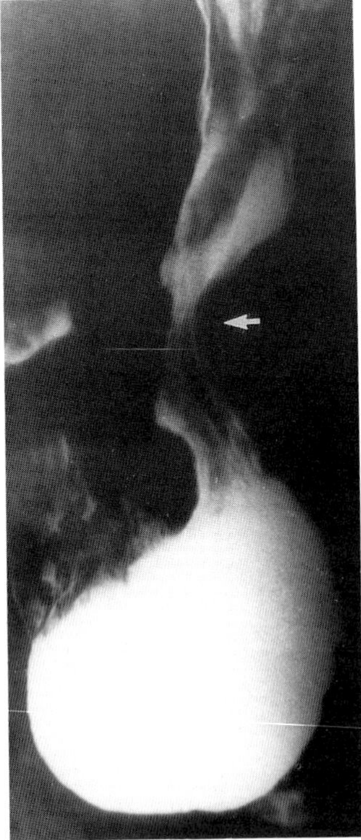

FIGURE 8.38. Multiple lesser curvature ulcers with spasm of the opposite wall (arrow).

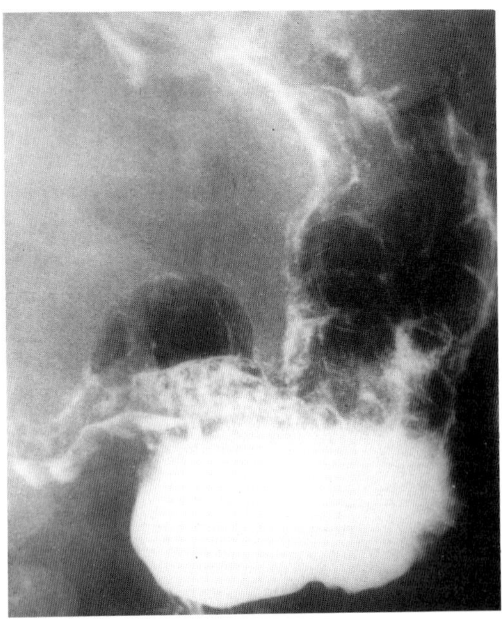

A

FIGURE 8.39. Penetrating lesser curvature ulcer of the gastric antrum. (A) Crater is much deeper than the expected wall thickness with layering of air, secretions, and barium in the crater.

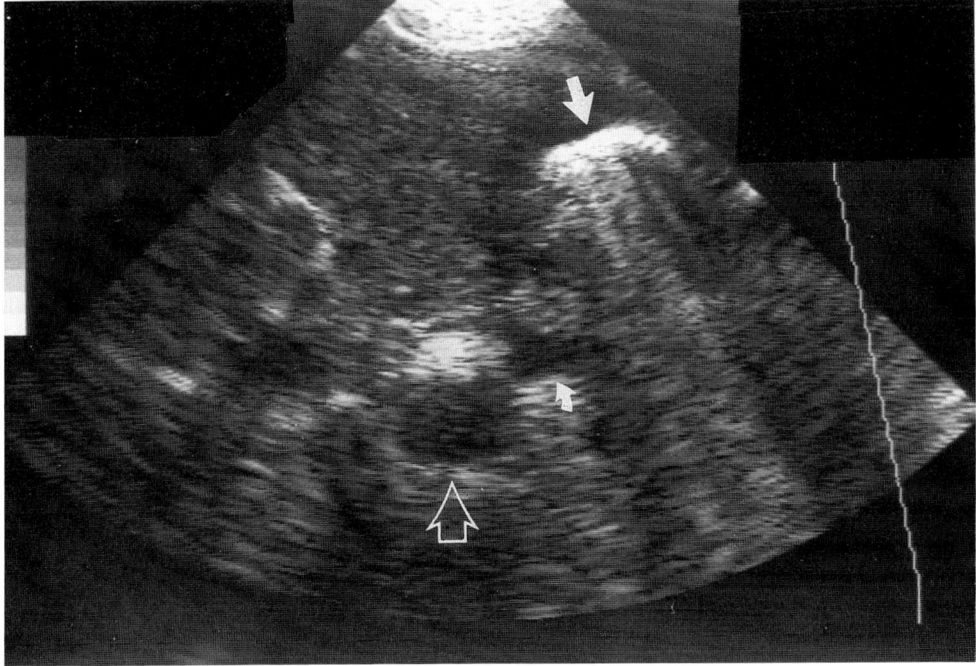

B

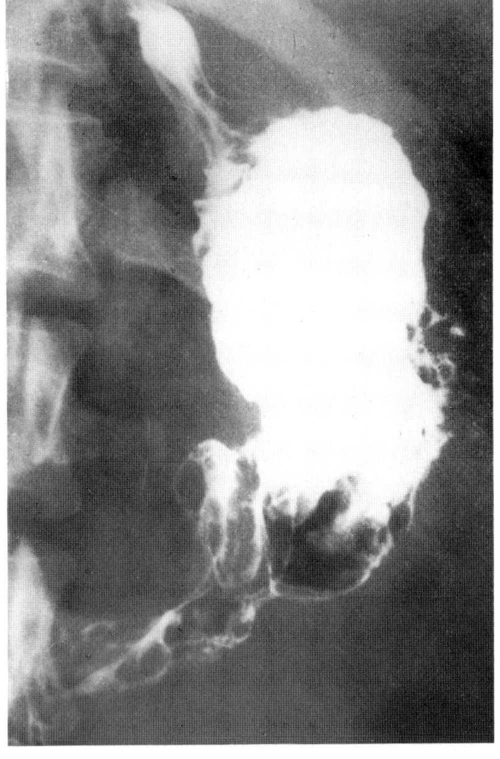

C

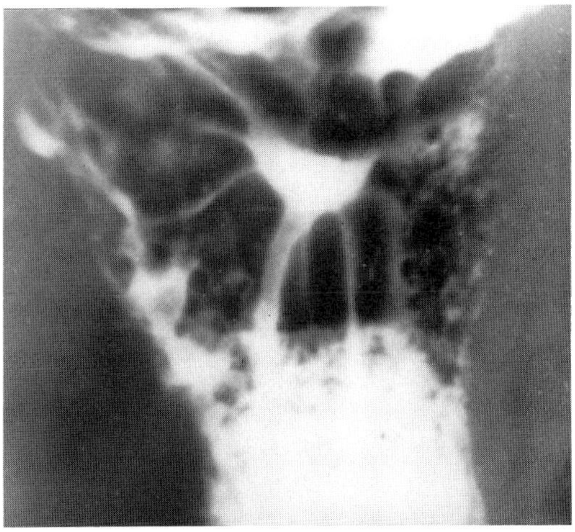

D

FIGURE 8.39. *continued.* Penetrating lesser curvature ulcer of the gastric antrum. (B) Ultrasound presentation of air within the ulceration (white closed arrow). Aorta (open arrow) celiac axis (curved arrow). (Courtesy of W.L. Wells, MD, Louisiana State University, New Orleans.) (C) Benign gastric ulcer penetrating into the gastrohepatic ligament with shortening of the lesser gastric curvature. (D) Chronic peptic ulcer with radiating folds.

or oval collection of barium surrounded by a smooth and regular collar of edema (Fig. 8.40) and radiating folds. Shown in profile, a gastric ulcer lies outside the inner contour of the gastric wall. If the areae gastricae can be seen around the ulcer, they are enlarged or have normal dimensions.

On occasion large gastric ulcers may be seen by CT and ultrasound (Fig. 8.39B).

INDIRECT SIGNS

The radiologic diagnosis of a peptic ulcer cannot be definitely established without demonstrating an ulcer crater. However, indirect radiologic signs may indicate that an ulcer is present but not clearly identified because of a shallow crater, or filling with mucus, necrotic tissue, blood clots, or food remnants.

Localized spasm may be present on the gastric wall opposite the crater (Fig. 8.38), and propagation of peristalsis can be impaired in the region of an undetected ulcer. If any indirect sign is present, it is reasonable to repeat the examination after several days or to perform endoscopy.

COMPLICATIONS

Perforation. Perforations of the stomach and duodenum occur in 2–4% of patients with peptic ulcer disease. Duodenal ulcers perforate more commonly than gastric. Perforation is more likely to occur in males than females (in a ratio of 12:1). An ulcer may freely perforate into the peritoneal cavity (*perforatio libera*) or into a closed space formed by adhesions (*perforatio tecta*). An ulcer may penetrate into an adjacent anatomical structure such as the pancreas or lesser omentum. Pneumoperitoneum is present in more than 80% of patients with perforation, and radiographic water-soluble contrast medium can appear outside of the stomach lumen at the site of perforation (see chapter 5, about acute abdomen, pages 157-160). Infections resulting from perforations of the posterior wall of the stomach seldom cause diffuse peritonitis.

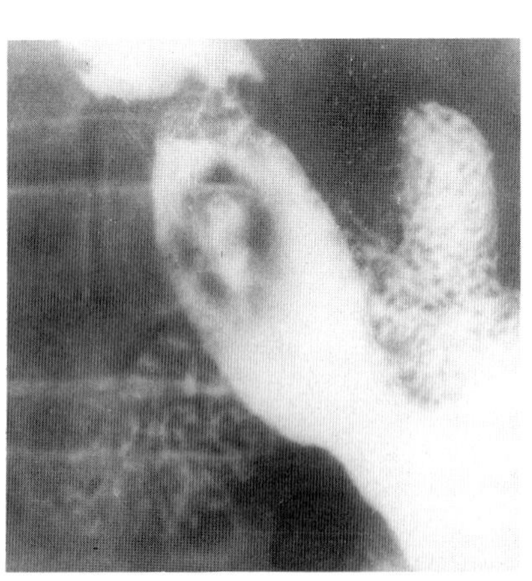

A

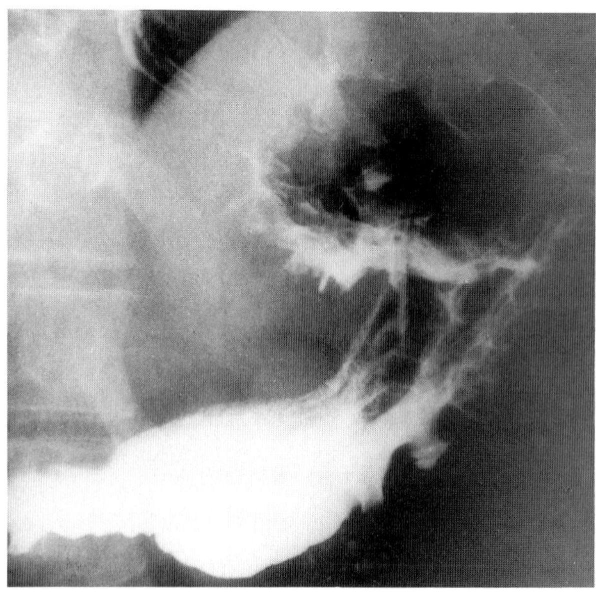

B

FIGURE 8.40. Benign ulcer with a mound of edema. (A) Antral. (B) Greater curvature.

Bleeding. Peptic ulcers of the stomach and duodenum are the most common causes of upper gastrointestinal bleeding. Massive bleeding results more frequently from a duodenal ulcer. Fatal hemorrhage may occur when a blood vessel is eroded. With suspected upper gastrointestinal bleeding, a *no-touch technique* of examination is used. Palpation and compression of the stomach are avoided.

Double-contrast examination reveals the site of a bleeding ulcer in 80% of patients by demonstrating one or more of the following signs: a clot in the ulcer, an artery at the bottom of the ulcer, or disturbances of contrast medium flow in the region of actively bleeding ulceration. However, endoscopy reveals a primary site of bleeding from the upper gastrointestinal tract in 93% of patients and facilitates treatment by means of photocoagulation. Vasopressin administration through an angiographic catheter will also stop the bleeding in a majority of patients.

Obstruction. Obstruction may result from scarring during peptic ulcer healing, but the frequency of obstruction can be decreased by medical treatment (Fig. 8.41). With minimal obstruction of the pylorus or the duodenal bulb, the stomach is dilated and deep peristaltic waves may be seen with retention of gastric contents. With higher degree of obstruction the stomach is hypotonic, filled with secretions and food remnants, and without peristaltic activity. Benign stenoses cause gradual obstruction of the gastric outlet with a tendency toward more dilatation than with malignant conditions. Ulcer scarring may result in an hourglass deformity of the stomach and may resemble indentation by the costal margin of the spleen, or by tumorous and inflammatory infiltration of the gastric wall.

Malignant Degeneration. Opinions are divided on malignant transformation of a gastric peptic ulcer. Carcinoma of the stomach developed in 3.4% of patients thought to have chronic peptic ulcer, and malignant cells first appearing at the peptic ulcer margin. Malignant ulcer may, but need not always, assume radiographic characteristics of a malignant growth.

HEALING OF PEPTIC ULCER

Peptic ulcer cure depends more on the depth of the crater and fibrotic changes than on the dimensions of the area affected. Radiologic signs of improvement are:

1. Reduction in depth of the crater.
2. Change in shape of the ulcer.
3. Decrease in the ulcer surface area.
4. Decrease in surrounding tissue reaction.

Propagation of peristalsis becomes restored. Data on the frequency of peptic ulcer scars differ, and their radiographic detectability lies between 50% and 90%. Postulcer scars may present as folds radiating from a shallow recess or by a stellate appearance without indentation of the gastric wall (Fig. 8.42). However, depressions without radiating folds, and linear scars with or without converging folds may also be found. Abundantly developed scar tissue may result in deformity of the stomach and obstruction.

Standard medical treatment of gastric peptic ulcer results in healing in four to eight weeks. Therefore, observation of the results of treatment is recommended after that period. It is easier to follow healing of a gastric peptic ulcer than a duodenal ulcer, since fibrotic changes are more pronounced in the duodenum.

Differential Diagnosis of Gastric Peptic Ulcer. Peptic ulcer should be differentiated from:

1. Ulcerated carcinoma,
2. Accumulation of barium between normal gastric rugae,
3. Gastric diverticula,
4. Benign tumors with central necrosis and subsequent ulceration
5. Choristoma of the pancreas.

BENIGN NEOPLASMS

Only 5–10% of gastric tumors are benign. They cause uncharacteristic clinical signs. The appearance of benign tumors depends on which layer the tumor originates from, and on tumor consistency and dimensions. Benign tumors are of either epithelial or mesenchymal origin. They result in negative filling defects on sin-

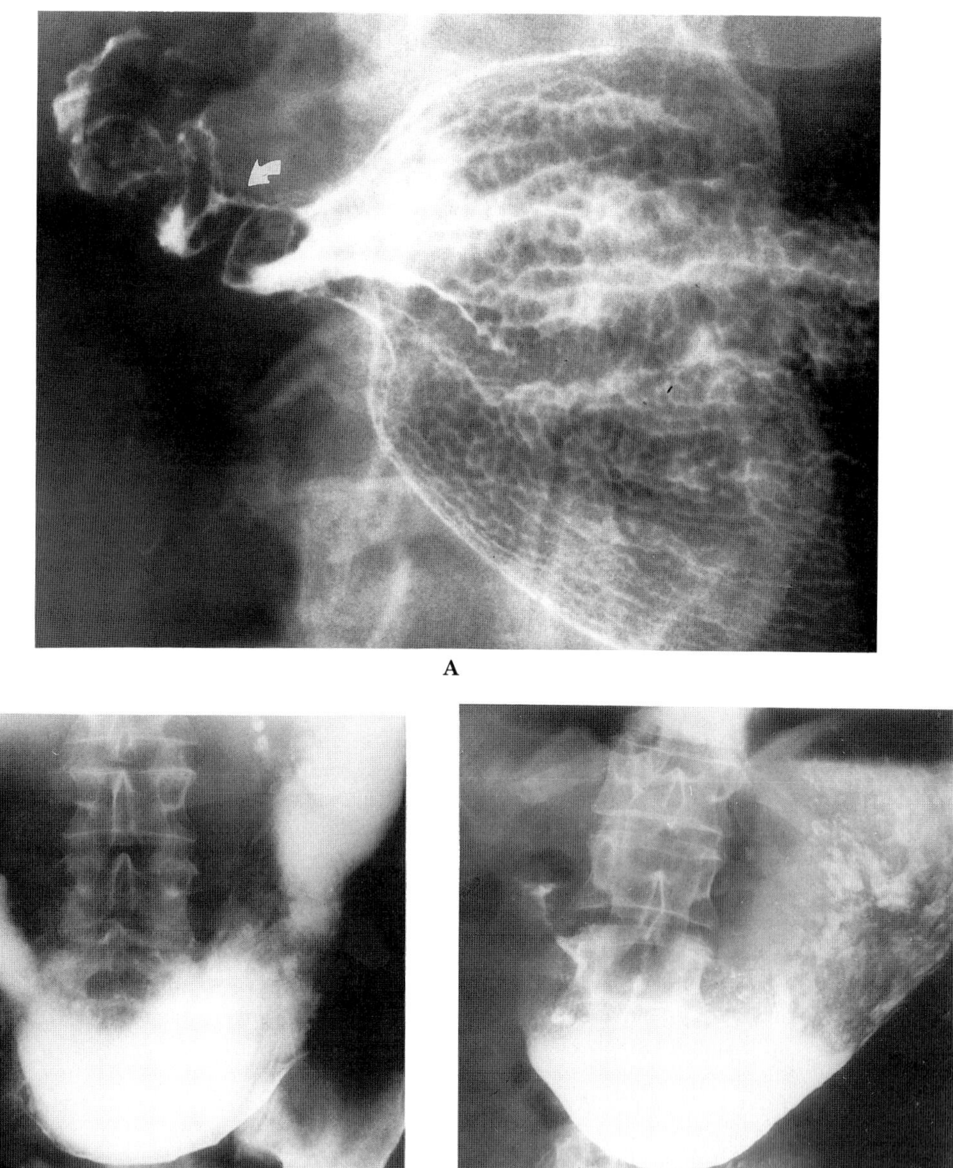

A

B

C

Figure 8.41. (A) Postulcer pyloric stenosis (arrow). (B, C) Postulcer gastric outlet obstruction.

gle-contrast examination, and double-contrast studies reveal regularly formed masses which protrude into the gastric lumen without destroying mucosal relief. The rugae may be pushed aside or may go around the tumor. Pliability of the adjacent gastric wall may be preserved or altered. Benign gastric neoplasms often cannot be distinguished from malignant. Consequently, endoscopy with biopsy is necessary for diagnosis. Heterotopic pancreatic tissue may resemble an ulcerated benign submucosal tumor.

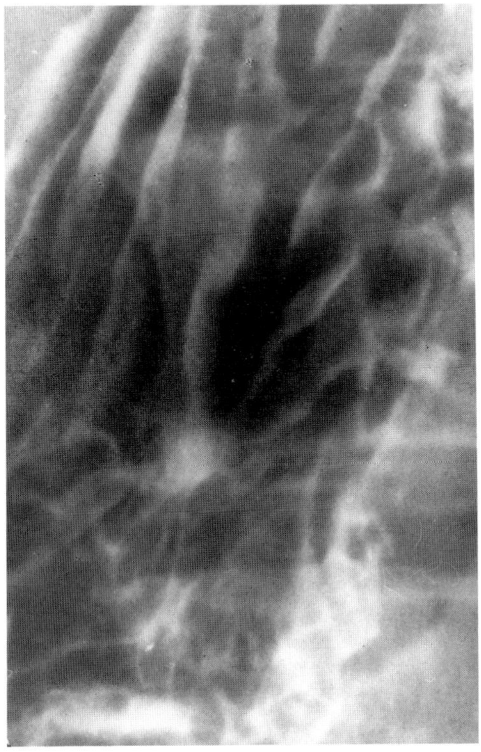
A

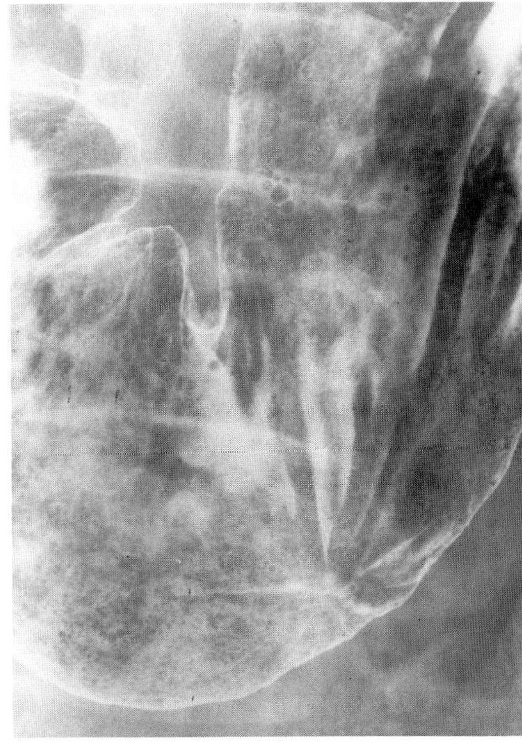
B

FIGURE 8.42. Postulcer scars. (A) Folds converging toward a shallow recess of the gastric wall. (B) Scar visible as radiating folds.

NEOPLASMS OF EPITHELIAL ORIGIN

Polyps. The term polyp originally denoted a pedunculated excrescence of mucosa, but has been extended to include all mucosal outgrowths. The majority of gastric polyps are sessile. Adenomas, hyperplastic formations, early polypoid type I carcinoma or sarcoma, and other tumors of the submucosa may present as polyps.

The majority of gastric polyps are hyperplastic, regeneratory, and clinically asymptomatic formations. They are postinflammatory lesions and do not represent true neoplasms; therefore, they do not undergo malignant degeneration. Hyperplastic polyps are multiple, smaller than 1 cm in diameter, and smoothly surfaced. They may arise in any portion of the stomach, but the majority are antral lesions (Fig. 8.43).

Polypoid adenomas are true neoplasms, and may be larger than 1 cm in diameter. The surface is either smooth or irregular (Fig. 8.44). Malignant transformation occurs in 40% of adenomas. The nature of a polyp cannot be distinguished by macroscopic examination without histologic analysis. Polyps larger than 1 cm in diameter should be removed and analyzed histologically.

With regard to gastric polyps:

1. Radiologic studies reveal gastric polyps in 1.7% of unselected patients while endoscopy reveals polyps in 3.9%.
2. Solitary polyps are common in the gastric antrum, most commonly representing regenerative, hyperplastic formations. Polyps larger or smaller than 2 cm in diameter are most often hyperplastic. Multiple polyps less than 1 cm in diameter are practically al-

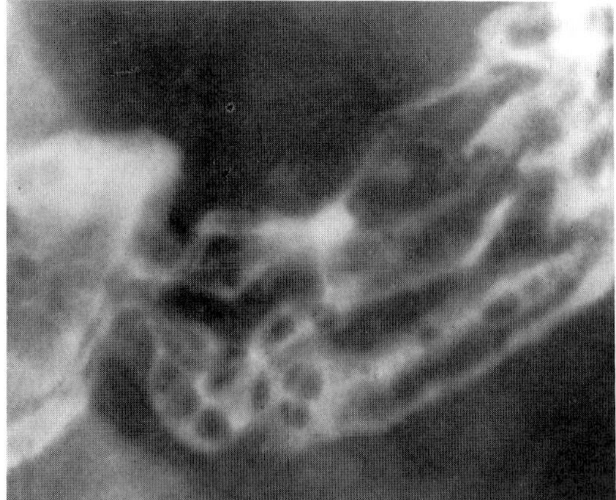

A

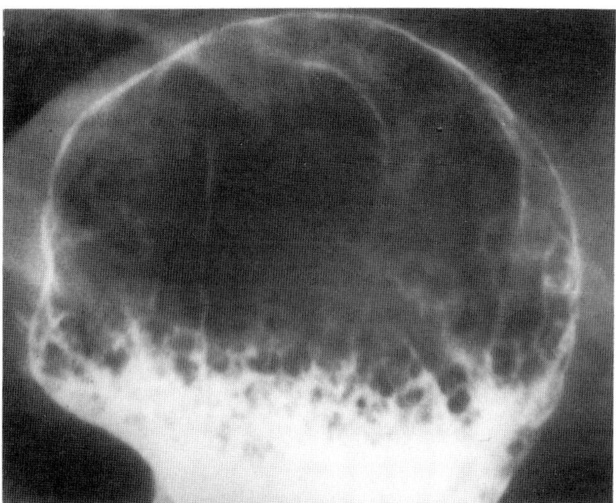

B

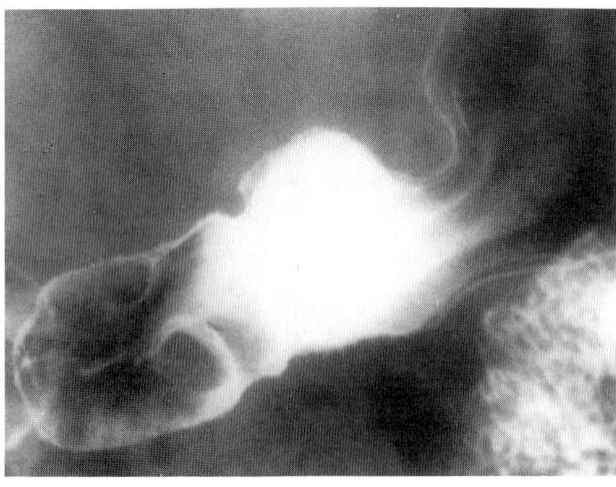

C

FIGURE 8.43. (A) Multiple small hyperplastic gastric polyps. (B) Freely movable air bubbles. (C) Large hyperplastic antral polyps.

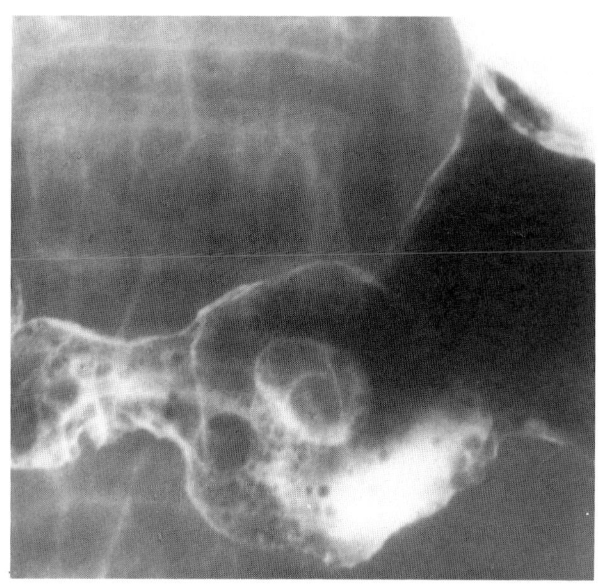

A

Figure 8.44. (A) Multiple adenomatous antral polyps. (B) Adenomatous polyp near the cardia (arrow). (*Figure continued on overleaf.*)

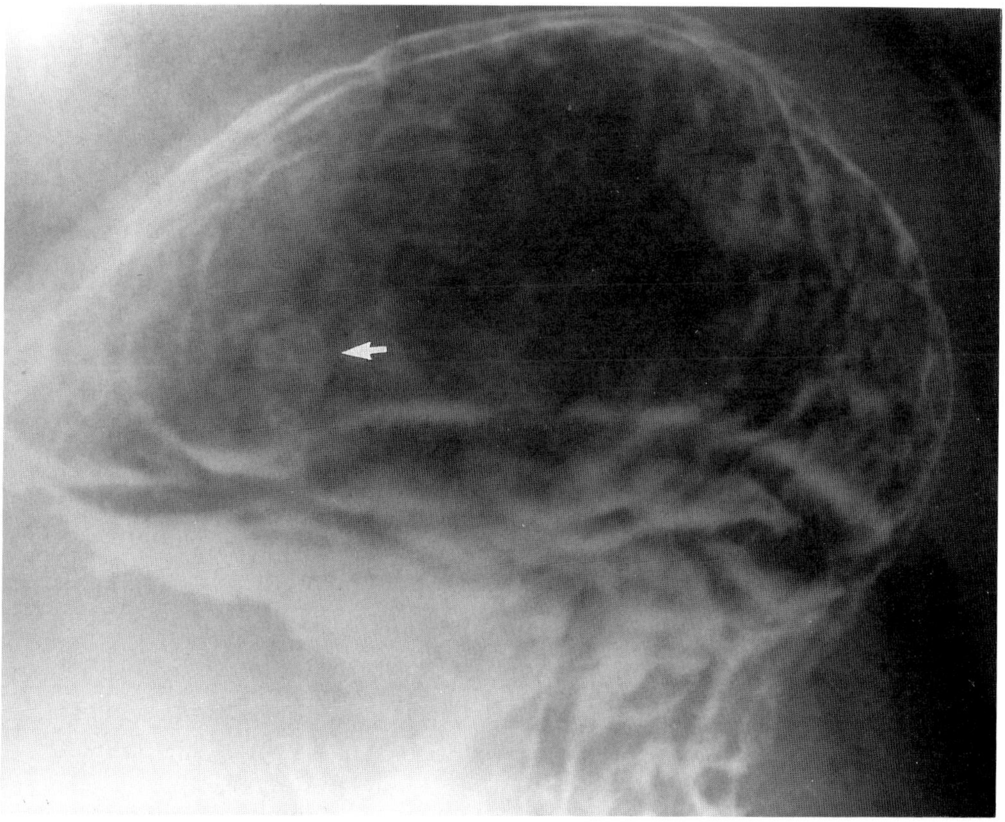

B

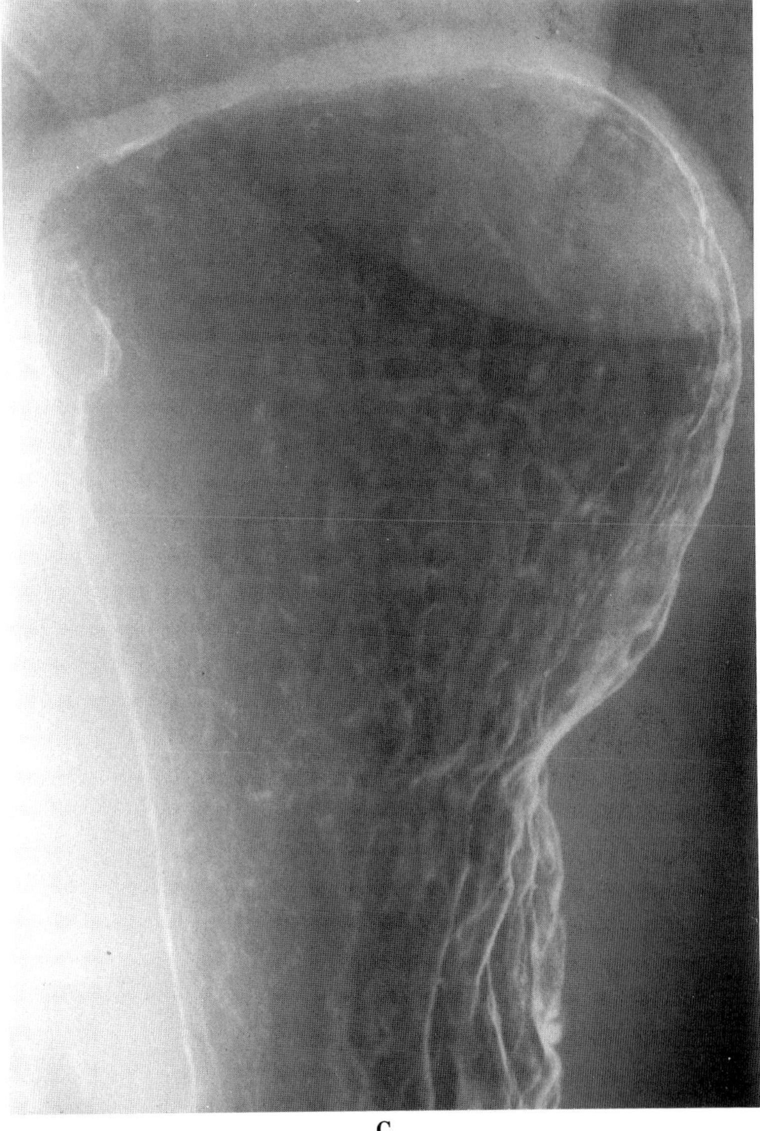

C

Figure 8.44 *continued.* (C) Adenomatous polyp near the cardia.

ways hyperplastic. A synchronous finding of hyperplastic and adenomatous polyps is infrequent.

3. In contrast to colorectal polyps, biological properties of gastric polyps do not correlate with their dimensions.
4. Gastric adenomas have low malignant potential and do not frequently undergo malignant transformation.
5. Early gastric carcinoma exceptionally presents as a small polypoid outgrowth.

Double-contrast examination is the method of choice for detection of gastric polyps. Simultaneous presence of polyps and carcinoma is uncommon; therefore, surgery is unnecessary for the treatment of gastric polyps.

Unfortunately, accurate radiographic differentiation of benign polyps from primary and secondary malignancies is impossible. Radiologic characteristics of benign and malignant gastric polypoid tumors are presented in Table 8.3. However, listed characteristics have only relative value. Polyps also need to be differentiated from gas bubbles (Fig. 8.43B).

TABLE 8.3. SIZE, GROWTH, AND SURFACE TEXTURE OF BENIGN AND MALIGNANT GASTRIC POLYPS

	BENIGN	MALIGNANT
Size	<1 cm	>2 cm
Growth	slow	rapid
Surface	often smooth	often uneven

NEOPLASMS OF MESENCHYMAL ORIGIN

Leiomyoma. Leiomyomas originate, as a rule, from the main muscular layer of the gastric wall. They represent about 10% of all gastric tumors and are more common in females. Covered by submucosa and mucosa, only about one-quarter of the myoma protrudes into the lumen (Fig. 8.45). The overlying mucosa and the tumor are frequently ulcerated. Gastric rugae swing in an arcuate manner over the tumor, or may be pushed aside by the leiomyoma

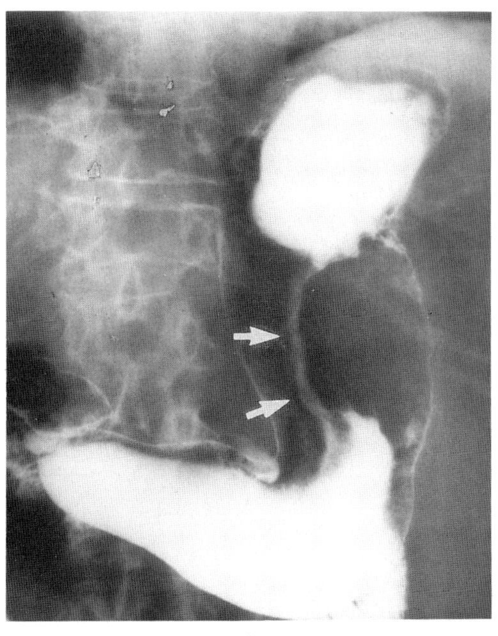

A

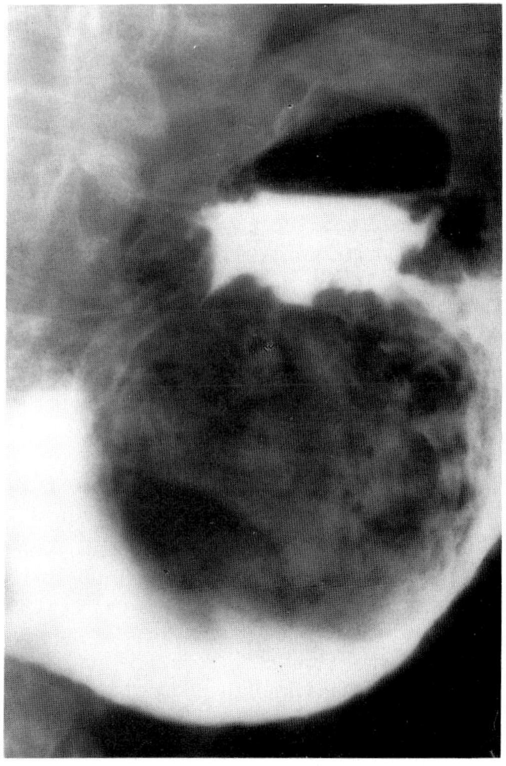

B

FIGURE 8.45. Gastric leiomyoma. (A) Large posterior wall mass (arrows). (B) Leiomyoma occupying almost the entire gastric lumen. Barium study. (*Figure continued on overleaf.*)

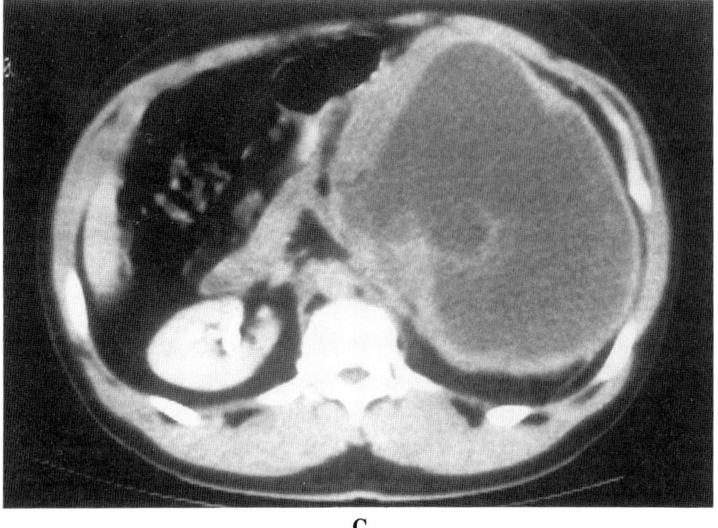

C

FIGURE 8.45 *continued.* Gastric leiomyoma. (C) CT examination.

mass. Differentiation from other submucous gastric tumors is not always certain.

Leiomyoblastoma. Leiomyoblastoma is an epithelioid leiomyoma with radiographic properties identical to those of a leiomyoma. Leiomyoblastomas are distributed as follows: 41% are confined to the gastric wall, 23% protrude into the lumen, and 26% grow immediately under the serosa. The remaining 10% resemble a dumbbell with the longitudinal axis perpendicular to the gastric wall. Approximately 30% of leiomyoblastomas are ulcerated.

Neuroma. Neuromas represent only 0.5% of gastric neoplasms. They arise from cells of the submucous and myenteric nervous plexuses and can be found in any portion of the stomach with a predilection for the antrum. They tend to ulcerate much the same as other mesenchymal gastric tumors. Unless ulcerated, neuromas are oval and smooth surfaced. About 5% of neuromas undergo malignant transformation. They cannot be distinguished radiologically from a very rare choristoma of the pancreas.

Lipomas, fibromas (Fig. 8.46), and *hemangiomas* are very uncommon benign gastric tumors. They manifest radiologically as an expansile submucosal formation.

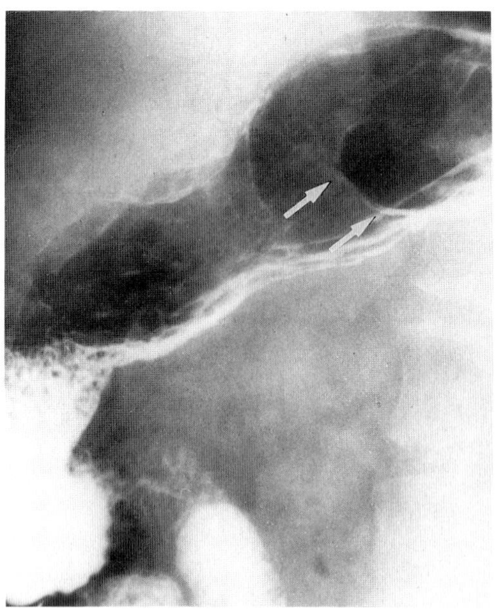

FIGURE 8.46. Fibroma of the gastric fundus (arrows).

MALIGNANT NEOPLASMS

Malignant gastric tumors are either epithelial or mesenchymal in origin.

MALIGNANCIES OF EPITHELIAL ORIGIN

Gastric Carcinoma. Carcinoma is the most common gastric tumor. It primarily affects elderly males, but may affect any sex at any age. Approximately 98% of gastric carcinomas are adenocarcinomas, but poorly differentiated carcinomas can also be found. Over the last three decades the prevalence of gastric carcinoma has decreased in Western countries. Prior to that period, gastric carcinoma was, next to bronchogenic carcinoma, the second most common fatal malignancy. The five-year survival rate in patients with gastric carcinoma is still only 10% since early diagnosis is established in only 40–50% of patients.

Atrophic gastritis, alone or associated with pernicious anemia, is a precancerous condition. The malignant potential of gastric adenomas is much lower than colonic, but malignant alteration can occur.

A scout film of the abdomen may reveal a tumor of the fundus protruding into a gastric lumen filled with air. Lack of peristalsis, inaccessibility to palpation, and prominent rugal pattern, make the fundus the most difficult portion of the stomach to find a small tumor. Each bizarre-shaped gastric fold should be straightened by graded compression or palpation to allow an estimation of gastric wall pliability. However, mucosal relief is best shown by double-contrast studies.

Carcinoma may arise in any portion of the stomach, but it is most common in the pyloric antrum (60%). Microscopic structure and macroscopic appearance are not in correlation.

Gastric carcinoma can present as a polypoid lesion protruding into the gastric lumen, an infiltrative, scirrhous neoplasm affecting deeper

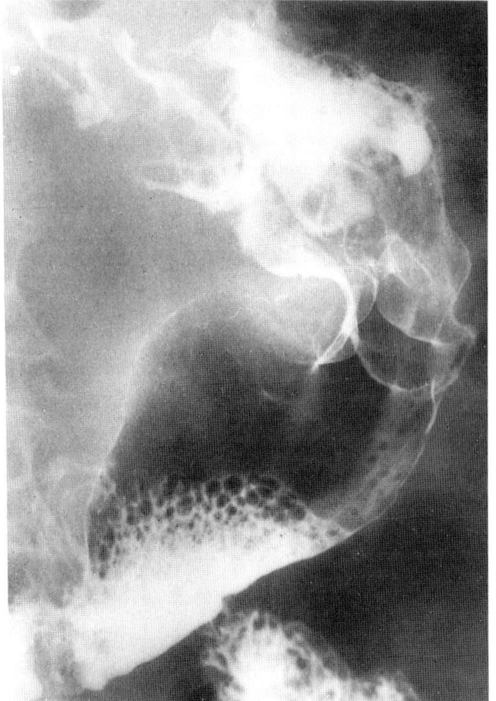

A

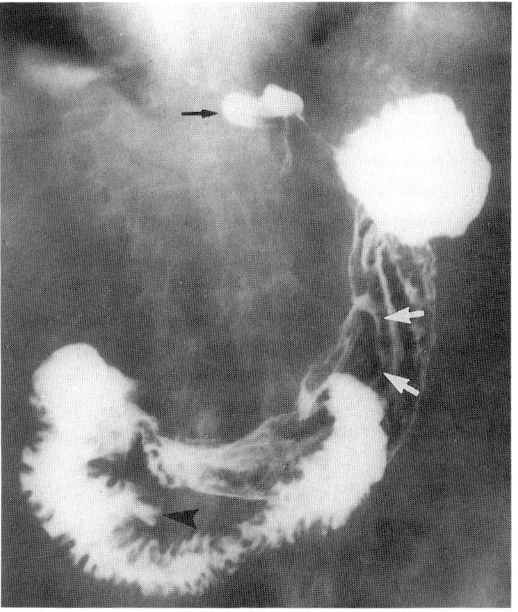

B

FIGURE 8.47. Polypoid gastric carcinoma. (A) Of the fundus affecting the body. (B) Of the gastric body (white arrows). Incidental hiatus hernia (black arrow) and duodenal diverticulum (arrowhead).

layers of the wall, or a malignant ulcer resembling a volcano. The first two comprise 80% of gastric carcinomas.

The radiologic appearance of a *polypoid* carcinoma is limited to the luminal surface of the mass. The surface of the neoplasm is commonly irregular with the mucosal relief destroyed (Figs. 8.47 and 8.48). In an early period the carcinoma may present as widening of the gastric rugae. If a gastric rugal fold widens by only one-third wider in diameter, over a length of at least half a centimeter, an impression of vary-

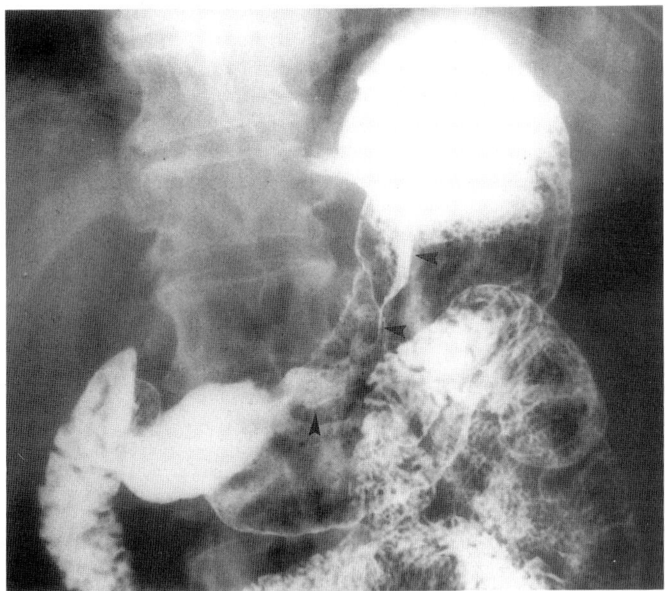

A

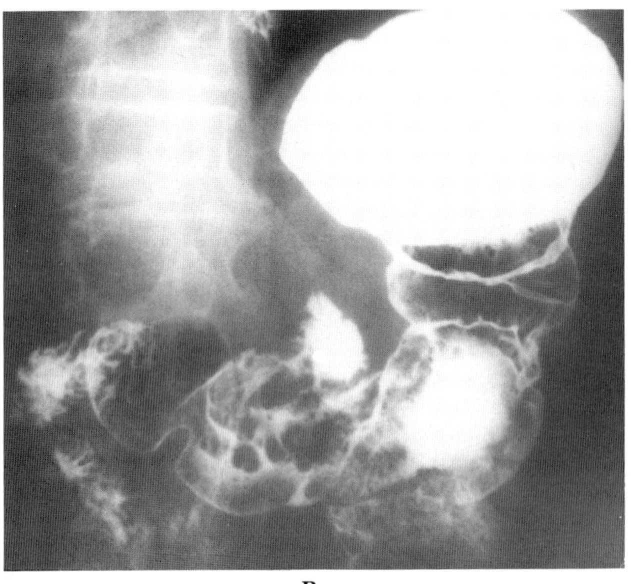

B

Figure 8.48. Polypoid gastric carcinoma. (A) Presents with a thin white line on the nondependent wall (arrowheads). (B) Negative (black) defect on the dependent wall.

ing caliber folds results. In the region of a tumor, wall pliability is diminished or disappears. A crater in the tumor will collect barium.

An *infiltrative* carcinoma may affect either the entire stomach, or only a segment, causing a pronounced desmoplastic reaction. Severe affection of the wall results in *linitis plastica* with narrowing of the gastric lumen (Figs. 3.44 and 8.49), and effacement of gastric folds. However, the rigidity of the wall may be the only finding (Fig. 8.50). Scirrhous carcinoma should be differentiated from Crohn's disease and corrosive gastritis. Crohn's disease affects the stomach infrequently and does not affect the stomach exclusively. An appropriate history eliminates any question of a corrosive lesion.

A *malignant ulcer* has a wide-mouthed crater with irregular contours and rigidity of the adjacent wall (Fig. 8.51). A peptic ulcer of the stomach infrequently undergoes malignant transformation, but a carcinoma often ulcerates. The base of a benign ulcer is the last area affected by malignant alteration, which starts at the edge of the mucosa near the crater. An advanced carcinoma cannot always be classified as to a particular macroscopic type.

Early gastric carcinoma does not infiltrate the wall deeper than the submucosa. A large dimension of the affected area and the presence of metastases in regional lymph nodes are not inconsistent with early gastric carcinoma. The diagnosis is established by histologic analysis of the resected specimen. The five-year survival rate in patients with resected early carcinoma depends on the microscopic type of the tumor, and can be higher than 90%. *Carcinoma in situ*, an intraepithelial carcinoma, is confined to the epithelium, and does not penetrate the basement membrane. Early carcinoma, limited only to mucosa, recurs less frequently than one affecting the submucosa, invading blood vessels, or metastasizing into regional lymph nodes.

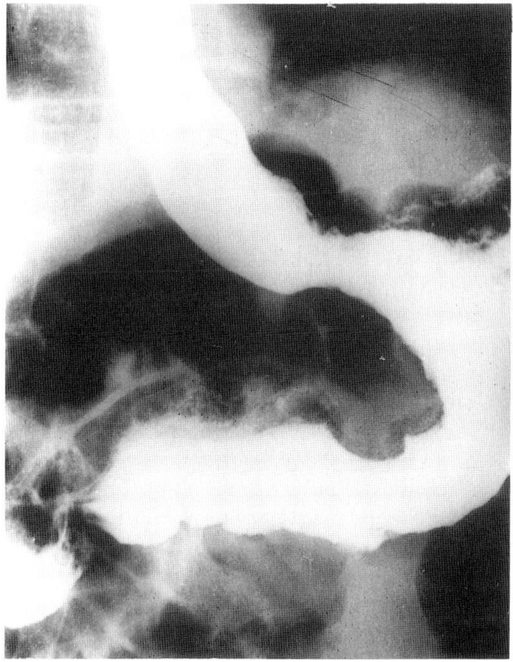

A

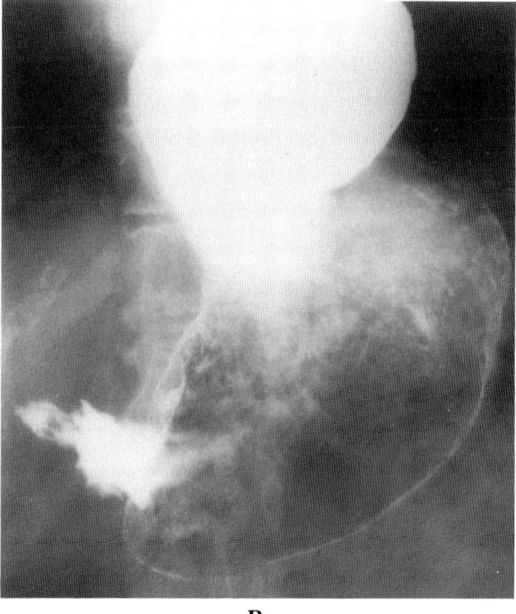

B

FIGURE 8.49. Infiltrative, scirrhous gastric carcinoma. (A) Affecting the entire stomach. The cardia is not narrowed, but the esophagus is dilated. (B) Affecting the antrum. Incidental hiatus hernia of the stomach.

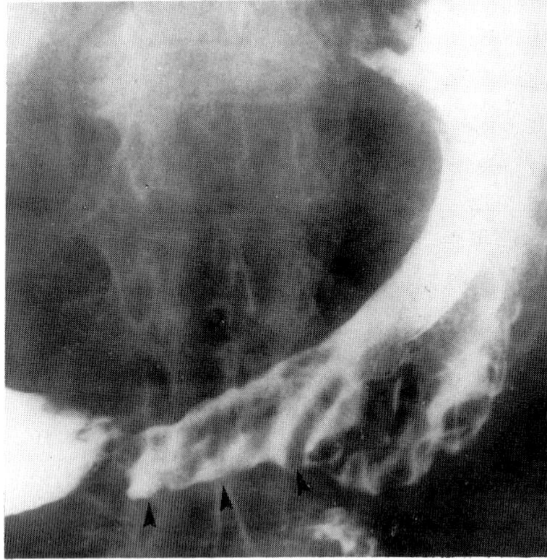

A

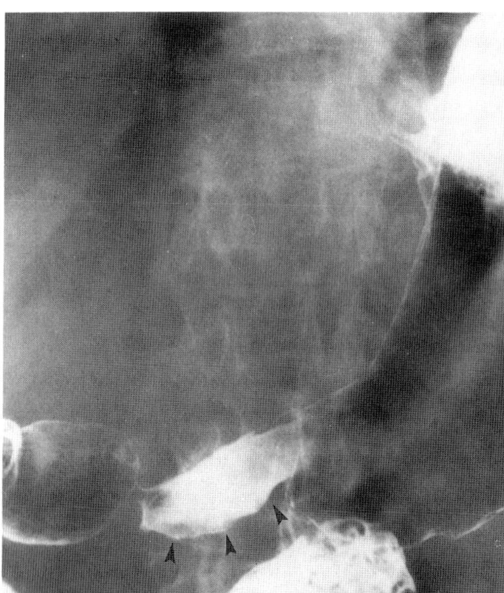

B

FIGURE 8.50. Intramural extension of antral carcinoma with loss of wall compliance (arrowheads). (A) Straightening of the greater curvature on single-contrast study. (B) Unchanged appearance on hypotonic double-contrast study.

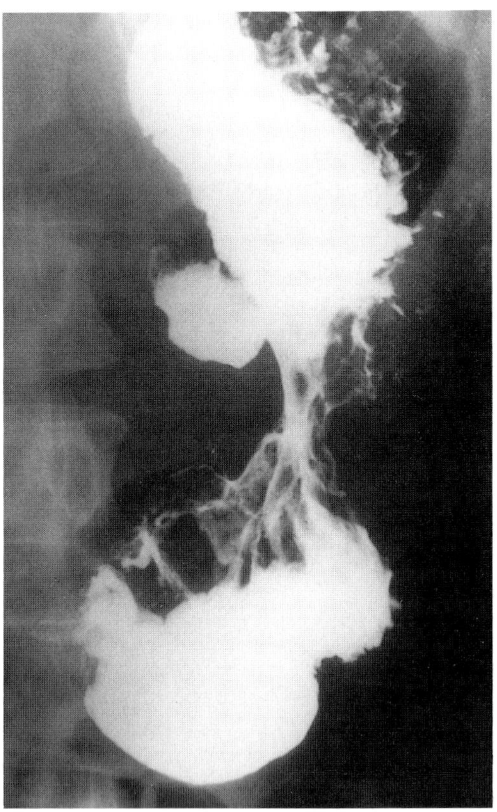

FIGURE 8.51. Ulcerated gastric carcinoma in two different patients. (A) Barium studies.

Double-contrast examination and endoscopy allow high diagnostic accuracy for an early gastric carcinoma. Clinical symptoms are highly nonspecific and may suggest a peptic ulcer.

Patients at risk for gastric carcinoma are generally older than 45 years, particularly those with atrophic gastritis and pernicious anemia, or with a familial history of gastric carcinoma. An early carcinoma is most often located along the lesser curvature of the stomach, and is not a separate entity. Double-contrast studies can reveal the macroscopic type of gastric carcinoma (Diagram 8.4). Type I is an exophytic carcinoma, rarely protruding more than 5 mm above the mucosal surface. Type II is an infiltrating carcinoma. In type IIa there is a discrete elevation on the mucosal surface. Type IIb, being a flat lesion, can be diagnosed only by endoscopy. Type IIc is a mucosal recess resulting from a shallow malignant ulcer, and type III is a mucosal ulcer. The difference between types IIc and III is the greater depth of the latter. Approximately 70% of early gastric

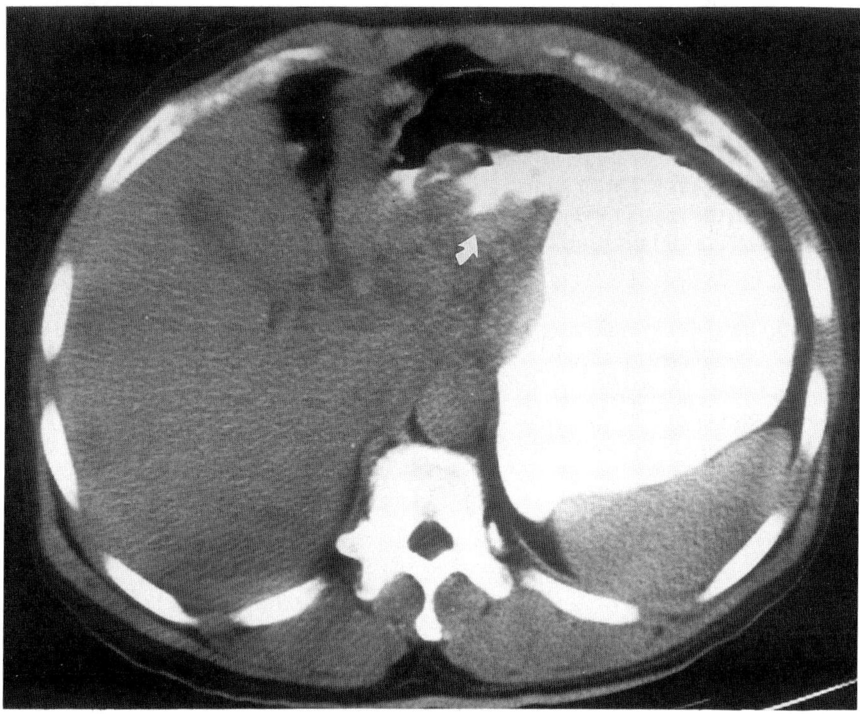

FIGURE 8.51. *continued.* Ulcerated gastric carcinoma in two different patients. (B) CT examination (arrow).

carcinomas belong to type III. Hopefully, these cause symptoms similar to those of a peptic ulcer, allowing early discovery.

Operable carcinoma of the stomach, regardless of its dimensions, spares adjacent structures and is without distant metastases. Block-resection including macroscopically unaffected lymph nodes is possible. As long as the submucosa is not affected, gastric carcinoma is not likely to metastasize.

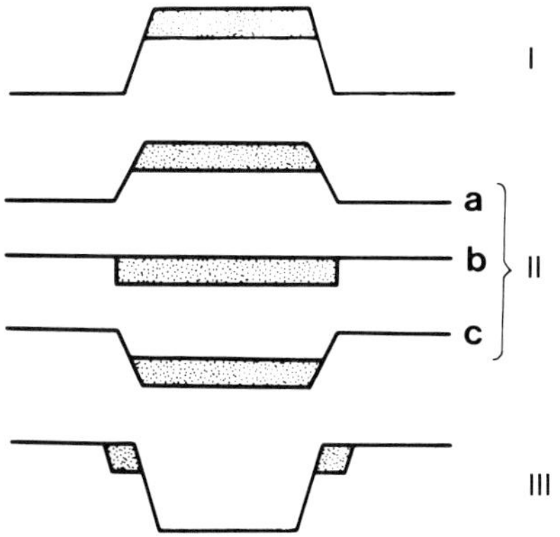

DIAGRAM 8.4. Forms of early gastric carcinoma.

Measured by CT, the normal gastric wall outside the region of the cardia is 2–5 mm thick, with 10 mm being the upper normal limit. After gaseous distension 3 mm is a normal upper limit. In gastric carcinoma the wall is thickened and the probability of transmural spread correlates directly with the wall thickness. Extension of the carcinoma into the regional lymph nodes can be diagnosed with a sensitivity of 67% and a specificity of 61%. The inability of CT examination to detect metastases in lymph nodes of normal size contributes to low sensitivity. Computed tomography, ultrasound (US) and magnetic resonance imaging (MRI) can readily demonstrate liver metastases of gastric carcinoma.

Multifocal gastric carcinoma cannot always be differentiated radiologically from lymphoma.

Differential Diagnoses of Gastric Carcinoma. *Polypoid carcinoma* must be differentiated from enlarged gastric rugae, benign tumors, lymphoma, and gastric varices. Variations in the rugal pattern account for radiologic "pseudolesions" which imitate neoplasms. Inflammatory pseudotumors may simulate neoplasms so that differentiation is difficult or even impossible. The imprint of the costal arch, spleen, pancreas, left lobe of the liver, heart, and enlarged lymph nodes onto the wall of the stomach may resemble a tumor mass. Impingement on the gastric wall can be detected by CT.

Infiltrating carcinoma should be differentiated from ulcer scars, corrosive lesions, adhesions, and antral muscular hypertrophy ("antral gastritis"). *Linitis plastica* usually cannot be differentiated radiographically from breast carcinoma metastases and gastric lues.

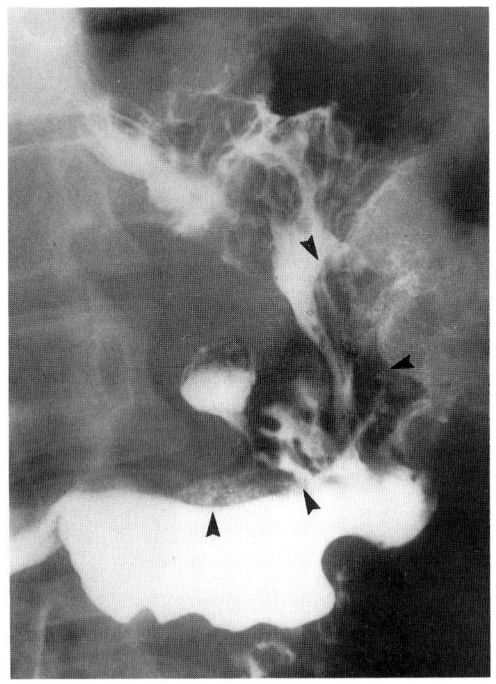

Figure 8.52. Large mound of edema surrounding a benign lesser curvature ulcer (arrowheads). Spasm of the opposite gastric wall.

Benign versus Malignant Ulcers. Uncharacteristic gross pathologic features of peptic ulcer or ulcerated carcinoma can make it impossible to radiologically distinguish benign from malignant ulcer with accuracy. Endoscopic biopsy is diagnostic. However, a series of characteristics such as radiating folds can suggest the nature of the lesion and can negate the need for endoscopy.

The *site* of the lesion is of little importance since benign and malignant ulcers are both often situated along the lesser curvature. It cannot be proved that ulcers along or adjacent to the greater curvature are more frequently malignant. Benign ulcers along the proximal segment of the greater curvature are not common. Ulcerations of the fundus are commonly malignant.

The *dimensions* of an ulcer have little relevance in deciding whether the ulcer is benign or malignant; however, malignant ulcers are usually more superficial within the area occupied.

The *morphology* of an ulcer may suggest its biological behavior. A benign ulcer is surrounded by a regular collar of edema and is located in the center of the mound (Fig. 8.52). The edges of a benign ulcer gradually taper into the normal gastric wall, and rugae can be seen entering the margin of an ulcer or merging into the ulcer mound (Fig. 8.53). A malignant ulcer tends to sit on the mass eccentrically, and has an irregular, nodular margin.

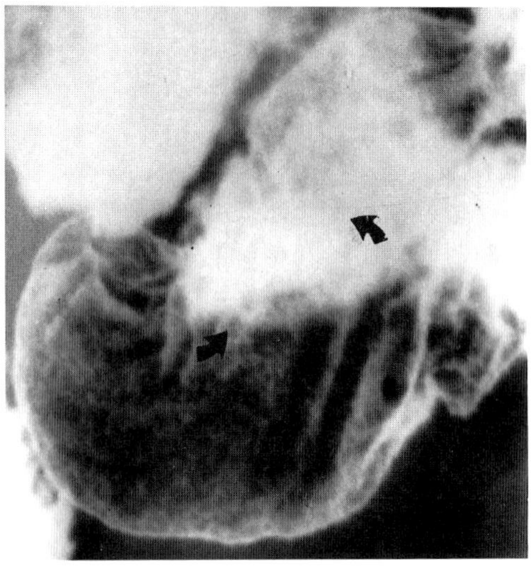

Figure 8.53. Large, oval crater of a benign gastric ulcer on the dependent, posterior wall is almost completely obscured by barium (arrows). Gastric folds are entering the margin of the ulcer.

Hampton's line, a sign of benign ulceration, is a lucent line that is 1 mm wide and of variable length (Figs. 8.37 and 8.54). It separates the ulcer crater from the gastric lumen and is formed by undermined mucosa.

Carman's sign results from the profile projection of an ulcerated gastric carcinoma (Fig. 8.55). The ulcer projects into the tissue mass that protrudes into the gastric lumen.

Benign and malignant ulcers frequently impair propagation of peristaltic waves. At fluoroscopy the rigid portion of the wall, an area approximately 1 cm wide surrounding a benign ulcer, floats like a raft on the waves. In carcinoma, the affected area tends to be larger. Postulcerous pyloric obstruction caused by scarring results in more pronounced gastric distension than carcinoma.

As a result of digestion of malignant lesions by gastric secretions, peptic ulcer can be seen in 3% of gastric carcinomas, lymphomas, or metastatic deposits. With treatment, such an ulcer may heal incompletely. However, after three weeks of medical therapy a benign ulcer will heal significantly, and will usually heal completely in five to eight weeks. Complete healing is proof of benignity since malignant ulcers fail to heal entirely with medical therapy. While benign ulcers regularly heal more completely and in a shorter period of time than peptic ulcers in malignant tissues, chronic benign ulcers may show only slow improvement. Repeated endoscopies with biopsy during the course of healing can rule out or confirm malignancy. Therapeutic results alone should not be considered absolute in differential diagnosis.

The properties of benign and malignant ulcers are presented in Table 8.4.

Carcinoid. Carcinoids cannot be reliably differentiated from other gastric neoplasms. They originate from the gastric mucosa and commonly develop an ulcer. Their biological properties do not differ from those of carcinoids in other portions of the alimentary canal (see chapter 10 on carcinoid of the small intestine,

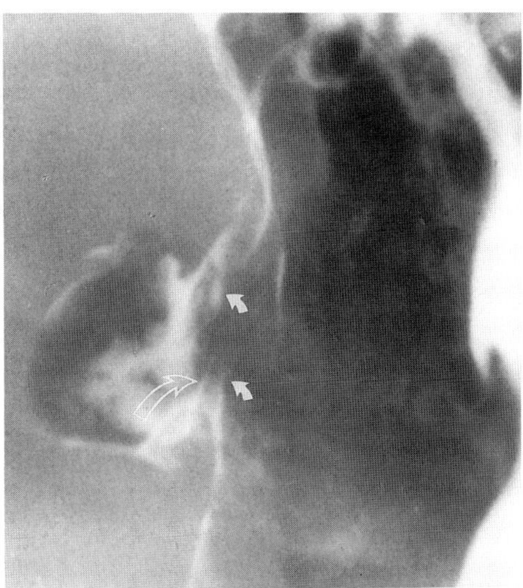

FIGURE 8.54. Hampton line created by undermined gastric mucosa in a benign, peptic ulceration (arrows).

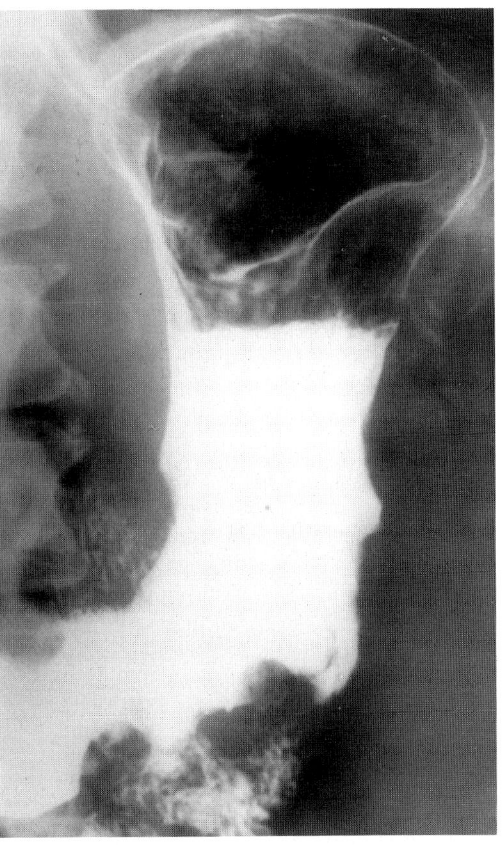

FIGURE 8.55. Ulcerated gastric carcinoma.

Table 8.4. Radiologic Properties of Benign and Malignant Gastric Ulcers

	Benign	Malignant
Location	Not relevant	Not characteristic, fundic ulcers are usually malignant
Shape	Regular, round, or bean-shaped	Irregular, linear
Size	Not relevant	Not relevant
Hampton's line	Yes	No
Periulcer edema	Yes	No
Irregular edge	No	Often
Mucosal relief preserved to the edge of an ulcer	Yes	No
Radiating folds	Yes	No
Carman's sign (ulcer within a mass)	No	Yes
Rigid wall	Limited to 1 cm radius	Yes

Yes = present; no = absent.

pages 382–388). The prognosis in patients with carcinoid is better than in patients with carcinoma.

Malignant Mesenchymal Neoplasms

Lymphoma. The incidence of lymphoma is second to that of carcinoma among malignant neoplasms of the stomach. It represents 76% of all malignant mesenchymal gastric tumors. The stomach and small bowel are also affected in 15% of patients with extragastrointestinal lymphoma. Of all alimentary canal organs, the stomach is most often affected by either primary or secondary lymphoma. Males are two to three times more commonly involved than females.

Primary and secondary lymphomas affecting the alimentary canal are, as a rule, non-Hodgkin's. The B-lymphocyte type lymphomas are the most frequent and the histiocytic type the least frequent. Alimentary canal lymphoma should be considered primary when Dawson's criteria are fulfilled:

1. Superficial lymph nodes are not enlarged.
2. White blood cell and differential counts are within normal limits.
3. No enlargement of lymph nodes is seen on chest roentgenograms.
4. At CT or laparotomy only regional lymph nodes may be enlarged.

Primary lymphoma cannot be differentiated from secondary by radiologic means. Besides such factors as histologic type and tumor spread, determining whether the tumor is primary or secondary is also important. Prognosis is better with primary lymphoma than with secondary lymphoma or carcinoma of the stomach.

Radiologic examinations may not differentiate lymphoma from other malignant gastric neoplasms. This is important for treatment and prognosis. Basic features of gastric lymphoma include an intraluminal mass, polypoid formation, nodular thickening of rugae, and diffuse widening of folds (Figs. 8.56 to 8.58). Any tumor can be ulcerated. Although all of these findings are somewhat nonspecific, the single most important feature of gastric lymphoma is the bulky tumor mass which does not significantly decrease stomach capacity.

Lymphoma affecting the stomach results in increased thickness of the gastric wall. It may not be possible to differentiate adenocarcinoma and gastric lymphoma on the basis of CT findings alone.

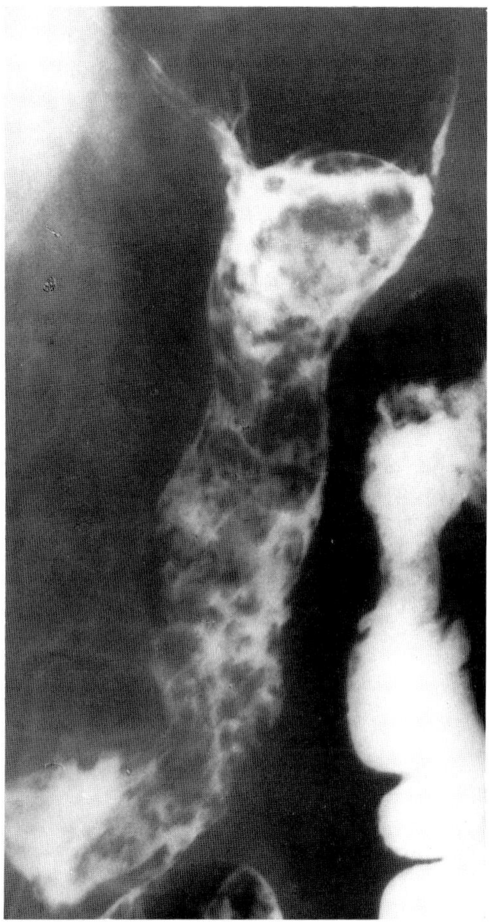

Figure 8.56. Gastric lymphoma resembles multiple polypoid lesions. Note prolonged stasis of barium in the stomach. The colon is filled with barium, while the stomach did not empty its contents.

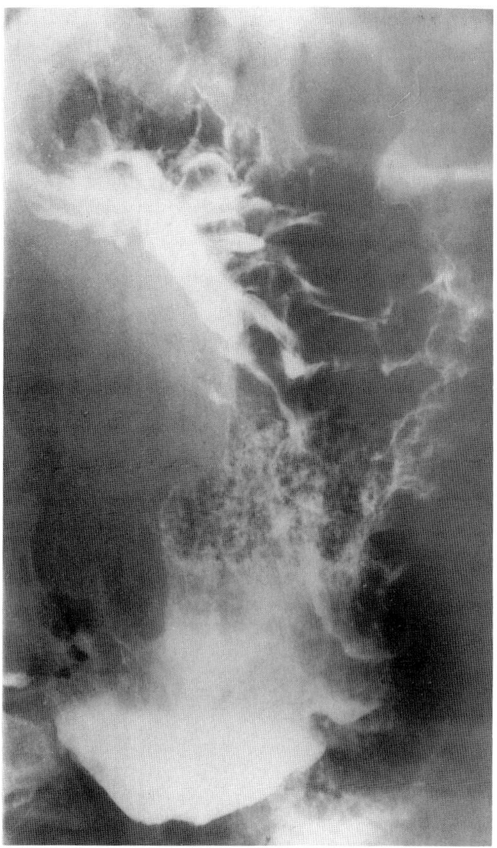

Figure 8.57. Gastric lymphoma. (A) Barium study. (*Figure continued on overleaf.*)

The macroscopic appearance of lymphoma does not correlate with microscopic structure. Hodgkin's lymphoma of the stomach resembles a polypoid carcinoma and undergoes necrosis. However, it is exceptionally rare. In contrast to characteristically monotopic carcinoma, gastric lymphomas are multifocal. In younger individuals, lymphoma is more common than carcinoma.

Pseudolymphoma results from chronic inflammation. Radiographic signs are identical to those of lymphoma. Giant gastric folds are not likely to be distinguished on radiographic grounds from those which are seen in Zollinger-Ellison syndrome and gastric mucosal hyperplasia. Even food remnants in the stomach may resemble lymphoma infiltration but are, in contrast to tumor, freely movable (Fig. 8.63E.) Lymphoma is therefore confirmed by endoscopy with biopsy.

Sarcoma. Gastric sarcomas are infrequent neoplasms manifested by circumscribed tumor masses, or more commonly, by extensive infiltration of the wall. As with other mesenchymal malignant tumors of the stomach, sarcomas change the properties of the wall by infiltrating the lamina muscularis mucosae, and/or the main muscular layer and intramural neural plexuses.

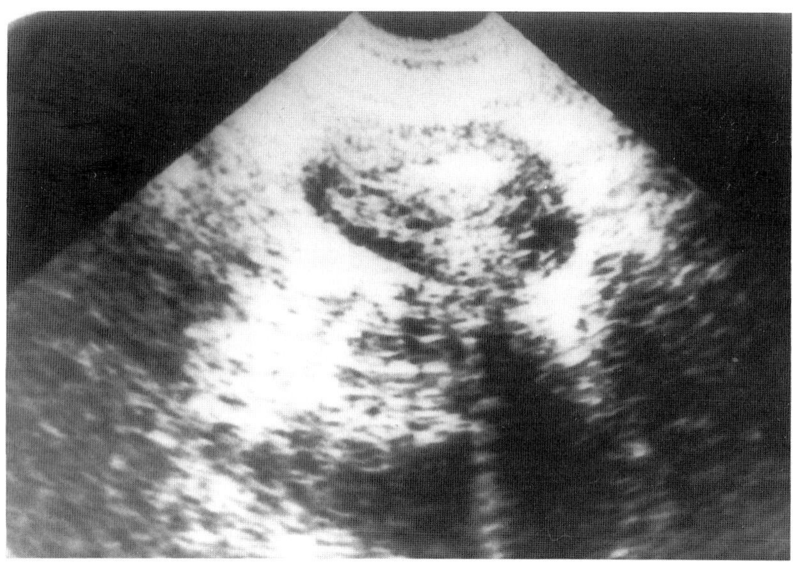

Figure 8.57. *continued.* Gastric lymphoma. (B) Ultrasound examination.

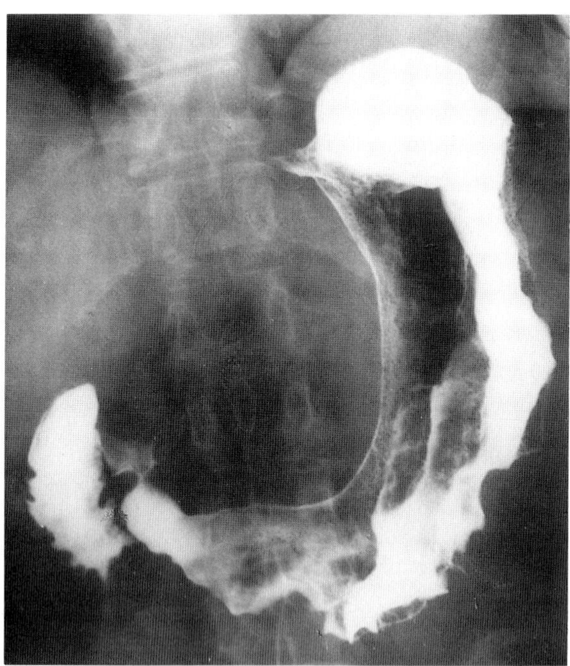

Figure 8.58. Gastric lymphoma. (A) Barium study demonstrates widened rugae.

The stomach may harbor myosarcoma (Fig. 8.59), liposarcoma, or fibrosarcoma. Malignant neural tumors also have properties of a sarcoma.

In patients with AIDS, the stomach, particularly the antrum, may be involved by *Kaposi's sarcoma*. Nodular lesions with or without central umbilications are seen (Fig. 8.60).

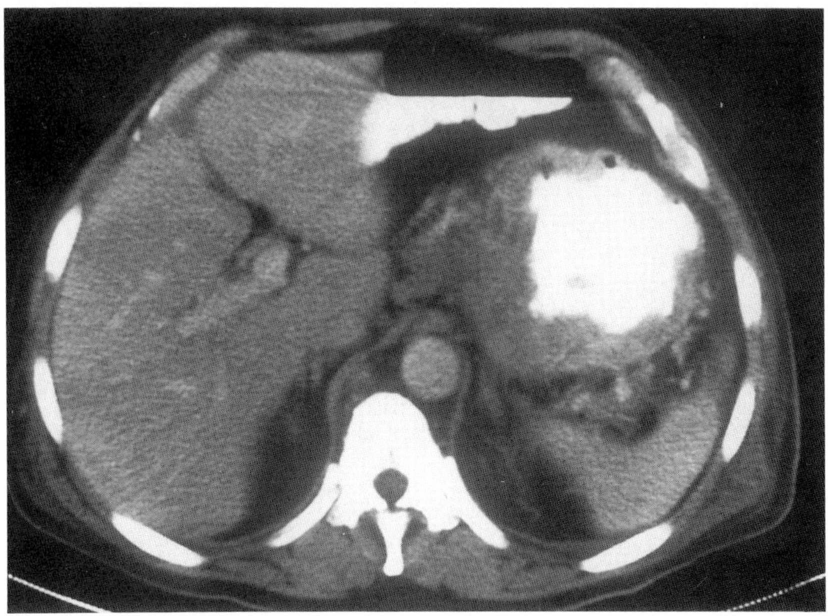

FIGURE 8.58. *continued.* (B) CT study demonstrates thickened gastric wall.

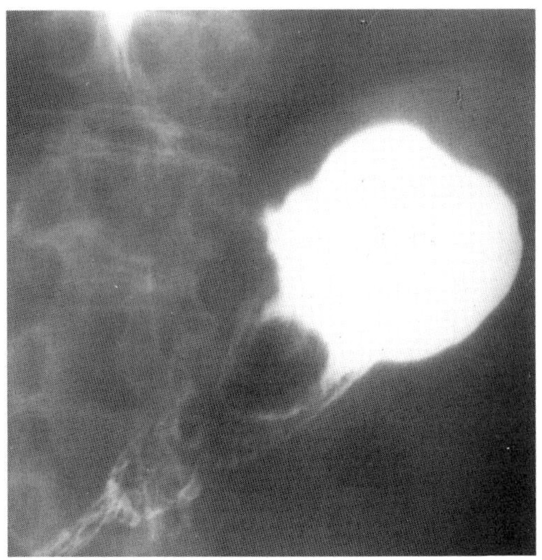

FIGURE 8.59. Recurrent leiomyosarcoma of the gastric remnant after Billroth I surgery.

Radiologic examination cannot distinguish between sarcoma, epithelial malignancies, and gigantic gastric folds of another etiology.

Leiomyosarcoma is an infrequent gastric neoplasm. The ratio of affected men to women is 2 to 1. These spherical or elliptical tumors in the main grow exogastrically. Calcification may be found within the tumor tissue. The average diameter of leiomyosarcomas at diagnosis is 15 cm (Figs. 4.35, 8.9B, and 8.59). Because the tumor and overlaying mucosa often undergo necrosis, contrast medium can be seen to accumulate in areas of ulceration. The tumor tends to invade adjacent anatomical structures, such as the lesser and greater omentum, and to metastasize to the liver. Metastases outside the abdomen are infrequent. In contrast to leiomyosarcoma, lymphoma does not undergo necrosis but does affect regional and retroperitoneal lymph nodes. The sarcomatous mass, as well as its propagation into adjacent structures and metastases to the liver, can be demonstrated by US, CT and MRI. Prognosis is better than for patients with adenocarcinoma.

METASTATIC MALIGNANCIES

Metastases to the stomach are unusual, and radiologic signs are nonspecific since metastases cannot be differentiated from primary gastric malignant neoplasms. Melanoma, carcinoma

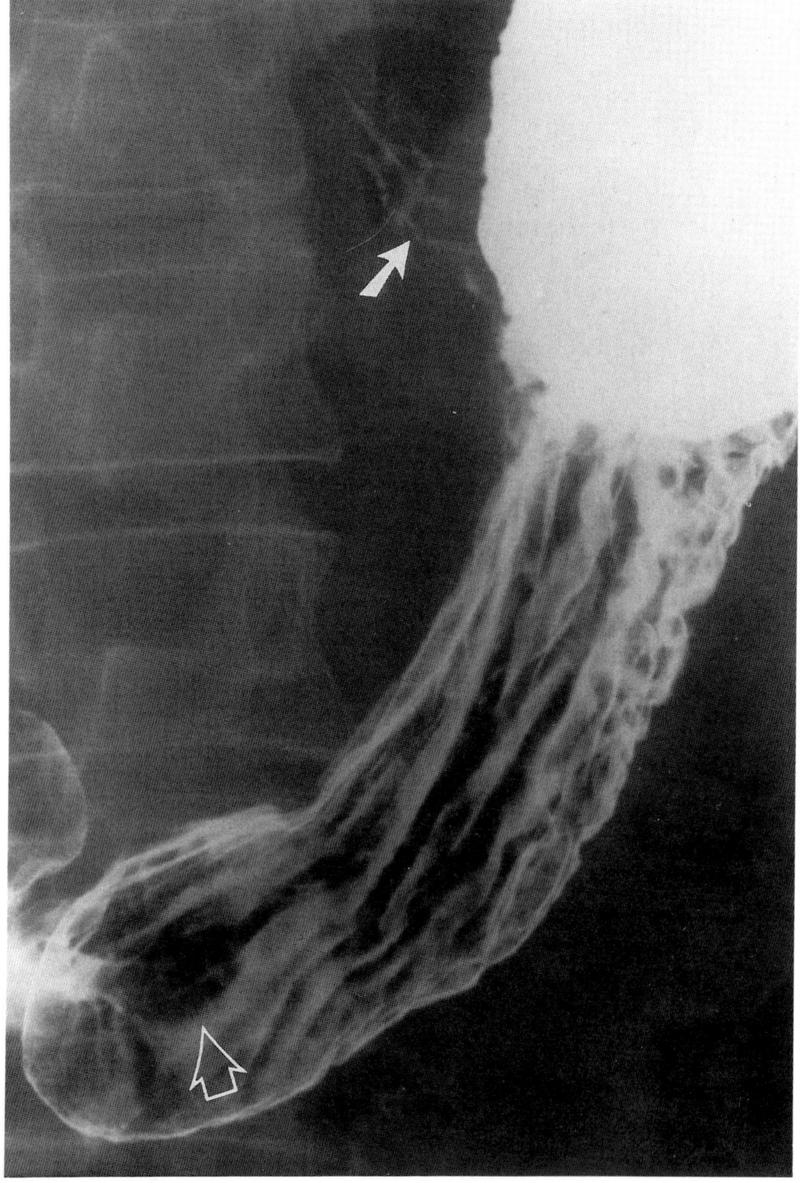

FIGURE 8.60. Multiple Kaposi's sarcoma foci in the gastroesophageal vestibule (closed arrow) and in the gastric antrum (open arrow).

of the lung, and breast carcinoma can lead to secondary tumors in the gastric submucosa. Since these tumors grow by infiltrating the mucosa, they destroy its relief. Other layers of the wall may also be affected.

In advanced stages, up to 7% of bronchial carcinomas metastasize to the stomach. Secondary bronchogenic carcinoma tends to present a bull's eye appearance similar to that of melanoma metastases (Fig. 8.61). In 20% of patients studied, advanced widespread carcinoma of the breast metastasized to the gastric wall,

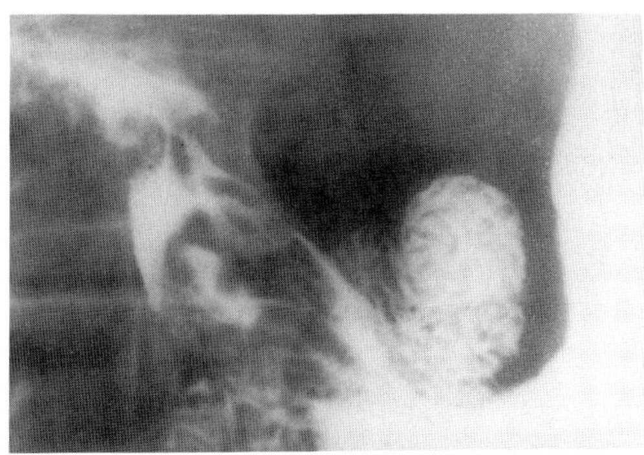

FIGURE 8.61. Ulcerated metastases of bronchogenic carcinoma involving the gastric antrum.

assuming a form of scirrhous carcinoma with relatively well preserved rugal relief (Fig. 8.62). In such instances, elasticity and pliability of the gastric wall are decreased and the curvatures are serrated.

FOREIGN BODIES IN THE STOMACH

Most foreign bodies enter the stomach by being swallowed (Fig. 8.63). However, some come through communications with adjacent hollow organs, for example, gallstones in patients with cholecystogastric fistula.

Some foreign bodies may form conglomerates called bezoars. The most common bezoars are phytobezoar and trichobezoar, the former being formed from plant fibers and the latter from hair (Fig. 8.63B).

Foreign bodies are freely movable and should be easily distinguished from organic lesions. Spherical conglomerates of viscous mucus may also resemble bezoars (Fig. 8.63C).

When a foreign body is fixed to the gastric wall, it may not be possible to differentiate it from an organic lesion. Food remnants and blood clots (Fig. 8.63D) are irregularly shaped and will change in position. Extensive food remnants may mimic diffuse lymphomatous infiltration on roentgenograms (Fig. 8.63E).

CORROSIVE GASTRITIS

Ingestion of acids, corrosive alkalies, and other caustic substances causes damage to the gastric wall. Examination should be performed with water-soluble contrast media although perforation rarely occurs. Edema of the mucosa with bleeding and ulcerations may occur. Gastric rugae are widened and tone becomes altered. Fibrotic changes cause decreased pliability of

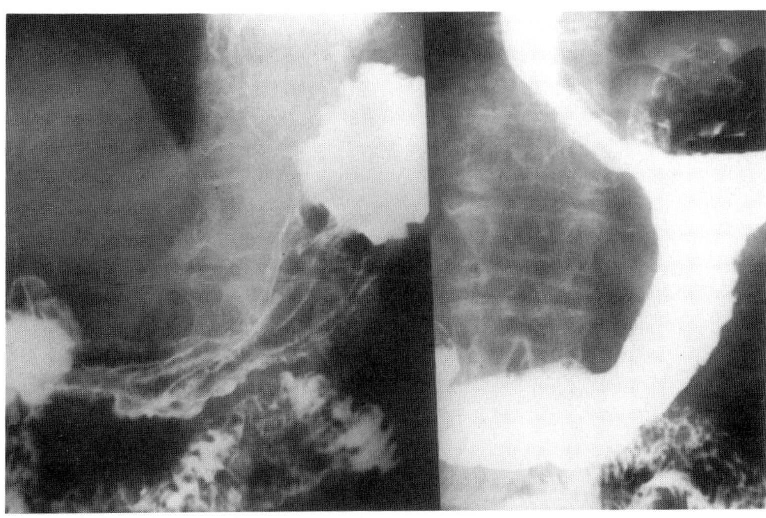

FIGURE 8.62. Metastatic breast carcinoma to stomach. Predominant submucosal growth with widened folds and loss of wall compliance.

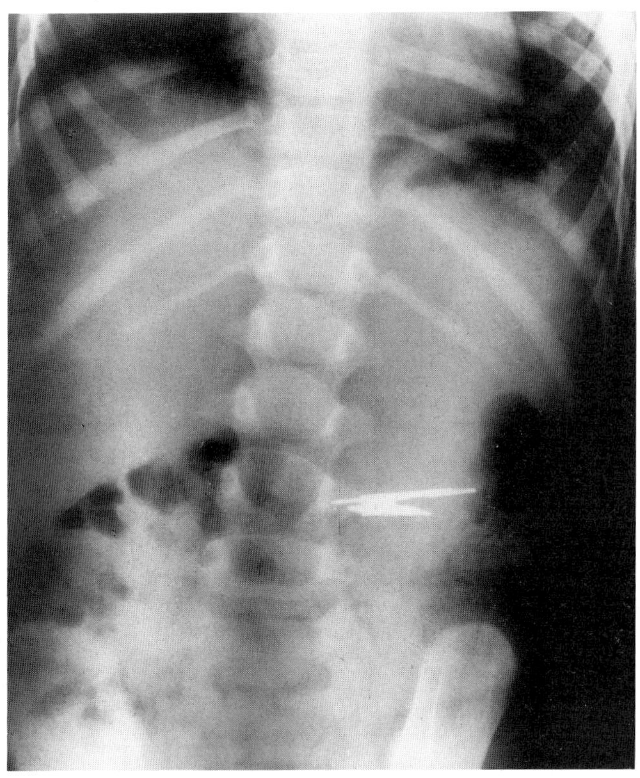

A

Figure 8.63. Gastric foreign bodies. (A) Small can opener. (B) Trichobezoar.

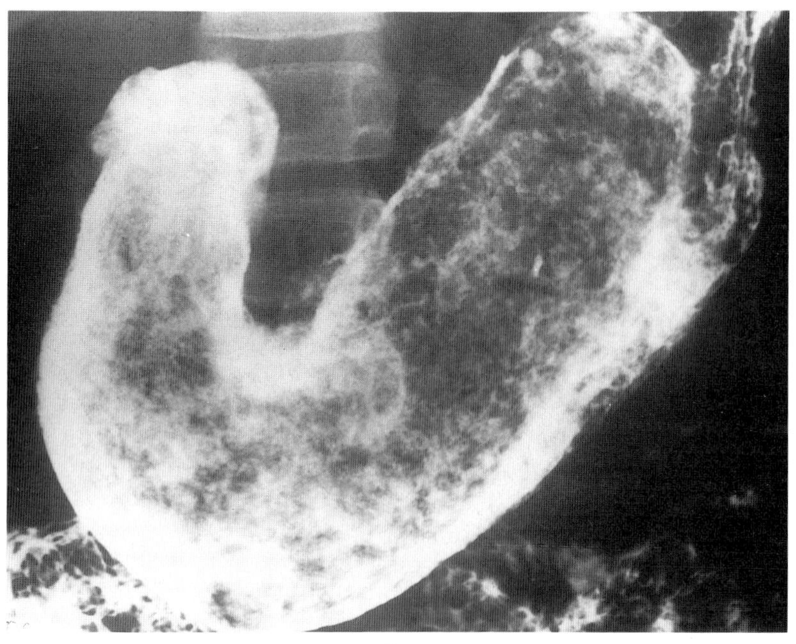

B

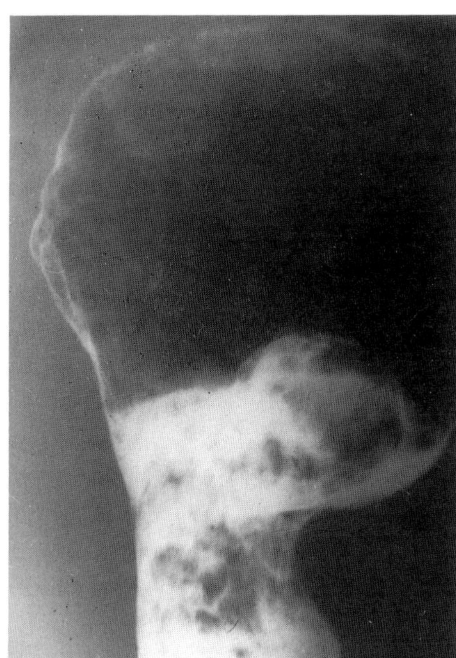

C

FIGURE 8.63 *continued.* Gastric foreign bodies. (C) Very thick mucus resembling a bezoar. (D) Blood clots in a partially twisted stomach. (E) Food remnants.

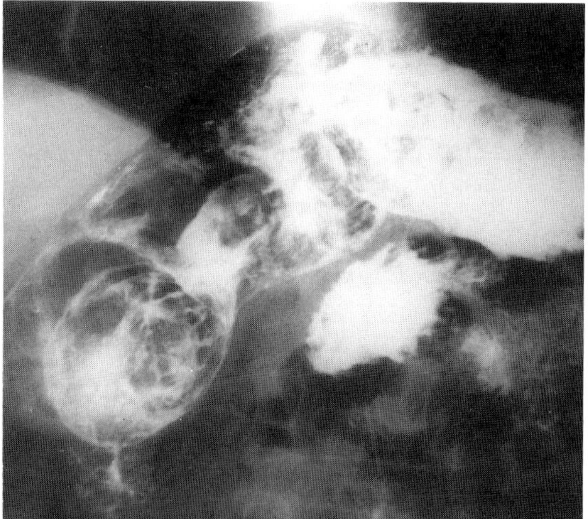

D

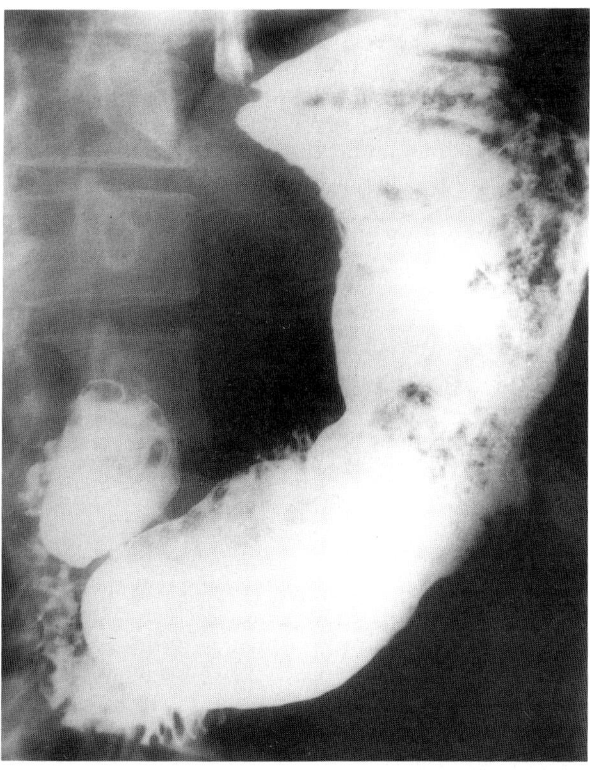

E

the wall and may resemble infiltrative carcinoma (Fig. 8.64).

THE POSTOPERATIVE STOMACH

Radiologic examination is useful in detecting the following:

1. Extent of resection.
2. Segments between which the anastomosis is created.
3. Method of anastomosis, for example, end-to-end.
4. Portions of the stomach wall that are anastomosed.
5. Relation to the colon (antecolic or retrocolic).

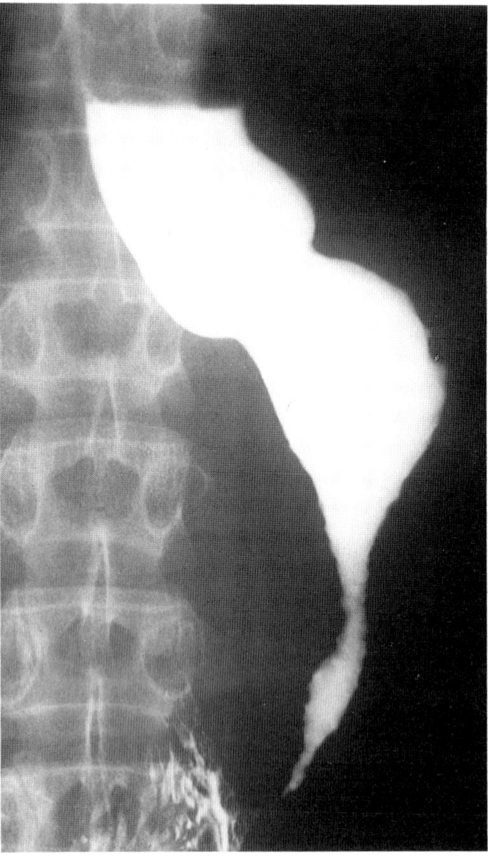

FIGURE 8.64. Corrosive gastric injury.

6. Direction of anastomosis with the small intestine (right-to-left or left-to-right).
7. Plane of anastomosis (horizontal or oblique).
8. Diameter of the stoma.
9. Direction of gastric emptying.
10. Rate of gastric emptying.
11. Length of proximal jejunal limb.
12. Evidence of vagotomy.

Barium examination is safe approximately 10 days following surgery. If postoperative bleeding or dehiscence of sutures has occurred, the examination should be performed using water-soluble contrast medium.

Edema, inflammation, scarring, and muscular contractions are important factors in evaluating the success of surgery. Following resection, the remaining segment of the stomach can be anastomosed to the intestine in an end-to-end, end-to-side, side-to-side, or side-to-end manner.

Oblique and lateral projections can determine the position of the stoma on the anterior or posterior wall of the stomach. The manner in which the loop of the small intestine is anastomosed, in an antecolic or retrocolic (through the mesocolon) manner, is readily demonstrated, along with dimensions of the stoma.

The anastomosed loop of the small intestine consists of proximal (afferent) and distal (efferent) arms. In right-to-left anastomosis, the proximal loop coming from the duodenum is anastomosed with the lesser curvature, and the distal loop leaves the greater curvature, an antiperistaltic or anisoperistaltic anastomosis (Diagram 8.5). In a left-to-right anastomosis, the relationships are reversed, an isoperistaltic anastomosis (Diagram 8.6).

The rate of emptying of the remaining stomach may be tested by administering solid food mixed with barium. Postoperative complications occur more often when the afferent arm is long. The direction of gastric emptying depends on the obliquity of the anastomosis. Therefore, gastric resection should include a generous portion of the lesser curvature.

In patients with malignant gastric tumors, any portion of the stomach may be resected. In patients harboring peptic ulcers, particularly in the duodenum, secretion of HCl and pepsin needs to be diminished. The majority of fundic glands secreting HCl and pepsin are situated in the fundus and body of the stomach. In the re-

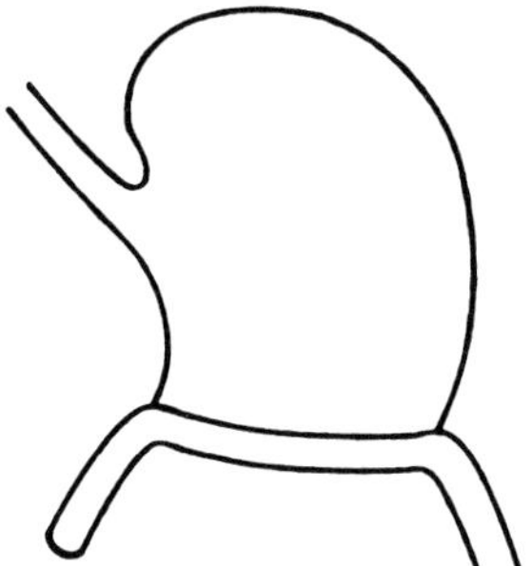

DIAGRAM 8.5. Right-to-left anastomosis.

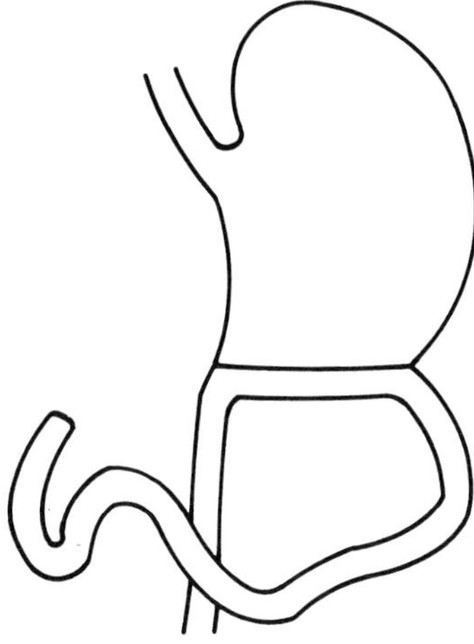

DIAGRAM 8.6. Left-to-right anastomosis.

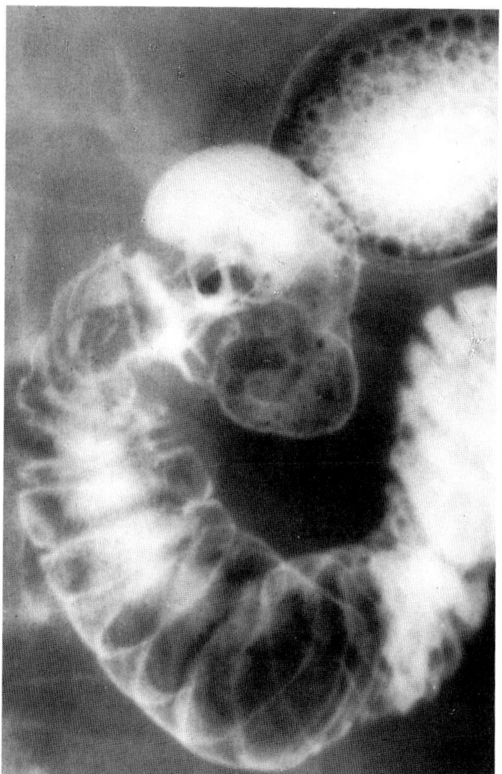

FIGURE 8.65. Pyloroplasty.

gion of pyloric glands, that is, in the antrum, gastrin is released into the blood stream stimulating parietal cell secretion. Therefore, if acid secretion is to be prevented, three-quarters, or at least the distal two-thirds of the stomach, should be resected in order to lower gastrin secretion. Vagotomy decreases parietal cell activity and, in that way, indirectly decreases secretion of HCl. However, medical therapy is also successful in preventing HCl secretion.

GASTRIC SURGERY WITHOUT RESECTION

Bleeding or perforating ulcers can be *sutured* with typical postoperative scars being detected several months later. *Vagotomy* can be complete or *supraselective*, in which case, branches of the vagus nerve which innervate parietal cells are transected. Several months after vagotomy, motility of the stomach is restored completely. *Pyloroplasty* is a reparative plastic operation of the pylorus. It is performed when the pylorus has to be widened (Fig. 8.65).

There are many types of hiatus hernia repair from which to choose, depending on the surgeon's preference. To prevent gastroesophageal reflux and its complications, a Nissen fundoplication is usually performed. The lower esophageal segment and the gastric fundus are mobilized, the fundus is then wrapped around the esophagus (Fig. 8.66). In the Belsey-Mark IV procedure, the distal 4 cm of the esophagus is attached to the gastric fundus and the fundus with the esophagus is then attached to the di-

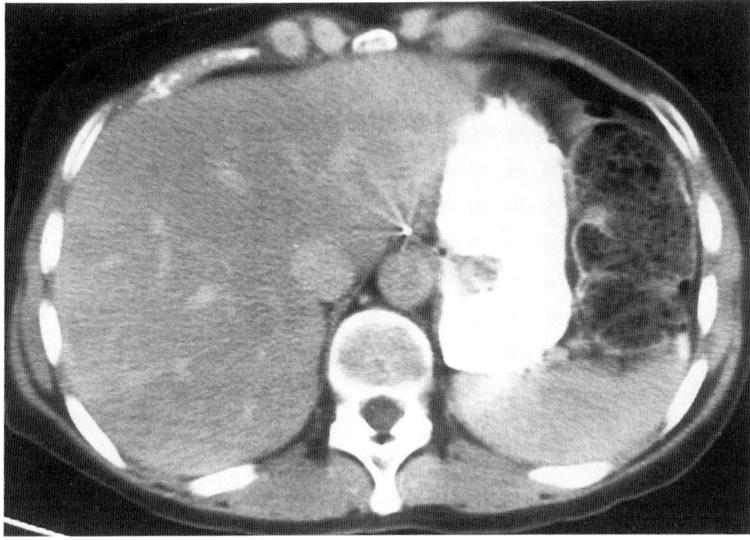

Figure 8.66. Nissen fundoplication resembling a tumor on CT examination.

aphragm. The single most important sign of a failed antireflux operation is persistent or recurrent gastroesophageal reflux (Fig. 8.67).

Gastroenterostomy refers to anastomosis of the stomach with a loop of small intestine (Fig. 8.68). The anastomosis is formed by connecting artificially created openings on the anterior or posterior wall of the stomach with the small intestine. A side-to-side anastomosis between the afferent and efferent limbs may also be created. In patients with peptic disease, recurrent peptic ulcers usually occur in the region of the anastomosis. Consequently this procedure is used mostly as a palliative procedure in patients with unresectable carcinoma of the pyloric region or pancreatic carcinoma. In patients with carcinoma of the duodenal papilla, choledochogastrostomy can be performed (Fig. 8.68B).

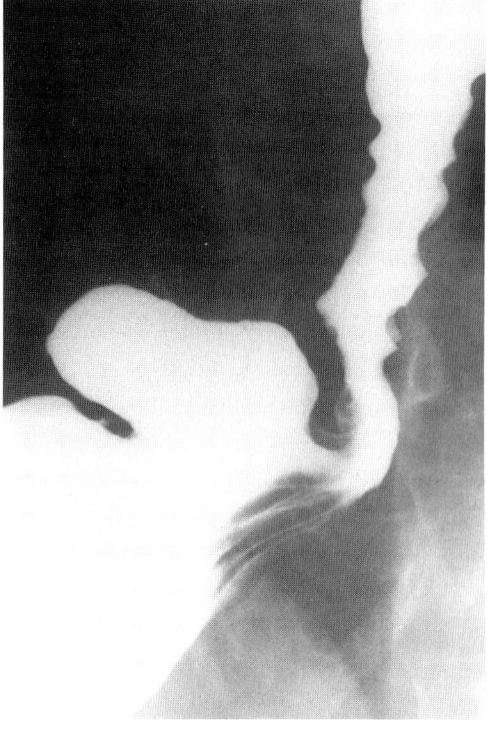

Figure 8.67. Failed Nissen fundoplication with gastric hiatus hernia, spontaneous gastroesophageal reflux, and reflux esophagitis.

Gastric Surgery with Resection

Several eponyms and synonyms are used for operations in which the stomach is resected. Only principal operations without modifications are described.

Billroth I (Diagram 8.7, Fig. 8.69) is partial gastrectomy with gastroduodenostomy. The distal portion of the resected stomach is anas-

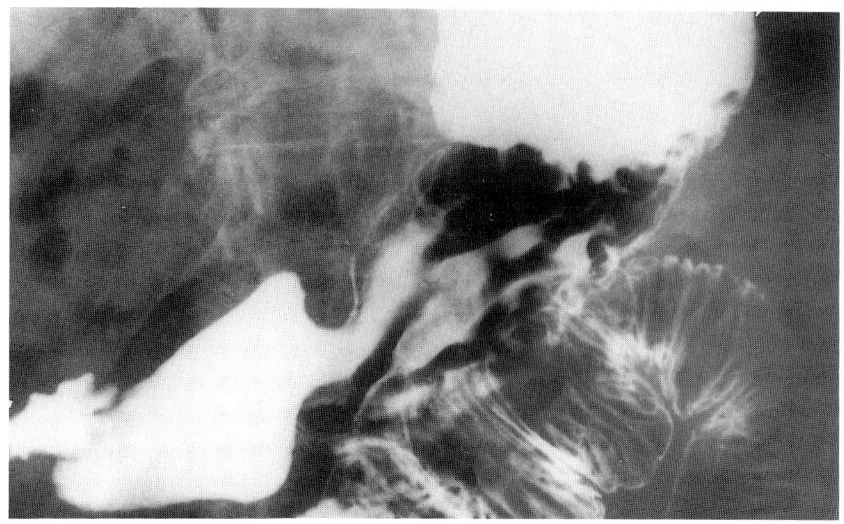

A

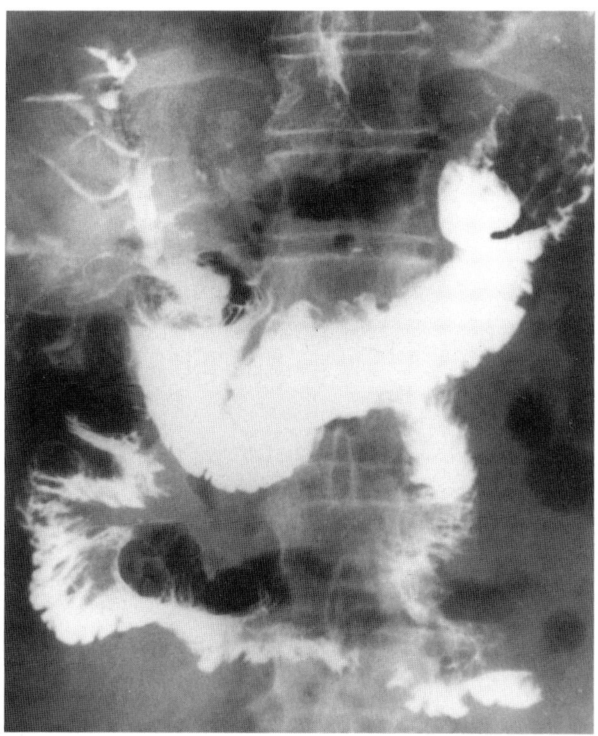

B

FIGURE 8.68. (A) Gastroenterostomy. (B) Gastroenterostomy with choledochogastrostomy.

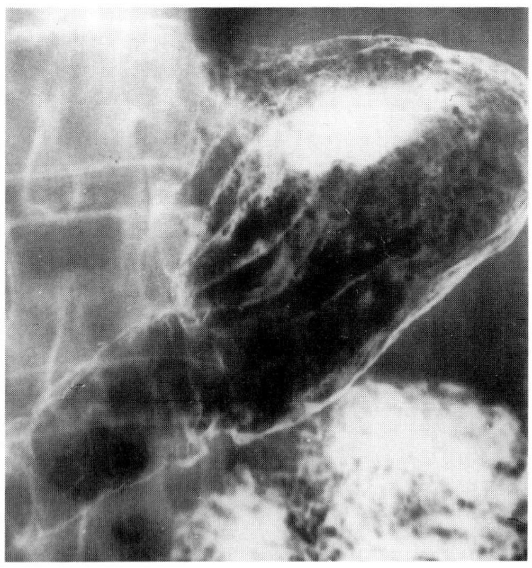

Figure 8.69. Billroth I gastric surgery. (See Diagram 8.7.)

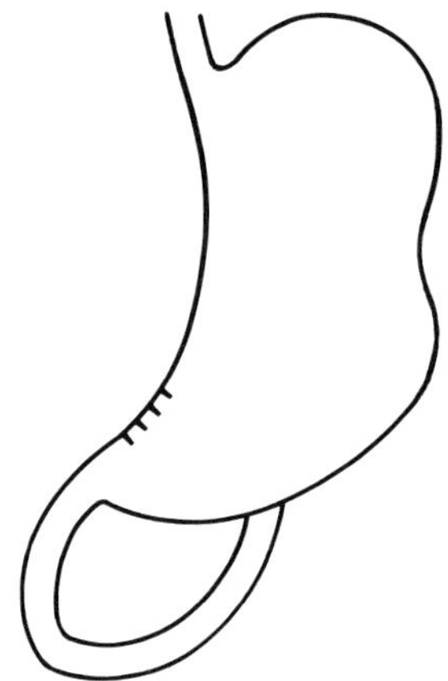

Diagram 8.7. Billroth I surgery.

tomosed with the suprapapillary portion of the duodenum. The proximal portion of the remaining duodenum often has a lower tone and can resemble a normal bulb. The finding can resemble microgastria. *Billroth II* is a partial resection of the stomach with gastrojejunostomy (Diagram 8.8 and Fig. 8.70). *Subtotal gastrectomy* (Diagram 8.9 and Fig. 8.71) is equivalent to a Billroth II procedure in which the gastric

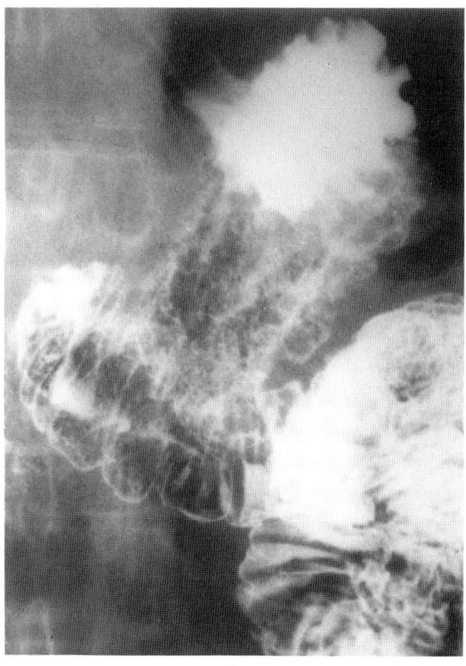

A

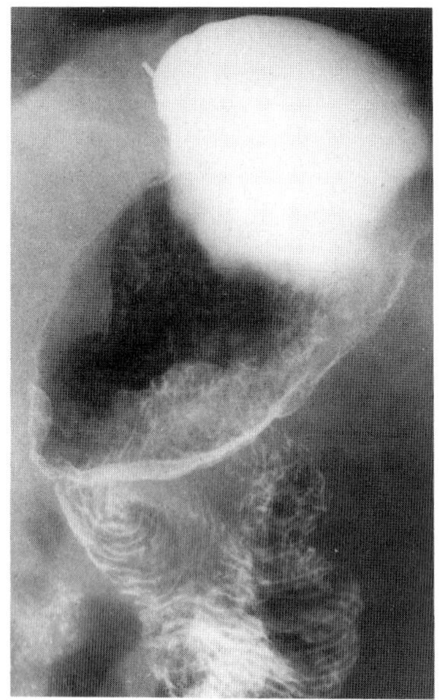

B

Figure 8.70. Billroth II gastric surgery. (See Diagram 8.8.) (A) Large gastric stump. (B) Transient intussusception of the ileum into the gastric stump. Side-to-side jejuno-jejunostomy. Postsurgical recurrence of carcinoma on the medial aspect of the stump.

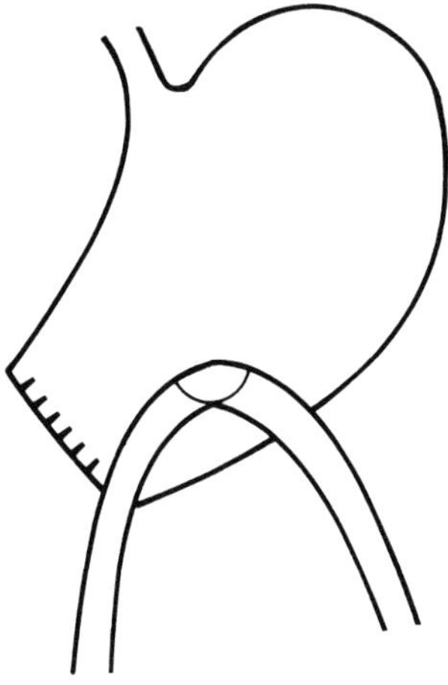

DIAGRAM 8.8. Billroth II surgery.

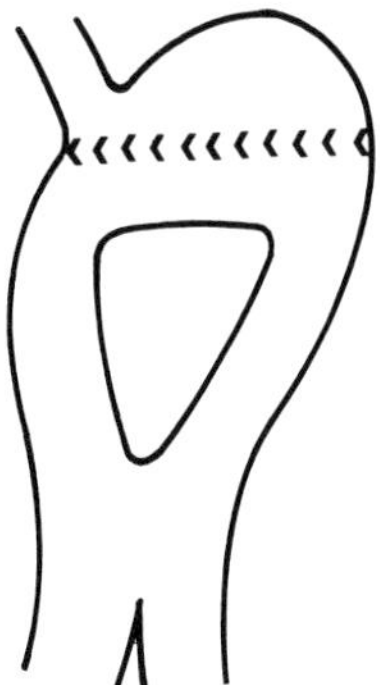

DIAGRAM 8.9. Subtotal gastrectomy with gastroenterostomy. Side-to-side jejuno-jenunostomy.

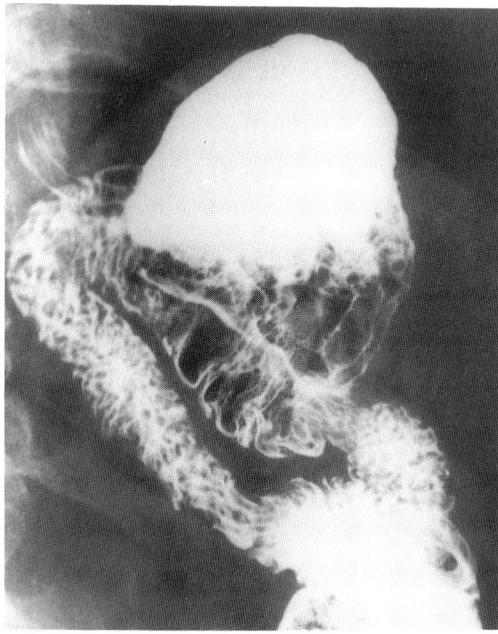

FIGURE 8.71. Subtotal gastrectomy. Side-to-side jejunal anastomosis. (See Diagram 8.9.)

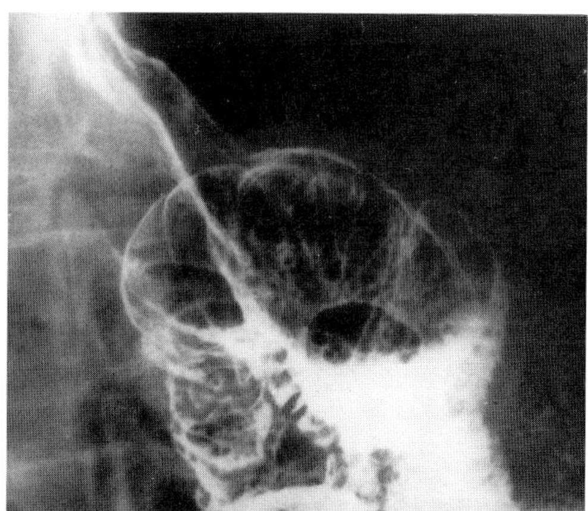

FIGURE 8.72. Esophagojejunostomy. (See Diagram 8.10.)

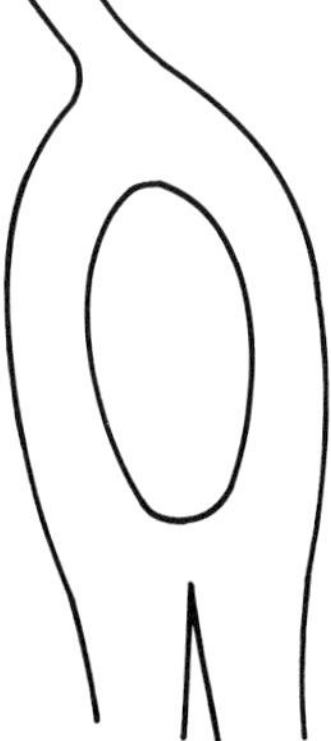

DIAGRAM 8.10. Gastrectomy. Esophagojejunostomy. Side-to-side jejuno-jejunostomy.

stump is the fornix of the stomach. In *total gastrectomy* esophagojejunostomy is performed (Diagram 8.10, Fig. 8.72). *Fundusectomy* is a resection of the fundus and major part of the body of the stomach. *Roux-en-Y procedure* is end-to-side jejuno-jejunostomy with or without anastomosis with the stomach, duodenum, esophagus, biliary tree, or pancreas (Diagram 8.11).

Gastropancreaticoduodenectomy (Whipple) is presented in Diagram 8.12 and Fig. 8.73. This is partial gastrectomy with retrocolic gastrojejunostomy and end-to-side choledochojejunostomy.

Postsurgical scars and folds resembling pockets between the sutures may be difficult to distinguish radiographically from tumorous processes and ulcers. Any suspicion of malignancy is an absolute indication for gastroscopy.

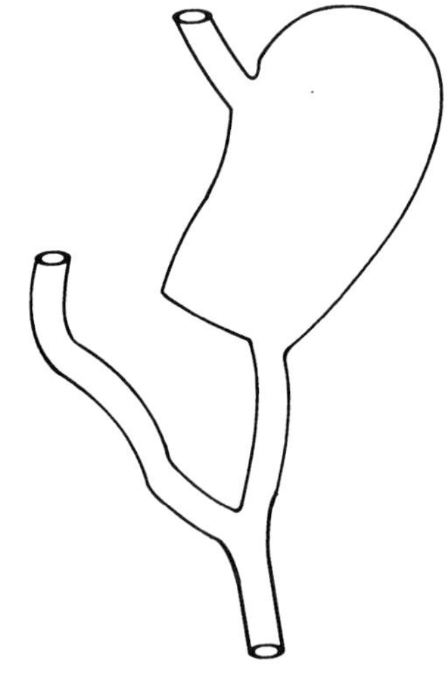

Diagram 8.11. Roux-en-Y surgery.

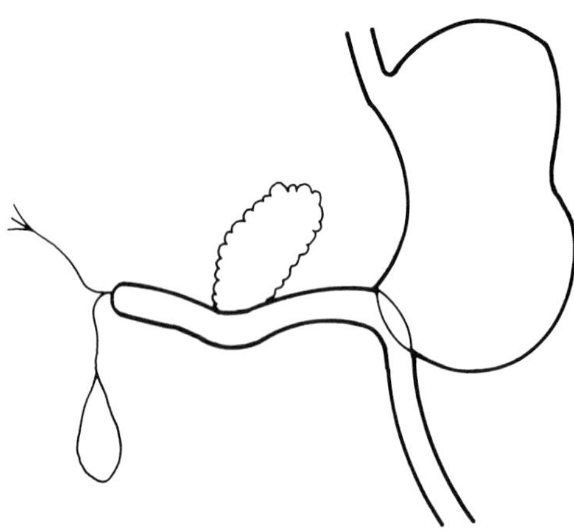

Diagram 8.12. Gastropancreaticoduodenectomy (Whipple).

Postoperative Complications

Radiologic examination can reveal and estimate postsurgical complications.

Bleeding. Postoperative hemorrhage may result from erosions, stress ulcer, dehiscence of sutures, inflammation, invagination of the small intestine into the gastric stump, or marginal ulcers. The flow of contrast medium may be disrupted over the site of bleeding.

Anastomotic Leaks and Ruptures. If leakage of gastric contents is suspected, water-soluble contrast medium should be used in order to detect contrast medium outside the gastric lumen. Rupture and dehiscence of sutures can lead to abscess and fistula, but diffuse peritonitis may also result.

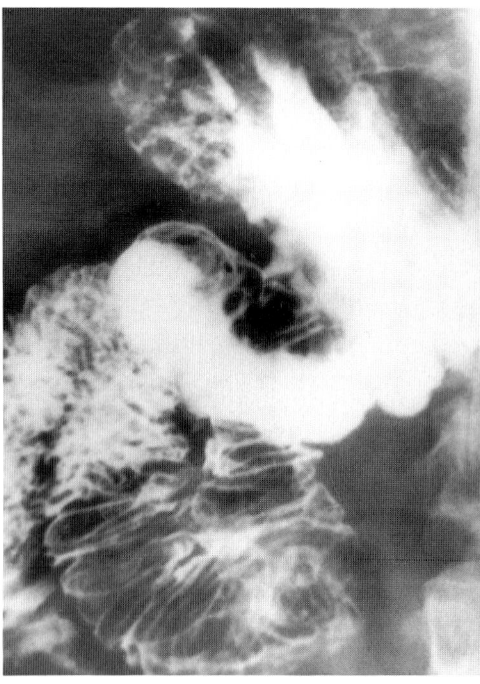

Figure 8.73. Whipple's operation. (See Diagram 8.12.)

Obstruction. Postsurgical obstruction may result from edema, hematoma, inflammation, or scar formation in the region of an anastomosis. Invagination of the small intestine into the stomach resembles a mushroom and can result in obstruction (Fig. 8.70B). The prolapse of thickened gastric mucosa into the small intestine may also cause obstructive symptoms. Obstruction may also develop at the site where the small intestine passes through the transverse mesocolon.

Acute Gastric Dilatation. Acute gastric dilatation, a component of the paralytic ileus syndrome, can be a rare postoperative complication. The stomach is extremely dilated by gas and secretions and fills the entire peritoneal cavity (Fig. 8.3).

Malabsorption. Malabsorption caused by resection of the stomach results from decreased absorption of micronutrients such as vitamin B12, reduced production of intrinsic factor, and disturbed metabolism of calcium. Malabsorption is particularly manifested after gastroileostomy.

Marginal Ulcers. Marginal ulcers are located near a gastrojejunostomy, especially when the antrum has not been resected. They are most common in the jejunum and may result in gastrocolic fistulae. Marginal ulcers result from hyperacidity; they are more common in patients with duodenal than with gastric peptic ulcer and are more frequent following Billroth II than Billroth I operations (Figs. 8.74 and 8.75). Their morphologic characteristics do not differ from peptic ulcers of any other location. Ulcers may also emerge on the gastric stump near the anastomosis.

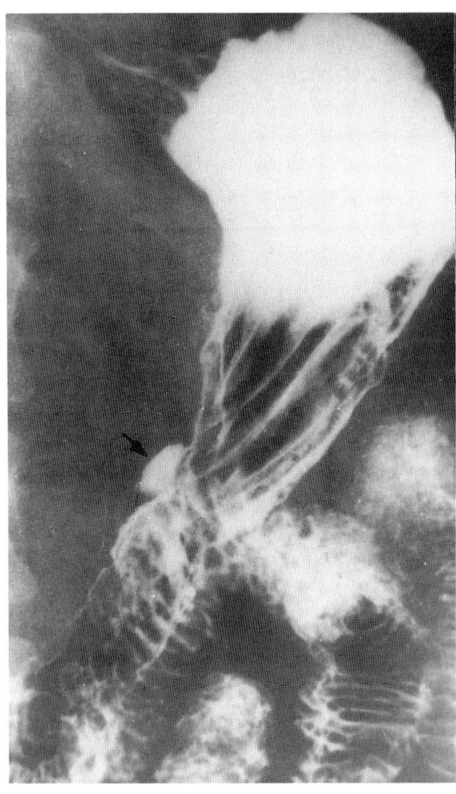

FIGURE 8.74. Billroth II resection. Peptic ulcer of the gastric stump adjacent to the anastomosis (arrow).

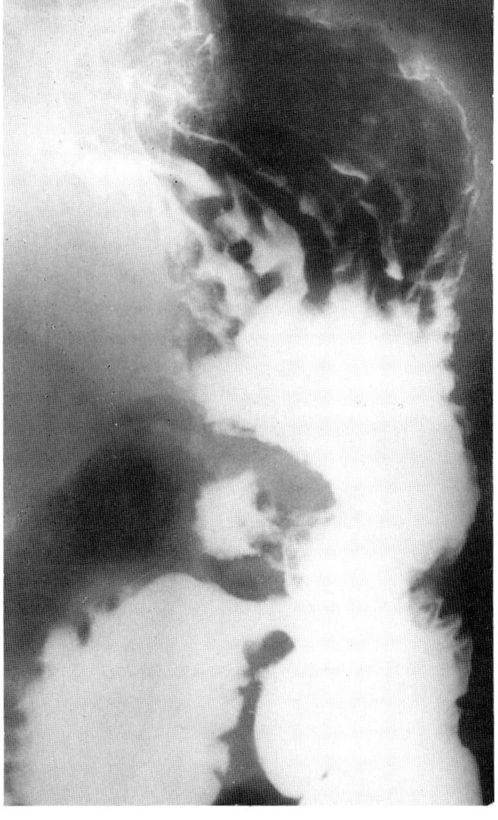

FIGURE 8.75. Marginal peptic ulcer following Billroth II surgery.

Postvagotomy Dysmotility. Peristaltic activity of the alimentary canal is often diminished for several months after vagotomy. Normal motor function is usually established after one year.

Postoperative Hiatus Hernia. Following gastric surgery, hiatus hernias appear more frequently than in the general population; they result from damage to the suspensory apparatus of the stomach (Fig. 8.76). If gastroesophageal reflux occurs, it may result in reflux esophagitis with all its complications.

Dumping Syndrome. Fast emptying of the gastric stump which results from loss of the storage function of the stomach predisposes the patient to dumping syndrome. Contents leaving the stomach are hypertonic compared to bowel contents. Transudation of fluid into the gut results in hypovolemia, and decreased blood volume causes vasomotor disturbances. An early dumping syndrome occurs approximately 10 minutes after a meal, and can last throughout the first year following surgery. A late dumping syndrome, a sequel of hypoglycemia, arises in the first hour after ingestion of food. Giving the patient only a barium suspension to drink will not provoke an accurate estimate of gastric emptying rate. Better results are obtained by adding solid food to the barium suspension.

Hypergastrinemia. When an operation such as gastroenterostomy excludes HCl from contact with the gastric antrum, hypergastrinemia results due to lack of normal inhibition by HCl. Parietal cells secrete excess HCl resulting in marginal ulcers.

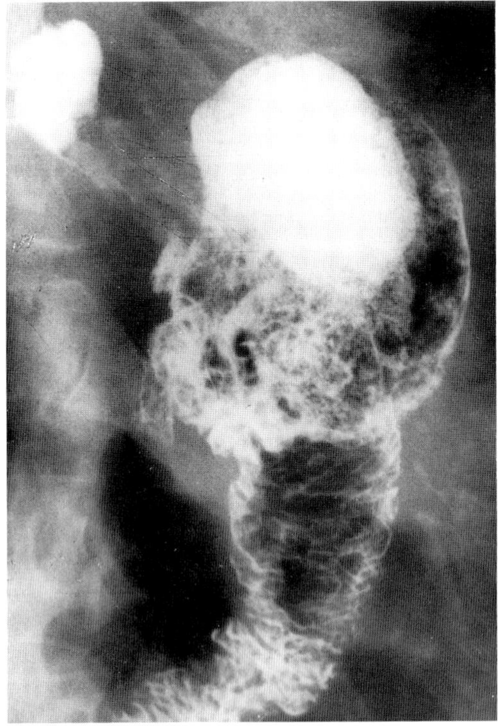

Figure 8.76. Billroth II surgery. Atrophic gastritis of the gastric stump and hiatus hernia. The afferent arm failed to fill with barium.

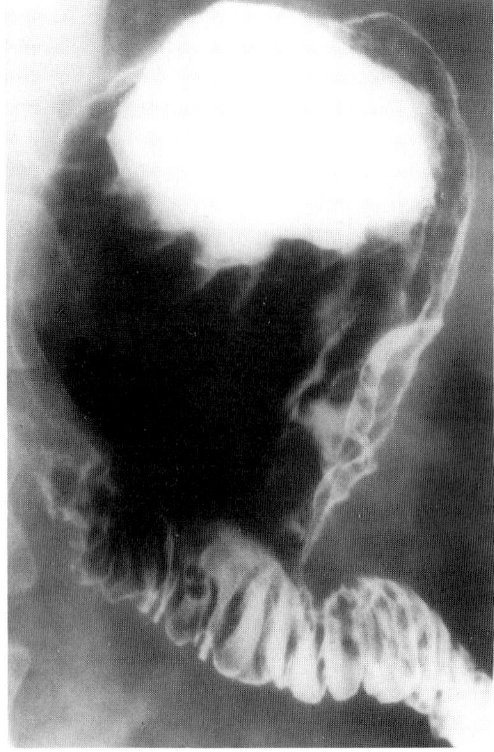

Figure 8.77. Primary carcinoma of the gastric remnant after Billroth II surgery.

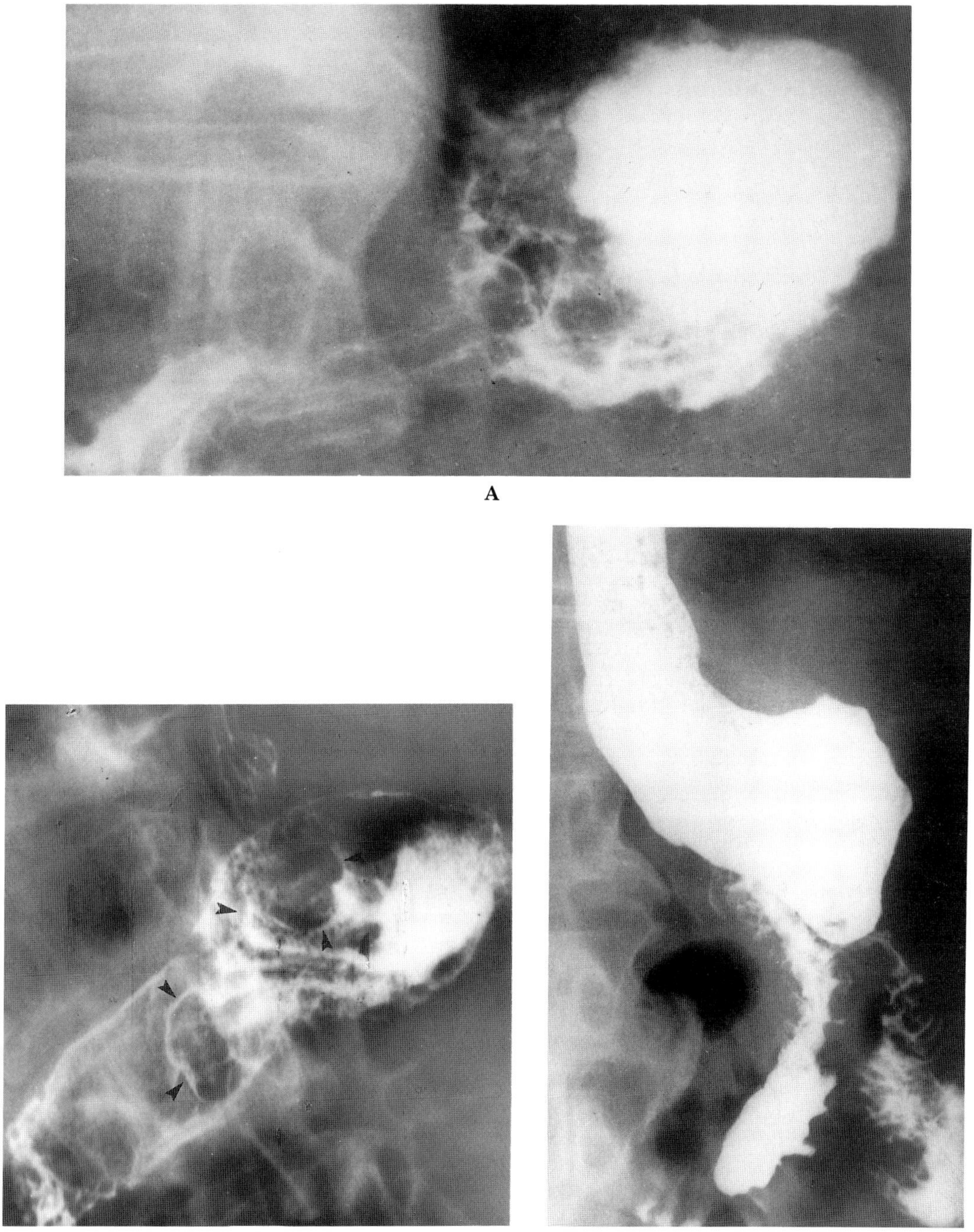

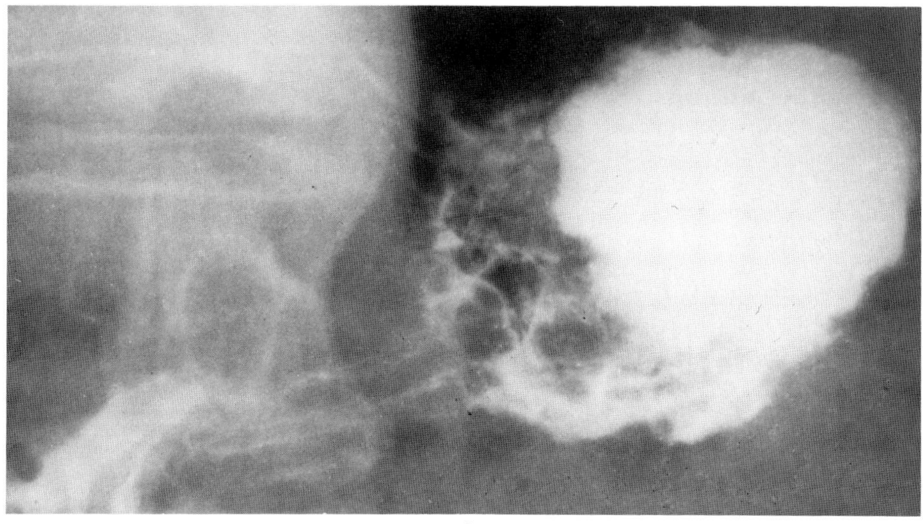

A

B

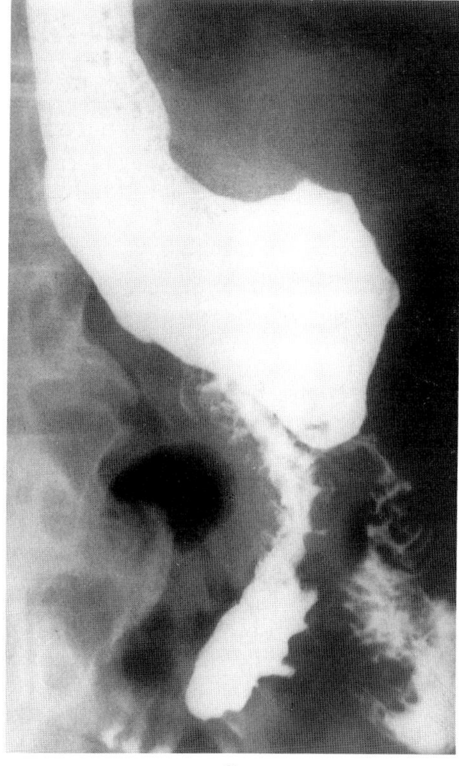

C

FIGURE 8.78. Recurrent carcinoma of the gastric stump. (A) After Billroth I surgery. Polypoid masses are adjacent to the anastomosis. (B) After Billroth I surgery. Multiple polypoid masses (arrowheads) and gastric hiatus hernia are evident. (C) After subtotal gastrectomy. Intramural tumor growth with sloping of the wall and dilatation of the esophagus without involvement of the cardia.

Afferent Loop Syndrome. This syndrome results from obstruction of the proximal portion of an afferent arm of the bowel after Billroth II type surgery. Reasons for obstruction include adhesions, too long an afferent arm, volvulus of the afferent arm, or left-to-right anastomosis. Symptoms results from the accumulation of bile, pancreas secretions, and bacteria, or associated toxins.

Postoperative Gastric Atrophy. The etiology of atrophic gastritis which may appear after gastric surgery is not clearly understood. Radiologic findings are identical to atrophic gastritis in patients without previous surgery, and are diagnosed using the same examination procedures (Fig. 8.76).

Primary Carcinoma of the Gastric Pouch. Postgastrectomy carcinoma may be primary or recurrent. Data on the prevalence and incidence of primary postgastrectomy gastric carcinoma are controversial. Radiologic signs of these tumors do not differ from carcinoma in an unresected stomach. The carcinoma is manifested by changes of mucosal relief, ulcer, rigidity of the wall and/or protruding mass (Fig. 8.77). The prevalence of primary gastric carcinoma is increased after resection for peptic ulcer. The risk of primary gastric pouch carcinoma is proportional to the time elapsed after surgery. This period is shorter in older patients.

Recurrent Gastric Carcinoma. The radiologic diagnosis of either a recurrent or primary gastric carcinoma of the gastric stump is difficult. Since a majority of gastric stumps are inaccessible to compression and lack peristalsis, double-contrast examination is preferred. Recurrent tumors may, but do not necessarily, assume the same morphology as the initial type of gastric carcinoma (Fig. 8.78). Scars may also mimic recurrent tumors. Intra-abdominal metastatic processes, in particular liver metastases and infiltration of the omentum, can be well visualized by US, CT, and MRI.

Arteriographic Evaluation of the Postoperative Stomach. Arteriographic examination may provide useful information in patients who bleed following gastric surgery. The site of bleeding may be shown in 74% of patients, and therapy can be administered. Iatrogenic arteriovenous fistulae and unintentionally ligated arteries may also be revealed.

Bibliography

Akerlund A. Ulcer niches with stopper-shaped vascular defect. Radiology. 1939;33:203.

Armington WG, Mann FA, Nelson JA. Cost-effective means of diagnosing and following benign and malignant gastric ulcers. Invest Radiol. 1985;20:171.

Bahk YW, Sung KY, Kim BK. Spicule or porcupine sign of primary gastric lymphoma – a correlative study of radiological findings with histology. Br J Radiol. 1984;57:265.

Balthazar EJ, Megibow AJ, Hulnick DH. Cytomegalovirus esophagitis and gastritis in AIDS. AJR. 1985;144:1201.

Balthazar EJ, Megibow AJ, Naidich D, Lefleur RS. Computed tomographic recognition of gastric varices. AJR. 1984;142:1121.

Birch CA. Primary sarcoma of the stomach. Br Med J. 1954;393:4884.

Blackledge G, Bush H, Dodge OG, Growther D. A study of gastrointestinal lymphoma. Clin Oncol. 1979;5:209.

Bluth I. Gastrointestinal carcinoid tumors. Radiology. 1960;74:573.

Bonfield RE, Martel W. The problem of differentiating benign antral ulcers from intramural tumors. Radiology. 1973;106:25.

Brady LW. Malignant lymphoma of the gastrointestinal tract. Radiology. 1980;137:291.

Bremer JL. Diverticula and duplications of the intestinal tract. Arch Path. 1944;38:132.

Brown CH, Moots MF. Multiple gastric carcinoma. Gastroenterology. 1954;26:846.

Brown WH, Davis J. Bezoar and its potential imitator. AJR. 1959;82:1041.

Burhenne HJ. Roentgen anatomy and terminology of gastric surgery. AJR. 1964;91:731.

Burrell M, Touloukian JS, Curtis AM. Roentgen manifestations of carcinoma in the gastric remnant. Gastrointest Radiol. 1980;5:331.

Calenoff L, Sparberg M. Gastric pseudolesions: roentgenographic–gastrographic correlation. AJR. 1971; 113:139.

Camp JD. Jejunal and gastrojejunal ulcer, their associated roentgenologic signs. JAMA. 1928;91:1436.

Camp WH. Carcinoid of the stomach. Radiology. 1955;65:753.

Cancelmo JJ. Interstitial gastric emphysema with report of a case. Radiology. 1954;63:81.

Carman MD. A new roentgen-ray sign of ulcerating gastric cancer. JAMA. 1921;77:990.

Caulas EM, Fildes. Radiopaque phytobezoar; case report. Radiology. 1953;60:261.

Christlieb AR, Schuster MM. Zollinger-Ellison syndrome: a clinical appraisal based on review of the literature. Arch Int Med. 1964;114:381.

Christoforidis AJ, Nelson SW. Radiological manifestations of ulcerogenic tumors of the pancreas: the Zollinger-Ellison syndrome. JAMA. 1966;198:511.

Craig O, Gregson R. Primary lymphoma of gastrointestinal tract. Clin Radiol. 1981;32:63.

Cronan J, Burrell M, Trepeta R. Aphthoid ulcerations in gastric candidiasis. Radiology. 1980;134:607.

Dawson IMP, Cornes JS, Morson BC. Primary malignant lymphoid tumors of the intestinal tract. Br J Surg. 1961;49:80.

Dekker W, Op den Orth JO. Early gastric cancer. Radiologia Clin. 1977;46:115.

de Lange EE, Slutzky V, Swanson S, Shaffer A Jr. Computed tomography of emphysematous gastritis. J Comput Assist Tomogr. 1986;10:139.

Doalgard JB. Volvulus of the stomach. Case report and survey. Acta Chir Scand. 1952;103:131.

Eklof O. Benign tumors of the stomach and duodenum. Acta Radiol Diagn. 1962;57:177.

Elliot GW, Walk M, Benz R. A roentgenologic study of ulcerating lesions of the stomach. AJR. 1957; 77:612.

Ellis K. Gastrojejunal ulcer. Radiology. 1958;71:187.

Evans JA, Delany F. Gastric varices. Radiology. 1953;60:46.

Evans JA, Weintraub S. Accessory pancreatic tissue in the stomach wall. AJR. 1953;69:22.

Evans KT. Oesophageal and gastric varices. Br J Radiol. 1959;32:233.

Farman J, Faegenberg D, Dallemand S, Chen CK. Crohn's disease of the stomach: the "ram's horn" sign. AJR. 1975;123:242.

Faulk DL, Anuras S, Christensen J. Chronic intestinal pseudo-obstruction. Gastroenterology. 1978; 74:922.

Feczko PJ, Halpert RD, Ackerman LV. Gastric polyps: radiological evaluation and clinical significance. Radiology 1985;155:581.

Feczko PJ, Halpert RD, Zonca M. Radiographic abnormalities in eosinophilic esophagitis. Gastrointest Radiol. 1985;10:321.

Fishman EK, Magid D, Jones B, Siegelman SS. Menetrier disease. J Comput Assist Tomogr. 1983;7:143.

Fork FT, Ekberg O, Haglund U. Radiology in primary gastric lymphoma. Acta Radiol Diagn. 1984; 25:481.

Gelfand DW, Ott DJ. Gastric ulcer scars. Radiology. 1981;140:37.

Gelfand DW, Dale WJ, Ott DJ. The location and size of gastric ulcers: radiologic and endoscopic evaluation. AJR. 1984;143:755.

Glickman MG, Szemes G, Loeb P, Margulis AR. Peptic ulcer of the pyloric region. AJR. 1971;113:147.

Golden R, Stout AP. Superficial spreading carcinoma of the stomach. AJR. 1948;59:157.

Gordon R, Laufer I, Kressel HY. Gastric polyps found on routine double-contrast examination of the stomach. Radiology. 1980;134:27.

Gorman B, Shaw DG. Congenital microgastria. Br J Radiol. 1984;57:260.

Gray RR, Louis ELSt, Grosman H. Crohn's disease involving the proximal stomach. Gastrointest Radiol. 1985;10:43.

Haller JO, Cohen HL. Hypertrophic pyloric stenosis: diagnosis using US. Radiology. 1986;161:335.

Hatfield M, Shapir J. The radiologic manifestations of failed antireflux operations. AJR. 1985;144: 1209.

Haudek M. Zur rontgenologischen Diagnose der Ulcerationen in der pars media des Magens. Munchen Med Wschr. 1910;57:1587.

Henry GW. Emphysematous gastritis. AJR. 1952; 68:15.

Hicks LM, Morgan A, Anderson MR. Pyloric stenosis: a report of triplet families and notes on its inheritance. J Ped Surg. 1981;16:939.

Hietala SO, Ghahremani GG, Crampton AR, Wirell M. Arteriographic evaluation of postsurgical stomach. Gastrointest Radiol. 1985;10:31.

Ike BW, Rosenbusch G. Gastrointestinal malignant lymphoma: roentgenographic features and pathologic and morphologic correlations. Diagn Imag. 1981;50:66.

Joffe N, Autonioli DA. Atypical appearances of benign hyperplastic gastric polyps. AJR. 1978;131: 147.

Johnson OA, Hoskins DW, Todd J, Thorbjarnarson B. Crohn's disease of the stomach. Gastroenterology. 1966;50:571.

Jordan GL Jr, Bolton BF, Heard JG, Waldron GW. Sarcomas of the stomach. Surg Gynecol Obstet. 1955;100:453.

Jordan GL, Barton HL, Williamson WA. A study of motility in the gastric remnant following subtotal gastrectomy. Surg Gynecol Obstet. 1957;104:257.

Kaplan IW, Shepard RM. Prolapse of the gastric mucosa into the duodenum. JAMA. 1951;147:554.

Katz ME, Blocker SH, McAlister WH. Focal foveolar hyperplasia presenting as an antral-pyloric mass in young infant. Ped Radiol. 1985;15:136.

Kenney PhJ, Brinsko RE, Patel DV. Gastric involvement in chronic granulomatous disease of childhood: demonstration by computed tomography and upper gastrointestinal studies. J Comput Assist Tomogr. 1985;9:563.

Keto P, Suoranta H, Tarpila S. Areae gastricae and gastritis in double-contrast barium meal. Fortschr Rontgenstr. 1979;130:576.

Kirklin BR. The meniscus complex in the roentgenologic diagnosis of ulcerating carcinoma of the stomach. AJR. 1942;47:571.

Kirsh TE. Benign and malignant gastric ulcers: roentgen differentiation. Radiology. 1955;3:357.

Klotz AP, Kirsner P. Mucus bezoar with partial gastric obstruction. Gastroenterology. 1955;28:124.
Kobler R. Prolapse of redundant gastric mucosa into the duodenum. Acta Radiol Diagn. 1950;33:69.
Kottler RE, Tuft RJ. Benign greater curvature gastric ulcer: the "sump-ulcer". Br J Radiol. 1981; 54:651.
Kreel L, Ellis H. Pyloric stenosis in adults: a clinical and radiological study of 100 consecutive patients. Gut. 1965;6:253.
Krone CL, Gelfand MD. Gastritis presenting as multiple polyposis of the stomach. Gastroenterology. 1969;57:703.
Laufer I, Trueman T, De Sa D. Multiple superficial gastric erosions due to Crohn's disease of the stomach. Radiologic and endoscopic diagnosis. Br J Radiol. 1976;49:726.
Lecomte P, Bruneton JN, Sicart M. Leiomyoblastoma of the stomach. Fortschr Rontgenstr. 1981; 135:57.
Lee KR, Levine E, Moffat RE, Bigongiari LR, Hemreck AS. Computed tomographic staging of malignant gastric neoplasms. Radiology. 1979;133: 151.
Lee S, Rutledge JN. Gastric emphysema. Am J Gastroenterol. 1984;79:899.
Levine MS, Creteur V, Kressel HY, Laufer I, Herlinger H. Benign gastric ulcers: diagnosis and follow-up with double-contrast radiography. Radiology. 1987;164:9.
Lorimer A, Penn L. Acute volvulus of the stomach. AJR. 1955;77:627.
Lukes RJ, Collins RD. New approaches to the classification of the lymphomata. Brit J Cancer. 1975; 31(suppl 2):1.
Lynn H. The mechanisms of pyloric stenosis and its relationship to preoperative preparation. Arch Surg. 1942;81:453.
Manolin RA, Avenarius DA. Inflammatory pseudotumors of the stomach. Diagn Imag. 1979;48:93.
Marshak RH, Friedman AJ. Carcinoids (argentaffinomas) of the stomach. AJR. 1951;66:200.
Marshak RH, Lindner AE, Maklansky D. Lymphoreticular disorders of the gastrointestinal tract. Roentgenographic features. Gastrointest Radiol. 1979;4:103.
Marshak RH, Lindner AE, Maklansky D, Gelb A. Eosinophilic gastroenteritis. JAMA. 1981;245: 1677.
Marshak RH, Maklansky D, Kurzban JD, Lindner AE. Crohn's disease of the stomach and duodenum. Am J Gastroenterol. 1982;77:340.
Martin JF, O'Brien TF, Holleman IL, Wall GH, Duque JL. The roentgenographic signs in atrophic gastritis and gastric atrophy. AJR. 1965;94:343.
Menetrier P. Des polyadenomes gatriques et leurs rapports avec le cancer de l'estomac. Arch Physiol Norm Pate. 1888;1:32.
Ming SC. Malignant potential of gastric polyps. Gastrointest Radiol. 1976;1:121.
Momoshima S, Imai Y, Sugino Y, Sekine Y, Kumakura K. Radiologic findings of linear gastric erosions. AJR. 1986;147:701.
Mountford RA, Brown P, Salmon PR, Alvarenga C, Neuman CS, Read EA. Gastric cancer detection in gastric ulcer disease. Gut. 1980;21:9.
Muhletaler CA, Gerlock AJ, de Soto L, Halter SA. Gastroduodenal lesions of ingested acid: radiographic findings. AJR. 1980;135:1247.
Mullin D, Shirkoda A. Computed tomography after gastrectomy in primary gastric carcinoma. J Comput Assist Tomogr. 1985;9:30.
Nathan MH, Newman A, Ochsner JL, Blum L. Sarcoidosis of upper gastrointestinal tract. AJR. 1960;84:275.
Nelson SW. The discovery of gastric ulcers and the differential diagnosis between benignancy and malignancy. Radiol Clin North Am. 1969;7:5.
Nevin NJ, Turner WW, Gardner HT. Early and late roentgenologic findings in corrosive gastritis. AJR. 1959;81:603.
Ochsner S. Benign ulceration on the greater curvature of the stomach. AJR. 1956;75:312.
Oi M, Oshida K. The association of esophageal and duodenal ulcers. Gastroenterology. 1959;86:57.
Oi M, Oshida K, Sugimura S. The location of gastric ulcer. Gastroenterology. 1959;36:45.
Ott DJ, Gelfand DW, Wu WC. Detection of gastric ulcer: comparison of single- and double-contrast examination. AJR. 1982;139:93.
Palmer ED. Chronic hypertrophic gastritis. Gastroenterology. 1954;26:496.
Pendergrass EP, Andrews JR. Prolapsing lesions of gastric mucosa. AJR. 1935;34:337.
Portman MV, Dunne EF, Hazard JB. Manifestations of Hodgkin's disease of the gastrointestinal tract. AJR. 1954;72:772.
Press AJ. Practical significance of gastric rugal folds. AJR. 1975;125:172.
Riggs W Jr, Long L. The value of plain roentgenogram in pyloric stenosis. AJR. 1971;112:77.
Rigler LG, Kaplan HW. Pernicious anemia and tumor of the stomach. JNCI. 1947;7:327.
Rose C, Stevenson GW. Correlation between visualization and size of the areae gastricae and duodenal ulcer. Radiology. 1981;139:371.
Salter RH, Gill DK, Girdwood TG, McNeil RH, Athey G. Gastric ulcer: is endoscopy always necessary? Br Med J. 1978;282:2097.
Samuel E. Gastric diverticula. Br J Radiol. 1955;28: 574.
Scatarige JC, Fishman EK, Jones B, Cameron JL, Sanders RC, Siegelman SS. Gastric leiomyosarcoma: CT observations. J Comput Assist Tomogr. 1985;9:320.
Schackelford RT, Wood S Jr, Boitnott JK. Primary

sarcomas of the stomach. Am J Surg. 1961;101: 292.

Schatzki R. Roentgenologic examination in patients with bleeding from the gastrointestinal tract. N Engl J Med. 1946;235:783.

Schumacher FV, Hampton AO. Radiographic differentiation of benign and malignant gastric ulcers. Clin Sympos. 1956;8:161.

Schwartz GE, Schafani SJA. Post-traumatic gastric stenosis due to perigastric adhesions. Radiology. 1985;154:4.

Seymour CT, Weinberg JA. Emotion and gastric activity. JAMA. 1959;171:1193.

Shirakabe H, Hayakawa H, Itai Y, Takeda N, Hosoi T. Comparison of X-ray, endoscopy and biopsy examination for the diagnosis of early gastric cancer. Jap J Clin Oncol. 1972;12:93.

Steiner PE, Maimam SN, Palmer WL, Kirsner JB. Gastric cancer: morphologic factors in five years survival after gastrectomy. Am J Path. 1948;24: 947.

Strode JE. Giant hypertrophy of gastric mucosa. Surgery. 1957;41:236.

Styles RA, Gibb SP, Tarshis A, Silverman ML, Scholz FJ. Esophagogastric polyps: radiologic and endoscopic findings. Radiology. 1985;154:307.

Swalm WA, Morrison LM. Gastroscopic and hystologic studies of the stomach with gastric and extragastric disease during life and autopsy. Am J Dig Dis. 1941;8:391.

Thoeni RF, Cello J. A critical look at the accuracy of endoscopy and double-contrast radiography of the upper gastrointestinal tract in patients with substantial UGI hemorrhage. Radiology. 1980;135: 305.

Thoeni RF, Gedgaudas RK. Ectopic pancreas: usual and unusual features. Gastrointest Radiol. 1980; 5:37.

Thoeni RF, Moss AA. The radiographic appearance of complications following Nissen fundoplication. Radiology. 1979;131:17.

Thompson G, Somers S, Stevenson GW. Benign gastric ulcer: a reliable radiologic diagnosis. AJR. 1983;141:331.

Thompson H. Gastritis in partial gastrectomy specimens. Gastroenterology. 1959;36:861.

Vade AG, Jafri SZH, Agha FP, Vidyasagar MS, Coran AG. Radiologic evaluation of gastrostomy complications. AJR. 1983;141:325.

Ugarkovic B, Tezak S, Plavsic B, Agbaba M. A case of bizarre liver form variation. Clin Nucl Med. 1986;12:461.

Wang CC, Petersen JA. Malignant lymphoma of the gastrointestinal tract: roentgenographic considerations. Acta Radiol Diagn. 1956;46:523.

Yamada E, Nakazato H, Koike A, Suzuki K, Kato K, Kito T. Surgical results for early gastric cancer. Int Surg. 1974;59:7.

Yamada T, Ichikawa H. X-ray diagnosis of elevated lesion of the stomach. Radiology. 1974;110:79.

Chapter 9

Radiology of the Duodenum

Food gradually passes in small portions from the stomach into the duodenum, where fluids are evacuated through the pylorus. Minced food is then mixed with gastric secretions.

The acidic contents of the stomach mix with alkaline pancreatic juices, bile, and secretions from intestinal glands. Subsequent changes in pH influence the properties of barium mixtures.

Pathologic changes are more prevalent in the duodenum than in the mesenteric small intestine, taking into account the length of both organs. Even considering the relative lengths of alimentary canal sections, peptic ulcers are substantially more frequent in the duodenal bulb. The duodenal bulb and peripapillary area are the most frequent sites of pathologic changes in the duodenum.

Signs of obstruction and perforation of the duodenum may be demonstrated by plain abdominal films and CT. However, data on the morphology of the duodenum are obtained mainly by barium studies. The majority of pathologic changes in the duodenum are well demonstrated by both single- and double-contrast methods.

FUNCTIONAL DISORDERS

Duodenal Tone

Congenital megabulb is extremely rare. The duodenal bulb results from physiologic hypotonia in the proximal duodenum. A megabulb is regularly shaped, hypotonic, and much larger than the duodenal bulb of healthy people, where it may measure up to 5 cm by 3 cm. Megabulb appears not only as a congenital condition, but may also be a consequence of disease in the hepatobiliary system and pancreas.

Congenital atonia of the entire duodenum is called *megaduodenum* (Fig. 9.1). The width of the *hypotonic* duodenum exceeds 3 cm. Peristaltic waves are less frequent than in patients with a normotonic duodenum.

Duodenal *hypertonia* is associated with more frequent peristaltic waves. In this case, the duodenal width is often less than normal. After administration of spasmolytics, signs of hypertonia disappear. The duodenal lumen may be narrowed as a result of a spasm or organic lesion, and organic stenoses may result from either inflammatory or malignant processes.

Although the duodenum is protected from ischemia by a dual arterial supply (celiac axis and superior mesenteric artery), ischemic lesions may rarely result in strictures. Functional obstructions can be distinguished from mechanical obstruction by the use of spasmolytics. Inflammatory lesions of the duodenum are often associated with spasm, resulting from stimulation of the autonomic nervous system.

Reflux of duodenal contents into the stomach results from contraction of the second portion of the duodenum when the pylorus is open. Mild regurgitation should be considered normal. The direction of evacuation for any section of the GI tract, including the duodenum, depends on pressure gradients which change with the contraction of muscles in the intestinal wall.

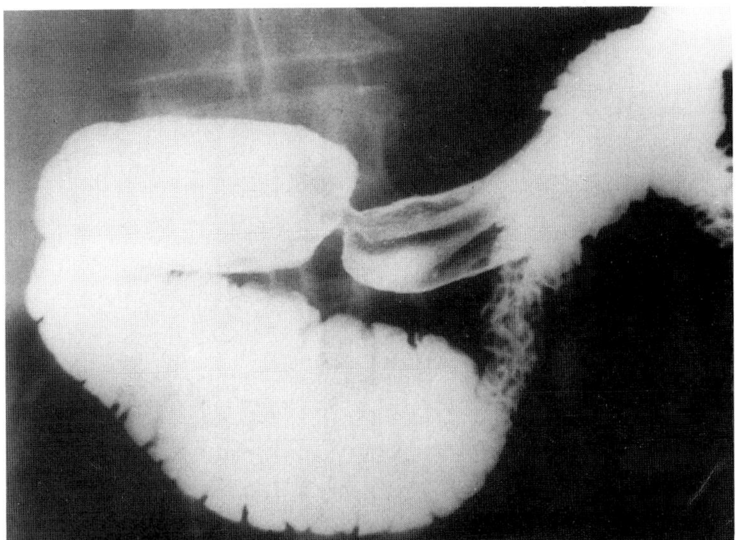

Figure 9.1. Congenital megaduodenum.

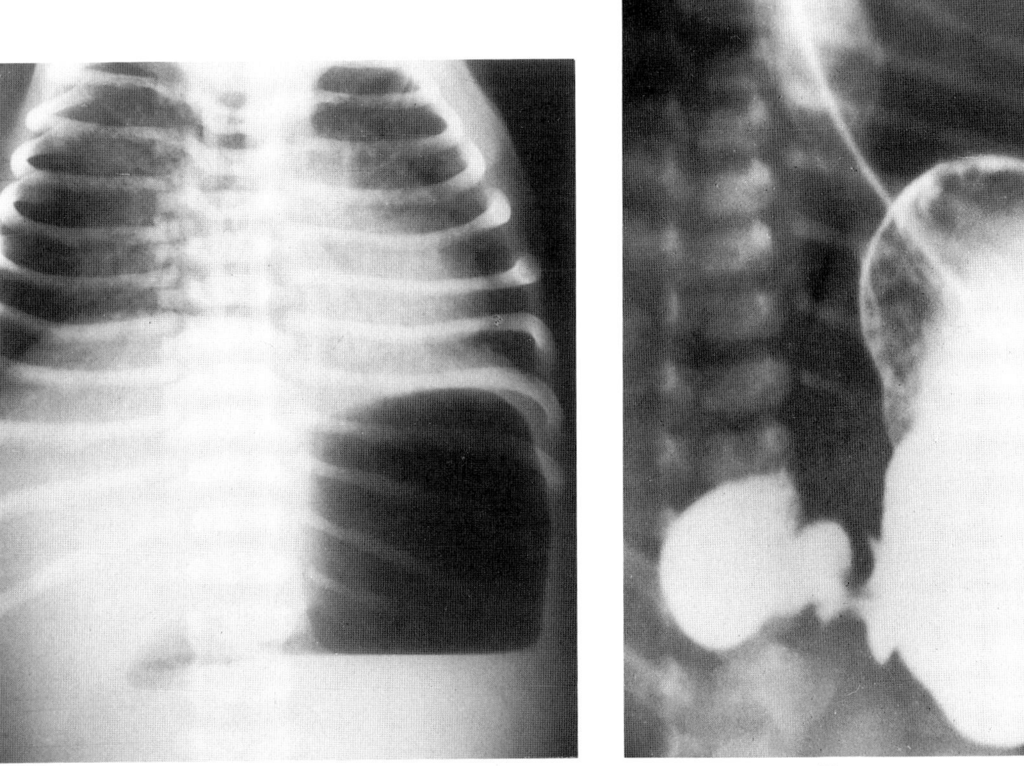

A B

Figure 9.2. Atresia of the first duodenal segment. (A) "Double-bubble" appearance on plain abdominal film. (B) Barium administered through a thin soft catheter was removed at the end of the examination.

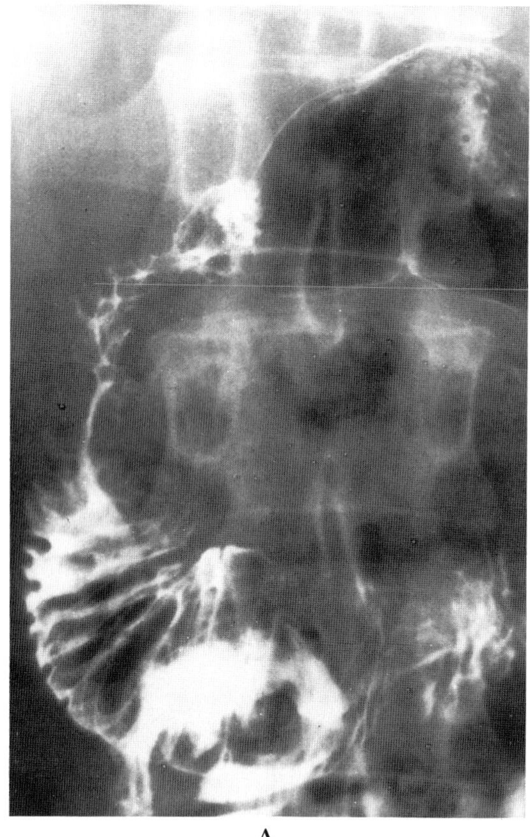

A

FIGURE 9.3. Annular pancreas. (A) Narrowed second portion of the duodenum. (B) Pancreatic duct in the uncinate process forming an annular pancreas (arrows) demonstrated by endoscopic retrograde cholangiopancreatography.

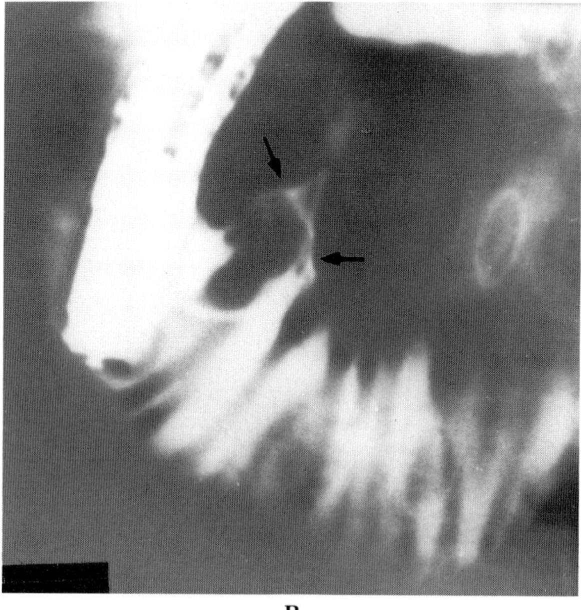

B

CONGENITAL MALFORMATIONS

Congenital *atresias* and *stenoses* of the duodenum are not rare. The duodenum is the most common site of intestinal atresia. Most frequently found with trisomy 21 (Down's syndrome), duodenal atresia presents on plain roentgenograms as a "double bubble" of a gas-distended stomach and dilated duodenal bulb (Fig. 9.2). Obstruction of the second or third duodenal sections results in two gas-fluid levels on plain abdominal films taken with the patient in a dependent position. Little or no gas is present distal to a stenosis of the alimentary canal. The site of obstruction can be exactly determined by positive or negative contrast examination. Duodenal narrowing may be caused by an excessively large, ring-shaped uncinate process of the pancreas, the *annular pancreas* (Fig. 9.3), which results from a persistent ventral embryonal bud of the pancreas. This portion of the pancreas has its own secretory canal. The mucosal surface of the duodenum is intact at the site of narrowing.

The anatomical course of the duodenum is variable (Fig. 9.4). The duodenum is located retroperitoneally between the superior duodenal flexure and the ligament of Treitz. The duodenum is mobile if this portion is not fixed by secondary peritoneum. If embryologic rotation of the duodenal loop does not occur, or if it remains incomplete, the course of the duodenal loop is atypical and may even be reversed.

Congenital membranes or webs are rare in the duodenum. Radiographically, membranes appear as transparent lines within the barium-filled duodenum. Optimal visualization is obtained by use of a double-contrast examination. Membranes may cause partial obstruction distal to the mucosal attachment because of a "windsock" phenomenon produced by peristalsis. External bands cause similar obstruction. Retroperitoneal attachment of the ascending colon compresses the duodenum when the cecum is malpositioned (Fig. 9.5).

Duplications in the duodenum are rare. When they communicate with the main duodenal lumen, they fill with barium and empty during contrast examination (Fig. 9.6). Noncommunicating duplications produce negative linear or spherical filling defects.

Duodenal *choristoma* is rare. Heterotopic gastric mucosa or pancreatic tissue may be seen (Fig. 9.7).

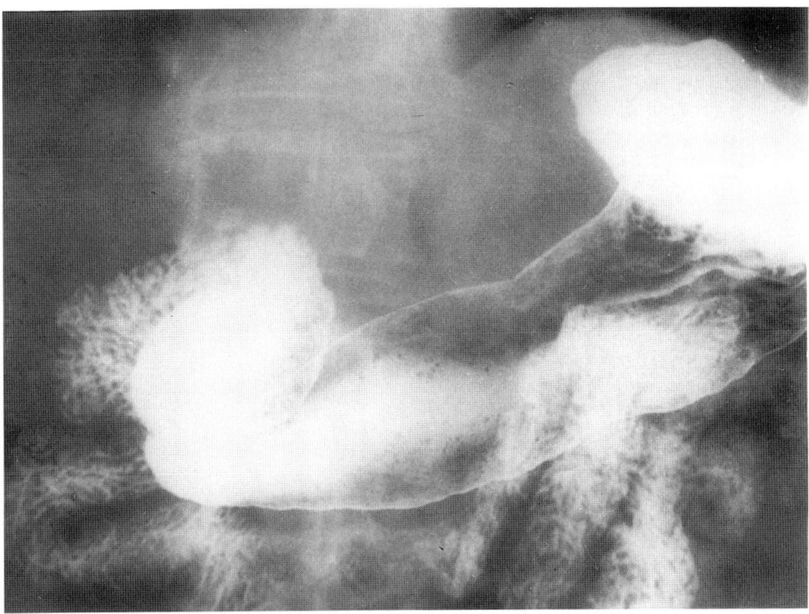

FIGURE 9.4. Mobile, nonfixed second and third portions of the duodenum.

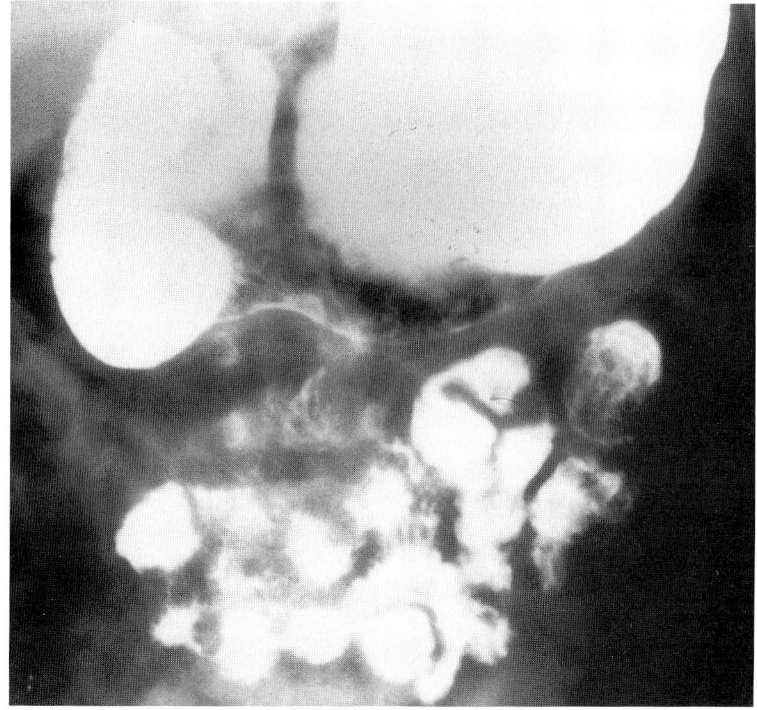

A

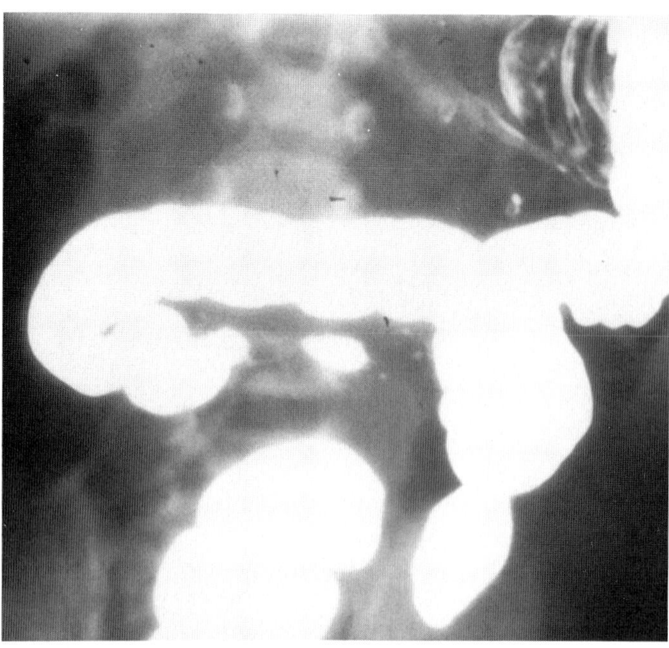

B

FIGURE 9.5. External band across the duodenum from a malpositioned cecum. (A) Duodenal obstruction. Peroral barium study. (B) Malposition of the cecum and ascending colon. Barium enema.

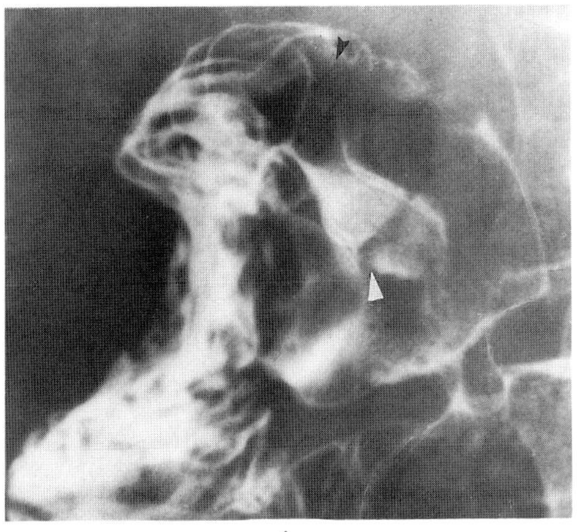

A

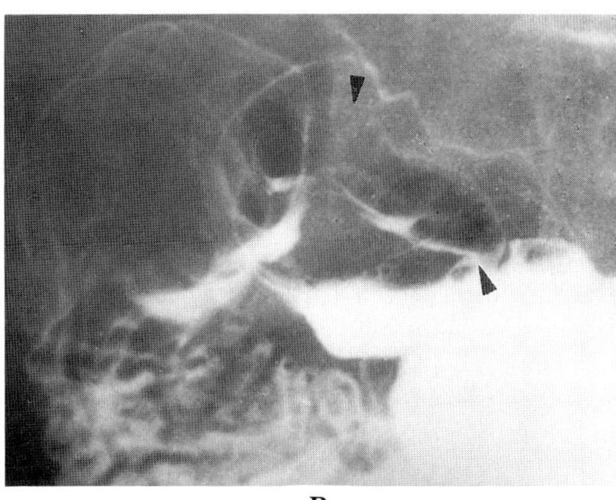

B

FIGURE 9.6. Duplication of the duodenal bulb communicating with the main lumen (arrowheads). (A) Filled with barium. (B) Subsequently emptied.

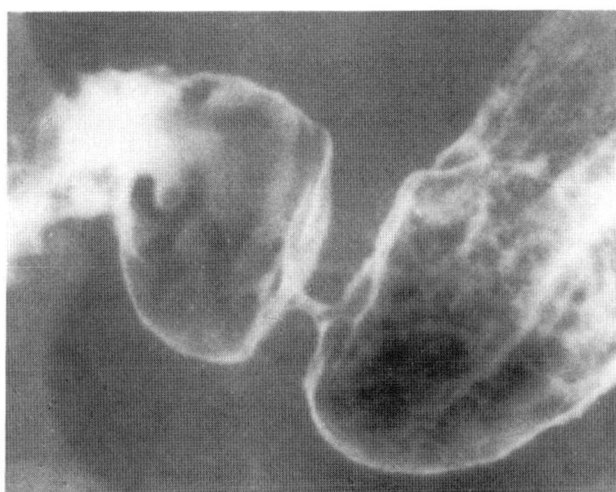

FIGURE 9.7. Heterotopic pancreatic tissue (choristoma) in the duodenal bulb.

DIVERTICULA

Duodenal diverticula are found in 1–2% of upper gastrointestinal series. The majority are acquired, since congenital diverticula are extremely rare. Congenital diverticula are true diverticula, whereas acquired diverticula are, as a rule, false. The former are found predominantly in the proximal section of the duodenum. True diverticula cannot be separated from false by radiologic examination. They

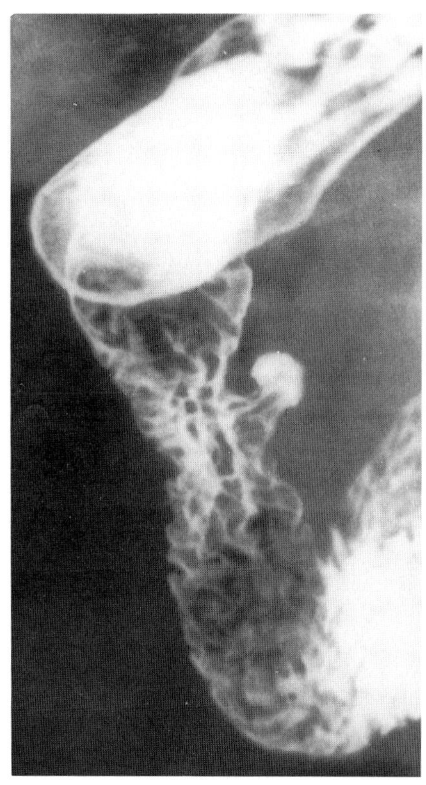

FIGURE 9.8. Diverticulum of the medial contour of the descending duodenum. Mucosal folds are seen within the diverticulum.

manifest as depressed lesions, positive defects of the contrast column. Acquired diverticula show a predilection for the concave side of the descending and inferior horizontal sections of the duodenum (Figs. 9.8 and 9.9). Mucosal folds enter diverticula through a diverticular neck. In contrast to ulcers, diverticula can change size and shape during examination.

An inverted diverticulum, as opposed to a diverticulum without this complication, is radiologically indistinguishable from a duodenal neoplasm with a central ulceration.

Uncomplicated diverticula are clinically silent. Rarely, very large diverticula may cause symptoms by compressing adjacent anatomical structures. Complications of diverticula include perforation, bleeding, formation of internal fistulas, abscesses, and formation of enteroliths.

INTRALUMINAL DIVERTICULA

An intraluminal diverticulum is composed of a membrane which creates a pocket, opened on the proximal side and closed distally (Diagram 9.1). An intraluminal diverticulum originates from the inner wall of the descending duodenum. The diverticular wall is thin and coated on both faces by duodenal mucosa (Fig. 9.10).

EXTRINSIC MASSES

Any section of the first portion of the duodenum may be compressed by the gallbladder (Fig. 9.11). The common bile duct traverses the posterior aspect of the proximal duodenum. If dilated, it can create a linear, well-demarcated

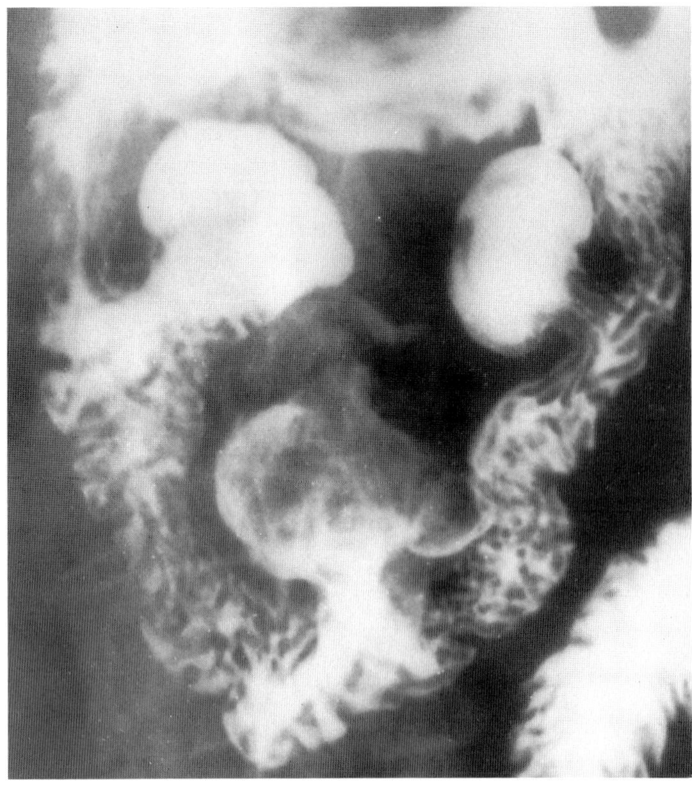

FIGURE 9.9. Multiple diverticula on the concave aspect of the duodenal sweep. Negative defects in the diverticular lumen are retained food.

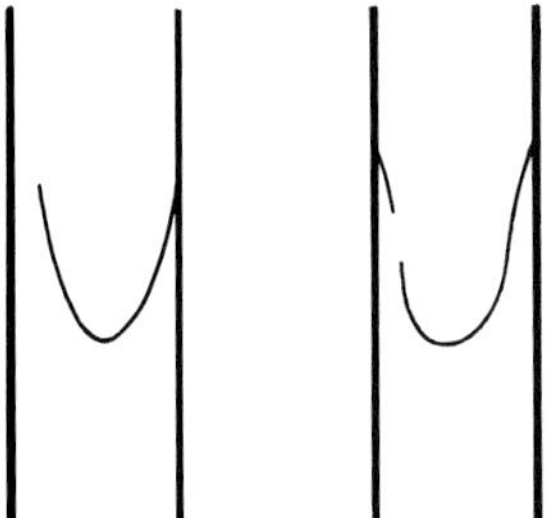

DIAGRAM 9.1. Intraluminal diverticulum of the duodenum. There is an opening in the proximal segment of the membrane.

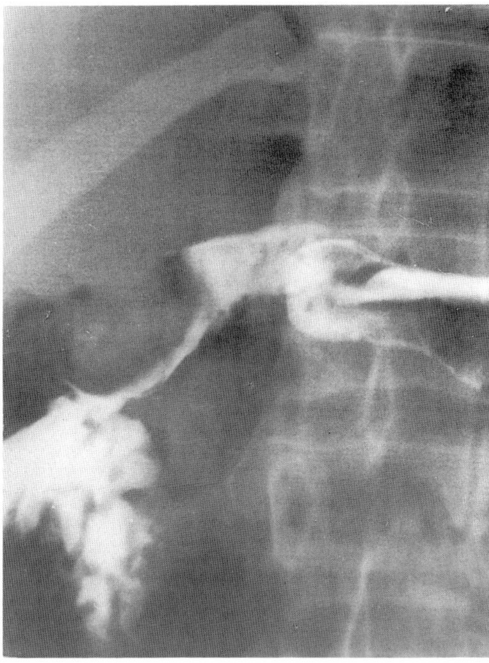

FIGURE 9.11. Impression on the first section of the duodenum by the gallbladder.

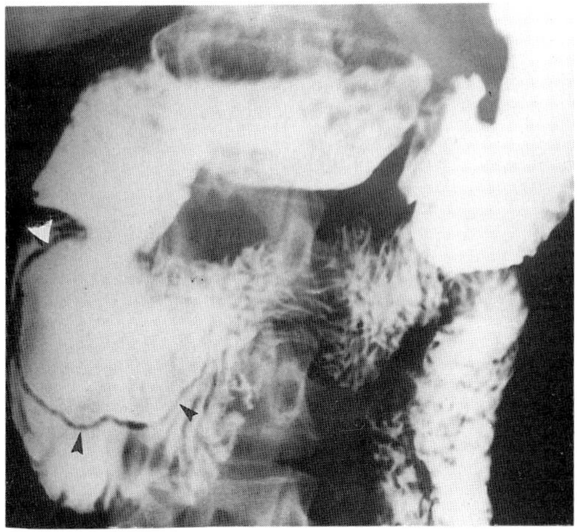

FIGURE 9.10. Intraluminal duodenal diverticulum. The radiolucent line (arrowheads) is the wall of the diverticulum.

negative defect in the contrast-filled duodenum (Fig. 4.34).

The duodenal sweep is enlarged in diameter in patients with a mass in the head of the pancreas (Fig. 9.12). Plicae conniventes on the medial portion of the C-loop may be distorted, serrated, flattened, or even effaced. At fluoroscopy, irregular contractions and spasm of individual duodenal segments may sometimes be observed. Enlargement of the head of the pancreas, particularly in patients with malignant

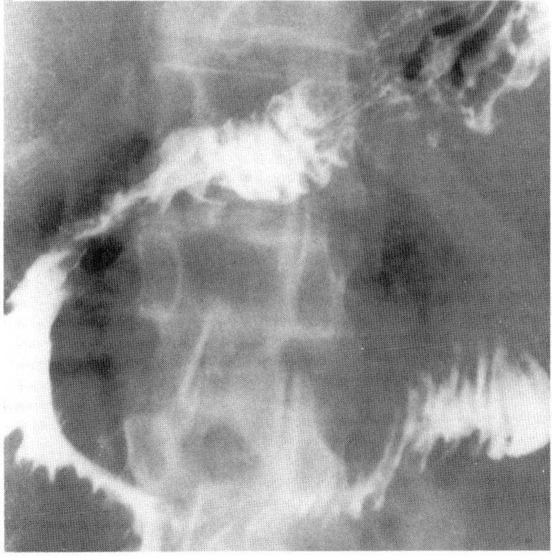

FIGURE 9.12. Pancreatitis. Widening of the duodenal sweep by an enlarged pancreas due to pancreatitis with impingement of the greater gastric curvature.

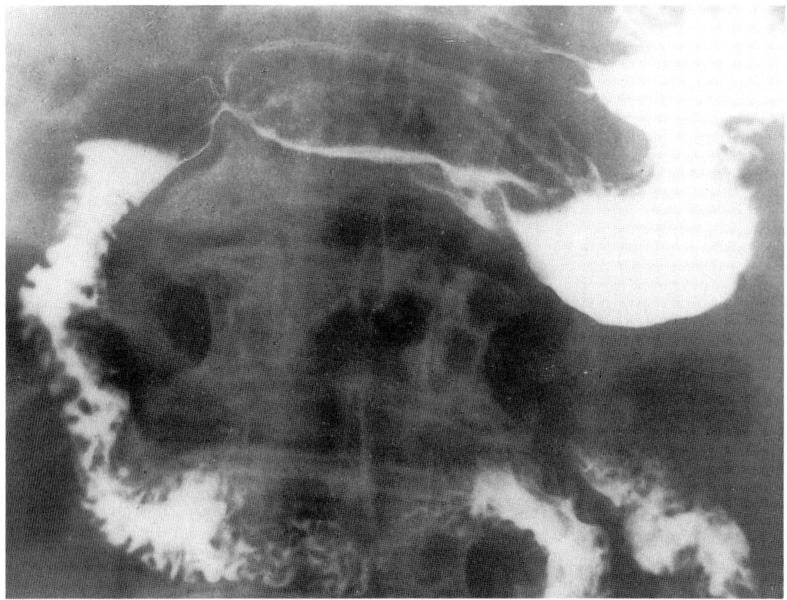

FIGURE 9.13. Carcinoma of the head of the pancreas. Widened duodenal C-loop with the second portion resembling a reverse "3" shape. Elevated gastric antrum.

neoplasms, creates a reverse "3" shape known as Frostberg's sign (Fig. 9.13). This configuration is due to reduced mobility in the region of the papilla.

Enlargement of the right kidney by hydronephrosis or neoplasm may cause medial deviation of the second portion of the duodenum.

DUODENAL OBSTRUCTION

Obstruction distal to the superior duodenal flexure may result in proximal distension of both the duodenum and the stomach with the formation of two gas-fluid levels—one in the duodenal bulb and another in the stomach. Postinflammatory bulbar stricture is the most frequent cause of duodenal obstruction and is due to repeated exacerbations of peptic ulcer disease.

Obstruction of the duodenum may be caused by either mural or intrinsic compression (e.g., diverticulum), or intraluminal pathology (Fig. 9.14). Classic radiologic and US examinations are of equal efficiency in demonstrating duode-

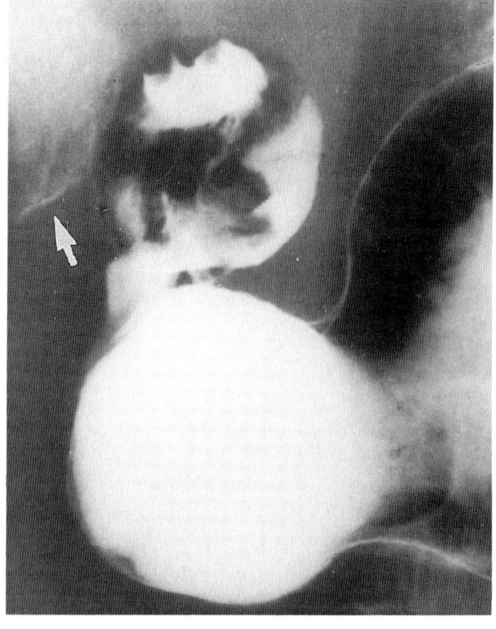

FIGURE 9.14. Duodenal bulb filled with prolapsed gastric mucosa. Radiopaque calculus in the gallbladder (arrow).

nal obstruction due to volvulus of the small intestine.

Partial or complete obstruction of the duodenal bulb may also be caused by large gallstones eroding into the duodenum with resultant impaction (Fig. 9.15).

The ligament of Treitz is a common site of duodenal obstruction, of which duodenal and pancreatic carcinoma may be causes (Figs. 9.16 and 9.17). Other causes are hernias in duodenal recesses, metastases in lymph nodes (Fig. 9.18), and compression by adjacent anatomical formations.

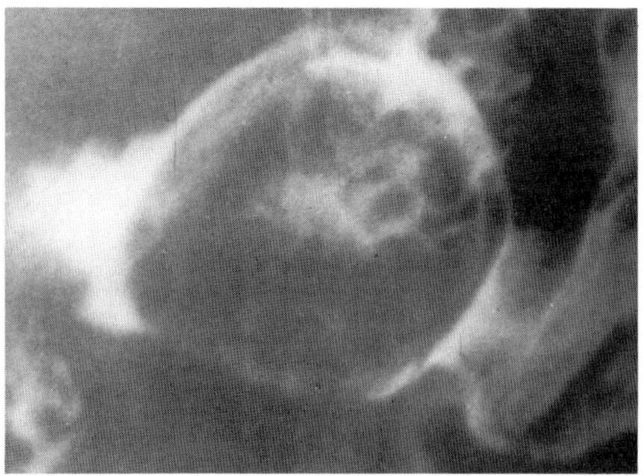

FIGURE 9.15. Large gallstone fills the duodenal bulb.

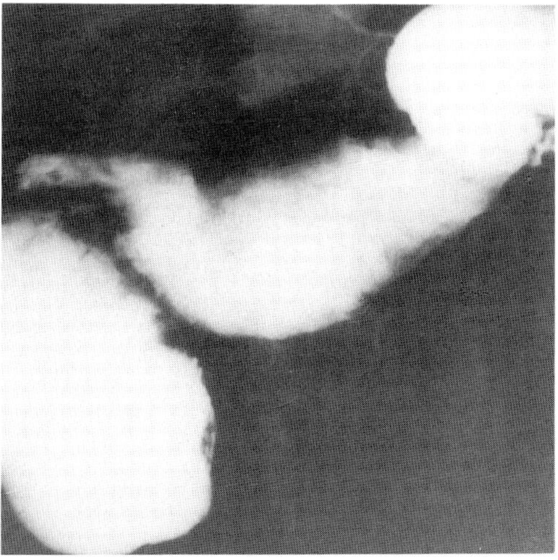

FIGURE 9.16. Complete obstruction of the third portion of the duodenum by annular carcinoma.

Signs of duodenal ileus may result from thrombosis of the superior mesenteric artery, cholecystitis, or pancreatitis.

SUPERIOR MESENTERIC ARTERY SYNDROME

Superior mesenteric artery syndrome is characterized by intermittent incomplete obstruction in the third portion of the duodenum. Rapid loss of body weight and subsequent disappearance of retroperitoneal fat may lead to compression of the duodenum between the superior mesenteric artery and the aorta. This condition is characterized by an acute angulation between these two blood vessels. The degree of obstruction may vary considerably, depending on the quantity of retroperitoneal adipose tissue and the patient's position. Restitution of adipose tissue is followed by the

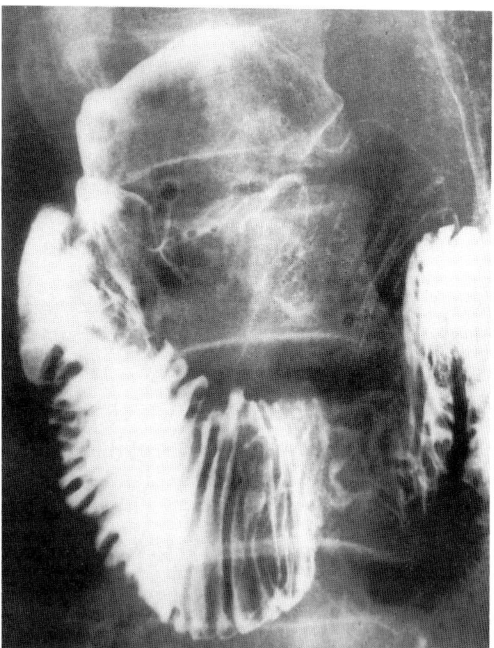

FIGURE 9.17. Pancreatic carcinoma infiltrates the third portion of the duodenum.

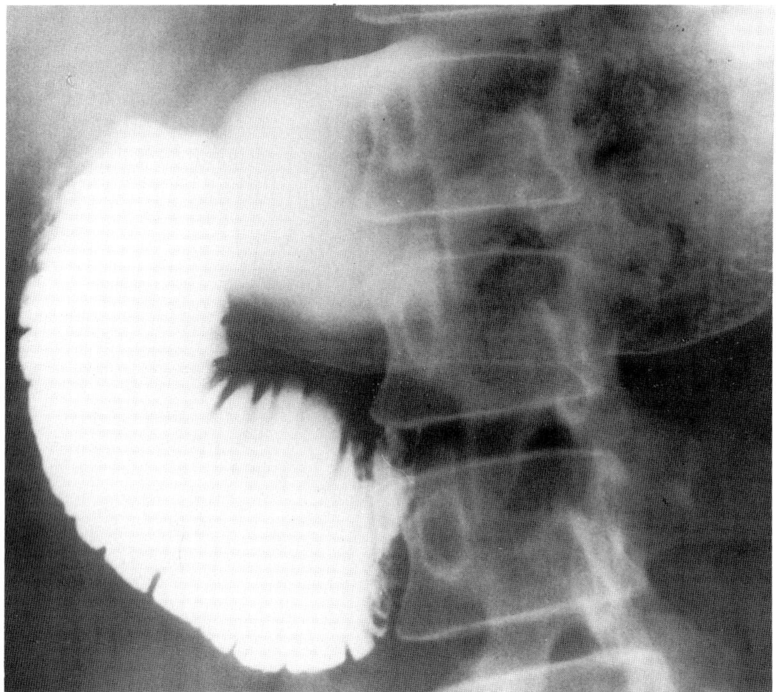

Figure 9.18. Obstruction in lymph nodes of the duodenojejunal junction, from metastatic carcinoma of the uterus.

spontaneous disappearance of symptoms. When the patient is placed on a horizontal table in a knee-chest position, the small intestine and mesentery with blood vessels shift toward the anterior abdominal wall, decreasing the degree of obstruction.

The onset of symptoms coincides with the appearance of a strip-like defect on the barium-filled inferior duodenum, located at the site of superior mesenteric artery crossing. Proximal sections of the duodenum are distended (Fig. 9.19). Peristalsis of the proximal duodenum propagates contents in both proximal and distal directions. In the early phase of the obstruction, as well as when patency is reconstituted, the duodenum may not be substantially dilated (Fig. 9.19C).

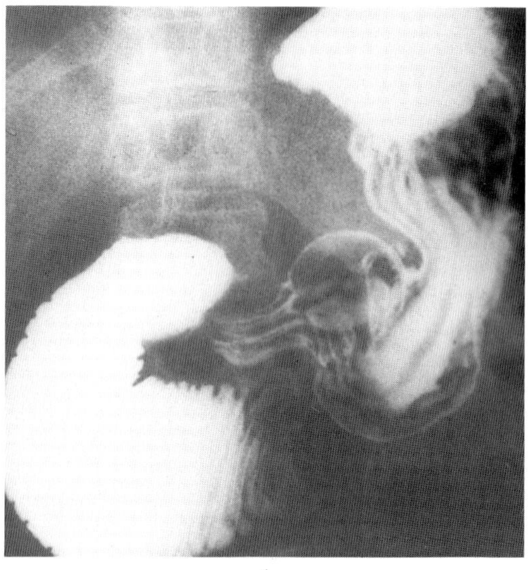

A

Figure 9.19. Superior mesenteric artery syndrome. (A) Almost complete obstruction of the third portion of the duodenum.

VARICES

Patients with portal hypertension may have varices of pancreatico-duodenal and right gastric veins. On barium studies varices appear as

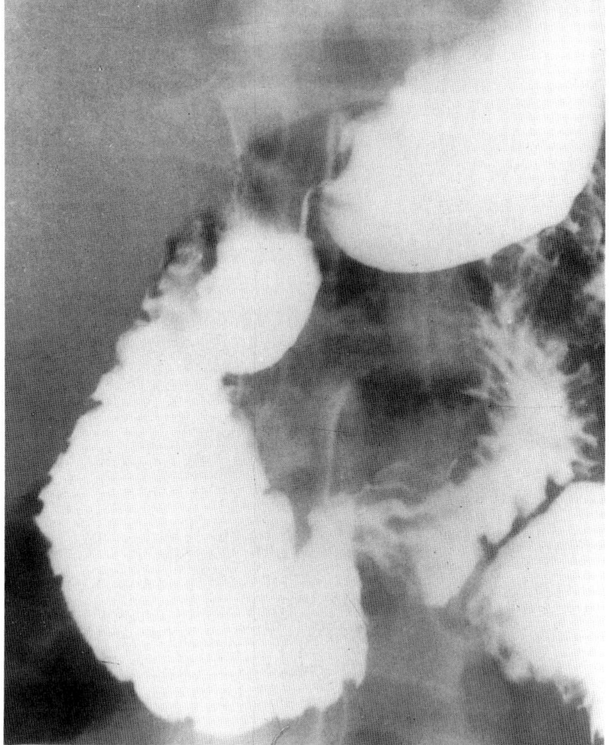

B

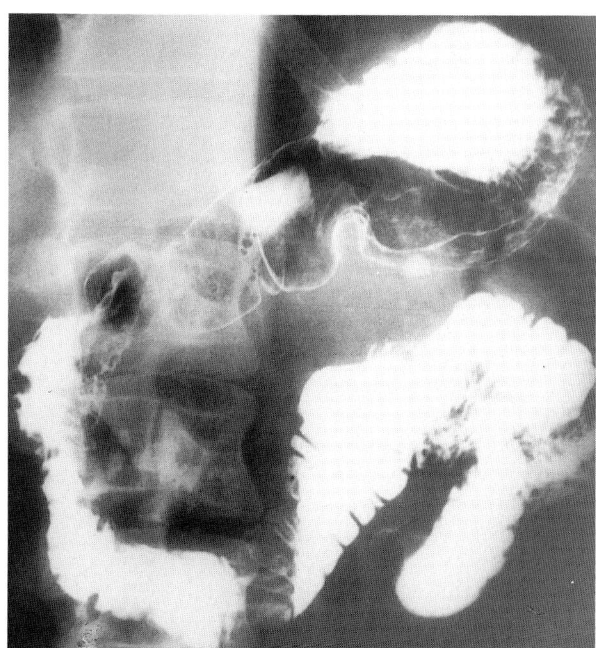

C

FIGURE 9.19 *continued.* Superior mesenteric artery syndrome. (B) Typical impression on the third portion of the duodenum with proximal distension. (C) Typical defect created by superior mesenteric artery without proximal dilatation.

spherical or serpiginous filling defects in the bulb and other sections of the proximal duodenum. Varices are best filled with blood in the prone position (Fig. 9.20).

Varices of the duodenum should be distinguished from enlarged Brunner's glands, benign neoplasms, prolapsed gastric polyps and/or prolapsed thickened gastric folds into the duodenal bulb, foreign bodies, and parasites. Varices are filled with blood and empty in various stages of an upper gastrointestinal series. Therefore, their radiographic appearance is inconstant. Differentiation from duodenal angiomas is not possible by conventional radiologic means.

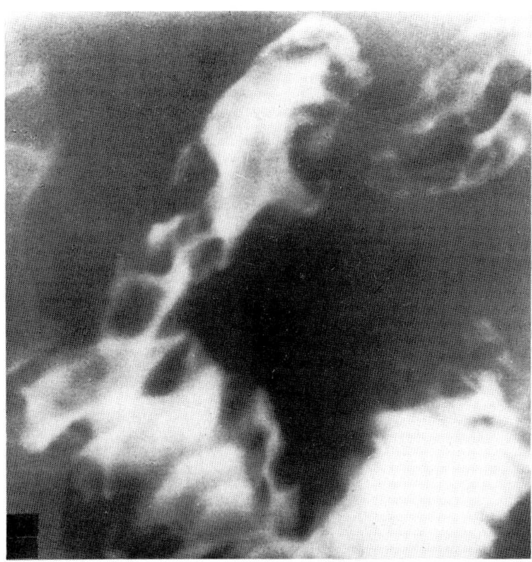

Figure 9.20. Varices of the duodenum and gastric antrum.

DUODENITIS

Duodenitis is twice as common as peptic ulceration of the duodenum, but it causes upper gastrointestinal symptoms in the same number of patients. There is a high correlation between endoscopic and histologic findings in patients with duodenitis. Based on endoscopic findings, duodenitis may be divided into the following stages:

1. Early stage – erythema of the mucosa, swelling of the duodenal folds and, at times, nodular thickenings of the folds.
2. Intermediate stage – small hemorrhagic areas in the mucosa.
3. Advanced stage – mucosal hemorrhage, erosions, and bleeding ulceration.

Careful multiphasic radiologic investigation may confirm the diagnosis of duodenitis with relatively high accuracy (Fig. 9.21). Duodenitis results in mucosal folds thicker than 5 mm, nodular thickenings of duodenal folds, erosions, and deformity of the duodenal bulb. Compared with endoscopy, the radiographic sensitivities for the detection of individual signs of duodenitis are: edematous folds (72%), nodular thickenings of duodenal folds (48%), deformations of the duodenal bulb (26%), and erosions (11%). The sensitivity of the radiologic examination when all signs are considered equals 80%, which is approximately the same as in the radiologic detection of peptic ulcer disease. The specificity of the radiologic examination is 76%. Mucosal erosions appear to be the least sensitive radiologic sign because they are found endoscopically in only 20% of affected patients.

Single-contrast and double-contrast techniques give equivalent results in the diagnosis of duodenitis. The sensitivity of radiologic detection increases with progression of the disease. Considering all four signs, the sensitivity of the radiologic method in detecting different stages of duodenitis is: first stage (72%), second stage (81%), and third stage (91%).

Most errors in radiologic diagnosis of duodenitis occur when only one sign is considered, for example, thickened folds. Patients with duodenitis usually do not have duodenal ulcers or hyperacidity.

Hyperplasia of Brunner's glands and nodular lymphatic hyperplasia of the duodenum should not be omitted from the differential diagnosis (Table 9.1). Occasionally, multiple tumors may resemble duodenitis (see the section about duodenal tumors, pages 342–343). Zollinger-Ellison syndrome, varices, tuberculosis, Crohn's disease, lymphangiectasia, and duodenal angiomas occasionally present with radiologic signs of duodenitis.

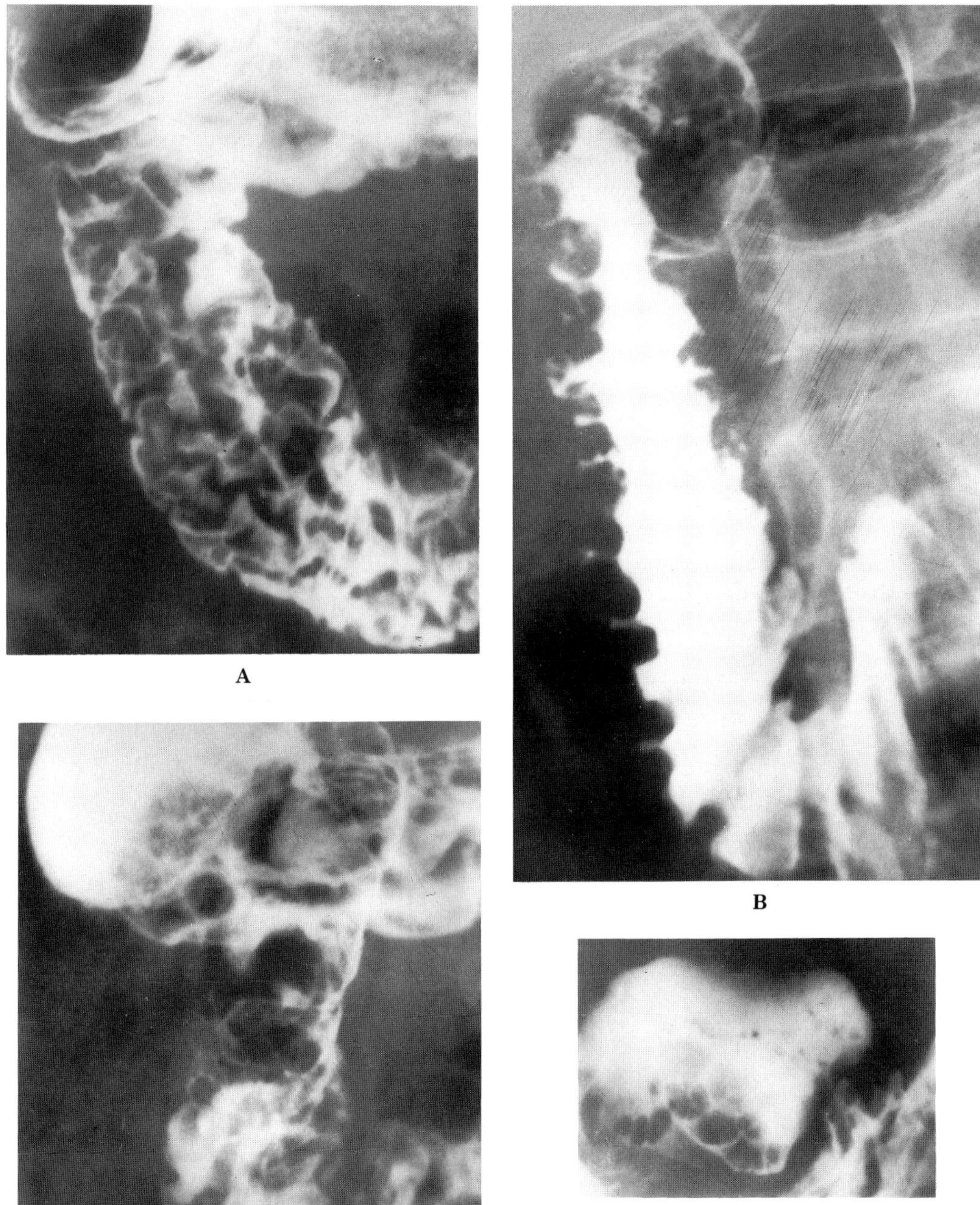

Figure 9.21. Duodenitis. (A) Widened folds with nodular lesions. (B) Thickened duodenal folds and erosions. (C) Nodular thickening of duodenal folds with multiple erosions. (D) Multiple erosions of the duodenal bulb near the greater curvature. Graded compression study.

TABLE 9.1. LESIONS PROTRUDING INTO THE DUODENUM

Enlarged Brunner's glands
Enlarged lymphatic follicles
Duodenitis
Polyps (adenoma, hamartoma, postinflammatory)
Varices
Celiac disease
Benign neoplasms
Malignant neoplasms

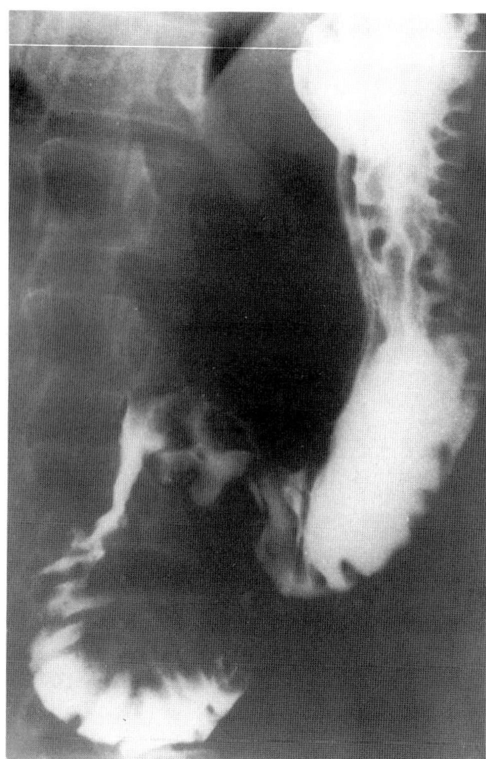

FIGURE 9.22. Crohn's disease. Stenosis of the duodenum with enlarged Brunner's glands. Primary involvement of the terminal ileum and colon.

GRANULOMATOUS INFILTRATION OF THE DUODENUM

The duodenum may be affected by Crohn's disease. Lesions are the same as in other segments of the digestive tube. The duodenum is particularly prominent in patients with extensive involvement of more distal segments of the alimentary canal. Initial changes of Crohn's disease, such as follicular lymphatic hyperplasia and aphthoid ulcers, finally culminate in deep longitudinal and transverse ulcers. Advanced phases are featured by strictures (Fig. 9.22).

Prolapse of gastric mucosa into the duodenum is discussed in chapter 8 (Fig. 9.23).

ENLARGED BRUNNER'S GLANDS

Brunner's glands are numerous in the submucosa of the suprapapillary portion of the duodenum, but their number is small in the distal duodenum. Brunner's glands may be enlarged due to hyperplasia, hypertrophy, or adenoma and are demonstrated as regular spherical projections of mucosa (Fig. 9.24). Radiologic methods cannot distinguish follicular lymphatic hyperplasia. In both conditions, the formations have been compared to buckshot. On barium studies, patients with atypical celiac disease may have hexagonal protruding defects in the duodenal bulb, up to 4 mm in diameter (Table 9.1). In addition, negative defects in the bulb may be due to ectopic gastric mucosa. *Genuine* defects of the duodenal bulb should be separated from prolapses of gastric mucosa. The latter are commonly reversible. Brunner's gland *adenomas* may be either solitary or multiple (Fig. 9.25). Giant adenomas have also been described exceeding 5 cm in diameter. *Mucocele* of a Brunner's gland is an extremely rare entity. It manifests as a soft tissue mass within the duodenal lumen.

PEPTIC ULCERS

In part, the etiology of peptic ulcer disease remains obscure. It has been firmly established that a duodenal peptic ulcer occurs only in the presence of HCl and pepsin, and gastric acid secretion is increased in a majority of affected patients. In contrast to a gastric peptic ulcer, duodenal peptic ulceration is accompanied by an increase of parietal cells in the gastric mu-

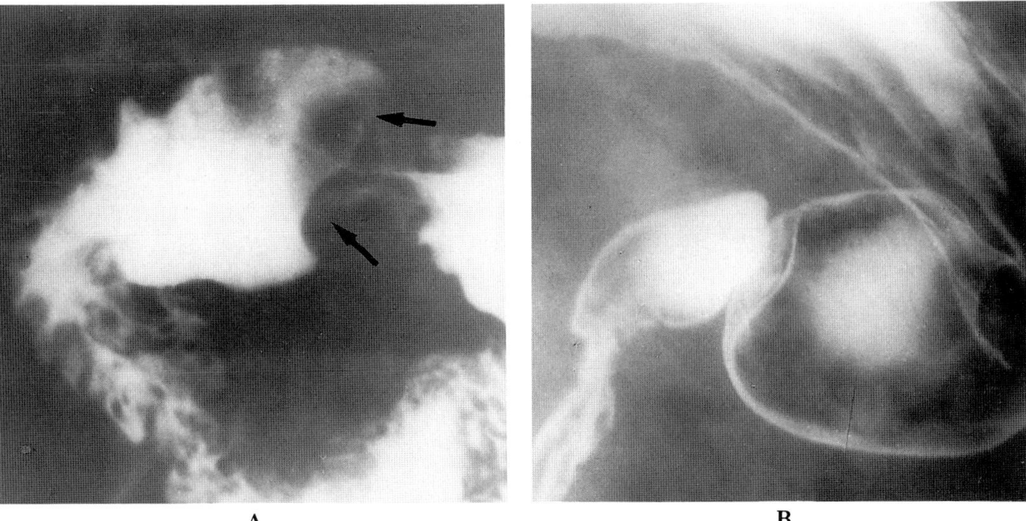

FIGURE 9.23. (A) Prolapse of the gastric mucosa into the base of the duodenal bulb (arrows). (B) Mucosa retracted back into the stomach.

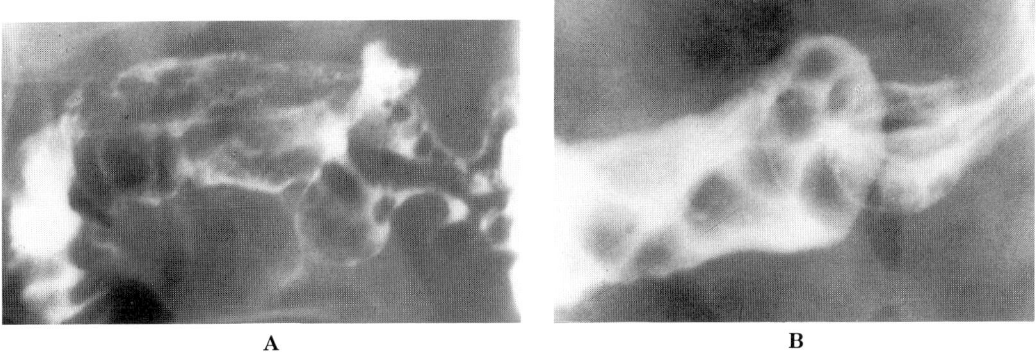

FIGURE 9.24. Enlarged Brunner's glands (A) with chronic peptic ulceration of the bulb and (B) in the duodenal bulb.

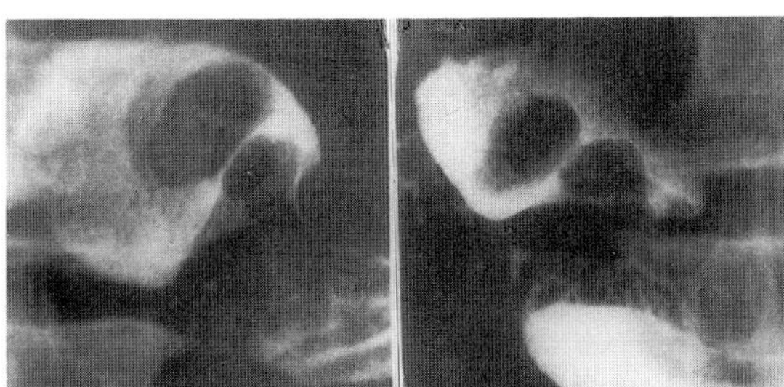

FIGURE 9.25. Two Brunner's gland adenomas in the duodenal bulb.

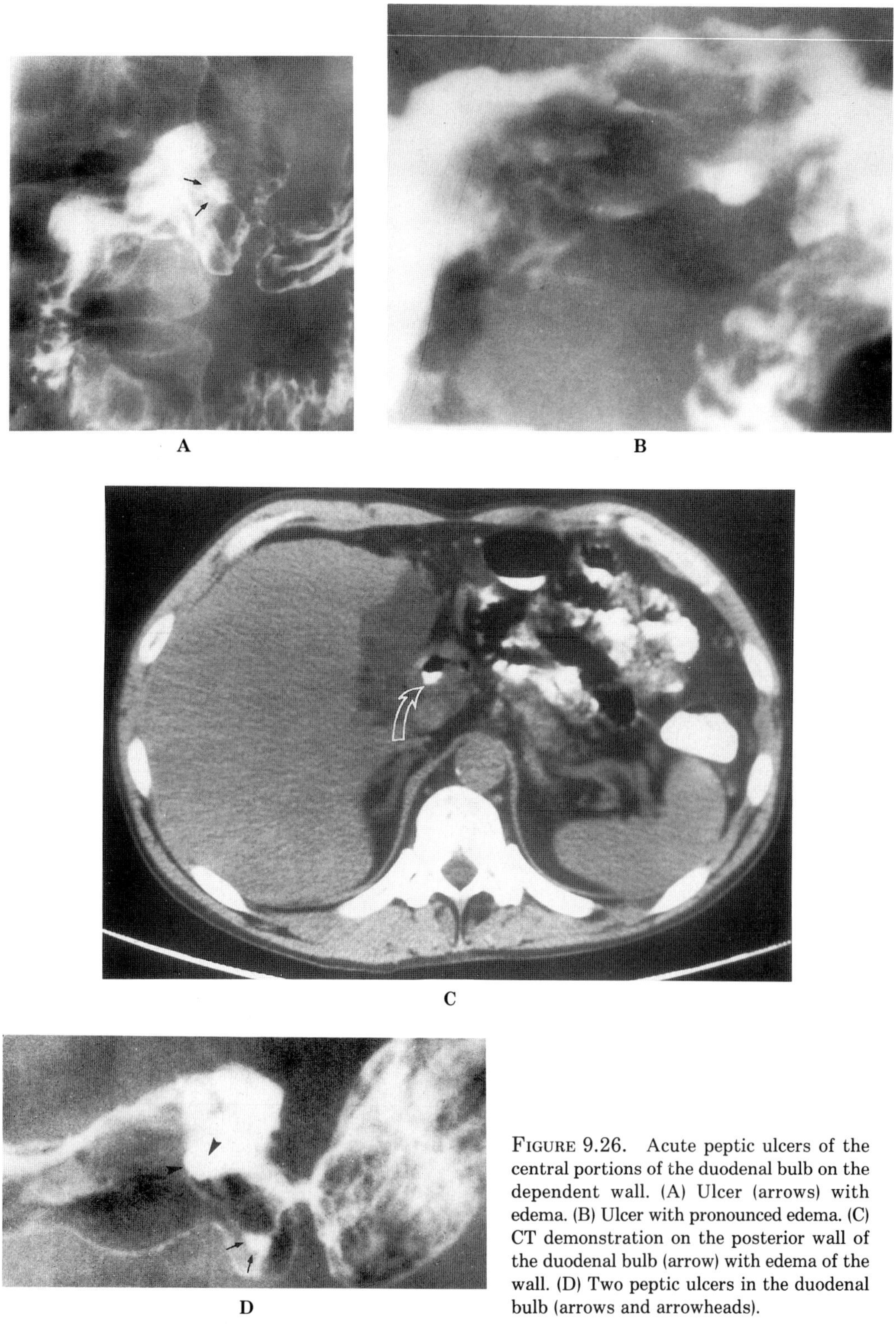

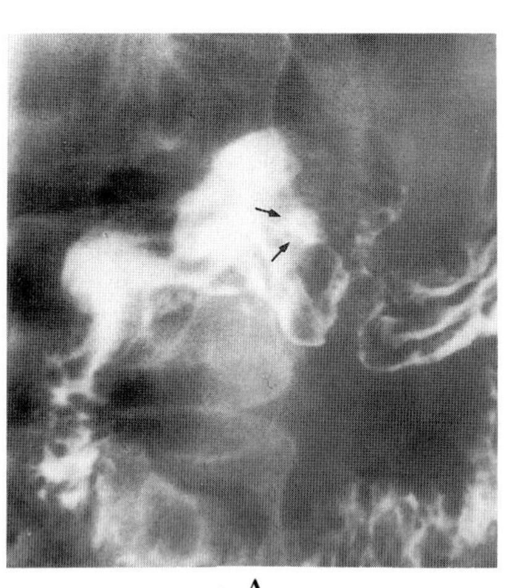

A

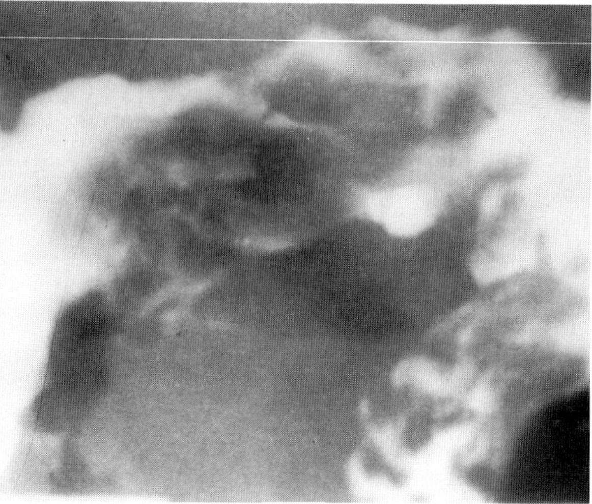

B

C

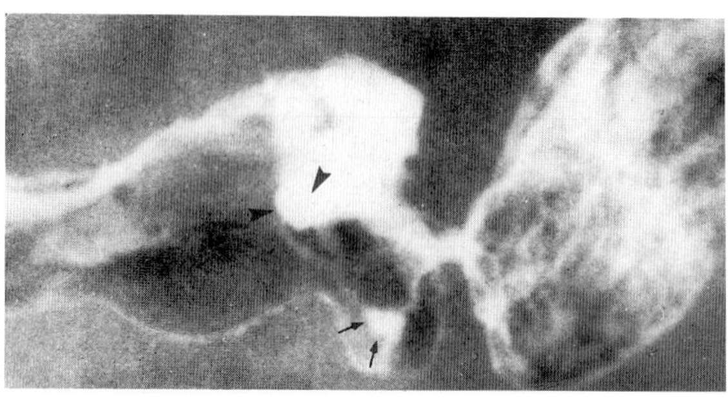

D

Figure 9.26. Acute peptic ulcers of the central portions of the duodenal bulb on the dependent wall. (A) Ulcer (arrows) with edema. (B) Ulcer with pronounced edema. (C) CT demonstration on the posterior wall of the duodenal bulb (arrow) with edema of the wall. (D) Two peptic ulcers in the duodenal bulb (arrows and arrowheads).

cosa. These parietal cells are the morphologic substrate for excessive secretion of HCl.

Duodenal peptic ulcer is almost three times as prevalent in family members of affected individuals as in an unselected population. Smoking is also a risk factor in duodenal peptic ulcer and, in addition, slows healing. Duodenal peptic ulcer is most often found in middle-aged patients, while gastric peptic ulcers are more often seen in the elderly. Pain caused by duodenal peptic ulcer occurs in the epigastrium about two hours after a meal and is relieved by food and antacids.

Approximately 95% of duodenal ulcers develop in the bulb. Pathologic changes evolve as follows: edema and infiltration, erosion, crater formation, and scarring. Scarring after a peptic ulcer is more pronounced in the duodenum than in the stomach. For this reason it is more difficult to monitor the evolution of a duodenal peptic ulcer than of a gastric peptic ulcer. Criteria for diagnosing gastric ulcers apply to duodenal ulcers as well. Duodenal peptic ulcer is featured by a crater deeper than the *lamina muscularis mucosae*. The crater is a direct radiologic sign of a peptic ulcer in any section of the digestive tube (Fig. 9.26). In contrast to a diverticulum, a mucosal fold never enters the niche of an ulcer nor does the ulcer change shape or size during the course of an examination (Fig. 9.27). The collection of barium remains constant. Separation of ulcers from "pseudodiverticula" (bulges of the wall adjacent to fibrotic change) is based on the same criteria. Namely, the duodenal wall adjacent to fibrotic change protrudes so as to resemble a diverticulum or large ulcer crater. However, unlike an ulcer, elasticity is preserved; therefore, pseudodiverticula change shape during an examination (Fig. 9.28). On single-contrast studies an ulcer presents as a positive defect in the barium column.

Interpretation of the double-contrast examination of an ulcer depends on whether the ulceration occurs on the dependent or nondependent wall. Oval and spherical ulcers seen *en face* on the nondependent wall are ring-shaped or crescent-moon-shaped collections of barium (Fig. 9.29). Dependent wall ulcers are demonstrated as barium accumulations (Fig. 9.30).

Duodenal ulcers are most frequently located in the center of either the anterior or posterior wall of the bulb. Duodenal ulcers may vary in dimension but most measure between 5 mm and 8 mm in diameter. An acute ulcer is often surrounded by a pale ring of edema (Fig. 9.26). Giant peptic ulcers of the duodenum exceed 2 cm in diameter and bleed quite frequently.

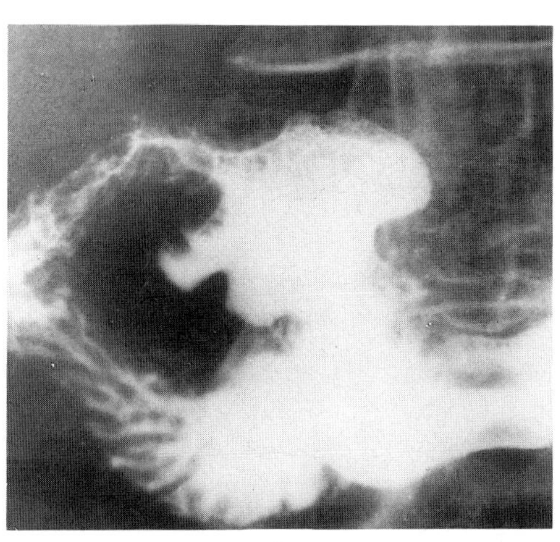

A

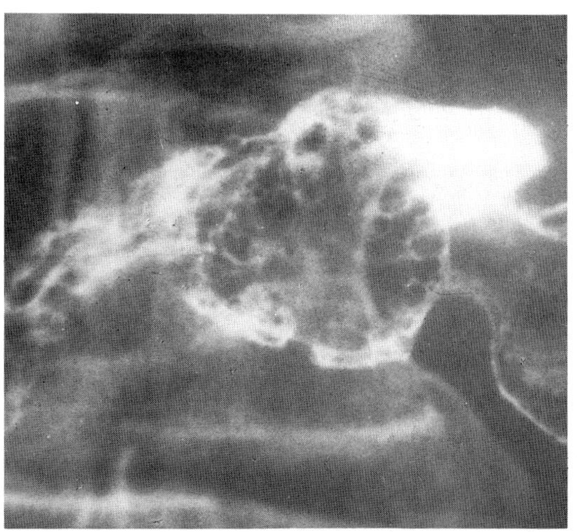

B

Figure 9.27. Transient diverticulum of the duodenal bulb. (A) Protruding from the greater curvature. (B) Diverticulum is not evident on the next film in the sequence.

They are sometimes misinterpreted as a deformed bulb or diverticulum. Giant ulcers are seldom amenable to medical therapy, and are frequently subject to complications.

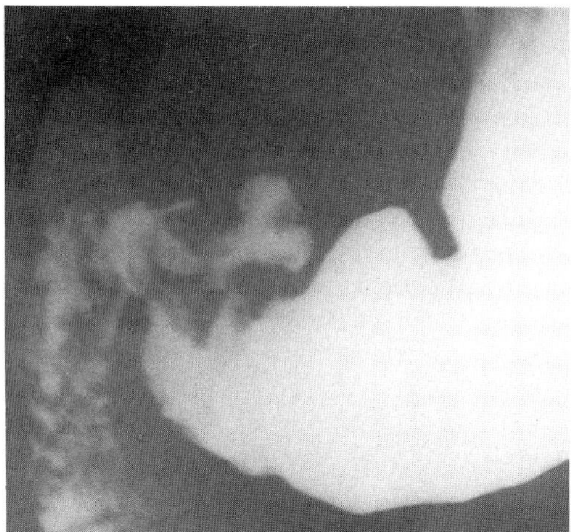

FIGURE 9.28. Deformity from scarring. Bulges of the duodenal bulb wall resemble an ulcer or a diverticulum. In contrast to ulceration, the deformity changes in dimension and shape during the examination.

Confidence in the diagnosis of duodenal peptic ulcer can be judged on three levels:

1. Low confidence. Barium collection seen in only one projection or appears to change in various projections.
2. Moderate confidence. Barium collection is visible in two or three projections.
3. High confidence. Barium collection is of constant shape and is seen in three or more projections.

In one study, when variabilities among examinees, ulcer dimensions, bulb deformations, and accuracy are taken into account, the overall positive predictive value in demonstrating duodenal peptic ulcers amounted to 57%. Individual predictive values among different radiologists varied between 47% and 70%. Higher sensitivity in the examination and interpretation of films is accompanied, as expected, by an increase in false-positive results and by a decrease in positive predictive value.

Since anterior and posterior walls of the duodenal bulb are seen in profile in a left anterior oblique position, this position is most suitable for the visualization of ulcers (see chapter 4, page 86). Ulcers on both lesser and greater curvature of the bulb are well demonstrated in

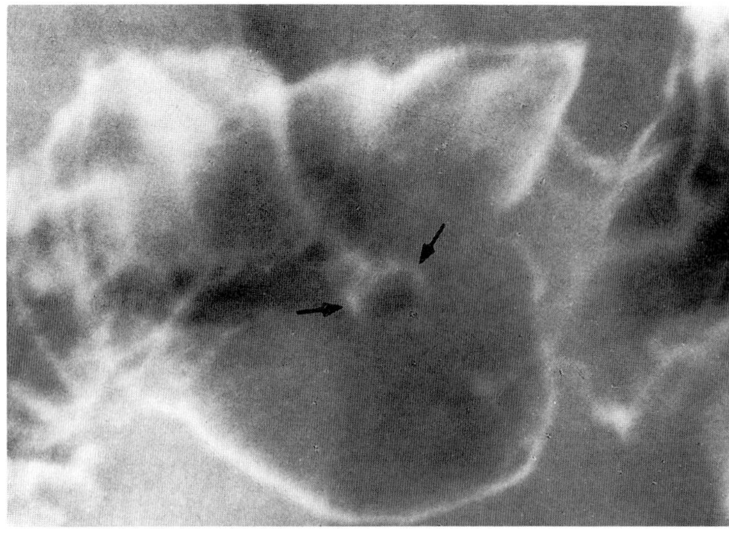

FIGURE 9.29. Peptic ulceration of the nondependent wall of the duodenal bulb presenting as a ringlike shadow empty of barium (arrows).

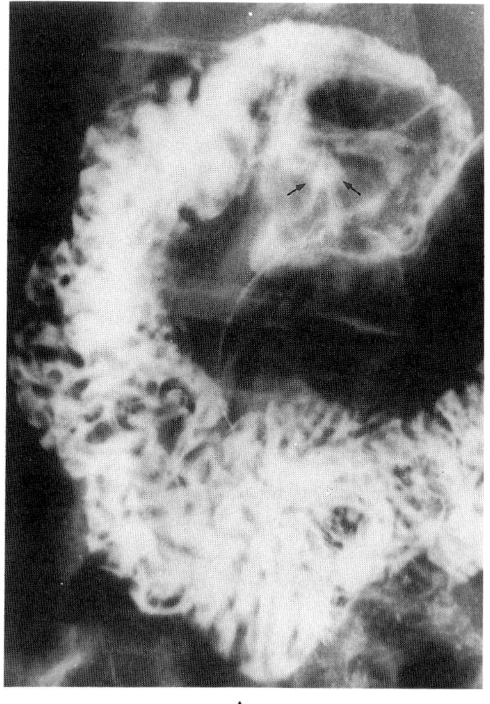

A

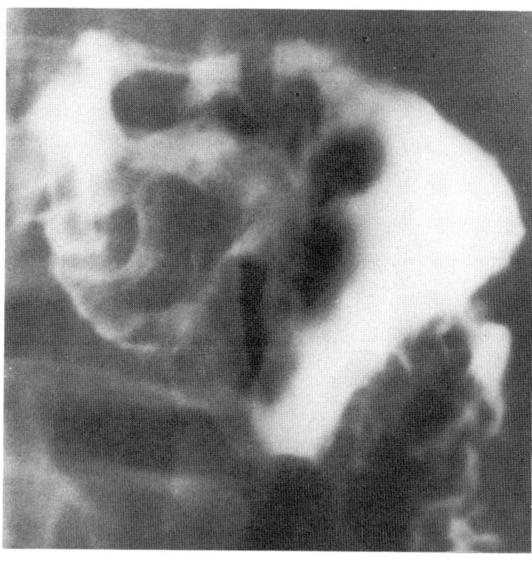

B

FIGURE 9.30. Chronic peptic ulcer of the bulb. (A) With converging folds (arrows). (B) With converging folds and edema.

a P-A position, or when the patient is slightly turned onto his left side (right anterior oblique projection).

Duodenal peptic ulcers may be either solitary or multiple (Fig. 9.26D). An acute duodenal ulcer often causes spasm of the pylorus and bulb; however, spasm may be absent. The shape of the bulb in patients with peptic ulceration may sometimes be very regular. A radiolucent defect at the bottom of the crater corresponds to a blood vessel or a clot within a bleeding ulcer.

A *chronic peptic ulcer* is surrounded by radiating mucosal folds (Fig. 9.30). During healing, fibrosis leads to bulb deformation (Figs. 9.28 and 9.31). The contour of the bulb is normally regular with the pylorus centrally placed at the base of the bulb. Irregularities of the duodenal bulb are, for the most part, consequences of scar formation, but may also be due to compression by adjacent anatomical structures or to spasm. Administration of spasmolytics enables a distinction to be made between deformities and spasticity changes. On a single-contrast examination, the most frequent cause of false bulb deformation is insufficient filling with barium. A truly deformed bulb can be pseudodiverticular-shaped. Sutures may leave permanent defects on the bulb (Fig. 9.32). Only appropriately cured shallow ulcers or first ulcerations can heal without deformity.

Peptic ulceration occurs twice as frequently in the duodenum as in the stomach. The ratio between males and females is four to one. The disease has a cyclic natural course with *recurrences* often appearing at the beginning and at the end of winter. Peptic ulcerations have the properties of a psychosomatic disorder. In newborns, duodenal ulcerations appear as a consequence of stress, although gastric ulcerations are more closely related to stress in adults. Ulcers occurring between the ages 1 and 15 years are probably etiologically and pathogenetically similar to peptic ulcers in adults.

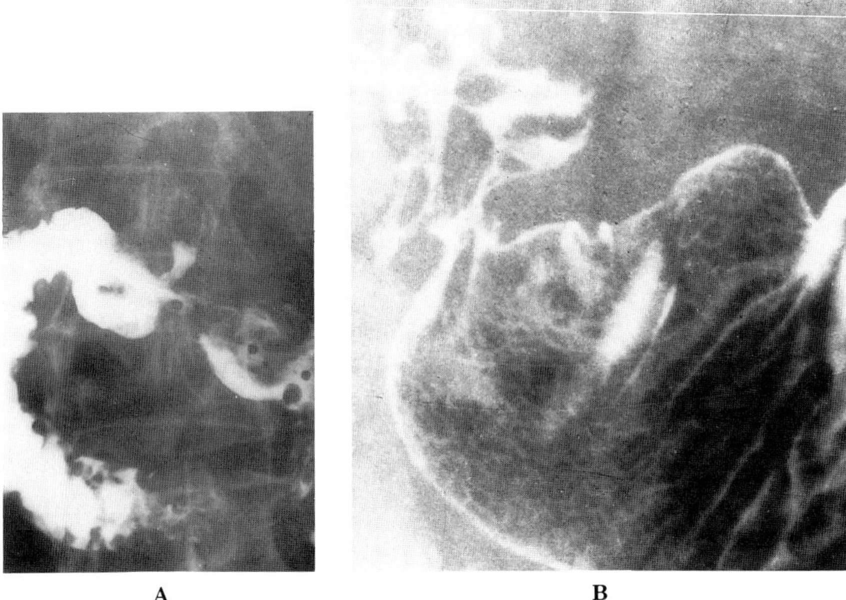

Figure 9.31. Postulcer deformity of the duodenal bulb. (A) On the lesser curvature. (B) Affecting the entire bulb.

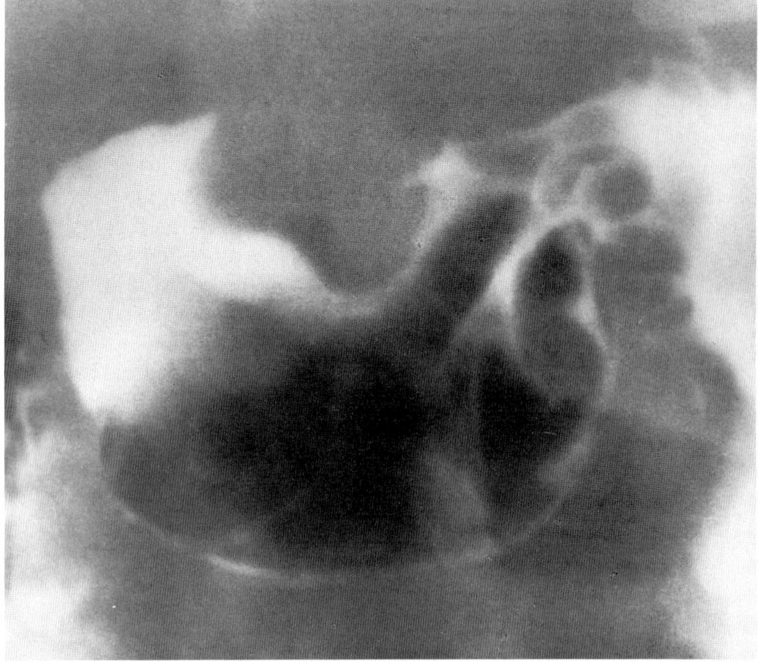

Figure 9.32. Suture ligation of a bleeding peptic ulcer results in deformity of the duodenal bulb.

Duodenal peptic ulcers do not undergo malignant alteration. Other complications, including bleeding, perforation, and obstruction are somewhat more frequent in the duodenum than in the stomach. The most common site of peptic ulceration is the anterior wall of the bulb. At the same time it is the most hazardous in regard to perforation. Signs of penetration are the same for both duodenal and gastric ulcers. The ulcer appears deeper than the apparent thickness of the wall. The crater may be filled with layers of barium, secretions, and gas.

POSTBULBAR ULCERS

Morphologic properties and clinical symptoms of postbulbar peptic ulcerations do not differ from those of bulbar lesions (Fig. 9.33).

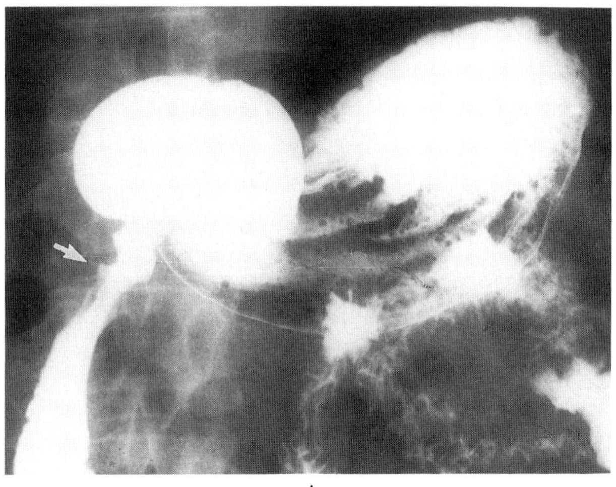

A

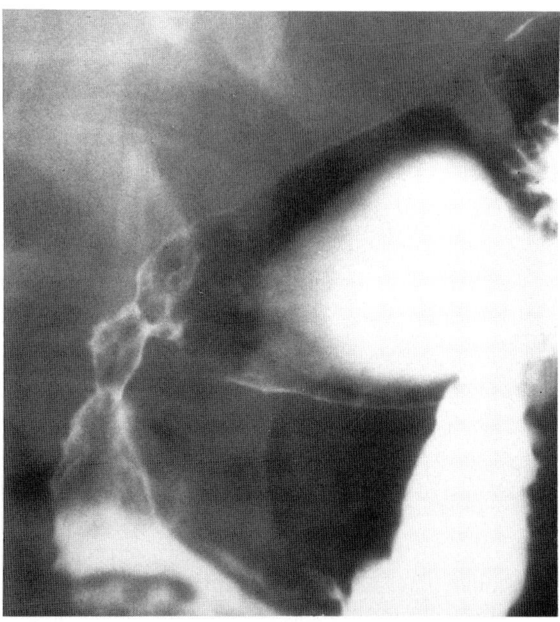

B

FIGURE 9.33. Postbulbar duodenal ulcer (A) on the convex aspect of the second segment (arrow). (B) Duodenal stenosis resulting from recurrent bulbar and postbulbar ulcers.

About 5% of peptic ulcers lie in the duodenum distal to the bulb, but peptic ulcers do not appear distal to the duodenal papilla. Postbulbar peptic ulcers are more often seen in patients with a short proximal duodenal segment. These are situated near the superior duodenal flexure, more frequently on the concave contour. Postbulbar ulcers bleed three times more often than bulbar, and between two and three times more often than gastric ulcers. This bleeding tendency can be attributed to the plentiful blood supply of the affected duodenal sections, as well as to deep ulcer craters.

DUODENAL HEMATOMA

Bleeding within the duodenal wall may be caused by blunt trauma or a tendency toward bleeding (thrombocytopathies, coagulopathies). Blunt trauma provokes bleeding in retroperitoneal, fixed duodenal sections. These segments cannot escape injury as well as mobile segments with an abundant mesentery. Approximately 70% of solitary duodenal hematomas result from blunt trauma. Separation of bleeding from morphologically similar pathologic changes, for example, lymphomas, is important.

There are various forms of bleeding within the intestinal wall:

1. Bleeding into the submucosa, characterized by truncated, widened duodenal folds (Fig. 9.34). Resultant transudate in the duodenal lumen dilutes the barium suspension.
2. Subserosal hematomas. These create oval, regular, and negative defects of the contrast column with distinct contours (Fig. 9.35). Circular folds are flattened or completely vanish.
3. Diffuse bleeding pervading all intestinal layers—a consequence of severe blood extravasation. "Aneurysmic" widenings of the intestinal wall, resembling lymphoma, appear as a result of a damaged intramural neural network.

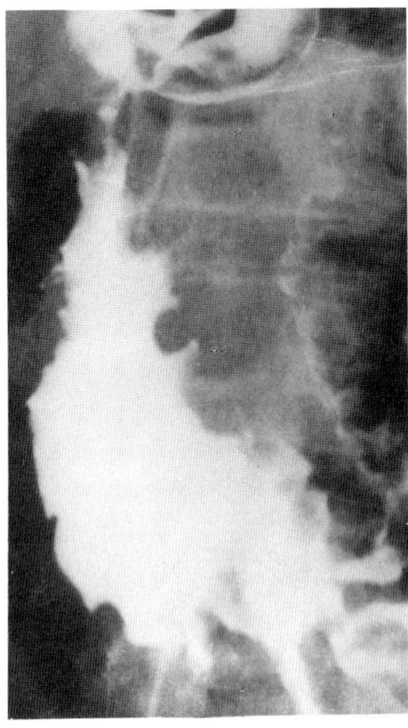

A

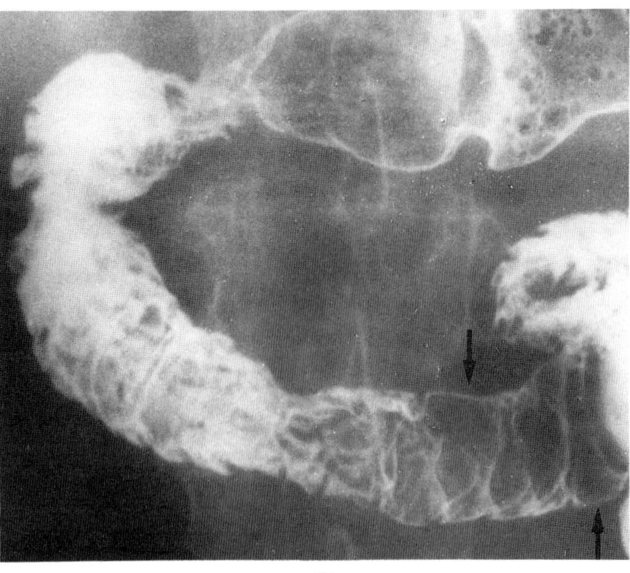

B

Figure 9.34. Hemorrhage into the duodenal wall. (A) Thickened duodenal folds. (B) Thickened folds in the distal duodenum (arrows).

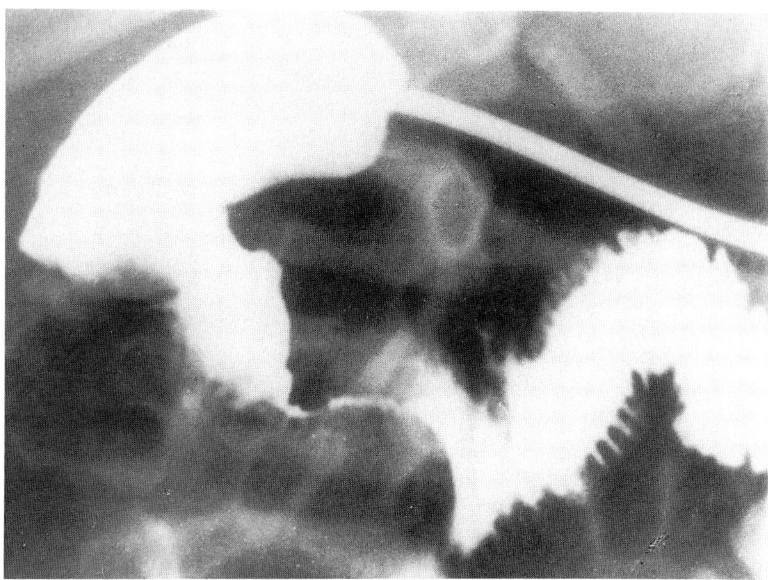

A

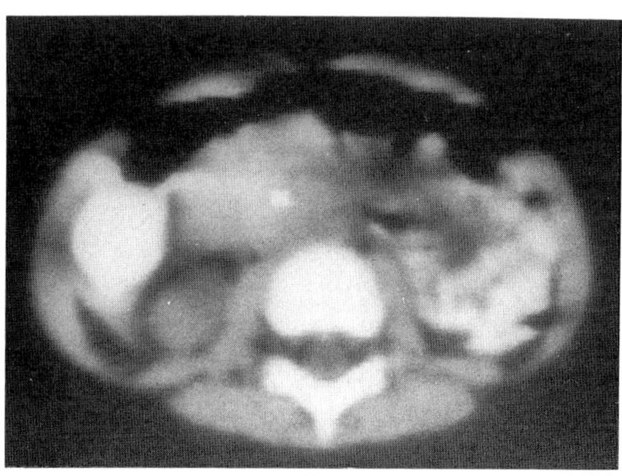

B

FIGURE 9.35. Large subserosal duodenal hematoma caused by blunt abdominal trauma. (A) Barium administered through the tube. (B) CT examination (cursor projects into the hematoma).

Unlike morphologically similar neoplastic lesions, hematomas are subject to resolution within several days or weeks. Therapy is therefore medical.

Radiologic findings in duodenal hematoma may resemble a coiled spring appearance. However, in at least one-third of patients with duodenal hematomas, radiologic findings are nonspecific.

At US, duodenal hematoma resembles pseudocyst of the pancreas. Differential diagnoses include cystic neoplasm, aneurysm, abnormality of the gallbladder, and perinephric abscess.

Computed tomography is more sensitive but less specific than US in diagnosing chronic duodenal hematomas. An acute hematoma has high attenuation values, whereas a chronic hematoma may closely resemble an abscess, necrotic tumor, or hemorrhagic pseudocyst of the pancreas.

Magnetic resonance imaging can accurately diagnose a duodenal hematoma. Three weeks after formation of a hematoma, the MRI finding will be specific. The lesion is seen surrounded by a ring with short T1 and long T2 relaxation time. Tissue-specific characterization can be demonstrated.

PROGRESSIVE SYSTEMIC SCLEROSIS

The duodenum affected by scleroderma has an intact mucosal surface and a widened lumen. Peristalsis is decreased; waves appear less frequently and have a lower amplitude.

Barium tends to stagnate in the duodenum. Similar signs may be present with superior mesenteric artery compression, metastases near the ligament of Treitz, adhesions, carcinoma of the pancreas, and Crohn's disease of the duodenum.

NEOPLASMS

Benign Neoplasms

Polyps of duodenal mucosa are not common, and are less common than prolapse of gastric polyps into the duodenum. *Adenomatous polyps* (Fig. 9.36) of the duodenal mucosa do not undergo malignant alteration and *adenomas of submucosal glands* are seldom seen (Fig. 9.25). Giant adenomas of Brunner's gland have been reported to cause symptoms of obstruction. When elevated, heterotopic gastric mucosa in the duodenum may resemble benign neoplasia.

Since clinical symptoms appear late, *leiomyomas* are usually diagnosed after they reach considerable size. They are spherical, hard in consistency, and clearly demarcated from the adjacent intestinal wall. These tumors are derived from the principal muscle layer and rarely from the muscularis mucosae. Because of hard consistency, duodenal peristalsis does not influence their shape (Fig. 9.37). The overlying mucosa may be ulcerated.

Hemangiomas and *lymphangiomas* are extremely rare in the duodenum and often appear as multiple submucosal tumors (Figs. 9.38 and 9.39). During peristalsis, the tumors seemingly diminish in size or even vanish because of the emptying of blood and lymph spaces, respectively. Since they cannot be mutually distinguished by radiologic means, distinction is made at endoscopy. Other benign mesenchymal tumors such as fibromas and lipomas are real rarities.

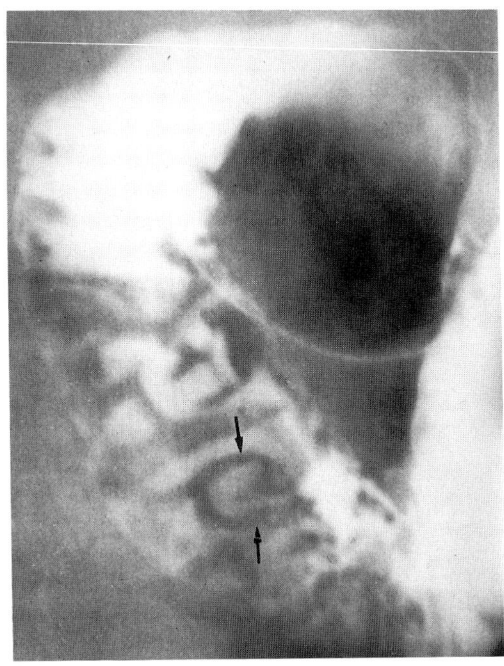

Figure 9.36. Polyp of the second portion of the duodenum (arrows).

Duodenal neoplasms should be radiologically distinguished from pseudotumors (hyperplastic gland, foreign bodies, etc.). The criteria for distinction of benign duodenal neoplasms from malignant are the same as in other sec-

Table 9.2. Duodenal Stenoses

Benign
Postulcerative
Recurrent pancreatitis
External compression (large diverticulum, enlarged pancreas)
Gallstone obstruction
Compression by superior mesenteric artery
Crohn's disease
Malignant
Carcinoma of the duodenum
Lymphoma (may also cause dilatation)
Pancreatic carcinoma
Metastases

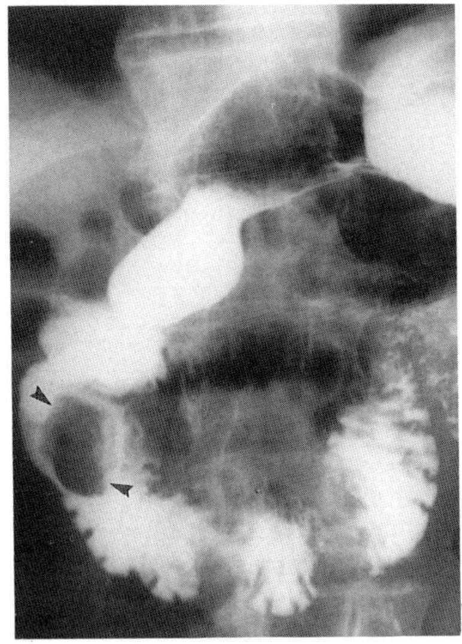

A

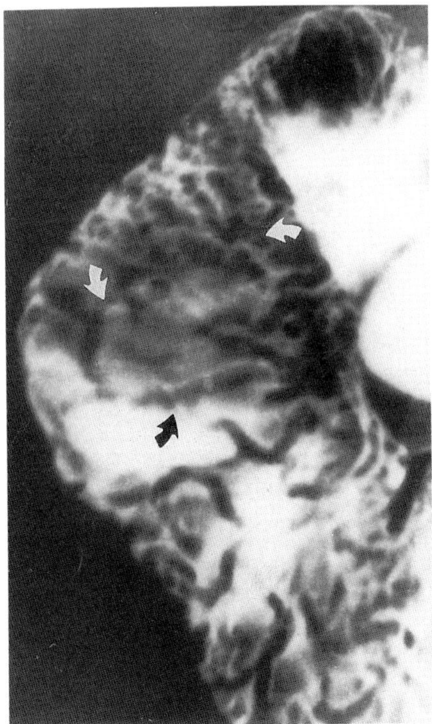

B

Figure 9.37. Leiomyoma of the second duodenal segment (arrowheads). (B) Leiomyoma of the posterior duodenal wall. Little mucosal change is caused by mainly extraluminal growth, resulting in faint radiographic defect (arrows).

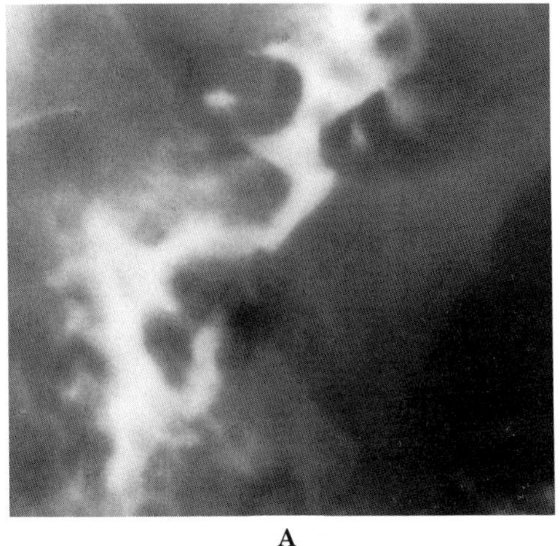

A

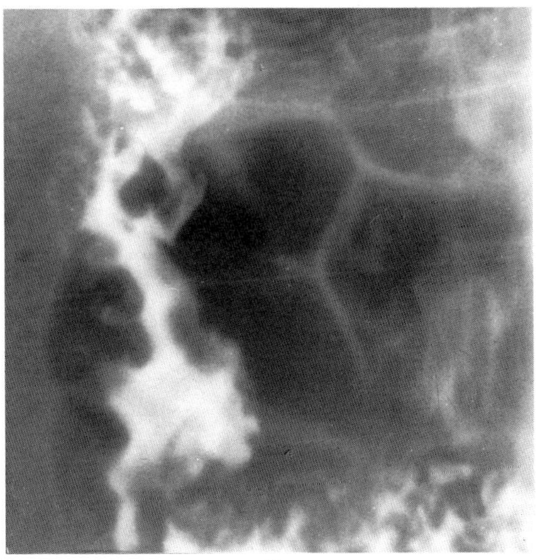

B

Figure 9.38. Duodenal hemangioma. (A) Masses protrude into the duodenal lumen. (B) Morphology changes on compression.

tions of the gastrointestinal tract. Malignant neoplasms destroy normal mucosal relief and create "shouldering" (Table 9.2).

Malignant Neoplasms

Malignant neoplasms of the duodenum are rare. *Carcinoma* occurs more frequently near the papilla (Figs. 9.40) and at the ligament of

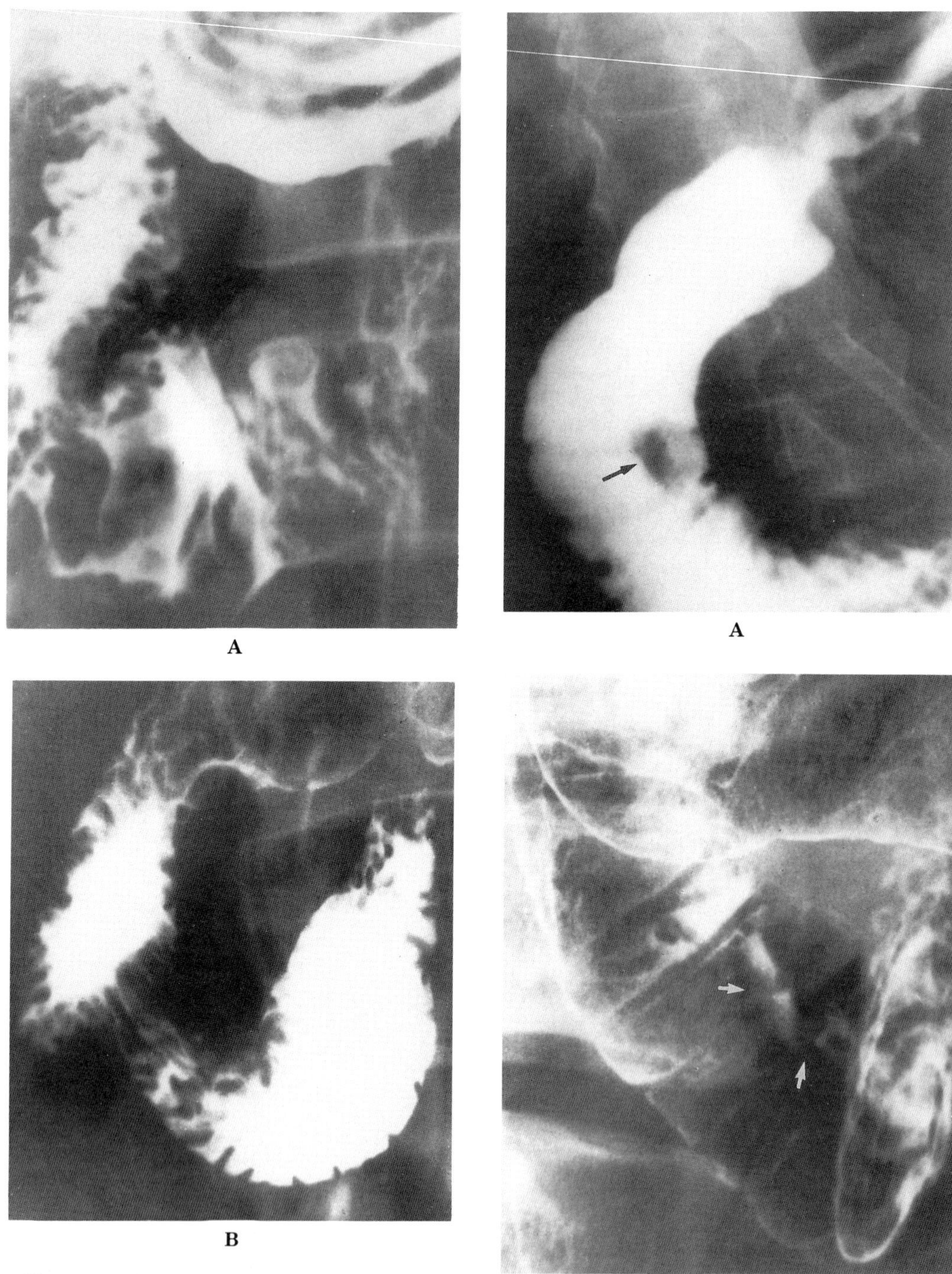

Figure 9.39. Duodenal lymphangioma. (A) Deformity of the third segment of the duodenum. (B) Deformity disappears with peristalsis. (Used by permission, Plavsic B, Jereb-Provic B. Radiologic and endoscopic diagnosis of duodenal angiomas. Acta Radiol Diagn. 1987;28:735.)

Figure 9.40. Polypoid carcinoma of the duodenal papilla. (A) Controlled compression study (arrow). (B) Double-contrast study in another patient (arrows).

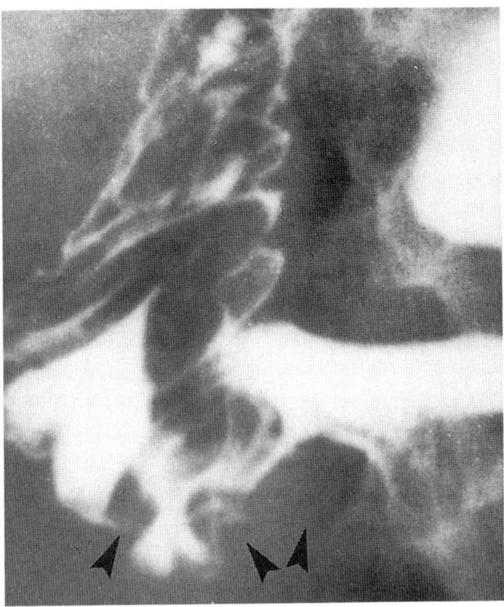

Figure 9.41. Polypoid carcinoma of the duodenum (arrowheads).

Treitz. Duodenal carcinomas most commonly assume one of three types of gross pathologic features: exophytic (Fig. 9.41), circumferential (Figs. 9.42), or volcano-like (ulcerated). As in other portions of the alimentary canal, however, combinations of these three basic types occur. Sometimes in advanced tumors it is impossible to attribute a particular tumor to a certain group. Ulcerated carcinomas are the most common. Carcinoma of the second segment of the duodenum may be suprapapillary, peripapillary, or intrapapillary. Duodenal carcinomas might be derived from heterotopic epithelium, such as choristomas of the pancreas and thyroid gland, or from gastric mucosa islets.

Carcinoma of the duodenal papilla (Fig. 9.40) is not of duodenal origin but originates from the epithelium of the bile duct or pancreatic duct. It is virtually impossible to radiologically distinguish duodenal carcinomas from other malignant tumors, benign neoplasms, or atypical granulomatous lesions. Separating duode-

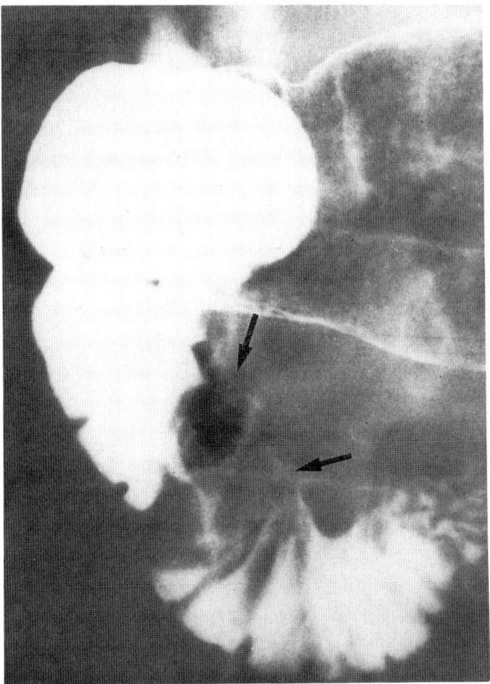

A

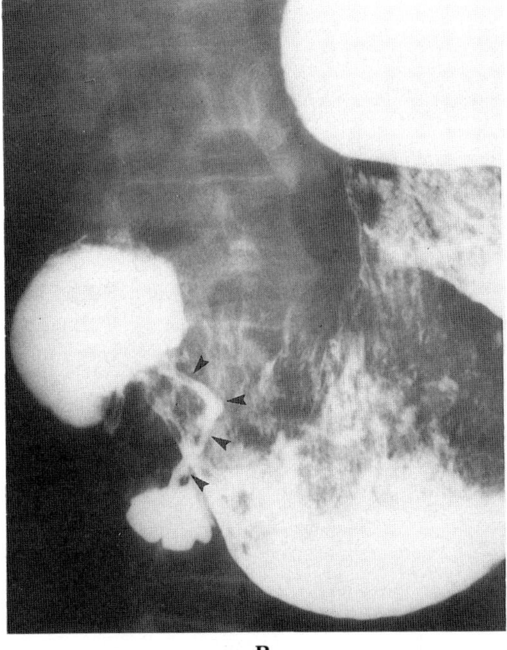

B

Figure 9.42. Annular carcinoma of the duodenum. (A) Affecting the inferior flexure (arrows). (B) Infiltrating the entire second segment (arrowheads).

nal carcinoma from pancreatic carcinoma, when the latter has penetrated the duodenal wall, may also be difficult (Figs. 9.17 and 9.45).

Cystic fibrosis of the pancreas may provoke radiologic signs similar to those of carcinoma of the second segment of the duodenum.

Carcinoids are rare in the duodenum. They may mimic either benign intramural submucosal tumors or ulcerated malignant neoplasms and metastasize into regional lymph nodes and liver. Patients bearing metastases may survive for a relatively long time, and patients without evidence of metastases often recover completely after surgical resection.

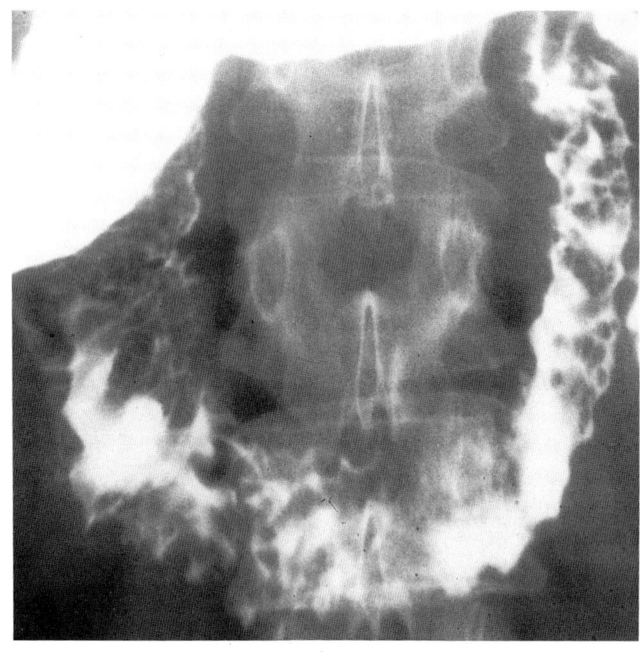

A

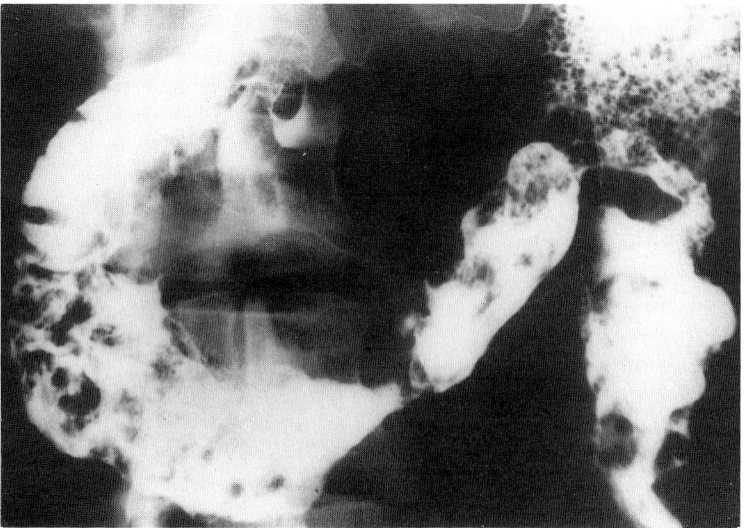

B

Figure 9.43. Lymphoma affecting the duodenum. (A) Nodular lesions with moderate distension of the lumen. (B) Masses protruding into the lumen with aneurysmal dilatations. The jejunum is also affected.

Lymphomas in the duodenum share morphologic features with similar tumors in the small intestine (see chapter 10). Radiologic findings depend on the mode of tumor growth. If the tumor is mainly intraluminal, numerous polypoid lesions are demonstrated (Fig. 9.43). Intramural growth is characterized by aneurysmal widening and a rigid duodenal wall. Lymphomas of retroperitoneal duodenal segments are difficult to remove by surgery. The overall prognosis is better with lymphoma than with carcinoma of the duodenum.

Leiomyosarcoma (Fig. 9.44) and other malignant mesenchymal tumors of the duodenum cannot be separated radiographically from other malignant neoplasms, except for lymphoma, which sometimes produces dilatation. Occasionally, leiomyosarcomas are difficult to distinguish from benign tumors. Malignant mesenchymal neoplasms may result from malignant transformation of benign tumors of the duodenum. Angiography demonstrates decreased vascularization of duodenal leiomyosarcomas compared to leiomyomas, which are usually smaller than leiomyosarcomas.

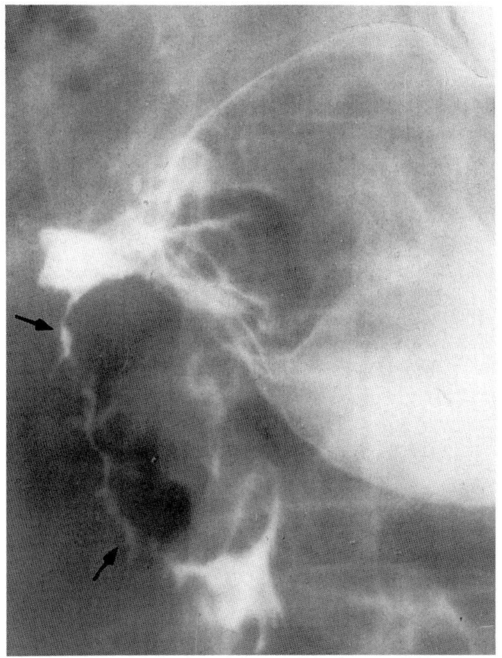

FIGURE 9.44. Leiomyosarcoma of the duodenum (arrows).

Metastatic neoplasms in the duodenum are not rare. In most instances, these completely resemble primary tumors (Table 9.2). Neoplasms of adjacent organs invading the duodenum are of about the same prevalence as primary malignant neoplasms of the duodenum. The latter may directly spread into the duodenal wall, and include pancreatic carcinoma (Figs. 9.17 and 9.45) and, less frequently, carcinomas of the biliary system, right kidney, and hepatic flexure of the colon. Carcinoma of the head of the pancreas can double the internal contour of the duodenal loop. In addition, it may form irregularities of mucosal relief in the duodenum, or stenosis of the duodenal lumen into a reverse "3" sign (Figs. 9.13 and 9.45). Carcinoma of the hepatic flexure of the colon may invade the duodenum destroying mucosal relief and creating stenoses. Rarely is the duodenum invaded by renal carcinoma. Magnetic resonance imaging and CT are helpful in diagnosing invasion of the duodenum by malignancies of adjacent organs. Only exceptionally is the duodenum a target for metastases of distant organs. This is most likely with melanoma.

DUODENAL PERFORATION

Approximately 10% of all perforations in the alimentary canal occur in the duodenum. Traumatic ruptures are caused by blunt trauma of the upper abdomen. As a rule the wall is lacerated at sites of duodenal fixation and cannot escape external compression. Unlike intraperitoneal ruptures, retroperitoneal perforation of the duodenum results in less pronounced clinical symptoms and physical findings. Air bubbles are demonstrated on plain abdominal films in one-third of patients with ruptures of retroperitoneal duodenal segments. These bubbles are often located near the psoas muscle or beside the kidneys, but may involve the mediastinum and even cause subcutaneous emphysema in the neck. If these findings are not observed on plain films, examination should be continued with water-soluble contrast medium.

DUODENAL FISTULAS

Duodenal fistulas are either internal or external. The latter may be postoperative or posttraumatic. Internal fistulas are pathologic communications with the biliary system after

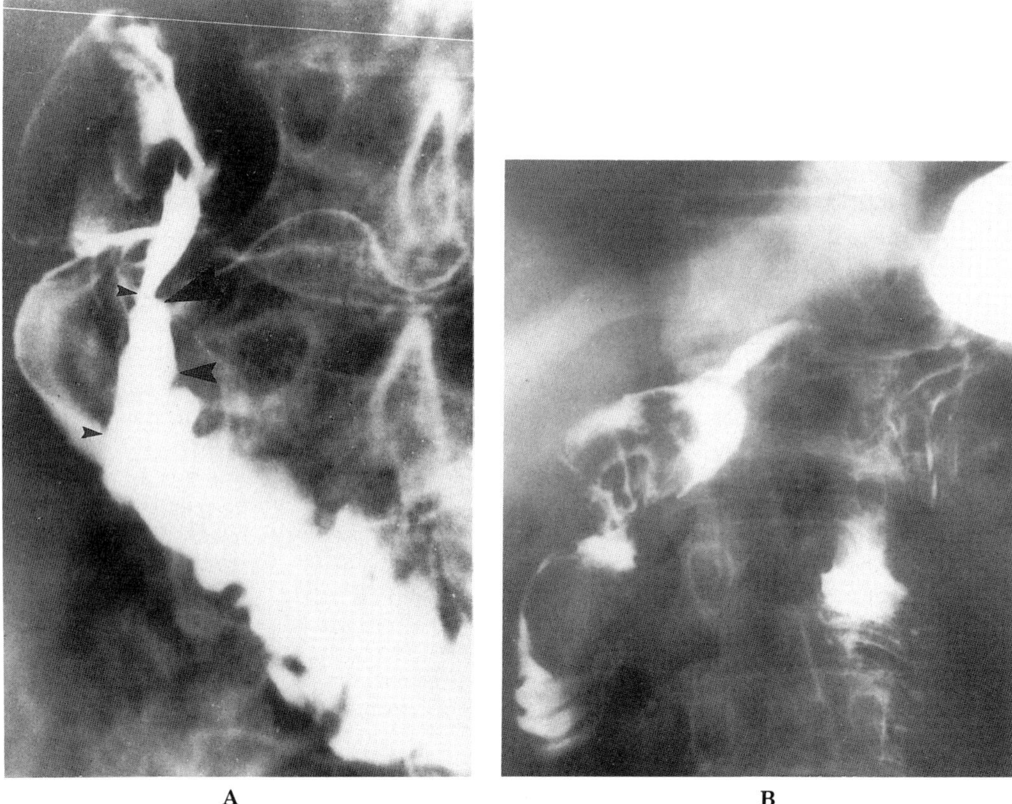

A B

Figure 9.45. Carcinoma of the pancreas infiltrating the duodenal wall. (A) Stenosis of the second portion (arrowheads). (B) Large masses protrude into the entire duodenum.

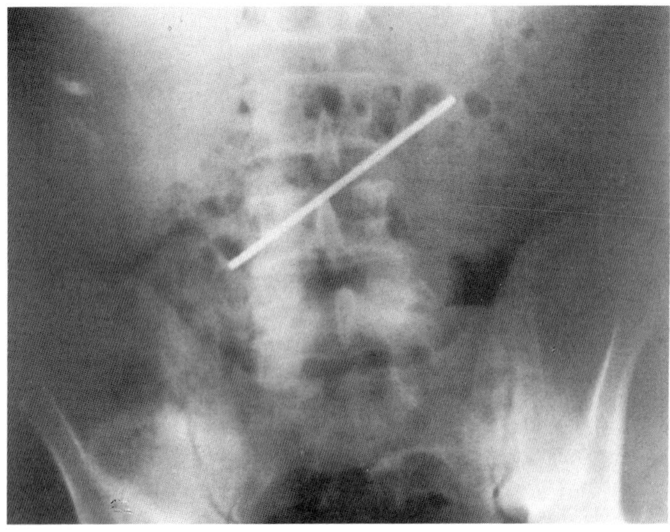

Figure 9.46. Swallowed welding rod. (A) Plain film.

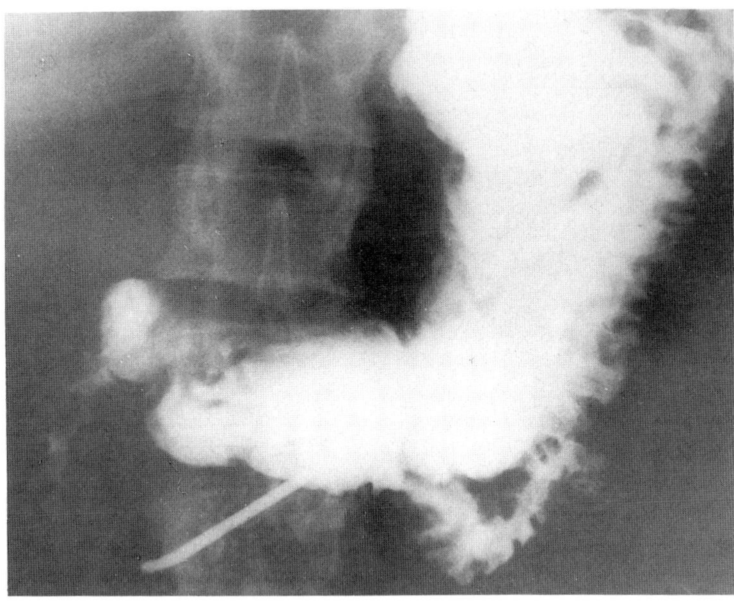

FIGURE 9.46 *continued.* Swallowed welding rod. (B) Water-soluble contrast medium localizes foreign body in the duodenum.

spontaneous expulsion of gallstones or after penetration of a peptic ulcer. Pneumobilia is seen on plain abdominal films. Because of its extremely low prevalence in the duodenum, Crohn's disease is unlikely to be the cause of fistula formation. Fistulas between the duodenum and the colon are, for the most part, created by infiltrating carcinoma of the colon (Fig. 11.49C).

FOREIGN BODIES

Foreign bodies enter the duodenum through the stomach (Fig. 9.46), or from adjacent hollow organs through a fistula. The pylorus rarely permits large foreign bodies to leave the stomach. Once in the small intestine, foreign bodies tend to lodge just proximal to the ileocecal valve, if they lodge at all.

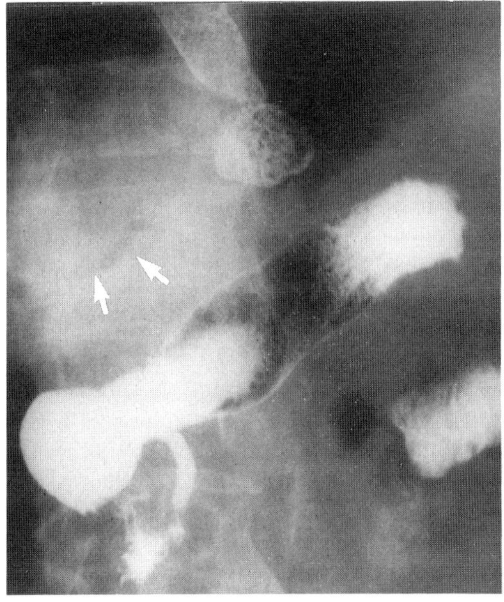

FIGURE 9.47. Common bile duct filled with barium on upper gastrointestinal series. Choledochoduodenostomy. Pneumobilia, gas in the biliary tree (arrows). Incidental gastric hiatus hernia.

THE POSTOPERATIVE DUODENUM

The common duct is sometimes demonstrated during upper gastrointestinal series following choledochoduodenostomy (Fig. 9.47). The anatomical relationships after removal of

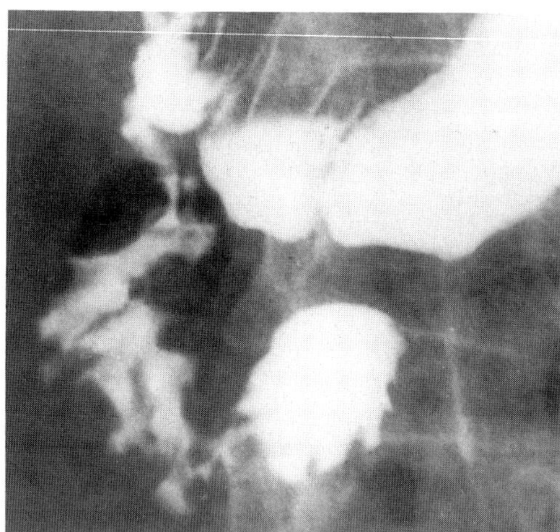

Figure 9.48. Surgery for pancreatic pseudocyst. Indentation of the second duodenal segment.

a pancreatic pseudocyst (Fig. 9.48) and after Whipple's operation are demonstrated in Diagram 8.12 and in Fig. 8.73.

Bibliography

Alberti-Flor JJ, Johnson AC, Dunn GD. Intraluminal duodenal diverticulum. Am J Gastroenterol. 1985; 80:500.

Anderson JR, Ernshaw PM, Fraser GM. Extrinsic compression of the third part of the duodenum. Clin Radiol. 1982;33:75.

Anderson JR, Mills J. Adult duodenal webs—a rare case of obstruction. Clin Radiol. 1984;35:223.

Akerlund A. Rontgenologische Studien uber den Bulbus duodeni mit besonderen Berucksichtigung des Ulcus duodeni. Acta Radiol. 1921;(suppl 1):1.

Berg HH. Die direkten Rontgensimptome des Ulcus duodeni and ihre klinische Bedeutung. Ergebn Med Strahlenfortschr. 1926;2:249.

Bergeg SN. Pseudotumors of the duodenal bulb. AJR. 1955;74:590.

Bergner LH, Gold E. Postbulbar peptic ulceration of the duodenum. Am J Gastroenterol. 1964;42:285.

Berman V, Goldberg MJ. Hyperplasia of Brunner's glands. Br J Radiol. 1950;32:241.

Brenner RL, Browk C. Primary carcinoma of the duodenum. Gastroenterology. 1955;29:189.

Cho KJ, Renter SR. Angiography of duodenal leiomyomas and leiomyosarcomas. AJR. 1980;135:31.

Clements JL, Roche RR. Carcinoid of the duodenum. A report of 6 cases. Gastrointest Radiol. 1984; 9:17.

Dodd GD, Fischer JS, Park OK. Hyperplasia of Brunner's glands. Report of two cases with review of the literature. Radiology. 1953;60:814.

Dodd GD, Nafis WA. Annular pancreas in the adult. AJR. 1956;75:333.

Faegenburg D, Bosniah M. Duodenal anomalies in the adult. AJR. 1962;88:642.

Felson B, Levin EJ. Intramural hematoma of the duodenum: a diagnostic roentgen sign. Radiology. 1954;63:823.

Fischer HW. The big duodenum. AJR. 1960;83:861.

Fisher JK. Mucocele of Brunner gland. Radiology. 1980;136:320.

Fontan AN, Rappaport M, Celeuer D, Piskorz E, Peralta CG, Rubio HH. Chronic nonspecific duodenitis (bulbitis). Endoscopy. 1978;10:94.

Gelfand DW, Dale WJ, Ott DJ, Wu WC, Kerr RM, Munitz HA, Chen YM. Duodenitis: endoscopic-radiologic correlation in 272 patients. Radiology. 1985;157:577.

Glaser GM, Margulis AR. Annular pancreas: etiology and diagnosis using endoscopic retrograde cholangiopancreatography. Radiology. 1979;133:303.

Gold RP. Medial indentation of the duodenal sweep by common bile duct dilatation. AJR. 1979;133: 233.

Gondos B. Duodenal compression defect and the "superior mesenteric artery syndrome." Radiology. 1977;123:575.

Gould RJ, Thorwarth WT. Retroperitoneal rupture of the duodenum due to blunt non-penetrating trauma. Radiology. 1963;80:743.

Gregg JA, Garabedian M. Duodenitis. Am J Gastroenterol. 1974;61:213.

Hahn PF, Stark DD, Vici LG, Ferrucci JT. Duodenal hematoma: the ring sign in MR imaging. Radiology. 1986;159:379.

Hayden CK, Boulden TF, Swischuk LE, Lobe TE. Sonographic demonstration of duodenal obstruction with mid-gut volvulus. AJR. 1984;143:9.

Jones B, Bayless TM, Hamilton SR, Yardley JH. "Bubbly" duodenal bulb in celiac disease: radiologic-pathologic correlation. AJR. 1984;142:119.

Jones WR, Davis JT, Hardy JD. Intramural hematoma of the duodenum: a review of literature and case report. Ann Surg. 1971;173:534.

Kaplan JW, Shepard RM. Prolapse of the gastric mucosa into the duodenum. JAMA. 1951;147:554.

Kirklin BR. A roentgenologic consideration of duodenitis. Radiology. 1929;12:377.

Kleinman PK, Brill PW, Winchester P. Resolving duodenal-jejunal hematoma in abused children. Radiology. 1986;160:747.

Langkemper R, Hoek AC, Dekker W, Op den Orth JO. Elevated lesions in the duodenal bulb caused by heterotopic gastric mucosa. Radiology. 1980; 137:621.

Lee CS, Mangala JC. Superior mesenteric artery compression syndrome. Am J Gastroenterol. 1978; 70:141.

Mandelson RM, Shepherd HA, Mitchell A. Inverted diverticulum mimicking an ulcerated duodenal tumor. Br J Radiol. 1984;57:426.

Marine R, Lattomus W. Cavernous hemangioma of the gastrointestinal tract. Radiology. 1958;70:860.

Nelson WI. Congenital diaphragm of the duodenum. Minn Med. 1947;30:745.

Ott DJ, Chen YM, Gelfand DW, Meshan I, Munitz HA, Kerr RM, Wu WC. Positive predictive value and examiner variability in diagnosing doudenal ulcer. AJR. 1985;145:1207.

Owen JP, Keir MJ. Duodenal loop widening in pancreatic diseases. Clin Radiol. 1978;29:635.

Peison B, Benisch B. Brunner's gland adenoma of the duodenal bulb. Am J Gastroenterol. 1982;77:276.

Phelan MS, Fine DR, Zantler-Munro PL, Hodson ME, Batten JC. Radiographic abnormalities of the duodenum in cystic fibrosis. Clin Radiol. 1983;34:573.

Plavsic B, Jereb Provic B. Radiologic and endoscopic diagnosis of duodenal angiomas. Acta Radiol Diagn. 1987;28:735.

Ritchie AC. Carcinoid. Am J Med Sci. 1956;232:311.

Scatarige JC, DiSantis DJ. CT of the stomach and duodenum. Radiol Clin North Am. 1989;27:689.

Stiennon OA. The anatomical basis for the epsilon sign of Frostberg. AJR. 1956;75:282.

Thompson WM, Cockrill H, Rice RP. Regional enteritis of the duodenum. AJR. 1975;123:252.

Vallance R, Peebles-Brown DA, Watkinson G. Duodenal ischaemia associated with atheromatous occlusion of the coeliac axis and superior mesenteric artery. Br J Radiol. 1983;56:136.

Weinberg PE, Levin B. Hyperplasia of Brunner's glands. Radiology. 1965;84:259.

Whitcomb JG. Duodenal diverticulum: a clinical evaluation. Arch Surg. 1953;88:275.

Wiot JF, Spiro E. Intraluminal diverticulum; a form of duplication. Radiology. 1963;80:46.

Chapter **10**

Radiology of the Small Bowel

The small bowel is the longest section of the gastrointestinal tube (5–6 m long). The surface area is extensive because of circular folds, intestinal villi, and microvilli on intestinal epithelial cells. This portion of the gastrointestinal tract is the most difficult to examine by radiologic means, and almost unapproachable by other methods. Since the small intestine is usually not completely emptied of chyme and mucus prior to examination, it is more difficult to interpret on subsequent roentgenographs.

In the distal small bowel, the lumen narrows and peristaltic movements are smaller in amplitude. The quantity of submucosal lymphatic tissue increases, as well as the amount of mucus in the lumen. Normal mucosal relief of the small intestine depends on contractions of lamina muscularis mucosae, hydration of the submucosa, and tone of the principal muscular layer. The width of the jejunum and terminal ileum varies from 2.5–3 cm and from 1.5–2 cm, respectively.

Although modern barium suspensions are relatively resistant to flocculation, prolonged close contact with the mucosal surface of the small intestine may cause unwanted flocculation of barium. For this reason, flow of barium during an examination should be accelerated for satisfactory demonstration of the internal surface of the small intestine.

The period of time measuring the passage of barium from the duodenum to the cecum is termed the *transit time*. In normal patients, it can normally vary from a half hour up to six hours. The *emptying time* of the small intestine is the sum of the transit time and the time required for complete evacuation of barium from the small intestine. The emptying time may be as long as nine hours.

Radiologic examination of the small intestine, when the transit time lasts more than four hours, yields poor results. The transit time may be shortened by the application of a large volume of diluted barium suspension, by adding ice to the contrast suspension, and by the use of drugs (see the section on pharmacoradiography, pages 78–80). Since the normal range is between a half hour and six hours, measuring transit time is of minor importance except in cases of extreme values. As barium may be retained in the stomach up to four hours, and as the range of the transit time is broad, simultaneous demonstration of the stomach and the entire intestine can be normal. Enteroclysis reduces transit time to only 10–15 minutes, and avoids any effect from differences in pH between the stomach and small intestine.

A plain abdominal film should be taken prior to barium administration. The barium suspension column in the small intestine is normally continuous. Attention should be paid to possible dilution or concentration of the barium suspension during the examination; however, concentration of barium in the distal ileum is a normal phenomenon (Fig. 10.1).

During fluoroscopic examination, the position and mobility of the intestinal loops are analyzed, as well as the width of the lumen and mucosal surface. The normal width of jejunal folds ranges from 2 to 3 mm. Pliability of the wall and peristaltic movements of the bowel should be observed, and pain on palpation

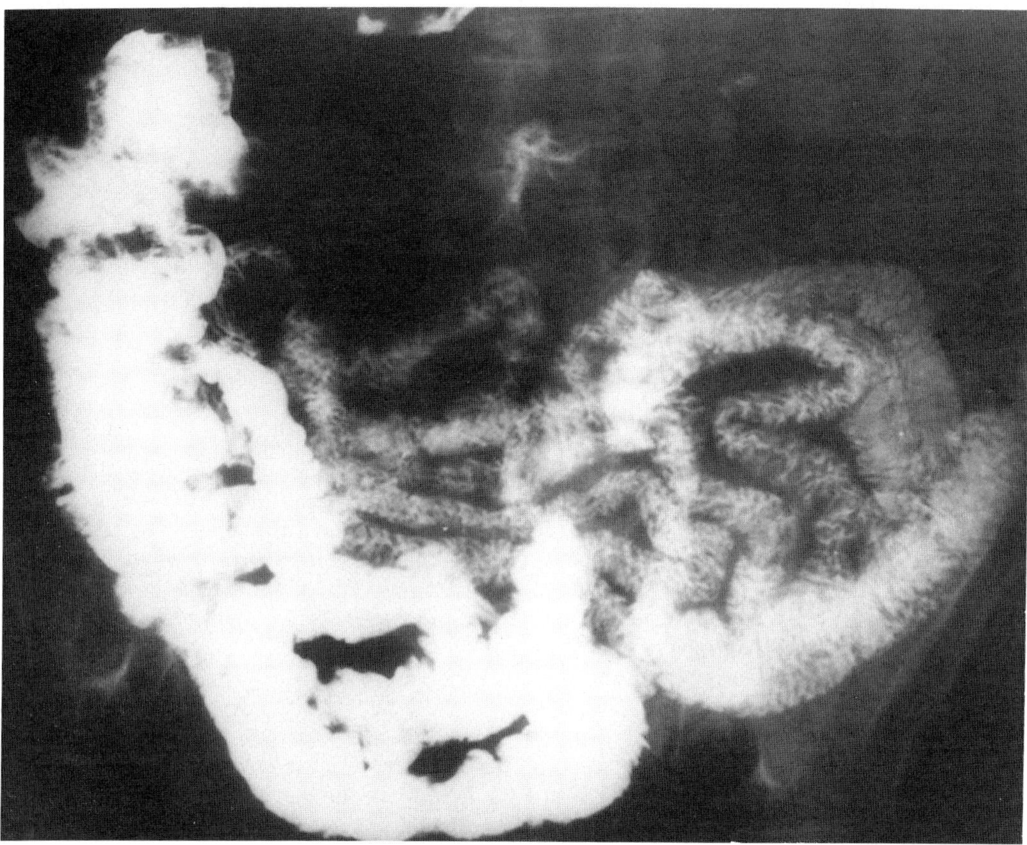

Figure 10.1. Follow-through small bowel study. Barium concentrated in distal small bowel and colon. Normal finding.

should be tested. Diseases of the small intestine may be diagnosed by observing abnormal contours and width of the lumen. The thickness of valvulae conniventes, their distribution and the possible presence of nodular changes on folds should be noted. Oral administration of barium does not convert a partial into a total bowel obstruction and therefore one should not hesitate to perform a small bowel follow-through examination in patients with partial small bowel obstruction.

FUNCTIONAL DISORDERS

The motility of the small intestine is estimated by measuring the transit time of a barium meal or radionuclide-labeled water. Manometry registers contractions, not propagation of contents.

As in other portions of the alimentary canal, the threshold of peristalsis is inversely proportional to muscular tone. Hypertonia and hypermotility are followed by a drop in the threshold of peristalsis and hurried transport of the small bowel contents. An increased volume of gastric contents also decreases the threshold of excitability and increases the amplitude of movements.

Spasm of individual intestinal segments is related to lesions such as inflammation, neoplasms, and foreign bodies. Parasympathetic stimulation may also provoke spasm of the small bowel.

Diffuse hypotonia of the small bowel accompanies intestinal malabsorption and hypothyroidism. However, the small intestine may be only segmentally distended. Causes of local distension may be either functional or organic. Organic causes include obstruction, lymphoma, scleroderma, amyloidosis, or intramural hematoma, among others (Table 10.1).

Ileus is characterized by a long-standing absence of intestinal motility. Contractions cease due to decrease of local and central reflexes. Stasis of intestinal contents results in the accumulation of gas and resultant dilatation of the bowel and stomach (see the section on ileus, page 154–157). Small intestine motility may be altered by diet, organic diseases of the alimentary canal, metabolic diseases, lesions of the central nervous system, psychological factors, and drugs.

Change in the dimensions of the mucosal folds, unless the mucosal pattern is altered, may result from differences in hydration between the mucosa and the submucosa and is also dependent on the tone of the principal muscular layer. Edema causes uniform thickening of mucosal folds.

GAS IN THE INTESTINAL LUMEN

The small intestine does not normally contain gas, with the exception of the duodenal bulb and terminal ileum. Moreover, the presence of gas in the lumen of the small intestine is of no pathologic significance in infants and bedridden patients. Apart from these situations, the presence of gas in the small intestine is considered abnormal. It may be caused by either obstruction, excessive air swallowing, ileus, or presence of gas-producing bacteria.

CONGENITAL ANOMALIES

The proximal three-fifths of the small intestine is jejunum and the remainder is ileum. The root of the mesentery extends from the duodenojejunal junction (ligament of Treitz) to the ileocecal valve. If embryological development is normal, the jejunum is located in the left upper and middle part of the abdomen, and the ileum is situated in the middle and lower, mainly on the right side of the abdomen.

Table 10.1. Causes of Dilatation of the Small Bowel

Causes
Distal obstruction
Nontropical sprue
Scleroderma
Pancreatic insufficiency with malabsorption
Lymphoma
Amyloidosis
Intramural hematoma

Aplasia and atresia of the small intestine are rare, particularly if there are multiple sites of involvement. A *duplication* may communicate with the main gut lumen. Noncommunicating duplication is referred to as an enterogenic cyst and exhibits signs of an extraluminal or submucosal mass on roentgenograms.

Malrotation

To understand the mechanism of malrotation, an awareness of the embryonic development of the alimentary canal is essential.

In *partial malrotation* the small intestine is located in the right hemiabdomen (Fig. 10.2) with the cecum in the right hypochondrium or to the left of the abdominal cavity. In *complete malrotation* (*mesenterium ileocolicum commune*), the colon is in the left and the small intestine in the right abdomen. There is a freely movable mesentery common to both small and large bowel (Fig. 3.6). Recognizing malrotation is important for the surgical approach to organs in the peritoneal cavity and, for example, in patients with atypical symptoms of appendicitis.

Diverticula

The prevalence of small intestinal diverticula at autopsy varies between 0.3 and 1.3%. The ratio of diverticula in the jejunum to those in the ileum is 3:1. Other data suggest that diverticula are seven times more common in the jejunum than in the ileum. The majority of small bowel diverticula are thought to be acquired.

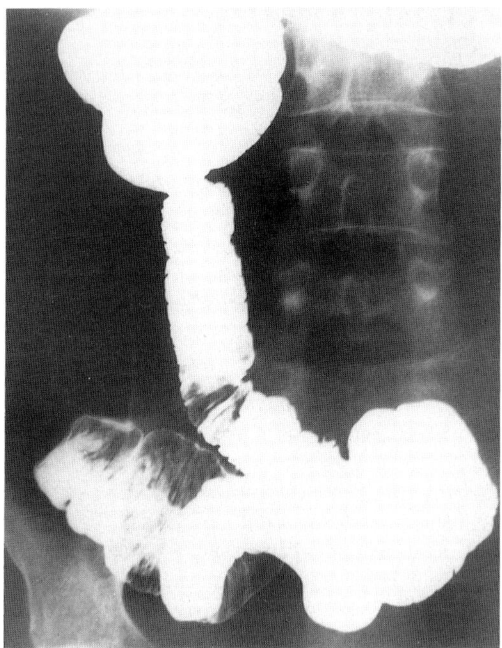

A

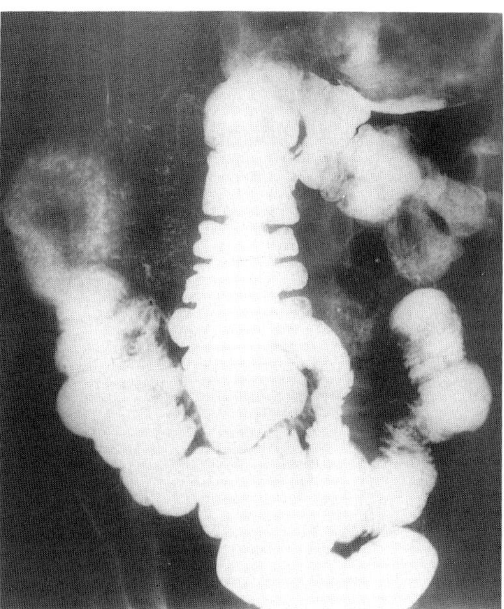

B

FIGURE 10.2. Partial malrotation. (A) Proximal jejunum is in the mid-abdomen. (B) Cecum and ascending colon in the mid-line. The small bowel is situated predominantly in the right hemiabdomen.

Enteroclysis, especially single-contrast enteroclysis, demonstrates diverticula more accurately than peroral barium studies. Diverticula are smaller in distal sections of the small intestine (Fig. 10.29). Unless complicated, they are clinically asymptomatic. Complications include diverticulitis, malabsorption, bleeding, and pseudo-obstruction (see the section on acquired diverticula of the small intestine, page 374).

Meckel's diverticulum, a remnant of the vitellinointestinal duct (Fig. 10.3), is located within 100 cm of the ileocecal valve. Meckel's diverticulum is an outpouching formation on the antimesenteric border of the small bowel. It may vary in size from a few millimeters in length and width to 10 cm in diameter. An autopsy series demonstrated a Meckel's diverticulum incidence of 0.2%. Unlike enteroclysis, follow-through examination rarely provides demonstration of Meckel's diverticulum. If covered by heterotopic gastric mucosa, it may be the site of peptic ulcer or adenocarcinoma. Ectopic gastric mucosa in Meckel's diverticulum is readily demonstrated by radionuclide studies (Fig. 4.90). Other complications of Meckel's diverticulum are bleeding, ulceration, perforation, intussusception, and volvulus. Approximately 2% of an unselected population have various remnants of the vitellinointestinal duct, including Meckel's diverticulum. Compli-

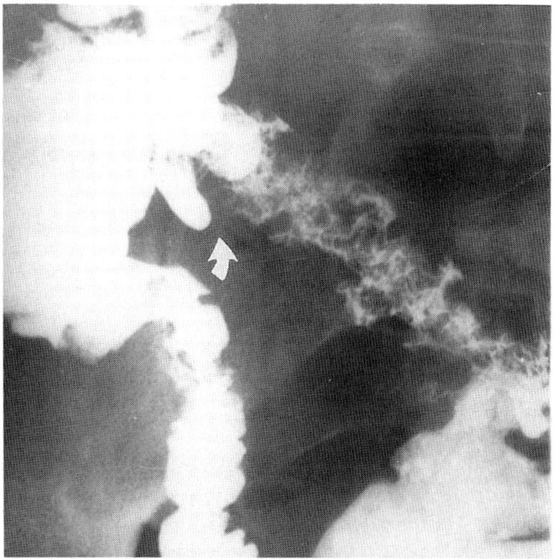

FIGURE 10.3. Meckel's diverticulum (arrow).

cations occur mostly in childhood, with bleeding and obstruction being the most common. With incomplete involution of the vitellinointestinal duct, a discrete solid band connects a Meckel's diverticulum to the umbilicus or gallbladder; its other end may even be free. This band may either compress the bowel, or cause a closed loop obstruction or volvulus. Obstruction is characterized by proximal distension of the bowel with gas-fluid levels.

ACQUIRED CHANGES OF SMALL BOWEL POSITION

A large volume of free fluid in the peritoneal cavity causes the separation of intestinal loops which appear as if they float, and have poorly defined contours.

A segment of small intestine may appear separated from adjacent barium-filled loops, as a result of a thickened mesentery such as occurs in Crohn's disease, lymphoma, and metastatic disease (Figs. 10.4 and 10.50). Pathology is suspected if a particular loop persists in position.

The position of intestinal loops may be altered due to extrinsic compression of adjacent anatomic structures. Gas in sections of the alimentary canal, or a mass such as a mesenteric cyst, may compress and displace the small intestine (Fig. 10.5). Large retroperitoneal masses also displace loops of the small intestine (Fig. 10.5C). The small intestine can be present in an internal or external hernia.

PNEUMATOSIS INTESTINALIS

Intestinal pneumatosis may occur in either of two forms, cystic or linear. Cystic intestinal pneumatosis is a disease of uncertain etiology. It affects both the small and large bowel and is often accompanied by stenoses of the gastrointestinal tract. Gas enters the intestinal wall through a defect in the mucosa. Bacterial growth is not likely to influence formation of cysts. Vesicles filled with gas may be seen on plain abdominal films as spherical transparencies. As a majority of cysts are subserosal, they do not significantly distort the contour of the barium-filled small intestine (Fig. 10.6).

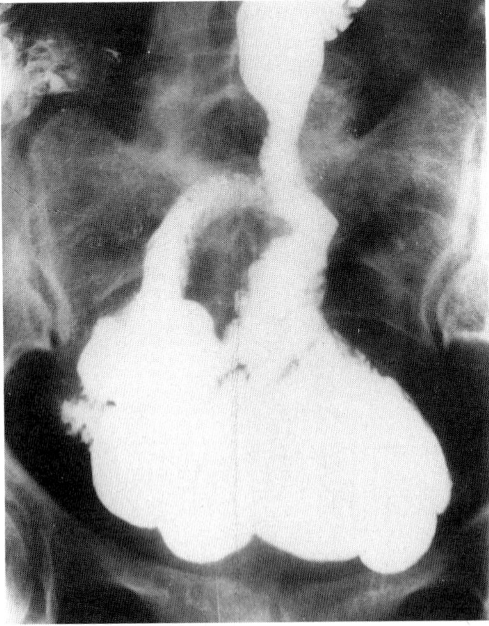

Figure 10.4. Lymphoma affecting the mesentery. Separated small bowel loops with identation of lateral contours.

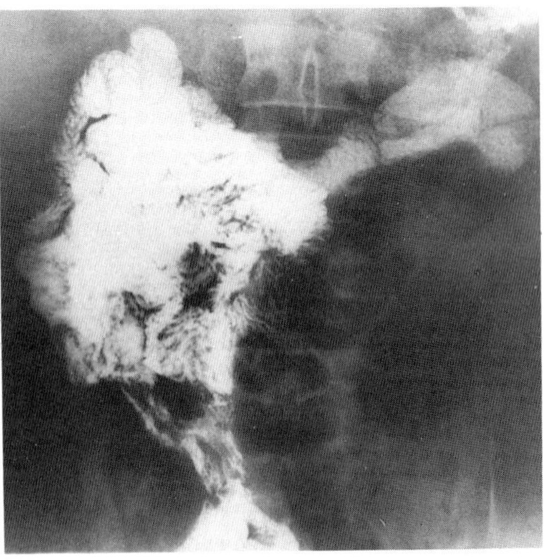

A

Figure 10.5. (A) Gas distended sigmoid colon displacing the small bowel.

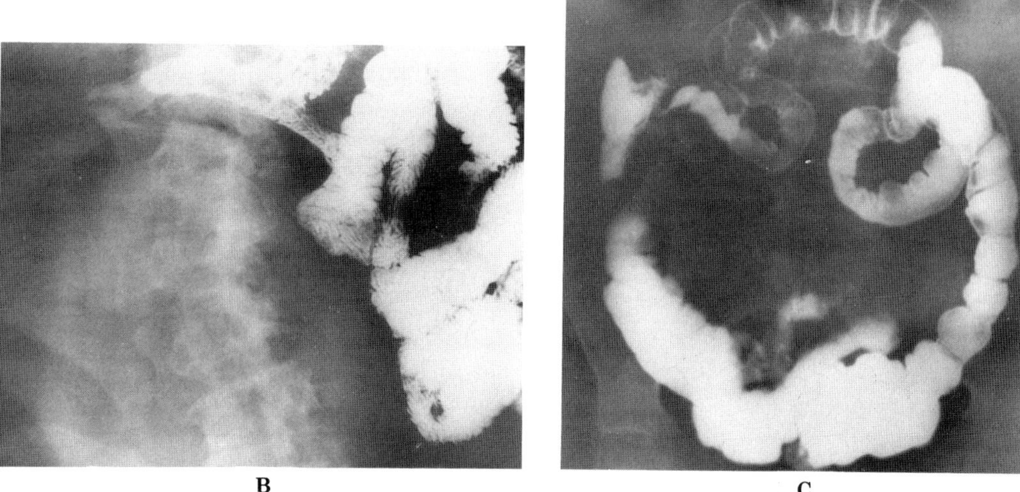

Figure 10.5 *continued.* (B) Gigantic mesenteric cyst displaces small bowel. Scoliosis of the spine. (C) Retroperitoneal and mesenteric lymphoma displacing the small and large bowel toward the periphery of the abdomen.

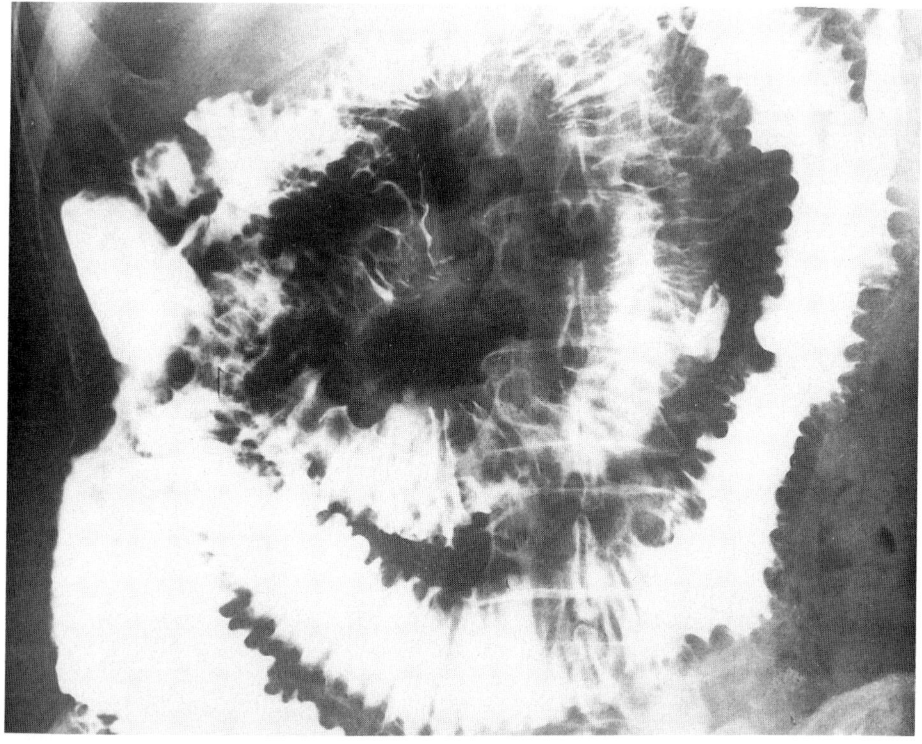

Figure 10.6. Pneumatosis intestinalis of the small bowel. Submucosal gas-filled cysts are evident.

When cysts are located deeper in the intestinal wall, distinction from granulomas or tumors is more difficult. Subserosal gas accumulations may perforate, resulting in pneumoperitoneum.

Both cystic and linear pneumatosis intestinalis develop in necrotizing enterocolitis and after abdominal surgery. Linear pneumatosis intestinalis may be an ominous sign resulting most commonly from intestinal ischemia. Transmural infarction, perforation, and peritonitis may result.

VARICES

Submucosal small bowel varices may be demonstrated in patients with portal hypertension by means of enteroclysis. They appear as serpiginous, sharply demarcated, inconstant filling defects. They are extremely rare in the small intestine; approximately 70 patients have been reported and almost all of them had portal hypertension. Varices may also occur in patients with occlusions of the superior mesenteric vein or as idiopathic varices of uncertain pathogenesis.

OBSTRUCTIONS

Alimentary tract obstructions most commonly occur in the small intestine, due to its narrow lumen and considerable length. *Complete obstruction* lasting 3–6 hours results in characteristic signs and symptoms (see the section on radiology of the acute abdomen, pages 147–154). *Partial obstruction* causes accumulation of gas and liquid proximal to the site of obstruction, but gas may also be seen in intestinal segments distal to the site of an obstruction. In partial obstruction, even large volumes of barium suspension do not increase the risk of conversion into a complete obstruction, and administration of barium is often followed by segmentation of the contrast column.

Meconium ileus occurs in infants with cystic fibrosis. The pancreatic ducts are dilated due to the accumulation of congealed secretions of abnormal composition. The impacted contents cause obstruction in the distal small intestine (Fig. 10.7). The mucosal surface of the small intestine is atrophic with narrow and shallow folds. Accumulation and stasis of se-

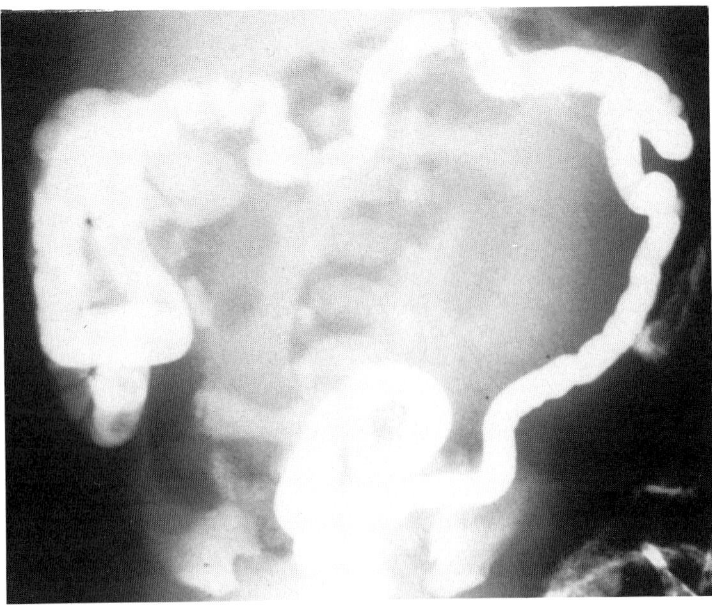

FIGURE 10.7. Meconium ileus. Microcolon is demonstrated by barium enema.

cretions in the respiratory system leads to atelectasis and pneumonia. Hyperosmolar contrast media such as Gastrografin have both diagnostic and therapeutic effects in patients with meconium ileus (see the section on radiographic contrast media, page 78).

Hernias often cause obstruction. External hernias are within the scope of physical examination, except diaphragmatic hernias which are best visualized by radiologic examination. External hernias include inguinal (Fig. 10.8A), obturator, umbilical, hernias through the linea alba, and diaphragmatic hernias. Unless obstructed, clinical symptoms do not occur. Intestinal loops filled with gas in the hernia sac indicate partial obstruction. When small intestinal loops in the hernia sac do not contain gas, and loops in the peritoneal cavity assume a reversed U-shape, with widened lumen and gas-fluid levels, the obstruction is complete and is caused by incarceration. Internal hernias occur when an intestinal segment protrudes into a recess in the parietal peritoneum. The small intestine may herniate into duodenal recesses, through the epiploic opening of Winslow into the lesser sac (Figs. 10.8B and C), or into paracecal or intersigmoid peritoneal recesses. Herniation into the pocket of Travers's space, between the ileocolic artery and its anastomosis with the last ileal artery, may occur. The most common internal hernias are paraduodenal hernias. Proximal small bowel loops are atypically placed in the epigastrium. Unless incarcerated, internal hernias are clinically asymp-

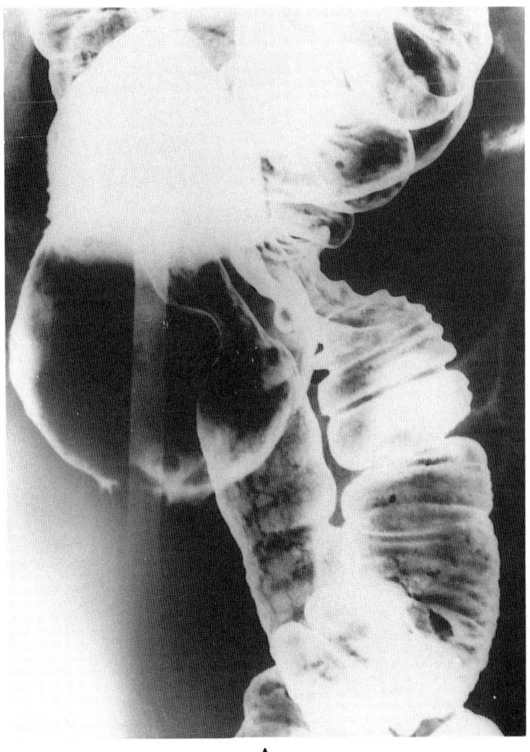

A

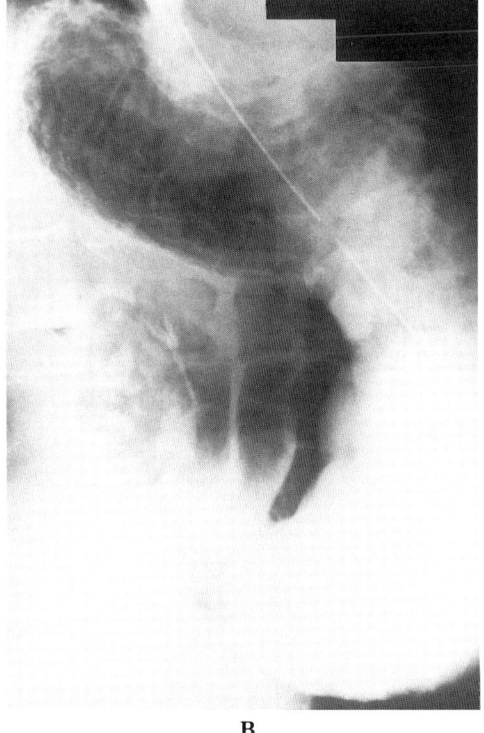

B

FIGURE 10.8. Abdominal hernias. (A) External hernia. Inguinal hernia of the small bowel. Double-contrast barium enema with filling of a portion of the small bowel. (B) Internal hernia. Herniation of the small bowel into the lesser sac. (*Figure continued on overleaf.*)

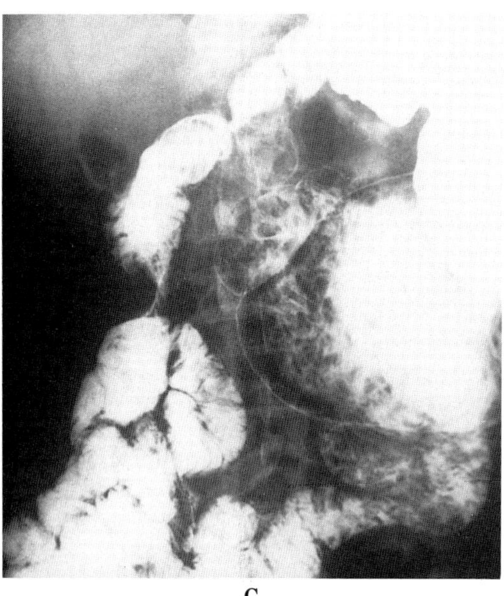

C

Figure 10.8 *continued.* Abdominal hernias. (C) Barium-filled small intestinal loops in the lesser sac.

tomatic, but an entrapped intestinal loop filled with barium may show decreased mobility on palpation.

Adhesions frequently cause both partial and complete obstruction of the small bowel. They may be congenital, postoperative, posttraumatic, or postinflammatory, and are demonstrated as radiolucent indentations (Figs. 10.9–10.12) or sharp angulations of the bowel, especially when the bowel is distended. Separation of intestinal loops by palpation may be impossible, and bowel motility may be decreased. Enteroclysis has proved to be effective in demonstrating both the level and cause of obstruction, whereas peroral examination may not clearly show adhesions. This is due to better distension by direct infusion of barium into the small bowel.

Obturations are caused by foreign bodies: enteroliths, gallstones, and matted balls of ascarids. Gallstones may penetrate into the duodenum or, less frequently, into the hepatic flexure of the colon (Fig. 10.13), and, if large enough, may obstruct the intestinal lumen. Af-

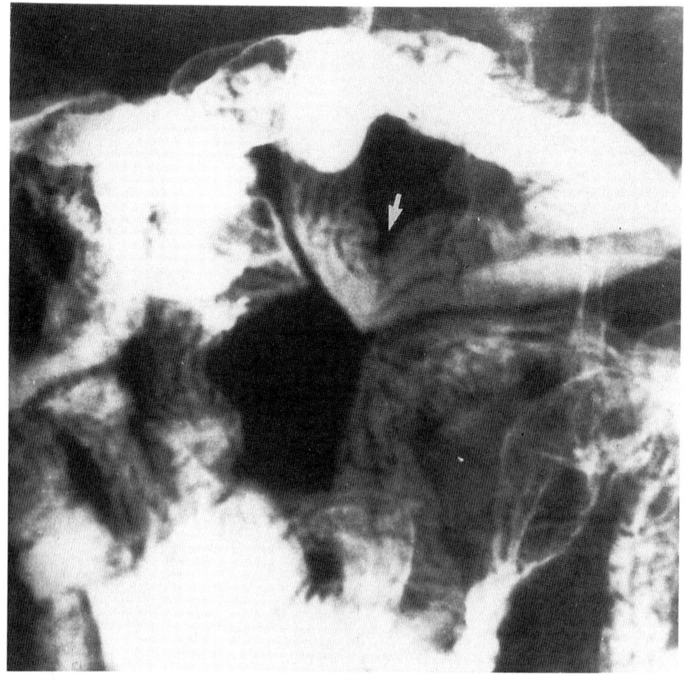

A

Figure 10.9. (A) Small bowel loop fixed by adhesion (arrow).

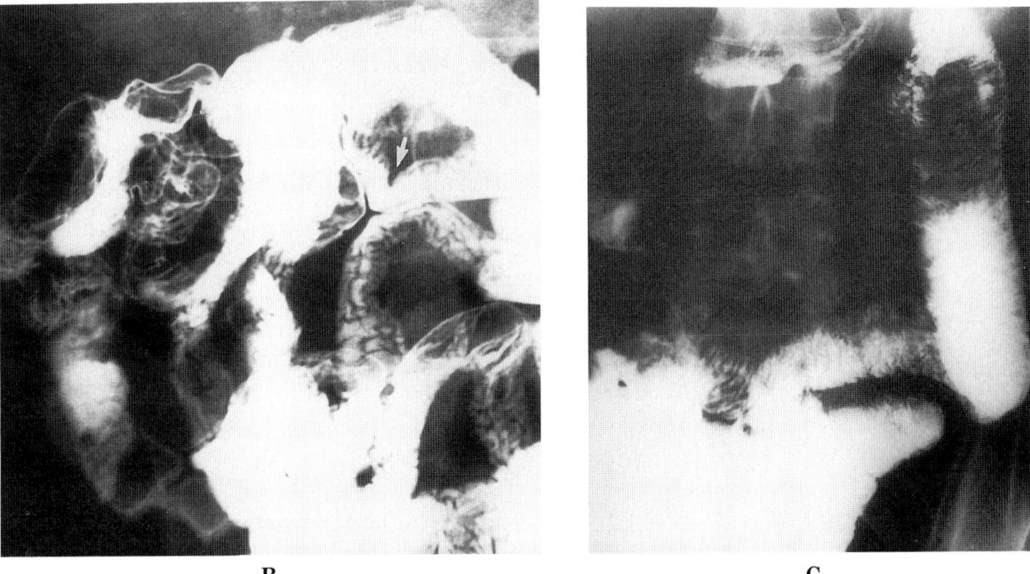

B C

FIGURE 10.9 *continued.* (B) Constant finding on follow-up film (arrow). (C) Partial obstruction resulting from adhesions. Dilatation of the intestinal lumen proximal to obstruction, with barium past the site of partial obstruction.

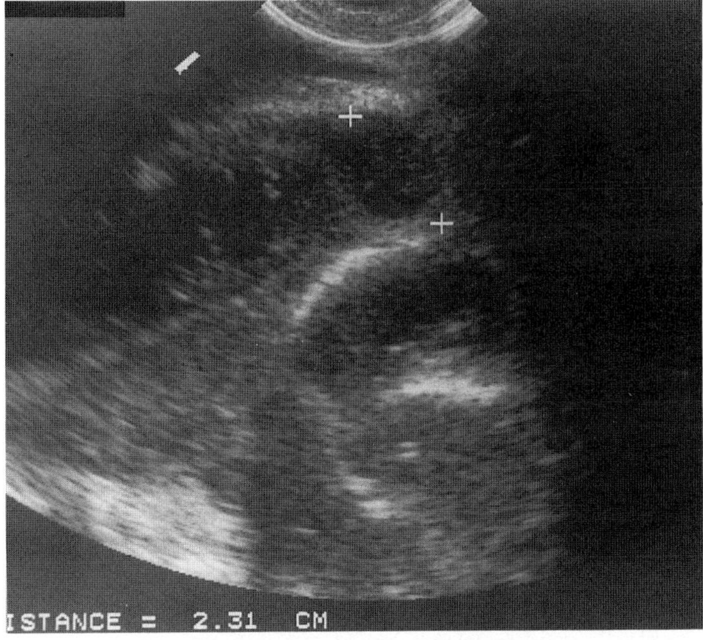

FIGURE 10.10. Ultrasound examination of thick-walled, small bowel loop distended from surgical adhesions, with bowel infarct. (Courtesy of W.L. Wells, MD, Louisiana State University, New Orleans.)

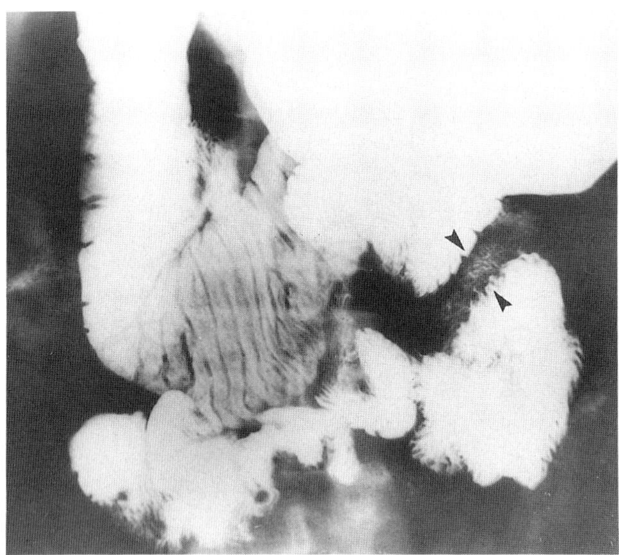

Figure 10.11. Linear transparency caused by adhesion (arrowheads). Significant proximal distension of bowel.

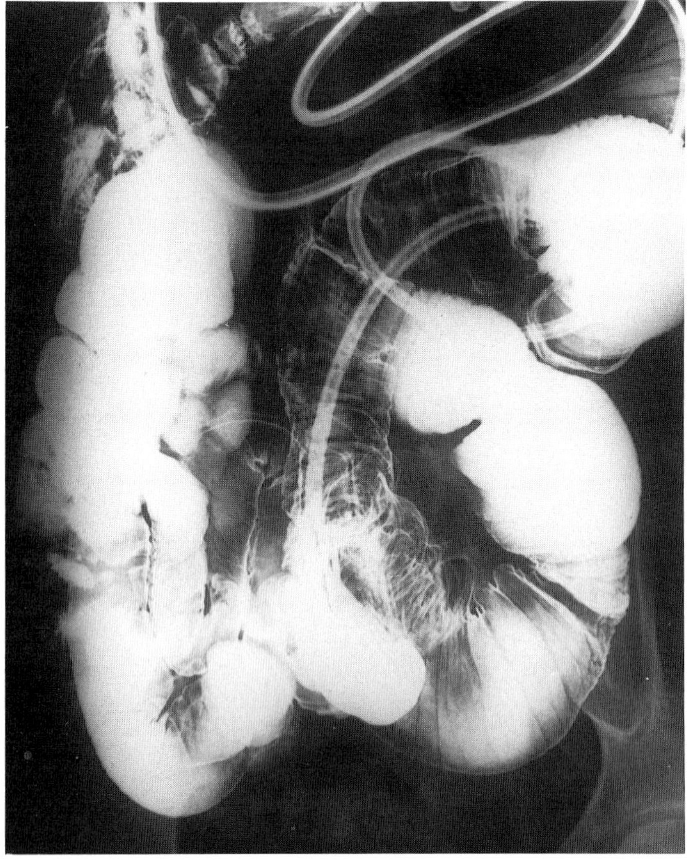

Figure 10.12. Adhesions in the terminal ileum with complete mechanical obstruction. Miller-Abbott tube is placed into the small bowel.

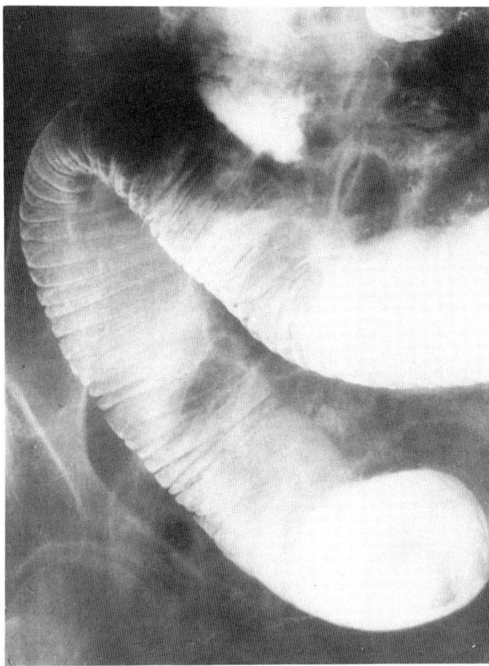

FIGURE 10.13. Small bowel obstruction by a gallstone.

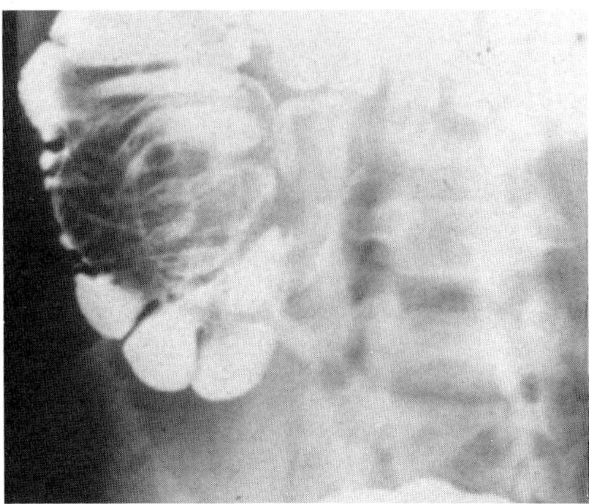

FIGURE 10.14. Ileocolic intussusception.

ter erosion of a gallstone into the gastrointestinal tract, gas can be visible in the bile ducts. Fistulas are appropriately visualized by barium suspension or by use of radionuclides.

Volvulus of the colon, particularly the sigmoid colon, causes obstruction more often than volvulus of the small bowel.

Intussusception or invagination is a telescopic protrusion of one segment of the gastrointestinal tract into the adjacent one. The slipped portion is the intussusceptum whereas the outer segment is the intussuscipiens. Intussusception is common up to the age of five, particularly in male children (Fig. 10.14). A polypoid tumor may be the leading mass for intussusception in adults. Common intussusceptions are ileoileal, ileocolic and colocolic. The causes of ileocecal intussusception may be hyperplasia of the mucosa and lymphoid tissue in the submucosa of the terminal ileum. Meckel's diverticulum may invert and prolapse into the small bowel causing intussusception or partial obstruction. If a complete obstruction lasts long enough, it can lead to necrosis of the intestinal wall due to compression of blood vessels (strangulation). If a plain radiogram of the abdomen reveals signs of obstruction, administration of contrast media may be contraindicated or to no avail.

After barium visualization of the site of an intussusception without strangulation, the lead point of the intussusceptum may be demonstrated. Penetration of barium between the intussusceptum and intussuscipiens creates a coiled spring appearance. The reduction of intussusception in children can be performed by a contrast enema if signs of peritonitis are absent. Ultrasound and CT also may demonstrate significant signs of intussusception:

1. Target sign of early intussusception (Fig. 10.15),
2. A mass with alternating low and high attenuation layers due to invagination of mesenteric fat and bowel wall, and
3. A reniform mass of edema in a strangulated loop.

Occlusion of mesenteric blood vessels is discussed in chapter 11.

ACUTE HEMORRHAGE FROM THE SMALL BOWEL

The site of acute gastrointestinal hemorrhage proves to be the small bowel in approximately 5% of patients. Etiologies include: vascular anomalies, primary and secondary

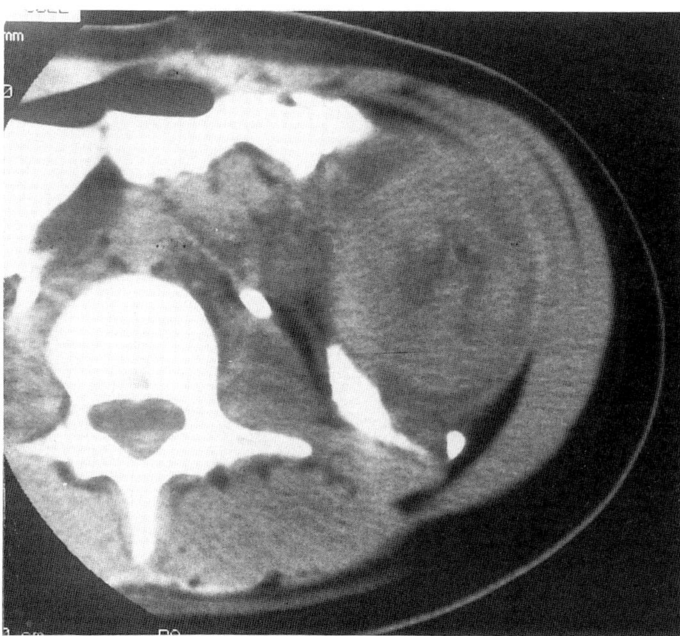

Figure 10.15. CT of jejuno-jejunal intussusception.

neoplasms, peptic ulceration, aortoenteric fistulas, and tuberculosis. After negative radiologic or endoscopic examination for a bleeding source in the upper gastrointestinal tract and colon, the site of bleeding from the small intestine can be confirmed by angiographic examination.

MALABSORPTION

Table 10.2 presents an etiologic classification of malabsorption syndrome. In a majority of patients the diagnosis must be established by small bowel biopsy.

Celiac disease and tropical sprue exhibit the same radiologic pattern. Dilatation of the bowel and thickenings of mucosal folds are associated with hypersecretion (Fig. 10.16). Due to unabsorbed food and mucus, even the most stable barium preparations are likely to flocculate.

Segmentation, fragmentation of the contrast column into amorphous collections, occurs in segments of the small intestine thickly coated with mucus (Fig. 10.17). A considerable amount of mucus forces barium sulfate particles out of suspension, a process termed flocculation, which may also result from motoric dysfunction of the small bowel. Segmentation due to excessive mucus, which may occur in normal children, cannot be distinguished from segmentation in pathological conditions. Segmentation occurs not only in the presence of mucus but also follows dehydration of contrast suspension, and the presence of fats and free

Table 10.2. Etiology of Malabsorption Syndromes

Diffuse lesions of small intestinal mucosa
Celiac disease
Adult celiac disease
Tropical sprue
Disaccharidase deficiency
Whipple's disease
Amyloidosis
Maldigestion
Deficiency of pancreatic secretions
Deficiency of conjugated bile acids
Diseases with defined pathologic lesions
Crohn's disease
Lymphoma
Scleroderma
Alimentary canal resection
Infection
Postsurgical intestinal obstruction

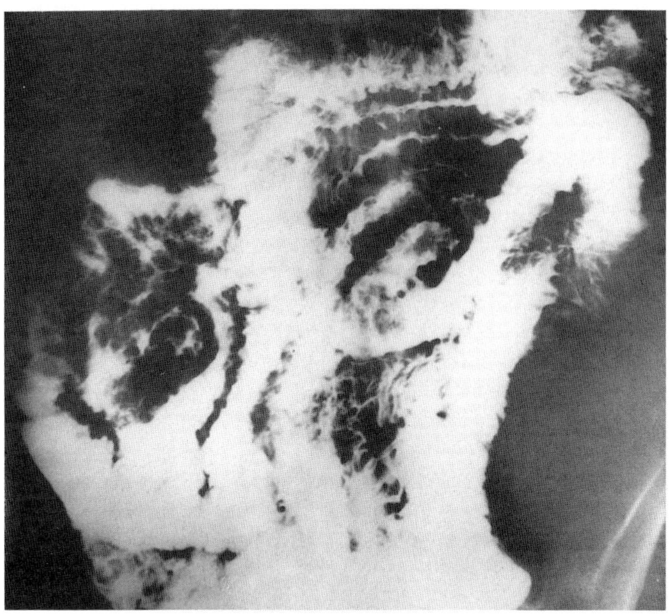

Figure 10.16. Celiac disease. Follow-through study.

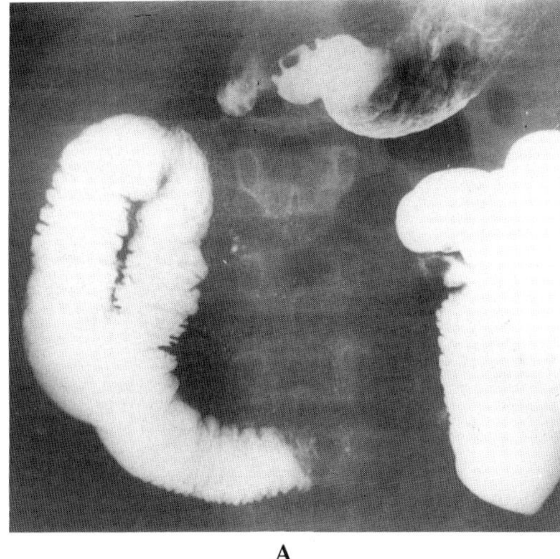

A

B

Figure 10.17. (A) and (B) Segmentation of barium sulfate in the small intestine.

fatty acids in the intestinal lumen. As a pathologic phenomenon, segmentation accompanies partial obstructions, bowel irritations, and malabsorption. Segmentation is seldom seen immediately after barium enters the small intestine, but occurs more often in the distal small bowel.

Dilatation of individual segments or of the entire small bowel is a very common finding in sprue and similar diseases. Dilatation becomes more prominent in severe forms of the disease. The width of the small bowel may exceed 4 cm. Dilatation throughout the entire length is also seen with distal obstruction, pancreatic insufficiency, and hypothyroidism. Segmental dilatation of the small bowel occurs with scleroderma.

Thickening of valvulae conniventes is a common radiologic sign of malabsorption. Diffuse, uniform swelling of valvulae conniventes is present with edema (Fig. 10.18), ischemia (Fig. 11.4) and, at times, hemorrhage into the small bowel wall, lymphangiectasia, and radiation enteritis. Small bowel edema occurs when the concentration of albumin in serum drops below 2 g/100 mL. Circular folds are irregularly thickened in celiac disease, Whipple's disease, and lymphoma.

The amount of secretions in the bowel lumen is taken into consideration, along with the width of the lumen and mucosal folds, to improve diagnoses of small bowel diseases, particularly in cases of malabsorption syndrome. *Hypersecretion* causes flocculation of barium. Moreover, if secretions are so excessive that they thickly cover the mucosal surface and fill spaces between mucosal folds, amorphous collections of barium in the center of the bowel lumen produce a "*moulage*" sign (Fig. 10.19).

Gluten-Induced Enteropathy in Children and Adults

Both diseases share the same pathogenic mechanisms but affect different ages. Changes result from hypersensitivity of the small bowel to the glutens in certain grains. Dilatation throughout the entire length of the small bowel is the most frequently observed radiologic sign (Fig. 10.20). Since enteroclysis normally produces distension of the small bowel, this sign is not significant in making a diagnosis. In patients with celiac disease, enteroclysis is successful only if a large volume of stable barium

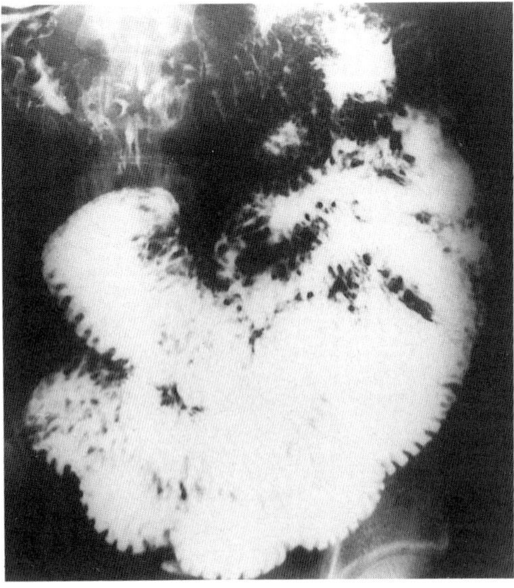

Figure 10.18. Small bowel edema. Uniform thickening of plicae conniventes.

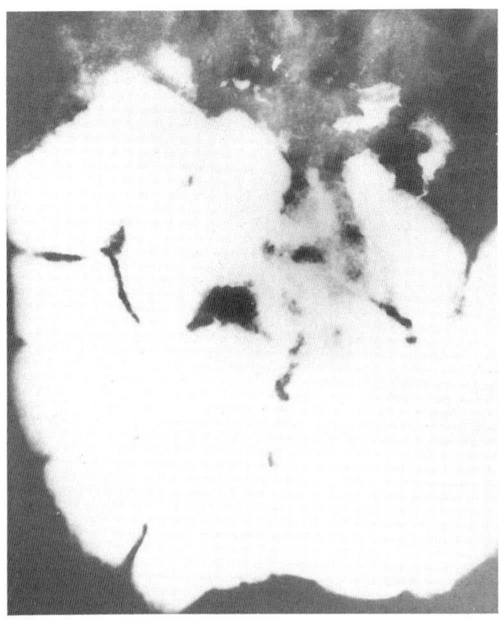

Figure 10.19. Celiac disease. Dilatation of the small bowel lumen. *Moulage* sign with segmentation of barium in the proximal small bowel.

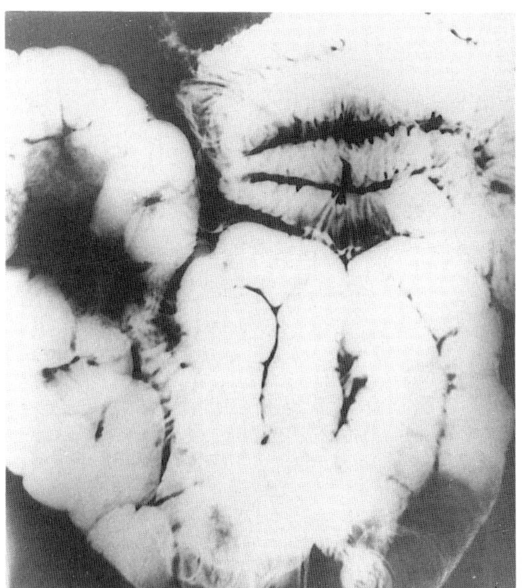

FIGURE 10.20. Celiac disease. Thickening of some plicae conniventes, others not evident (*moulage* sign). Distension of the small bowel.

suspension is given within the shortest possible time period. If methylcellulose solution is to be given, this should be done as quickly as possible, taking care to avoid vomiting.

Circular folds in patients with celiac disease are truncated and short, with increased separation, especially in the proximal jejunum. The finding of increased fold separation, or disappearance of folds, has not been met in conditions other than celiac disease. The average number of folds per 5 cm of proximal jejunum has been reported to be 6 in the group with celiac disease versus 10 in the control group. This is, at least partly, a consequence of bowel dilatation by unabsorbed food. Intestinal villi and microvilli vanish, and microscopically, inflammatory cells infiltrate the mucosa and submucosa. A *moulage* sign may also result from absence of mucosal folds (Fig. 10.19). The ileum assumes morphologic properties of the jejunum, with an increased number of circular folds in the ileum, a process called jejunalization (Fig. 10.21). These changes are believed to be

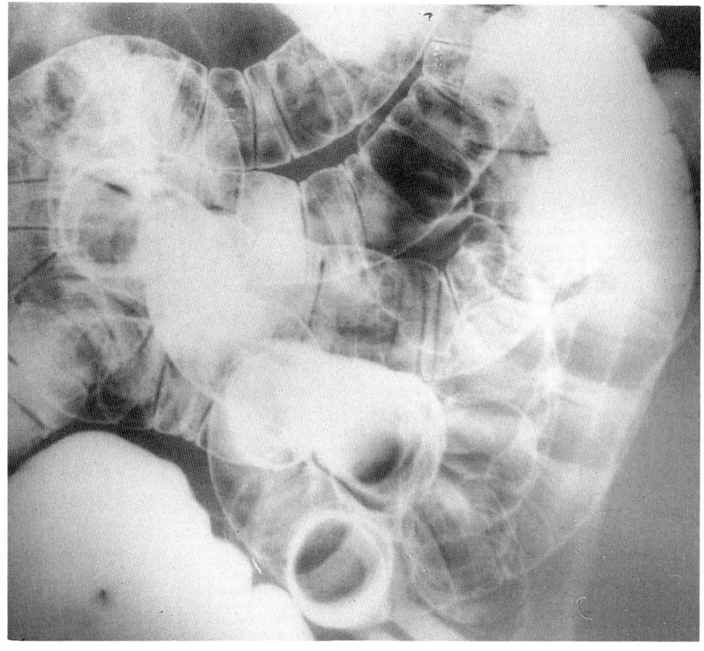

A

FIGURE 10.21. (A) Reduced number of circular folds (plicae conniventes) are evident in the small intestine of a patient with celiac disease. (*Figure continued on overleaf.*)

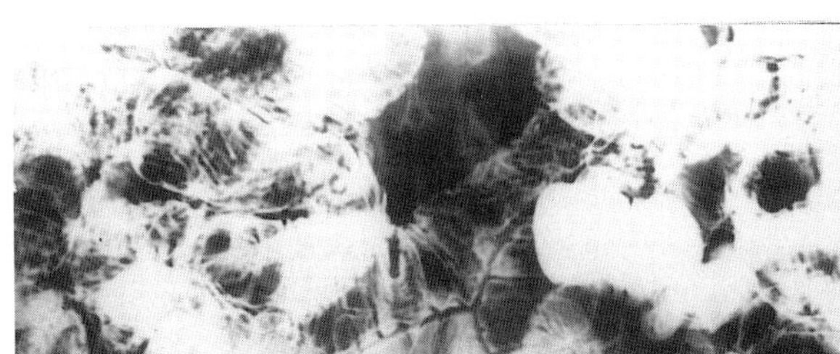

B

Figure 10.21 *continued.* (B) For comparison, normal number of circular folds in a healthy subject. (C) Increased number of circular folds in the ileum—"jejunalization" of the ileum.

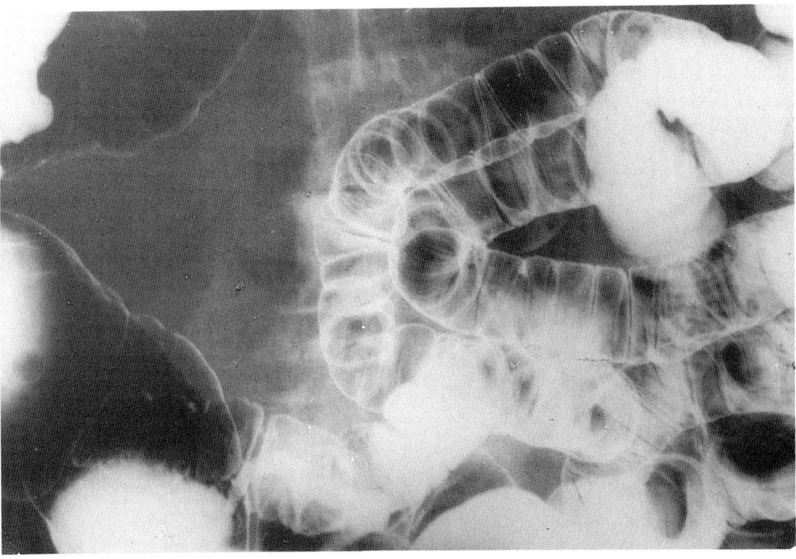

C

compensation for the long-standing atrophy of intestinal villi in the proximal section of the small bowel.

In patients with celiac disease, double-contrast enteroclysis can reveal polygonal or oval elevations of small bowel mucosa 1–2 mm in diameter. This appearance is the "mosaic pattern" described by endoscopists, and seen in scanning microscopy studies of celiac disease biopsy specimens (Table 10.3).

Besides dilatation of the small bowel, segmentation of the contrast column, as well as flocculation and dilution of barium, occur during the course of examination. Dilatation and flocculation are nonspecific signs of celiac disease in adults. Flocculation obscures more specific features of celiac disease and delays the recognition of complications. Lymphoma is the most serious complication of celiac disease, usually developing 10 to 20 years after the onset of symptoms. The diagnosis of celiac disease is confirmed by laboratory findings and biopsy of the jejunal mucosa.

Patients with long-standing celiac disease

TABLE 10.3. CAUSES OF NODULAR LESIONS OF THE SMALL INTESTINE

Nodular lymphatic hyperplasia
Crohn's disease
Lymphoma
Whipple's disease
Eosinophilic enteritis

who eat a normal diet or who have lost the favorable response to a gluten-free diet are placed at increased risk for alimentary canal malignancies. The histiocytic lymphoma is the most common malignancy among patients with celiac disease. Adenocarcinomas of the small bowel and esophagus are also more common in celiac disease. Enlarged mesenteric and para-aortic lymph nodes demonstrated by CT may reflect reactive hyperplasia and can regress on a gluten-free diet. However, when nodes do not decrease in size on CT, biopsy may be necessary to exclude lymphoma.

DISACCHARIDASE DEFICIENCY

Disaccharidases are enzymes, found in intestinal microvilli, that split disaccharides into monosaccharides, thereby allowing absorption. Lactase deficiency is most common, but sucrase-isomaltase and sucrase may also be deficient. If a disaccharide which cannot be enzymatically split is administered with the contrast suspension, the passage of barium through the small bowel is considerably accelerated, and the barium suspension is diluted, due to increased secretion into the intestinal lumen (Fig. 10.22). Patients with celiac disease have, in contrast, normal or prolonged transit time. Disaccharidase deficiency is not associated with swollen valvulae conniventes. Overall, this deficiency is extremely uncommon.

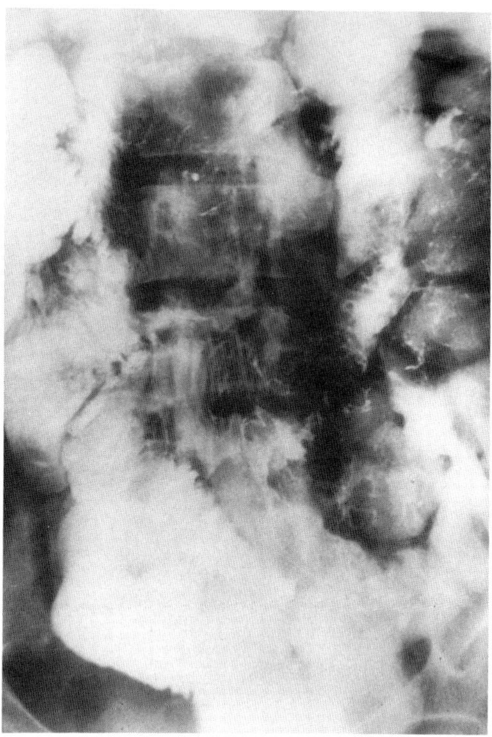

FIGURE 10.22. Malabsorption in lactase deficiency. Dilution of contrast medium with very shortened transit time occurred after addition of lactose to barium suspension.

WHIPPLE'S DISEASE

This disease is characterized by steatorrhea, abdominal pain, arthritis, and weight loss. Macrophages in the lamina propria of the intestinal mucosa and in mesenteric lymph nodes contain glycoprotein. Radiologic signs may resemble celiac disease (Fig. 10.23). Particularly constant changes are swollen valvulae conniventes which sometimes have altered architecture. Whipple's disease is amenable to antibiotic therapy, supporting an infectious etiology (Table 10.3).

AMYLOIDOSIS

Amyloidosis affects the small bowel as either a primary or secondary process. The secondary form accompanies pulmonary tuberculosis, malignant neoplasms, and chronic purulent inflammations. Valvulae conniventes of the small intestine are thickened, and their architecture is sometimes changed (Fig. 10.24). Intestinal amyloidosis cannot be reliably distinguished from intestinal lymphangiectasia, Whipple's disease, or early stages of lymphoma, by radiologic methods alone.

When pancreatic secretions are deficient, di-

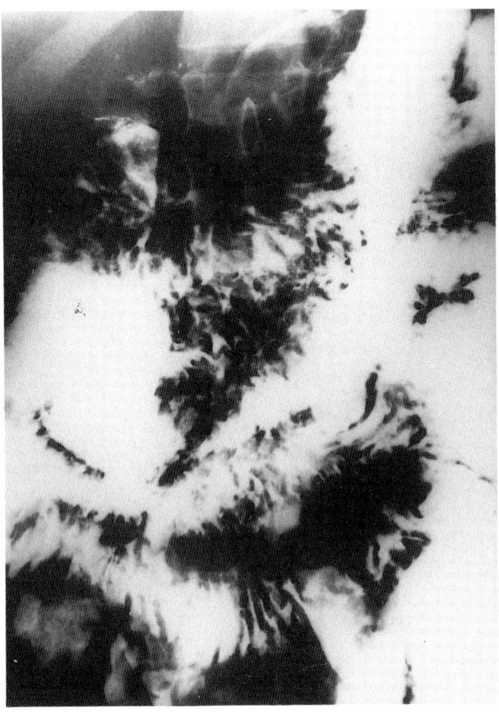

FIGURE 10.23. Whipple's disease. Thickened, irregular small bowel circular folds.

latation of the small bowel is accompanied by reduction in the number of plicae conniventes (Fig. 10.25).

SCLERODERMA – PROGRESSIVE SYSTEMIC SCLEROSIS

The small intestine is infrequently involved in patients with scleroderma. When affected, abnormalities are simultaneously present in the esophagus. The small bowel loops involved are distended and their motility is reduced. When longer segments are involved, transit time is prolonged. The mucosal surface remains unchanged (Fig. 10.26).

Scleroderma more often affects the duodenum than the small intestine. Patients with small intestine involvement are predisposed to diverticular formation on the antimesenteric aspect of the wall.

INTESTINAL LYMPHANGIECTASIA

In patients with intestinal lymphangiectasia (Gordon's exudative enteropathy), intestinal villi are widened as a result of defective lymphatic

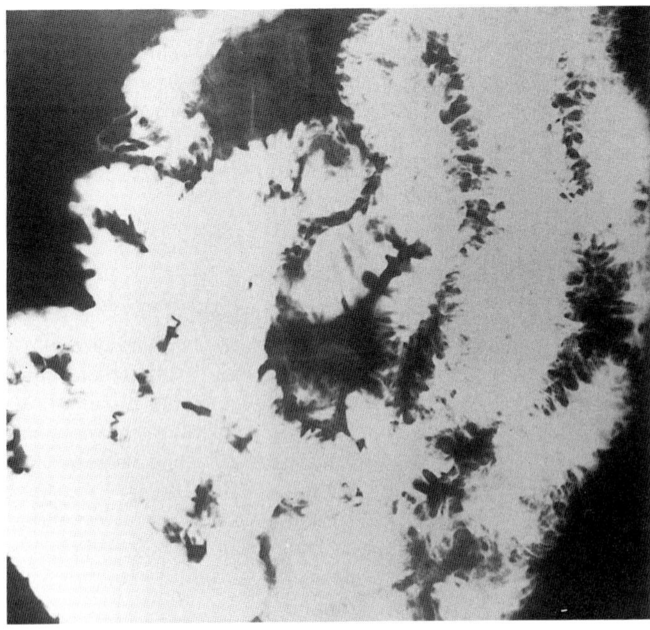

FIGURE 10.24. Small bowel amyloidosis. Thickened small bowel circular folds.

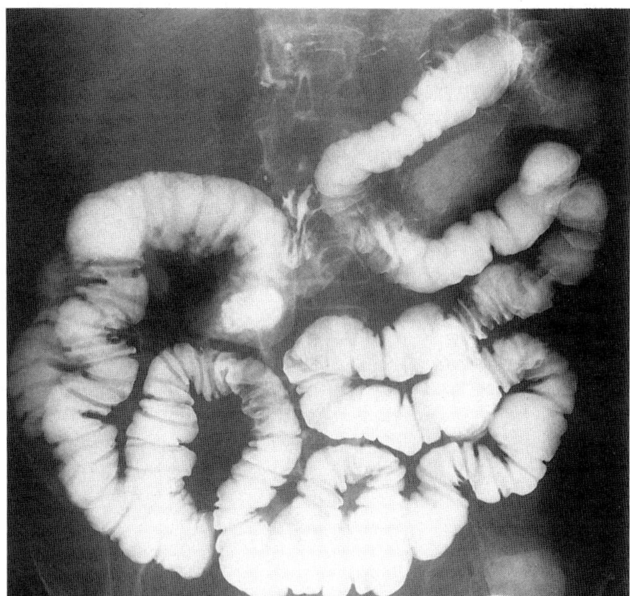

FIGURE 10.25. Pancreatic insufficiency. Distended small bowel lumen with reduced number of plicae conniventes.

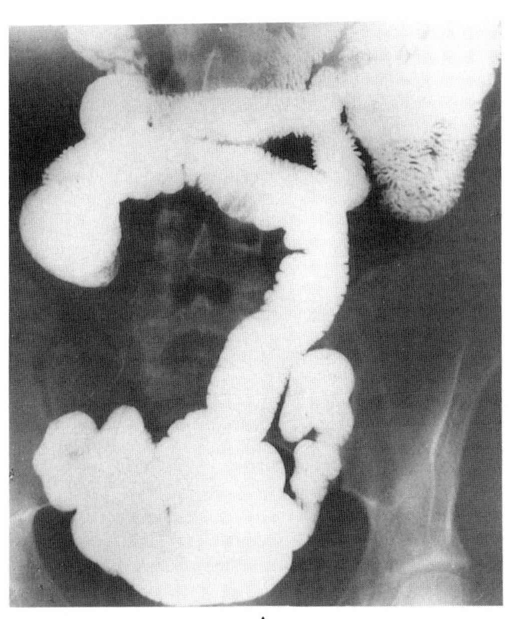

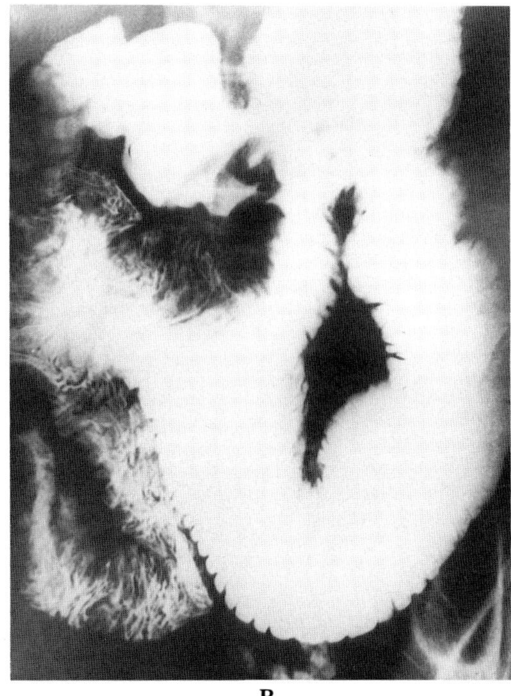

A B

FIGURE 10.26. Scleroderma. Mucosal relief is preserved. (A) Dilatation of a long jejunal segment. (B) Significant dilatation of the proximal jejunum.

development. The valvulae conniventes are truncated, and the intestinal lumen is moderately dilated. Radiologic findings resemble edema (Fig. 10.27). Barium may penetrate the intestinal wall through perforations in lymphatic vessels. The disease is one of the protein-losing enteropathies and results in malabsorption symptoms.

Radiation Enteritis

Aggressive radiotherapy for malignancies of the female genital organs or the urinary bladder may cause radiation damage to the intestine. The large intestine is affected more often because of its relative fixation and decreased mobility. Initial changes are characterized by edema of the wall, particularly pronounced in the mucosa (Fig. 10.28A). Ulcers may subsequently develop and finally adhesions with adjacent intestinal loops occur. Fibrosis with narrowing of the intestinal lumen can be seen after a few months (Fig. 10.28B). Although mucosal lesions remain clinically unapparent, radiologically detectable changes are often apparent (Table 10.4). Lesions of the small bowel may be expected after 45 Gy (4500 rad) exposure. Doses of 65 Gy cause substantial complications in 50% of patients within five years.

Chronic changes are usually visible from six months to two years after radiation exposure. However, this range may vary from three months to five years. Pathologically, submucosal edema is noted with fibrin exudation.

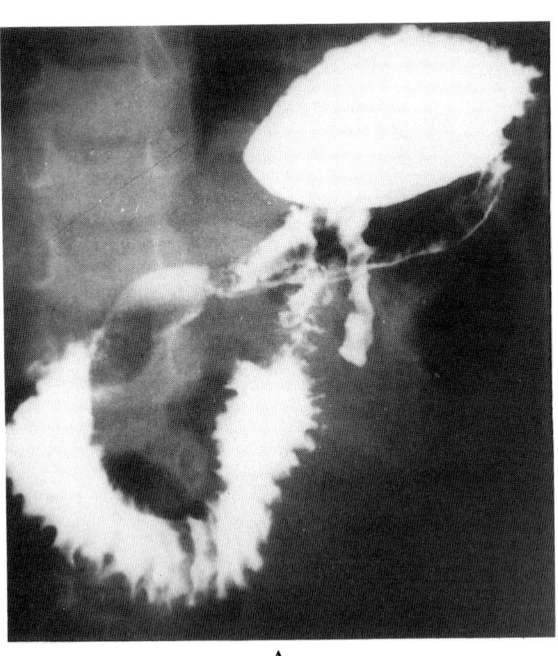

A

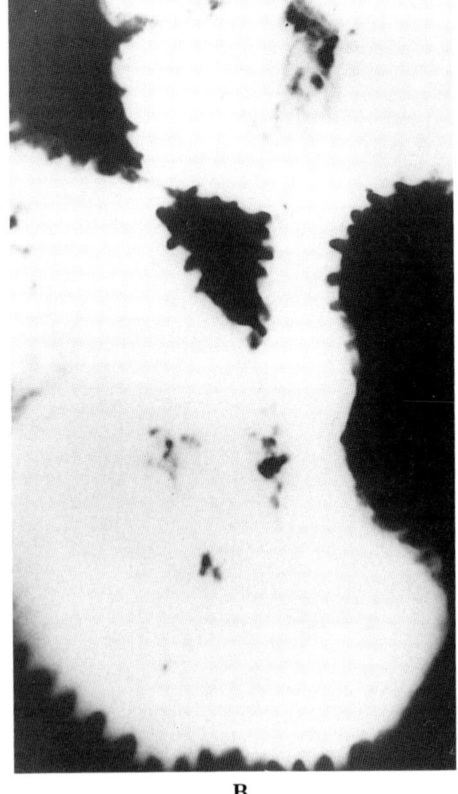

B

Figure 10.27. Intestinal lymphangiectasia (exudative Gordon's enteropathy) in a child. Equal widening of circular folds. (A) Involvement of the distal duodenum and proximal jejunum. (B) Jejunal disease.

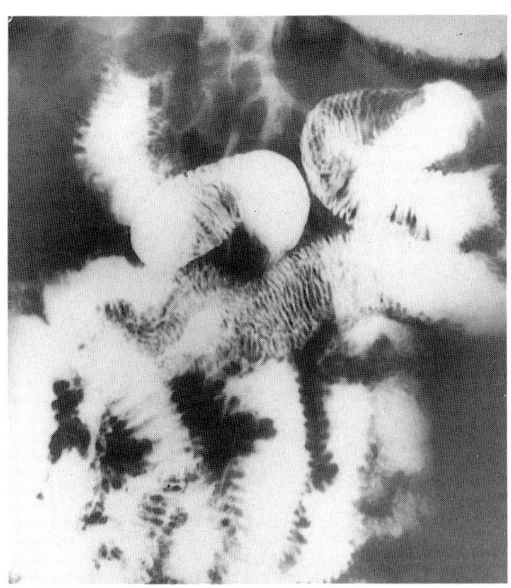

A

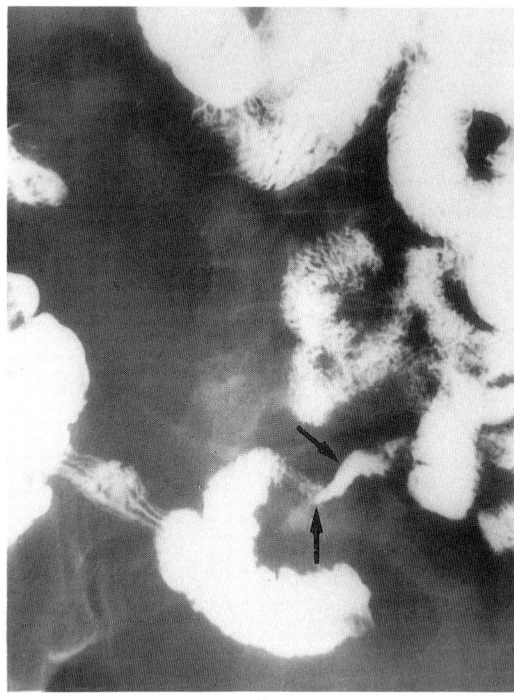

B

FIGURE 10.28. Radiation injury to the small bowel. (A) Acute changes in middle and distal sections of the small bowel. (B) Chronic changes with stricture formation (arrows).

Ultimately hyalinization and fibrosis may occur. The radiologic finding may resemble ischemia, early Crohn's disease, or intestinal lymphangiectasia.

PROTEIN-LOSING ENTEROPATHY

This group of entities includes:

1. Menetrier's disease, which, in addition to the stomach, may involve both the small and large intestine.
2. Exudative enteropathy (Gordon's enteropathy, intestinal lymphangiectasia) (Fig. 10.27).
3. Partial occlusions of the superior mesenteric artery.
4. Zollinger-Ellison syndrome. In addition to changes in the stomach and duodenum, Zollinger-Ellison syndrome may be also accompanied by changes in the small intestine. The second segment of the duodenum is widened and valvulae conniventes in the entire small intestine are thickened, with substantial hypersecretion in the mesenteric small intestine.

TABLE 10.4. EXAMPLES OF ACUTE AND CHRONIC RADIATION ENTERITIS

Acute
Thickened plicae conniventes
Hypersecretion
Erosions and ulcers
Fistulae
Chronic
Moderate
Thickened plicae conniventes
Decreased distensibility and motility
Severe
Ulcers
Long strictures
Fistulae
Obstruction

ACQUIRED DIVERTICULA OF THE SMALL INTESTINE

Acquired diverticula of the small intestine cannot be distinguished radiologically from congenital diverticula. Single-contrast enteroclysis better demonstrates diverticula than follow-through examinations. These saccular formations project outside the intestinal contour. The diverticular neck may be either narrow or wide, and mucosal folds are often demonstrated entering the diverticular lumen (Fig. 10.29). Unless complicated, diverticula are clinically asymptomatic.

SMALL BOWEL HEMATOMA

Bleeding into the small intestinal wall may be due to a bleeding diathesis, trauma, angiodysplasia, neoplasm, or ischemia. Hematomas are demonstrated as submucosal expansile formations (Fig. 10.30). They may assume a "picket fence" appearance or create a "stacked

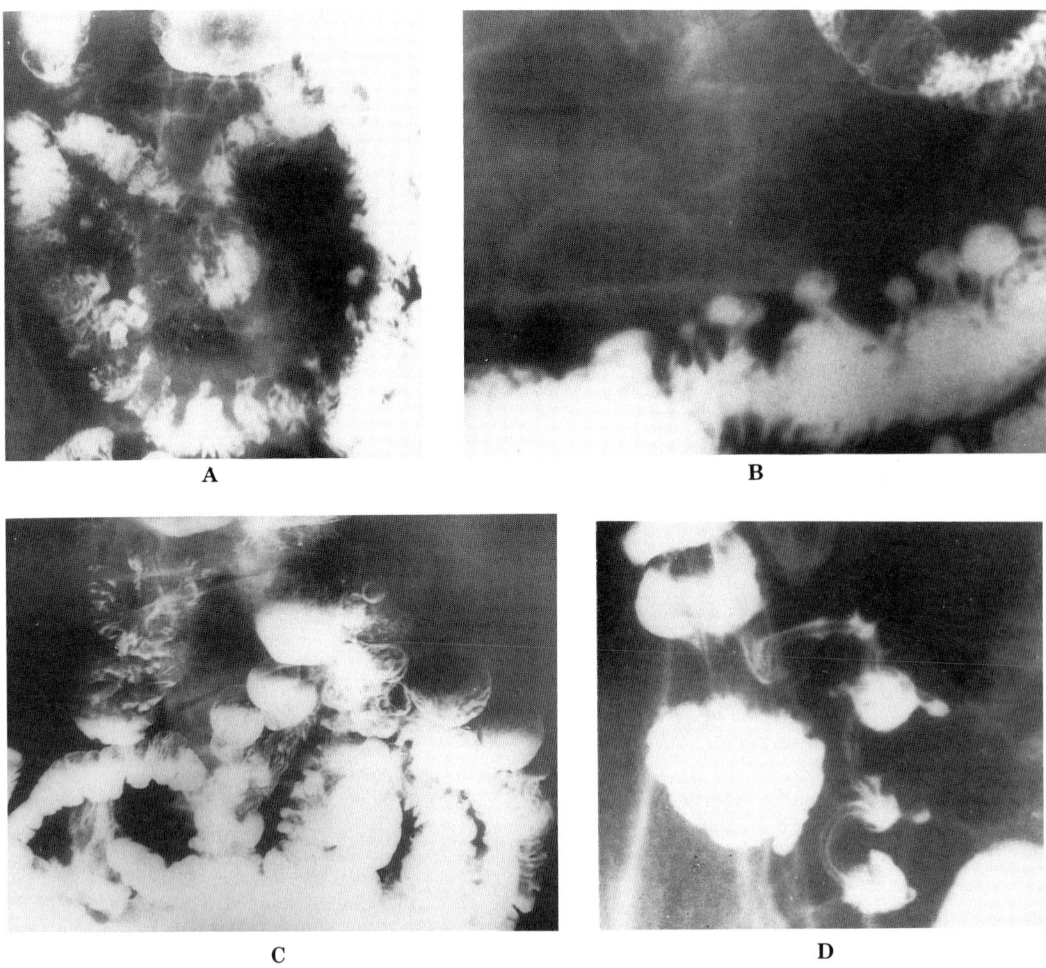

FIGURE 10.29. Multiple small bowel diverticula. (A) In the jejunum and the ileum. (B) Mucosal folds entering diverticula. (C) Very large and average size jejunal diverticula. (D) In the terminal ileum.

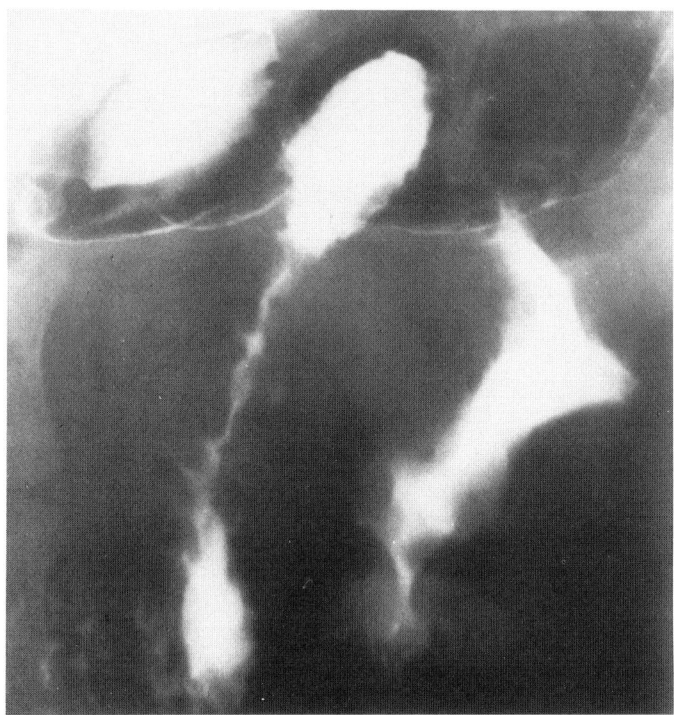

FIGURE 10.30. Coagulopathy and small bowel hemorrhage. Hematoma involving all layers of the proximal jejunum.

coin" sign of small bowel hemorrhage. Chronic stages are characterized by symmetric circumferential narrowing along with thickening of the intestinal wall. (See the section on bleeding into the duodenal wall, pages 340–342.)

GRAFT-VERSUS-HOST REACTION

Graft-versus-host reaction occurs after allogeneic bone marrow transplantation. The donor's lymphoidocytes react against tissues of the host such as liver, skin, and alimentary canal.

The *acute phase*, lasting up to 15 days after the onset of digestive tube symptoms, is characterized by edematous valvulae conniventes and by mucosal edema in the small bowel and, on occasion, in other sections of the gastrointestinal tract, such as the esophagus. The volume and flow of intraluminal fluid is accelerated (Fig. 10.31A). In the *subacute phase*, which can last up to 100 days after the onset of alimentary canal symptoms, tissue changes resemble those of the preceding phase, but are less intensive (Fig. 10.31B). Changes in the *chronic phase* are confined to the terminal ileum, where discrete narrowing may remain.

Examination by CT demonstrates thickening of the small intestinal and colonic walls, as well as of the mesentery. Barium studies and CT cannot accurately distinguish acute graft-versus-host disease from viral enterocolitis.

INFLAMMATORY DISEASES

ACUTE INFLAMMATIONS

Necrotizing Enterocolitis. Necrotizing enteritis and enterocolitis are mainly diseases of newborns, particularly those under two weeks

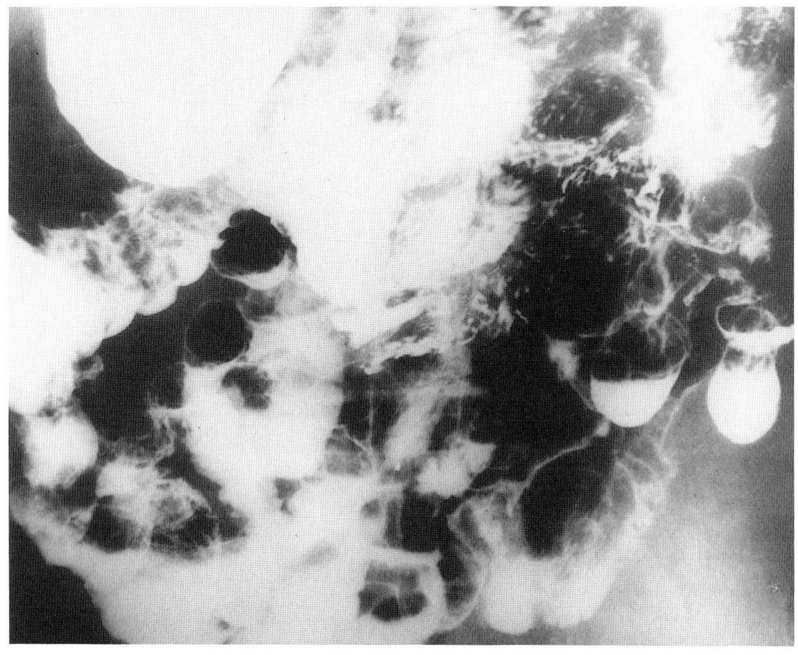

A

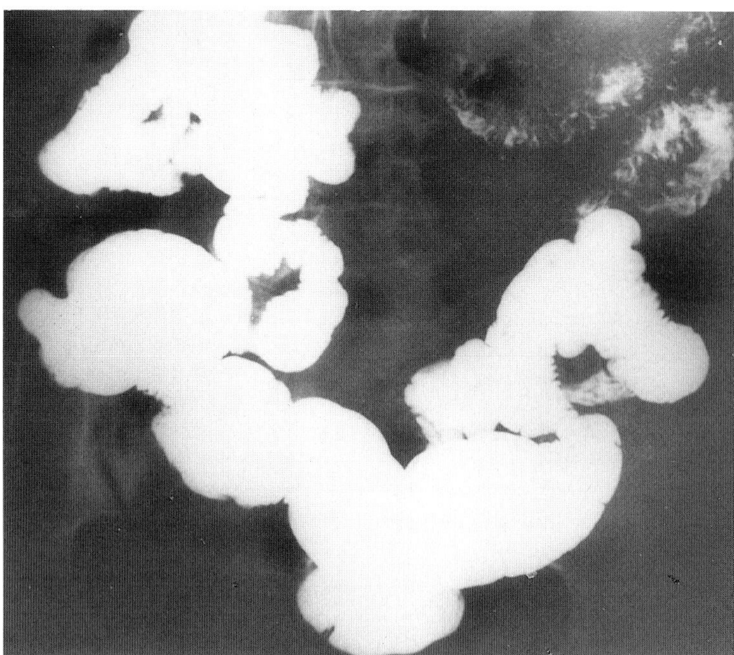

B

Figure 10.31. Graft-versus-host disease. (A) Acute phase. Dilatation and increased fluid content in the small bowel. (B) Late subacute phase. Dilatation of the small intestine with narrowing of plicae conniventes.

of age. Prematures and debilitated newborns are particularly susceptible. The conditions are a result of intestinal ischemia, often without overt arterial occlusion, and are probably related to vascular shunting to other vital organs. Similar findings can be seen when mesenteric vascular occlusion is accompanied by thrombi related to indwelling umbilical catheters. Early radiologic signs are ileus and ill-defined contours of the walls distended by gas; these are associated with the irregular accumulation of gas in various sections of the intestine (Fig. 10.32). Radiologic signs may precede clinical symptoms for a few hours.

Gas within the intestinal wall has been reported in 41% of patients and, in 16% of patients, gas is present in the hepatic portal veins. Subserosal cystic intestinal pneumatosis or linear gas collections may be found. The late phase corresponds to gangrene of the bowel and is commonly associated with linear intramural gaseous collection. Segments ranging from 10–20 cm in length may be involved.

A severe gangrenous form of ischemic colitis, referred to as necrotizing colitis, occurs in subjects over 60 years of age, associated with cardiac arrhythmia, hypotension, congestive heart failure and shock (see bowel ischemia). Surgery is indicated when there is perforation with accumulation of fluid in the peritoneal cavity, and in the late phase, in subjects with strictures. Signs of necrotizing enterocolitis in its chronic phase mimic Crohn's disease.

Chronic Idiopathic Ulcerative Enteritis. This form of enteritis is rare, and only 40 cases have been reported. It most often occurs in the fifth and sixth decade with a mortality rate approaching 75%. Abdominal pain, diarrhea, fever, and malabsorption dominate the clinical

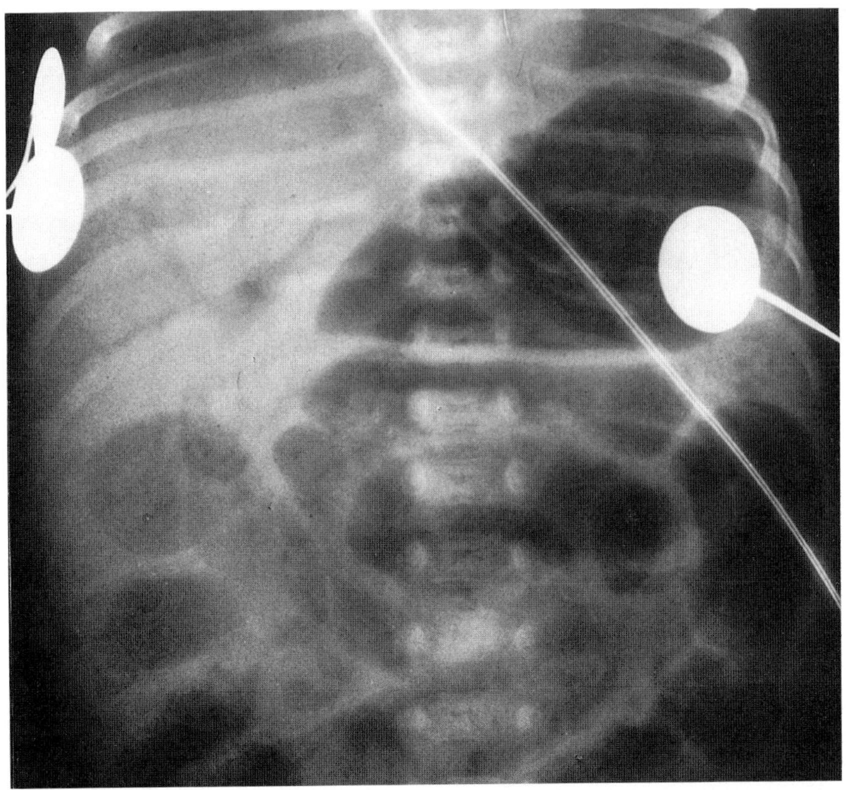

Figure 10.32. Necrotizing enterocolitis in a premature child. Ileus, linear intestinal pneumatosis, and gas in the portal vein.

picture. Peroral barium examination reveals distension of the small bowel, barium flocculation, segmentation of the contrast column, and ulceration. When perforations of the intestinal wall are revealed by plain roentgenography, barium administration is contraindicated. The chronic stage is characterized by strictures. Differential diagnosis includes Crohn's disease, lymphoma, celiac disease, tuberculosis, mycotic infections, typhoid fever, bacillary dysentery, Zollinger-Ellison syndrome, and ischemic disorders.

Chronic Inflammations

Chronic inflammatory diseases of the small intestine are accompanied by fibrotic changes and often by granulomas. Increased irritability of the small bowel is quite often seen. *Crohn's disease* is discussed in chapter 11.

Tuberculosis. Tuberculosis of the small intestine mainly occurs in patients with pulmonary tuberculosis. Tubercle bacilli demonstrate a predilection for the ileocecal area where they first invade intestinal glands and thereafter spread along the mucosa and submucosa (Fig. 10.33A). Both aggregated lymphoid follicles (Peyer's patches) and solitary lymphoid follicles are enlarged. Mucosal folds in the terminal ileum are swollen due to edema. Lymphoid follicles are ulcerated, and scars remain after healing. Tuberculosis is quite difficult to distinguish from Crohn's disease by radiologic examinations. However, patients with Crohn's disease often have more pronounced areas of

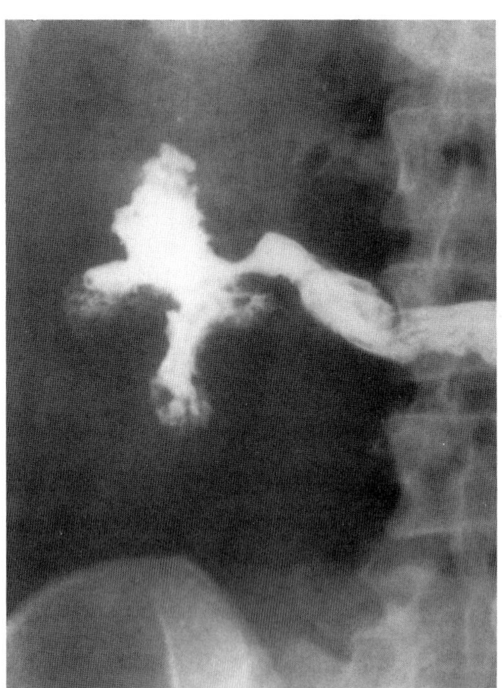

A

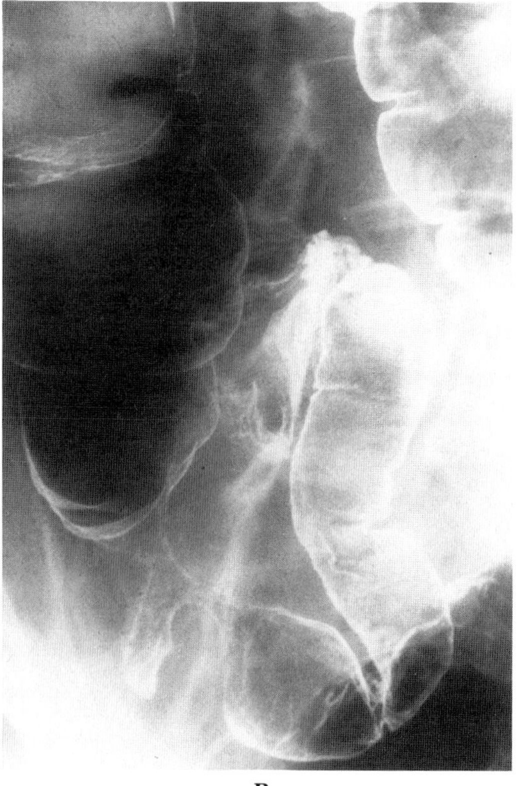

B

Figure 10.33. (A) Spasm of the cecum and terminal ileum in ileocecal tuberculosis. Discrete irregularities of bowel contour. (B) Stierlin's sign of ileocecal tuberculosis. A single lumen of ileum and ascending colon.

stricture formation and normal pulmonary status.

The distinction between strictures resulting from tuberculosis and those resulting from carcinoma, as well as other malignancies, is based on criteria listed in Table 3.1. Intestinal tuberculosis may assume either of the following macroscopic forms: ulcerative, hyperplastic, or pseudotumorous. Incidence of the latter two forms has decreased since infection by *Mycobacterium bovis* has become exceptionally rare.

Tuberculosis of the ileocecal area often exhibits Stierlin's sign: cecal spasm due to a pathologic process in the cecum. This appearance is due to barium passing directly from the ileum into the ascending colon (Fig. 10.33B).

INTESTINAL LYMPHOID HYPERPLASIA

Hyperplasia of both solitary and aggregated lymphoid follicles of the small bowel may be demonstrated by use of a double-contrast radiographic method of controlled compression studies. Intestinal lymphoid hyperplasia occurs in patients with hypogammaglobulinemia and dysgammaglobulinemia. Enlarged solitary lymphoid follicles are in most cases found in the distal small intestine, and are demonstrated as oval or spherical, regular, well-demarcated submucosal formations measuring 1–3 mm in diameter (Fig. 10.34). However, the jejunum and colon may also be involved.

Intestinal lymphoid hyperplasia is occasionally found in patients with scarlatina, diphtheria, yersiniosis, tuberculosis, and lymphoma. Enlarged lymphoid follicles are often the first detectable radiologic sign of Crohn's disease (Table 10.3).

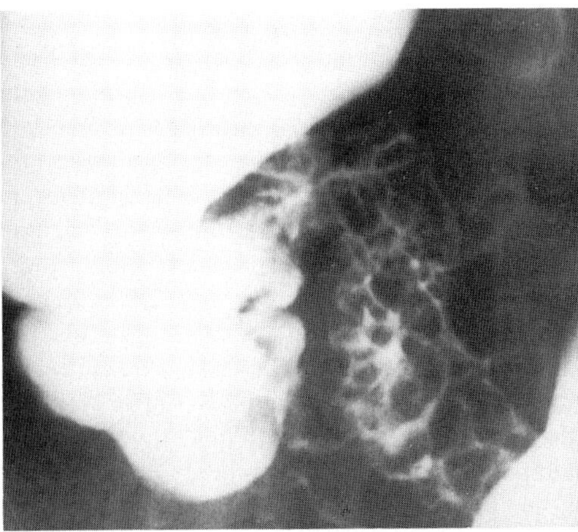

FIGURE 10.34. Lymphoid hyperplasia of the terminal ileum. Controlled compression study.

PARASITIC INFESTATIONS

Parasitic infestation of the small intestine does not always warrant radiologic examination. Intestinal parasites, however, may cause both specific and nonspecific radiologic signs.

Ascaris lumbricoides is evident on barium examination as elongated negative defects (Fig. 10.35A). When parasites ingest barium, their alimentary canal is demonstrated (Fig. 10.35B). They reside, in a majority of cases, in the middle section of the jejunum. A matted ball of ascarids may cause obstruction.

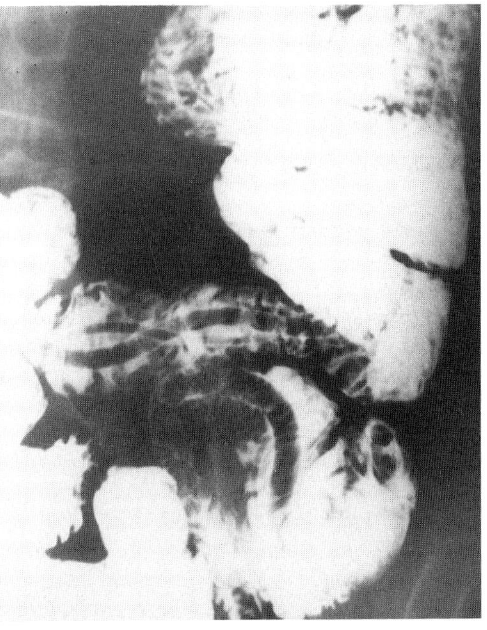

A

FIGURE 10.35. Parasitic infestations. (A) Ascariasis. Transparent linear defects in the small intestine. (*Figure continued on overleaf.*)

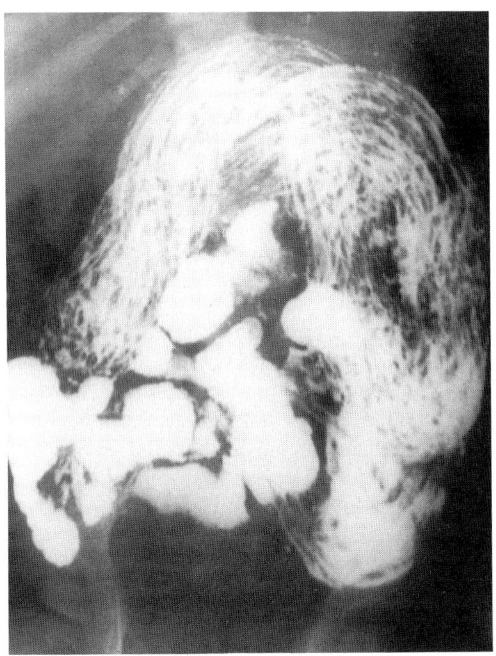

B

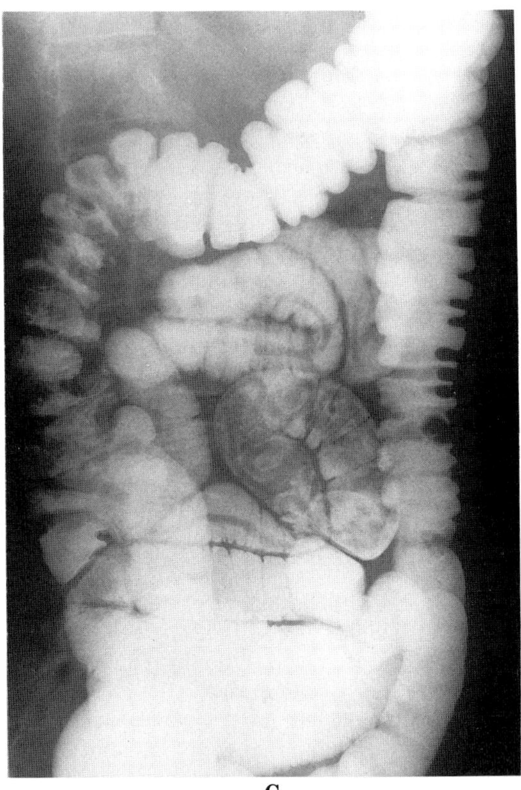

C

FIGURE 10.35 *continued.* Parasitic infestations. (B) A large number of ascarids have ingested barium with demonstration of their alimentary tract. (C) *Tenia saginata*—tapeworm in the small bowel.

Taenia solium and *Taenia saginata* (tapeworm) are less frequently demonstrated by radiologic examination than ascarids (Fig. 10.35C). In the duodenum, where scolices are attached, signs of irritation such as spasm are observed, along with irregularities of the mucosal surface. These parasites do not have an alimentary canal.

Ankylostoma duodenale and *Strongyloides stercoralis* penetrate into an organism through the skin. They invade the duodenal wall and mesenteric small bowel where they provoke a tissue reaction. Involved intestinal segments exhibit swollen valvulae conniventes, ulceration, and a widened lumen.

Infestations of the duodenum and proximal small intestine by *Giardia* result in thickening of the valvulae conniventes.

BENIGN NEOPLASMS

Benign neoplasms of the small intestine may be classified as: (1) *Intraluminal*—either on a stalk or sessile, (2) *Mainly intramural*, (3) *Subserosal* (exoenteric), or (4) *Combined morphology*—a combination of the above. Benign neoplasms, as well as malignant, may originate from any layer of the intestinal wall. Macroscopic features may refer to biologic properties of the particular tumor, yet distinction between malignant and benign neoplasms by radiologic means is usually unreliable. Benign neoplasms do not destroy mucosa. They have a regular shape and sharp contour but may be ulcerated, as in the case of leiomyoma and lipoma. The length of the mesenteric small bowel with its overlapping barium-filled loops makes detection more difficult. Palpation as well as an adequate number of radiographic projections during spot filming are of considerable importance. Accuracy is also increased by single- or double-contrast enteroclysis. Radiologic finding will be positive in 60–90% of subjects with benign neoplasms of the mesenteric small bowel.

Benign tumors may cause bleeding. Partial, or less frequently complete, obstruction can be provoked by intussusception or obliteration of the lumen by the tumor mass.

When benign neoplasms arise in the mucosa, they tend to protrude into the intestinal lumen. Subserosal and intramural tumors predominantly grow away from the lumen, and hence do not influence the contrast column until they assume large dimensions. Benign tumors of the small intestine may be either mesenchymal or epithelial in origin. Their prevalence increases in the distal direction.

Polyps may be hyperplastic, adenomatous, or hamartomatous. They appear as spherical, often pedunculated defects in the small bowel. Adenomatous polyps are epithelial tumors growing either solitary (Fig. 10.36), or in the context of polyposis syndromes. Adenomatous polyps may originate from Brunner's or Lieberkühn's glands. Early malignant transformation of these tumors cannot be assessed by radiologic methods. Multiple hamartomas may populate the small intestine of patients with Peutz–Jeghers syndrome.

Mesenchymal tumors include leiomyomas, lipomas, hemangiomas, lymphangiomas, fibromas, and rare neuromas.

Leiomyoma is the most common benign neoplasm of the small intestine (Fig. 10.37). The tumor grows predominantly subserosally, and the overlaying mucosa is often ulcerated. When a leiomyoma grows towards the lumen, it displaces valvulae conniventes. Malignant transformation is not always radiologically detectable.

Lipomas have the same prevalence as ade-

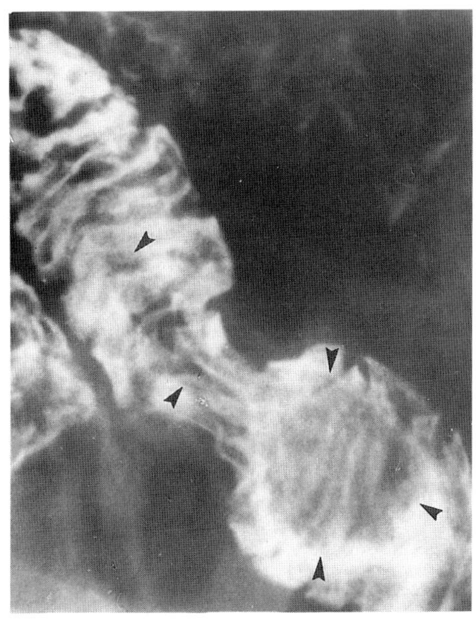

A

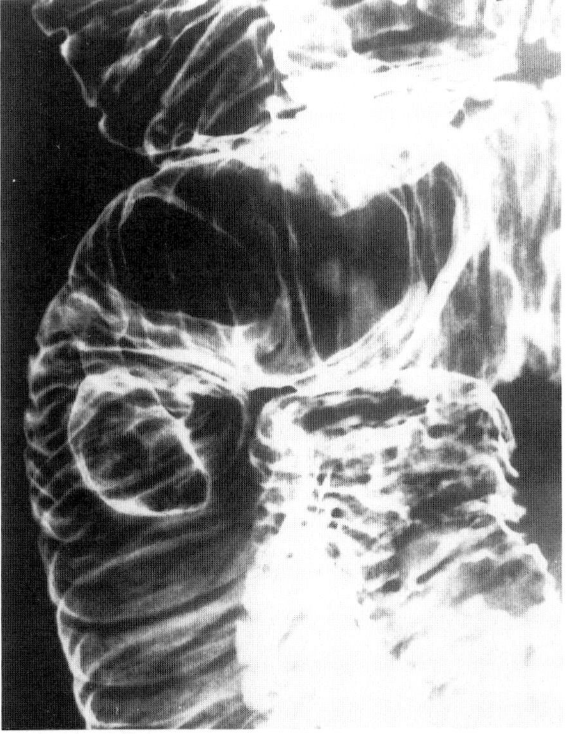

B

FIGURE 10.36. Adenomatous small bowel polyps on a stalk. (A) Controlled compression study. (B) Double-contrast (air contrast) enteroclysis.

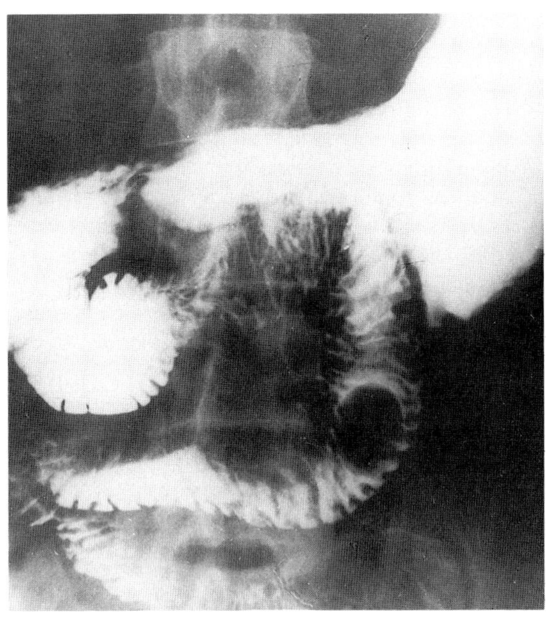

A

Figure 10.37. Small bowel leiomyoma. (A) In the jejunum. (B) Arteriographic study.

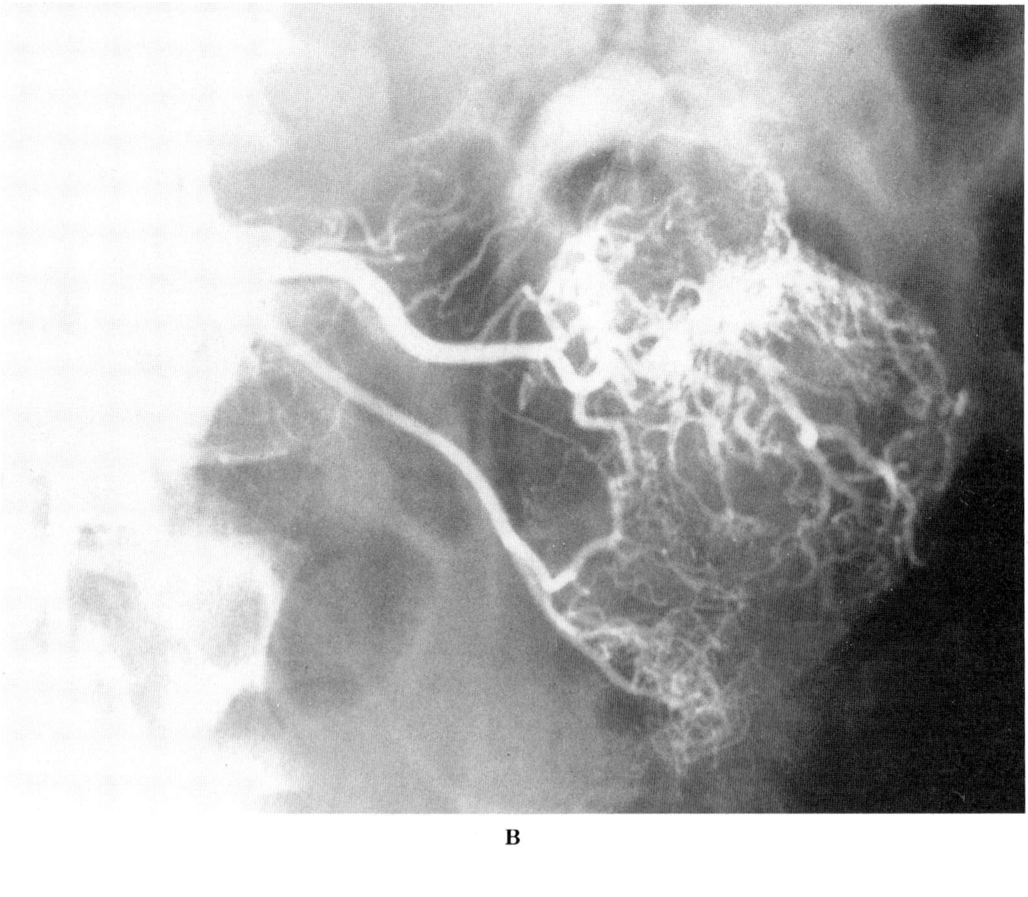

B

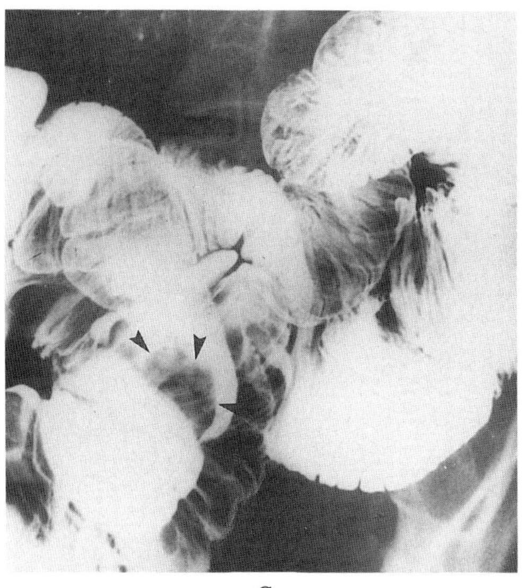

C

FIGURE 10.37 *continued.* Small bowel leiomyoma (C) In the proximal ileum (arrowheads) causing proximal distension.

nomatous polyps of the small bowel, comprising approximately 15–20% of small bowel neoplasms. They may be attached to the intestinal wall by a stalk or elevate overlying mucosa (Fig. 10.38). Subserosal lipomas have also been described. Solitary tumors are seen more often than multiple, the latter being termed lipomatosis. Lipomas are in most cases clinically inapparent. They consist of differentiated fat cells and are encapsulated. It may be hard to distinguish lipomas from other benign tumors of the small intestine by barium studies. As intestinal lipomas are of a fluid consistency, they tend to be more pliable than solid tumors such as leiomyoma. Computed tomography enables their differentiation from liposarcomas, since lipomas are homogenous in structure, while liposarcomas contain areas with higher attenuation values (Fig. 10.38B). However, malignant transformation does not occur in lipomas. Complications accompanying lipomas, as well as other benign neoplasms, are bleeding, intussusception, obstruction, and volvulus. A

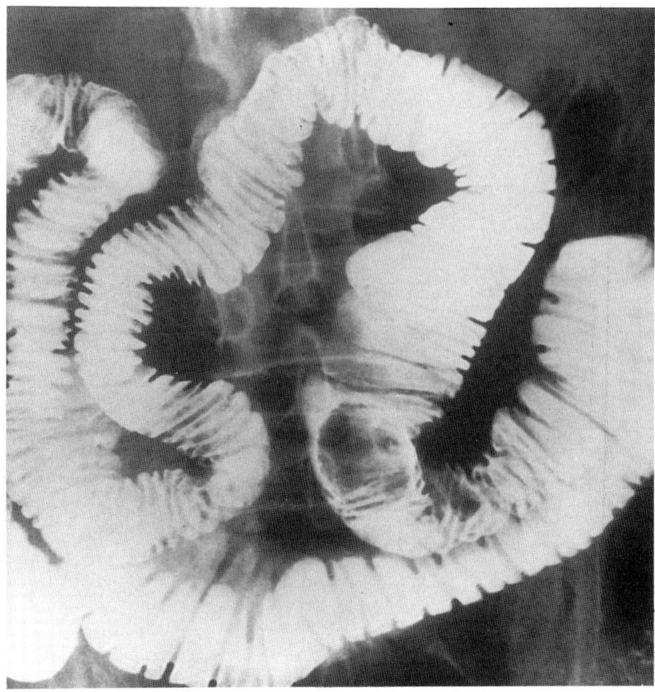

A

FIGURE 10.38. (A) Small bowel lipoma. Follow-through study. A soft round mass causing proximal distension. (*Figure continued on overleaf.*)

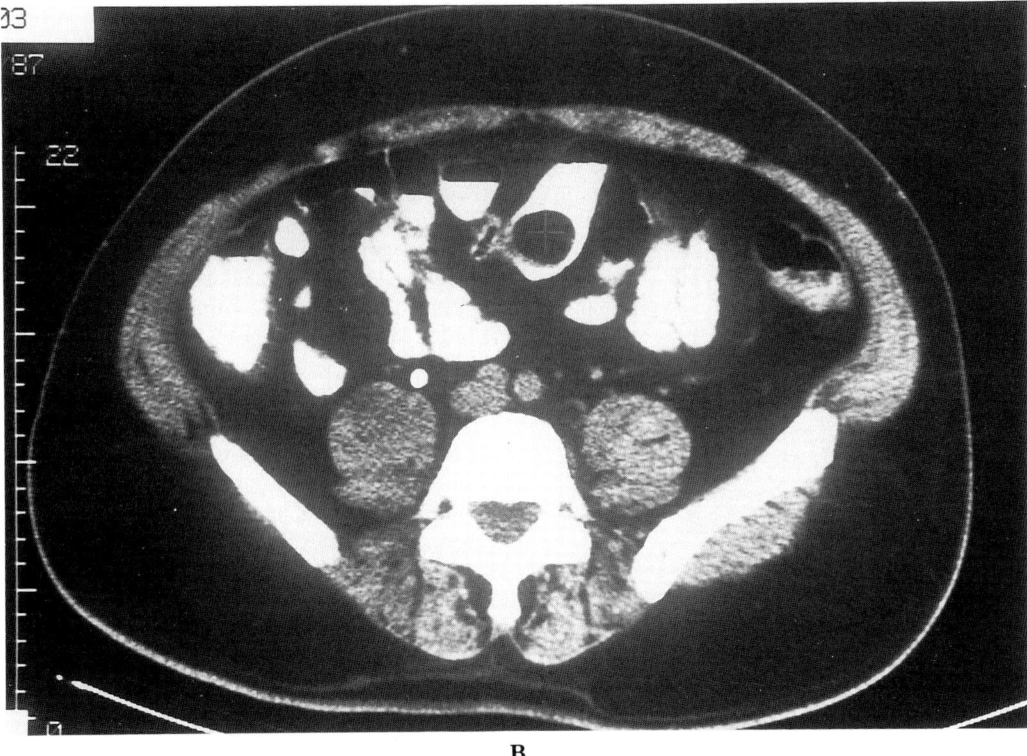

B

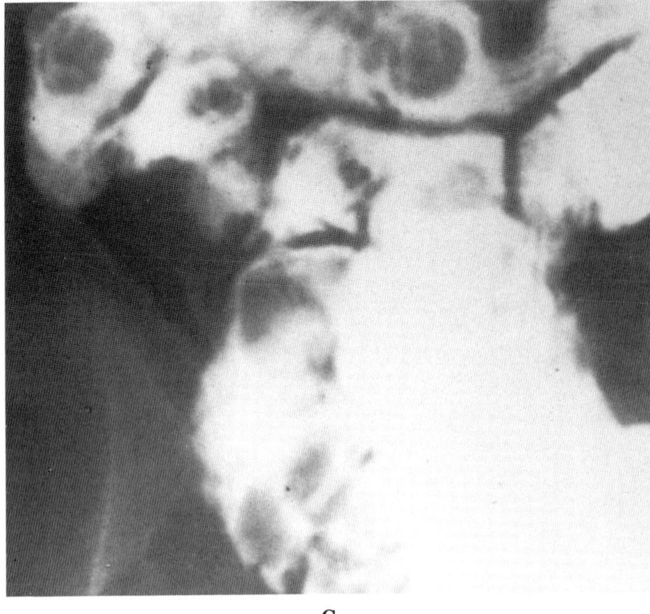

C

Figure 10.38 *continued.* (B) CT examination of (A). (C) Small bowel neurofibromatosis with multiple small bowel negative filling defects.

lipoma on a stalk may occasionally undergo torsion with subsequent alarming symptoms.

In patients with *neurofibromatosis*, the small bowel may be affected. Submucosal lesions create negative defects (Fig. 10.38C).

Hemangiomas and lymphangiomas are submucosal neoplasms that have a regular spherical or oval appearance. Their mutual distinction is not possible by radiologic means. Peristalsis or palpation can empty fluid from the neoplasm, causing the mass to diminish or seemingly to vanish.

Fibromas are rare in the small intestine and cannot be distinguished from other benign tumors by radiologic examination.

Distinguishing benign neoplasms from those that are malignant may cause considerable problems (Tables 10.5 and 10.6). Mobile gallstones, air bubbles, and mobile foreign bodies should be easily separated from neoplasms during the examination. However, impacted gallstones, unless associated pneumobilia is present, sometimes produce differential diagnostic difficulties.

TABLE 10.5. STENOSES OF THE SMALL INTESTINE

Inflammatory
Crohn's disease
Ischemic enteritis
Radiation enteritis
Eosinophilic enteritis
Neoplastic
Benign
Malignant

TABLE 10.6. SMALL INTESTINAL LESIONS WITH MALIGNANT APPEARANCE

Adenocarcinoma
Carcinoid (usually)
Lymphoma
Metastases

MALIGNANT NEOPLASMS

MALIGNANCIES OF EPITHELIAL ORIGIN

Carcinoma. Only 1% of alimentary canal carcinomas originate in the small intestine. Primary carcinomas of the small intestine have features similar to those of other gastrointestinal carcinomas. They assume one of three macroscopic forms: polypoid, annular, or ulcerated. However, combined characteristics are also possible. Macroscopic, and therefore radiologic, features of both primary and secondary carcinomas of the small intestine are similar. Gross pathologic features do not correlate with the histologic type of carcinoma. When the tumor grows into the intestinal wall, reactive fibrosis creates stenosis. A circumferential form of carcinoma is most frequent (Fig. 10.39A). The tumor occupies a short intestinal segment, most often not longer than 6 cm, with accompanying asymmetric stenosis. The transition between the neoplasm and the normal wall is abrupt, with overhanging margins, referred to as shouldering (Fig. 10.39B). Stenosis and decreased pliability of the wall lead to distension of proximal segments of the small bowel. When carcinoma grows in the direction of the serosa, it may resemble lymphoma in cases where destruction of intramural neuronal plexuses causes distension (Fig. 10.39C).

Approximately 50% of small bowel malignant neoplasms are carcinomas. They are the most common malignant neoplasm in the jejunum. Although carcinomas are less frequent than carcinoids, they are more likely to cause clinical symptoms. The association of ulcerative colitis and Crohn's disease with carcinoma of the small bowel is discussed in chapter 11. Small intestinal carcinoma is more prevalent in patients with the polyposis syndromes that bear adenomas. Moreover, patients with celiac disease, who are known to be placed at an increased risk for lymphomas of the small intestine and the mesentery, also have a higher prevalence of carcinomas in the small intestine.

Carcinomas of the small bowel cannot be reliably distinguished radiologically from granulomatous stenoses, benign polyps, or other benign tumors (Table 10.5). For this distinction, the same criteria are used as for other segments of the gastrointestinal tract (see the section on alimentary canal pathology, pages

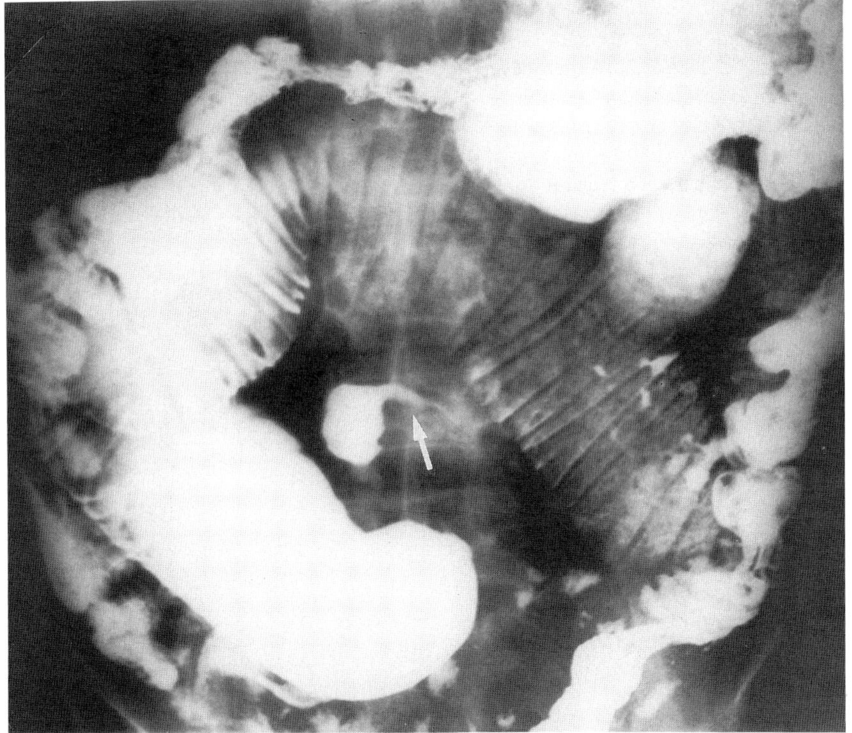

A

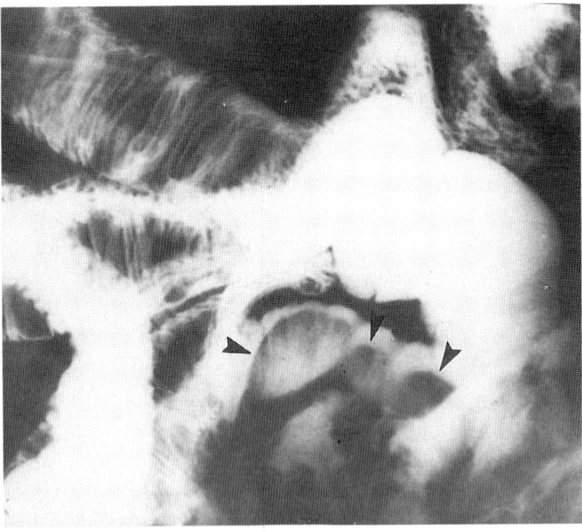

B

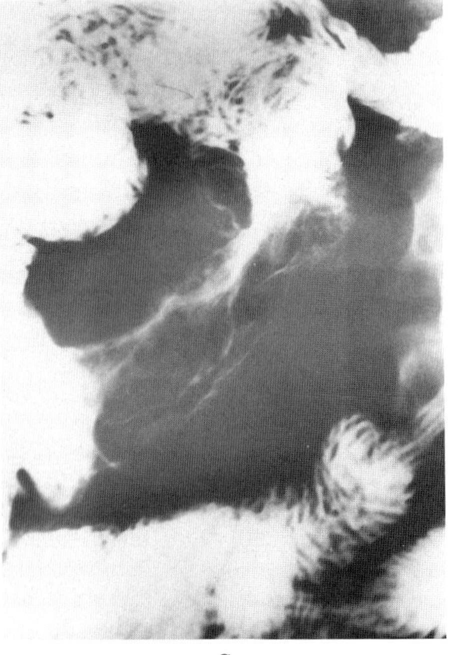

C

FIGURE 10.39. Small bowel carcinoma. (A) Stenosing, annular carcinoma (arrow), resulting in significant proximal dilatation of the bowel. (B) Polypoid carcinoma (arrowheads). Double-contrast enteroclysis. (C) Atypical carcinoma growth toward serosa destroys neuronal network resulting in dilatation in the region of the tumor.

55–58). Certain forms of small intestinal lymphoma have the same gross pathologic appearance as carcinomas (Table 10.6).

Small bowel wall thickness normally measures 2–3 mm, except in the terminal ileum, where 5 mm is regarded as the upper limit of normal. Neoplasms commonly present as eccentric wall thickenings and/or adjacent mesenteric masses. Findings are similar or identical to metastases of the small intestine.

Carcinoid. Carcinoids, or argentaffinomas, often exhibit macroscopic characteristics of malignant tumors, though their malignant potential is relatively low. The malignant potential is directly proportional to the dimensions of the carcinoid lesion. Carcinoids may infiltrate adjacent structures, metastasize into regional lymph nodes, and give rise to distal metastases. Long-term survival of patients with carcinoid is possible even with metastases in the liver. Some patients harbor carcinoids without clinical symptoms. Since carcinoids secrete serotonin, the excess of this neurotransmitter may stimulate alimentary canal motility, causing diarrhea. Carcinoid syndrome (flushing of the skin, cyanosis during the attack, tachycardia, diarrhea, attacks of bronchospasm, hypotension, edema, and ascites) is the first manifestation of the disease in only 4% of cases, because circulating serotonin is quickly converted into inactive metabolites. Carcinoid syndrome is more often seen in association with liver and/or lung metastases.

These tumors are relatively pliable and soft, and may extend either toward the lumen or toward the serosa (Fig. 10.40A). In most cases, equal proliferation in both directions influences radiographic demonstration. Carcinoids may assume gross pathologic properties of either benign or malignant tumors. In most cases, tumors are between 2 and 4 cm in diameter at the time of detection. Metastases are rare when the tumor's diameter does not exceed 1 cm. However, tumors above 2 cm in diameter metastasize in more than 80% of patients.

The angiographic pattern of the tumor vascularity in carcinoids is much the same as in carcinomas. There is a noncharacteristic vascularized tissue mass with a narrowing of individ-

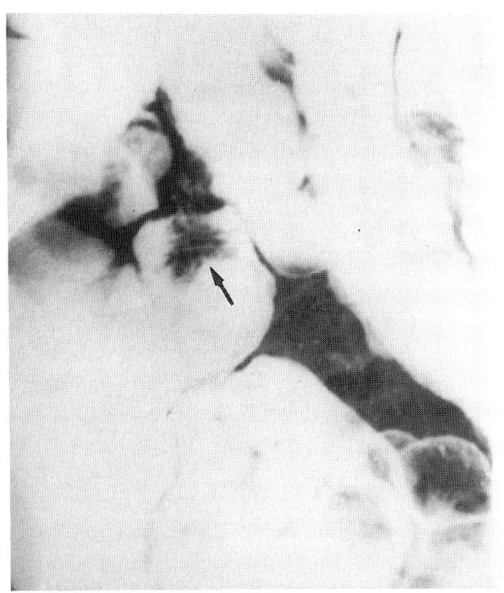

A

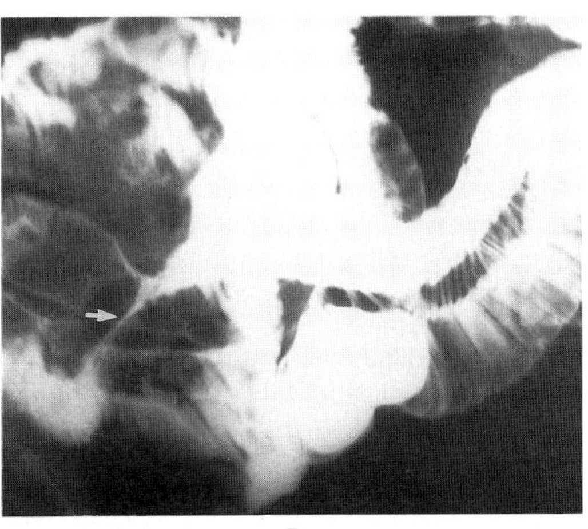

B

FIGURE 10.40. Carcinoid of the small intestine. (A) Polypoid (arrow). Follow-through barium studies. (B) Significant desmoplastic reaction (arrows).

ual arteries and poor demonstration of veins. The radiologic separation by barium studies from other neoplasms of the small intestine is not reliable, but the CT appearance can be quite characteristic. Carcinoids tend to provoke desmoplastic reaction of the associated intestinal wall and mesentery (Fig. 10.40B). Mesenteric lymph nodes are enlarged. Thickening of the intestinal wall and mesentery is readily demonstrated by CT. Intestinal obstruction, which accompanies rather advanced tumors, is a sequel to intussusception, to intramural growth associated with desmoplastic reaction, or to angulation of an intestinal loop.

Besides other small intestinal neoplasms, differential diagnosis includes Crohn's disease accompanied by stenoses and changes in the mesentery.

MALIGNANCIES OF MESENCHYMAL ORIGIN

Lymphoma. Lymphoma of the small intestine is not common. Only 5% of primary lymphomas arise in the alimentary canal. They are twice as frequent in males as in females. Secondary lymphomas are more common and do not show a predilection for age. Lymphomas are basically classified as Hodgkin's or non-Hodgkin's lymphomas. The latter variant is more frequent in the alimentary canal. According to Rappaport, non-Hodgkin's lymphomas may be classified as nondifferentiated, well-differentiated lymphocytic, poorly differentiated lymphocytic, and histiocytic. Other classifications consider lymphomas to be divided into nondifferentiated lymphomas, lymphomas of B or T cell types, and histiocytic types.

Primary intestinal lymphomas originate in the submucosa or in the lamina propria of the mucosa. Depending on the propagation of the tumor in the intestinal wall, several gross pathologic types can be distinguished. There are multinodular, infiltrating, polypoid, and transmural tumors with indentations and fistulas, as well as mainly mesenteric forms.

Radiologic signs cannot distinguish primary and secondary lymphomas without other clinical findings. However, Dawson's criteria, described in chapter 8 on gastric lymphoma (see page 296), separate primary from secondary lymphomas of the alimentary canal. Particular histologic types of lymphoma are indistinguishable on gross pathologic inspection. Similarly, radiologic examination does not enable separation of Hodgkin's from non-Hodgkin's lymphoma.

Radiologic properties of small intestinal lymphomas are determined by the specificities of tumor growth (Figs. 10.41 and 10.42). Aneurysmal widening with loss of mucosal relief is caused by intramural lymphoma growth that destroys neural plexuses. Infiltrated segments of small intestine are not able to readily transport intestinal contents. Symptoms of mechanical obstruction subsequently develop (Fig. 10.41A).

Nodular lymphoma of the small intestine is characterized by nodular outgrowths that protrude into the lumen (Fig. 10.43).

Alpha-chain disease involves the small intestine diffusely (Fig. 10.44). The intestinal wall is thickened and plicae conniventes are deformed with nodular outgrowths. This tumor can transform into immunoblastic sarcoma. Heavy-chain disease usually affects young people of the Mediterranean region and is therefore named Mediterranean lymphoma.

The frequency of primary lymphomas is higher in distal portions of the small bowel. This is probably related to the higher concentration of lymphoid tissue in the ileum. Primary lymphoma metastasizes to regional lymph nodes and other portions of the alimentary canal. Alimentary canal metastasis can be explained by the existence of a lymphocyte population recirculating in the alimentary canal.

Lymphomas are avascular tumors which displace adjacent blood vessels (Fig. 10.41C). Distinguishing small intestinal lymphoma from morphologically similar conditions may be difficult. In contrast to gastric lymphoma where radiologic accuracy reaches 79%, the diagnostic accuracy of small intestinal lymphoma is only 26%. About 65% of lymphomas of the small intestine cannot be distinguished from other neoplasms, Crohn's disease, tuberculosis, lymphangiectasia, celiac disease, and ulcerative nongranulomatous jejunitis. Differential diagnostic problems can also exist in patients with pseudomembranous enterocolitis, submucous bleeding, actinomycosis, and scleroderma.

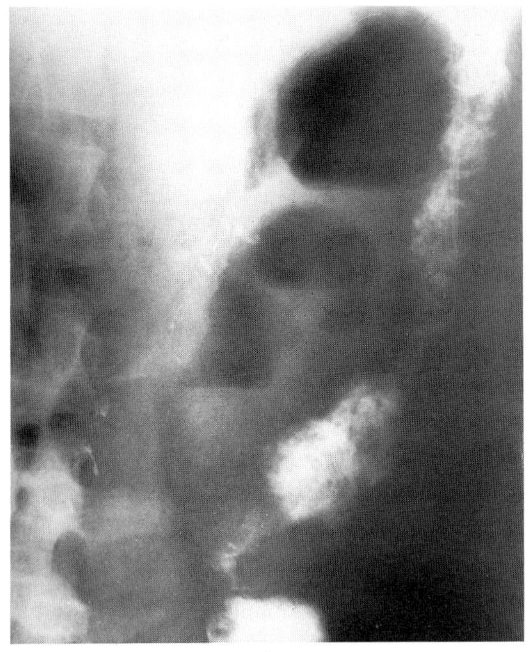

A

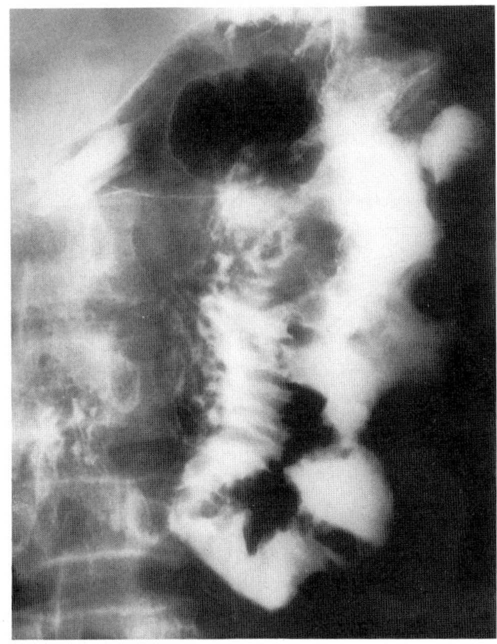

B

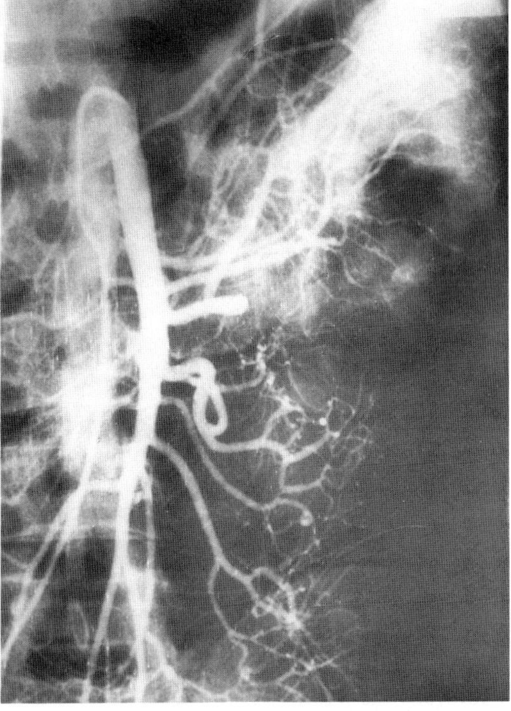

C

FIGURE 10.41. Small bowel lymphoma. (A) Gas-fluid levels in distended small intestinal loops affected by lymphoma. (B) Follow-through barium study. (C) Mesenteric arteriography demonstrates jejunal branches curving around avascular tumor masses.

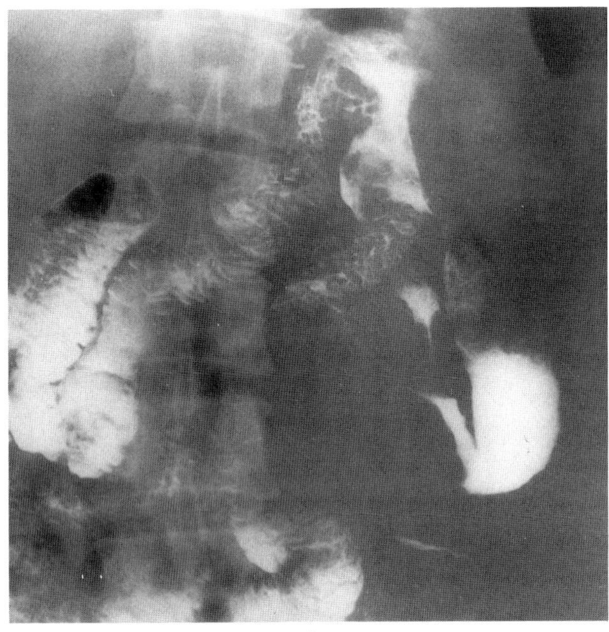

A

Figure 10.42. Small bowel lymphoma. (A) Alternating stenoses and aneurysmal dilatations of the affected bowel. Tumor masses protrude into the lumen. (B) Lymphoma affecting the mesentery separating small bowel loops.

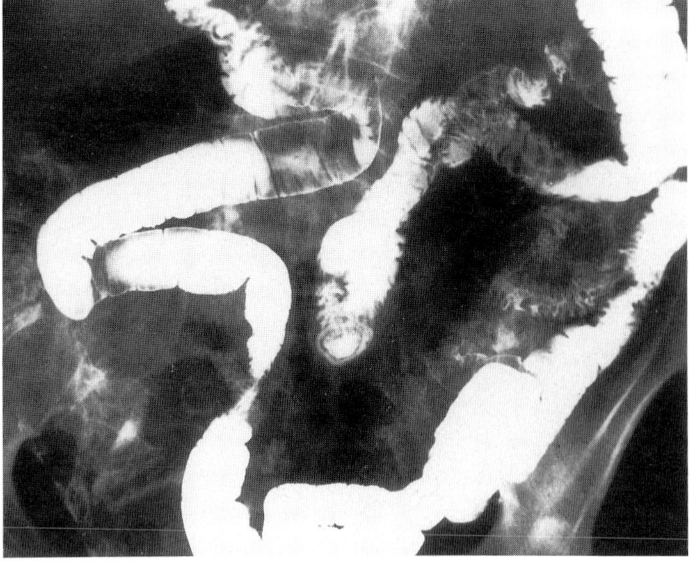

B

Leiomyosarcoma. This tumor may grow as a primary malignant neoplasm or may supposedly result from malignant alteration of a benign leiomyoma. It develops either in the principal muscular layer or in the lamina muscularis mucosae. A calcified tumor may be detected on plain abdominal films. Contrast radiography demonstrates spherical or oval

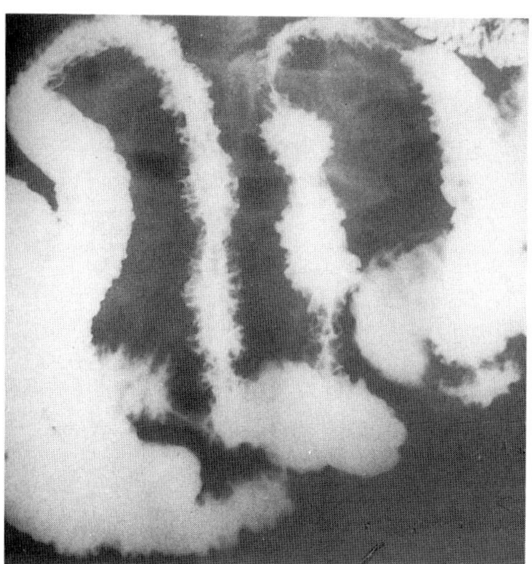

FIGURE 10.43. Nodular lymphoma of the small bowel.

neoplasms of hard consistency (Fig. 10.45). Examination by CT enhances demonstration of an exophytic lesion and can reveal metastatic deposits.

Leiomyosarcomas are larger than leiomyomas due to their more rapid growth and to loss of control of cell division. Both benign and malignant tumors derived from smooth muscles are often necrotic and ulcerated. In most cases, the overlying mucosa is ulcerated. Leiomyosarcomas tend to give rise to liver metastases.

Liposarcomas and fibrosarcomas are rare in the small intestine. Distinction from other tumors of the small intestine by radiologic means is usually not possible.

Mastocytosis may occur in any section of the alimentary canal. It is manifested in the small intestine by "bull's-eye" lesions, similar to those in melanoma metastases. However, the lesions may appear without ulceration (Fig. 10.46).

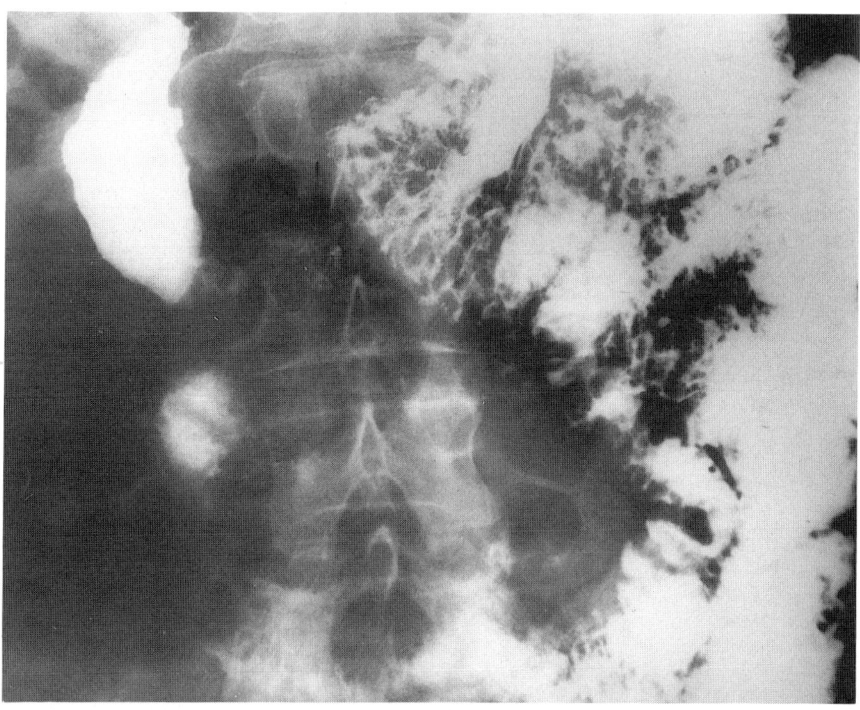

A

FIGURE 10.44. Heavy-chain disease (Mediterranean lymphoma). (A) Of the duodenum and jejunum. (*Figure continued on overleaf.*)

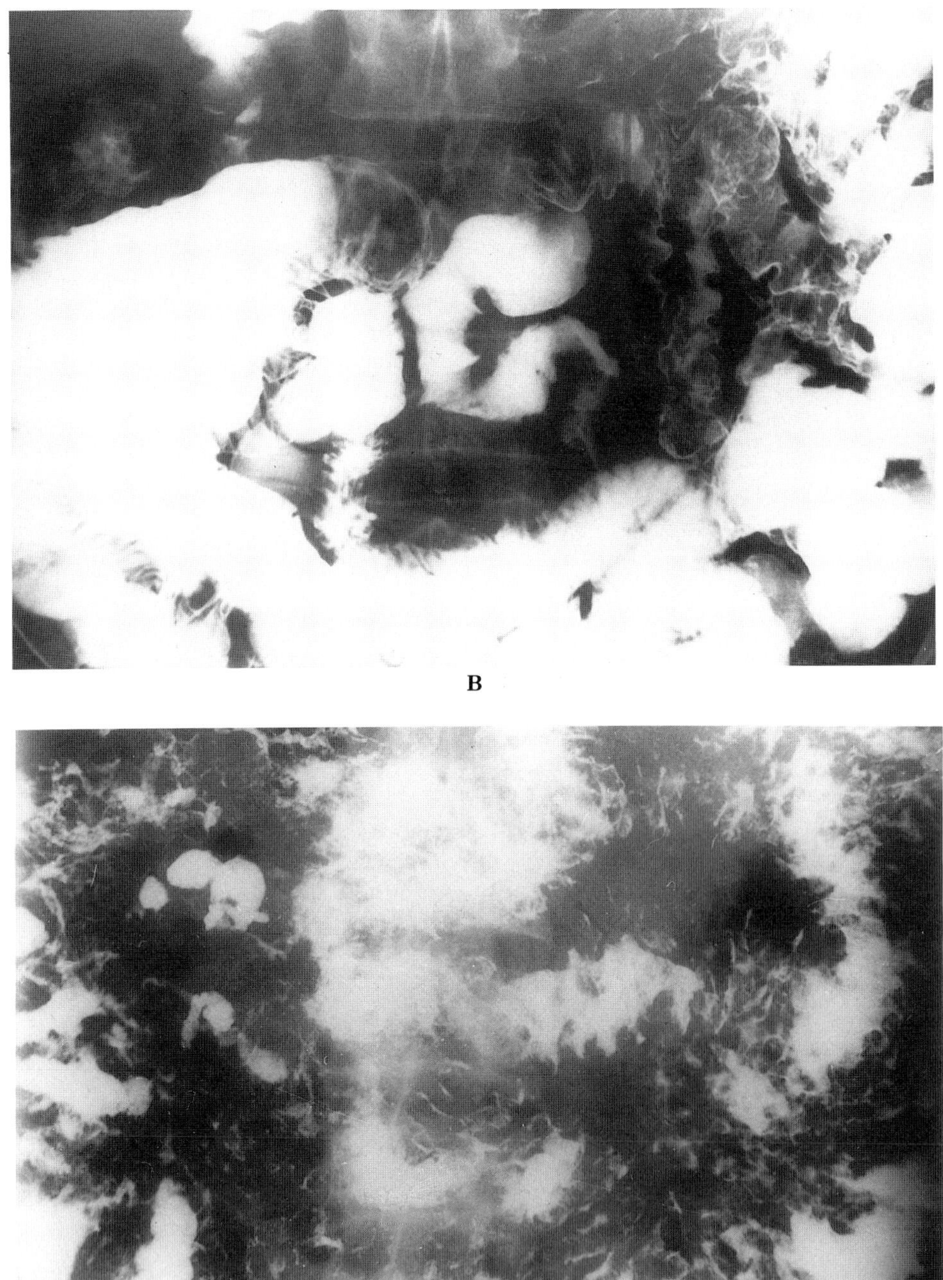

B

C

Figure 10.44 *continued.* Heavy chain disease (Mediterranean lymphoma). (B) Of the transitional small bowel. (C) Of the entire small bowel with complete loss of mucosal relief architecture.

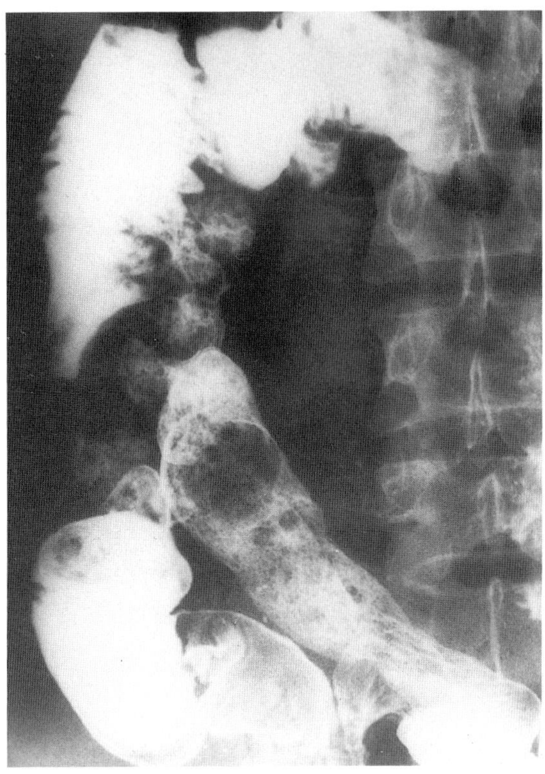

FIGURE 10.45. Leiomyosarcoma of the terminal ileum. Intense spasm of the cecum and ascending colon with proximal distension of small bowel.

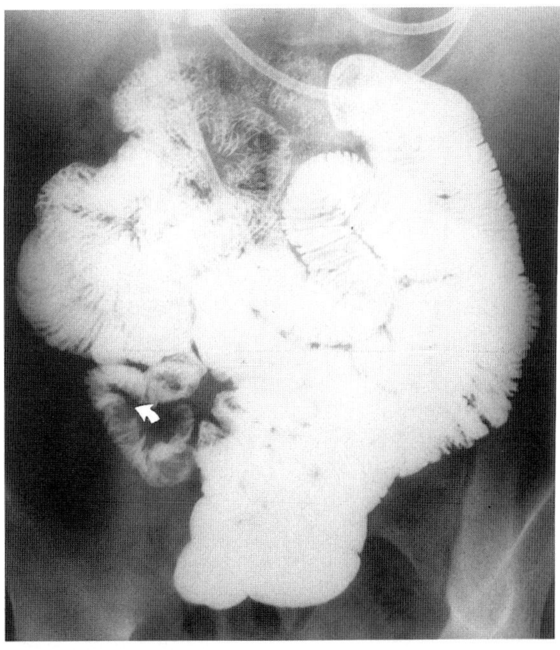

FIGURE 10.46. Mastocytosis in the ileum. Arrow indicates the largest lesion. Several smaller adjacent lesions are visible proximally. Single-contrast enteroclysis.

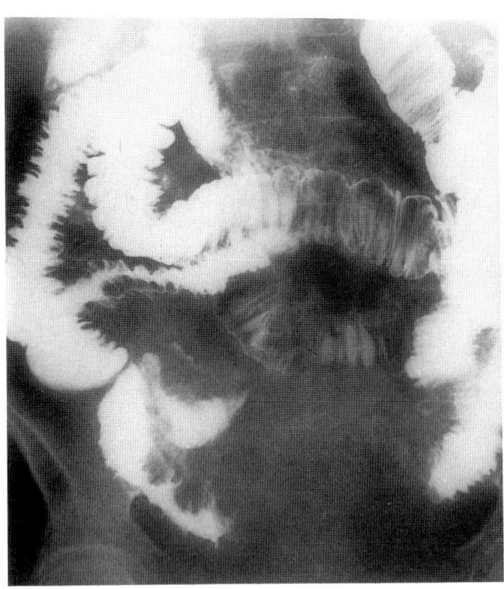

FIGURE 10.47. Ovarian carcinoma infiltrates the small bowel.

METASTATIC MALIGNANCIES

Approximately 10% of malignant neoplasms metastasize to the small bowel, particularly in their terminal stages. The prevalence of secondary neoplasms in the small intestine is equal to that of primary tumors. Even quite rare neoplasms, such as Merkel's tumor, derived from mechanoreceptive cells, metastasize into the small intestine. Metastatic carcinomas of the small intestine have the same morphology as primary carcinomas.

Mechanisms of involvement of the small intestine with secondary neoplasms are discussed in chapter 11. Malignant cell invasion into the peritoneal cavity results from direct invasion, embolic metastases, or peritoneal seeding. The small intestine is subject to invasion by neoplasms of the colon, uterus, ovary (Fig. 10.47), stomach, and other organs in the peritoneal cavity and retroperitoneal space. Intestinal obstruction is the most common sign (Table 10.7).

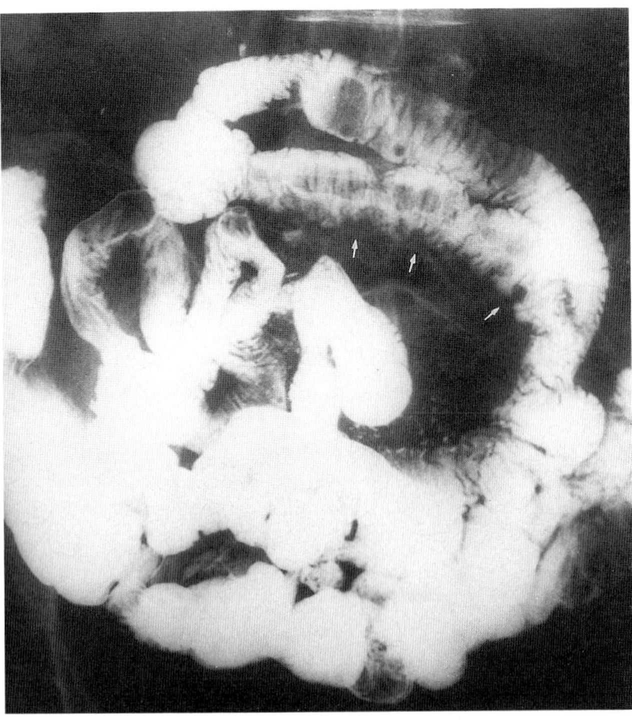

FIGURE 10.48. Submucosal hematogenous metastases of cutaneous melanoma to small bowel (arrows).

TABLE 10.7. SIGNS OF INVASION OF THE SMALL INTESTINE

Fixed and dislocated loops
Impressions on the wall
Irregular small intestinal contour
Destruction of mucosal relief
Eccentric stenosis
Partial or complete obstruction
Nodularity of the wall

Hematogenous and lymphogenous metastases of distant primary tumors are rarer than direct invasion from adjacent neoplasm. Embolic metastases of melanoma (Fig. 10.48), female genital carcinoma, bronchogenic carcinoma, and breast carcinoma (Fig. 10.49) are most often seen among secondary neoplasms of the small intestine. Melanoma metastases may, but need not, be ulcerated. Obstruction follows stenosis or intussusception. Secondary neoplasms in the mesentery separate the adjacent bowel loops (Fig. 10.50).

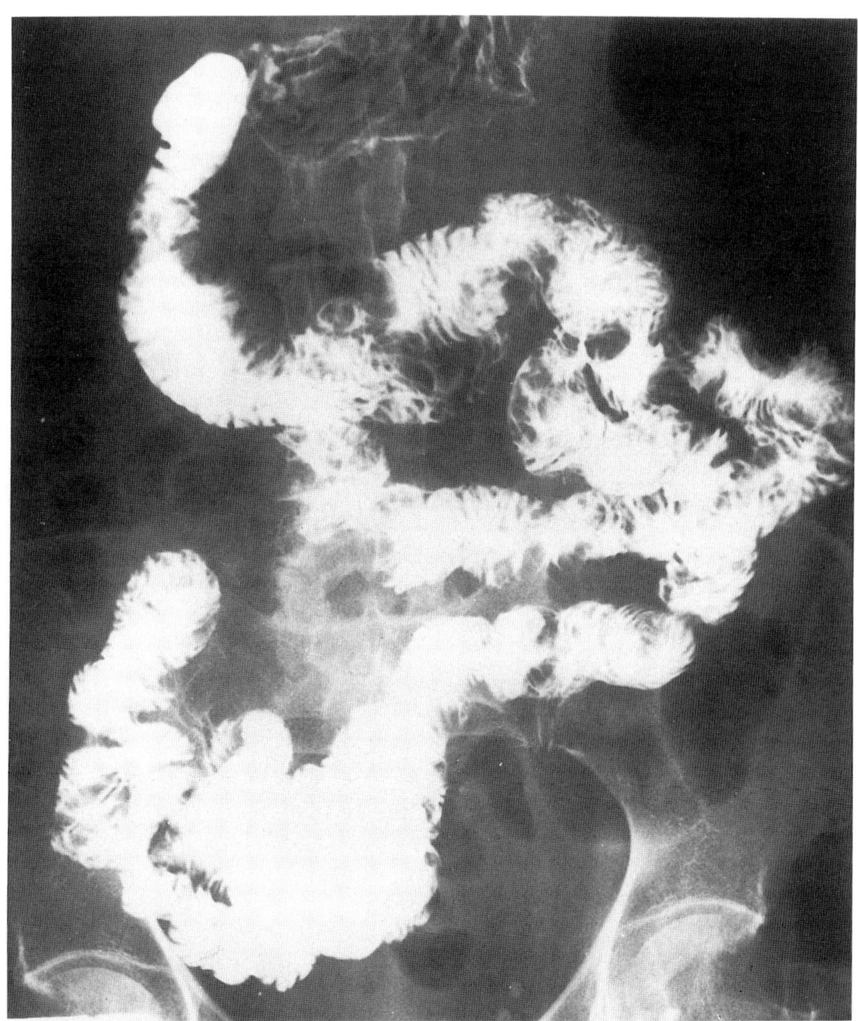

FIGURE 10.49. Submucosal, hematogenous metastases from breast carcinoma.

FOREIGN BODIES

Ordinarily, foreign bodies enter the small intestine from the stomach; some, such as gallstones, may enter through fistulas to the small intestine from adjacent organs. Fecaliths have properties of foreign bodies. Foreign bodies usually leave the gastrointestinal tract naturally. For instance, needles and pins move in a distal direction with the blunt end forward. However, foreign bodies may obstruct or impact in the intestinal wall.

INJURIES

Abdominal trauma may result in perforation of the mesenteric small intestine or in laceration of the mesentery with subsequent formation of a mesenteric hematoma. Subserosal accumulation of blood detaches the serosa from the muscular layer (Fig. 10.30) (see chapter 9 about the duodenum, page 340–342).

Hematomas in the intestinal wall can also result from hypocoagulability, as a side effect of anticoagulant therapy. Hematomas are demonstrated as submucosal masses or create a "stacked coin" appearance. Subsequent rupture of the small intestine results in pneumoperitoneum and ileus.

THE SMALL BOWEL IN CHILDREN

The transit time of barium in newborns may be longer than nine hours, without pathologic significance. In healthy children over the age of three, transit time can normally extend up to eight hours.

The presence of gas in the small bowel lumen in newborns should not be considered pathologic unless there is distension. A large volume of mucus in the small bowel of children commonly causes flocculation and segmentation of barium. Such findings are abnormal in adults, whereas they can be seen in otherwise healthy children.

In adolescents, instead of characteristic longitudinal folds in the terminal ileum, regular spherical or oval protruding negative defects may be observed. These are aggregated or solitary hyperplastic lymphoid follicles and need not indicate a pathologic process (Fig. 10.51).

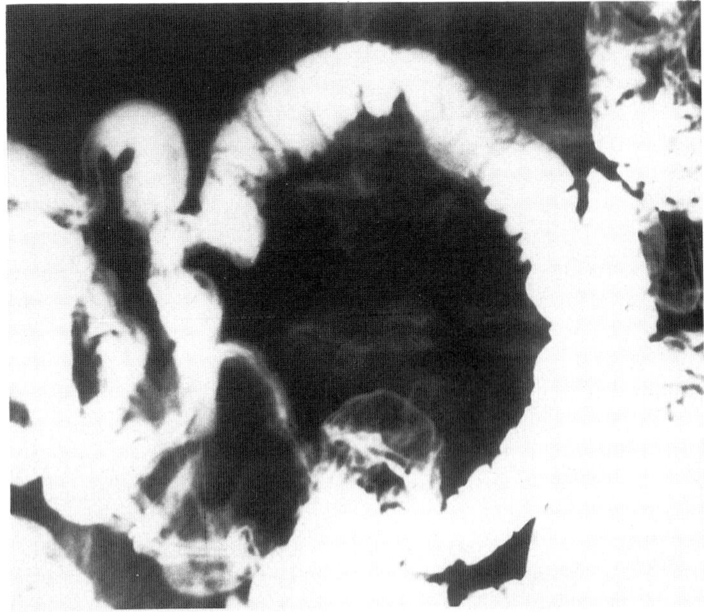

Figure 10.50. Chloroma metastatic to the mesentery. Separation of small bowel loops.

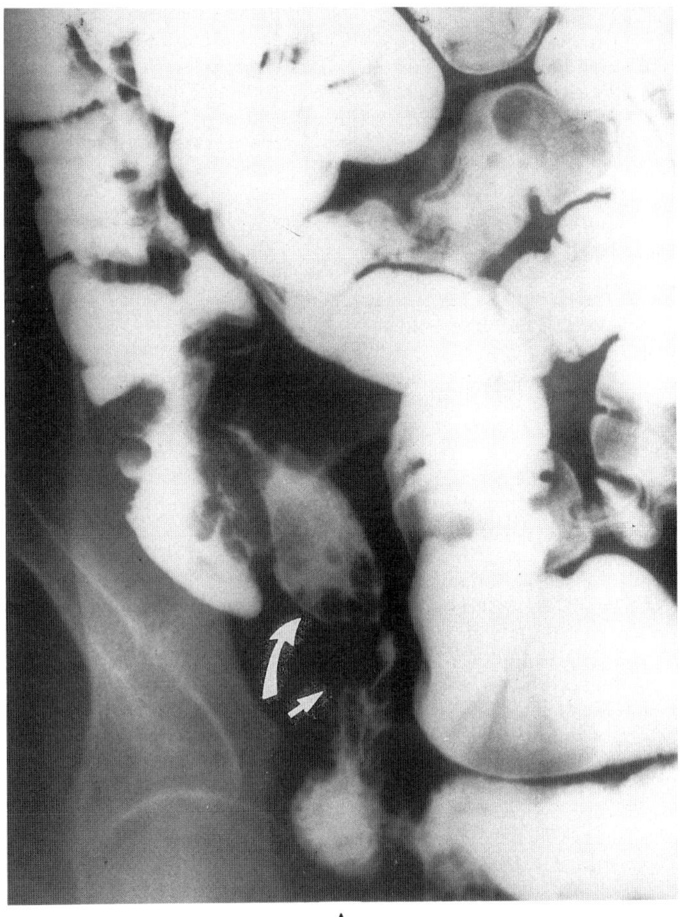

A

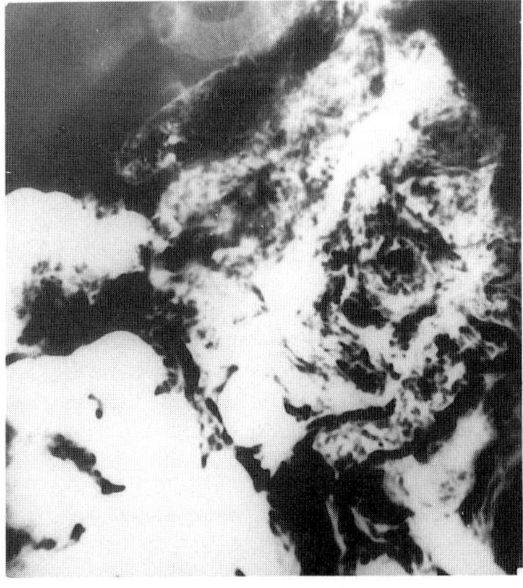

B

Figure 10.51. Lymphoid hyperplasia (A) in the terminal ileum (arrows) and (B) in the jejunum. Such appearance is not necessarily pathologic in children and adolescents.

Bibliography

Agarwal D, Scholz FJ. Small bowel varices demonstrated by enteroclysis. Radiology. 1981;140:350.

Anderson CM, Astley R, French JM, Gerrard JW. Small intestine pattern in coeliac disease. Br J Radiol. 1952;25:526.

Anderson RR, Geever EF. Intestinal pneumatosis. Am J Dig Dis. 1952;19:385.

Archer VW, Peterson CHH. Roentgen diagnosis of ascariasis. JAMA. 1930;39:1819.

Balthazar EJ. Carcinoid tumors of the alimentary tract, I:Radiologic diagnosis. Gastrointest Radiol. 1978;3:47.

Balthazar EJ, Hulnick D, Megibow AJ, Opulencia JF. Computed tomography of intramural hemorrhage and bowel ischemia. J Comput Assist Tomogr. 1987;11:67.

Benson GD, Kowlessar OD, Sleisenger MH. Adult coeliac disease with emphasis upon response to the gluten-free diet. Medicine (Baltimore). 1964; 43:1.

Blackberg B. Recurrent intussusception due to gastrointestinal polyposis in Peutz-Jeghers syndrome. Acta Chir Scand. 1960;119:45.

Blum L, Nathan H. Radiographic findings in Whipple's disease. South Med J. 1959;52:1428.

Bodart P, van Trappen G. Radiologic differences between ileocecal tuberculosis and Crohn's disease. Am J Dig Dis. 1961;6:604.

Boijsen E, Reuter SR. Mesenteric angiography in the evaluation of inflammatory and neoplastic disease of the intestine. Radiology. 1966;87:1028.

Bora JG, Friedman AC, Wesler E, Hopens TA, Wytock DH. Adaptation of the ileum in non-tropical sprue: reversal of the jejunoileal fold pattern. AJR. 1985;144:299.

Bowman PG. Primary carcinoma of the jejunum and the ileum. Ann Intern Med. 1944;20:779.

Brilley CA, Jackson DC, Johnsrude JS, Mills SR. Acute gastrointestinal hemorrhage of small bowel origin. Radiology. 1980;136:317.

Brown A, Carty H. Segmental dilatation of the ileum. Br J Radiol. 1984;57:371.

Bryk D. Strangulating obstruction of the bowel: a reevaluation of radiographic criteria. AJR. 1978; 130:835.

Caroline DF, Herlinger H, Laufer I, Kressel HY, Levine MS. Small bowel enema in the diagnosis of adhesive obstructions. AJR. 1984;142:1133.

Cockey BM, Fishman EK, Jones B, Siegelman SS. Computed tomography of abdominal carcinoid tumor. J Comput Assist Tomogr. 1985;9:38.

Collins SM, Hamilton JD, Lewis TD, Laufer I. Small bowel malabsorption and gastrointestinal malignancy. Radiology. 1978;126:603.

Craig O, Gregson R. Primary lymphoma of the gastrointestinal tract. Clin Radiol. 1981;32:63.

Dawson IMP, Cornes JS, Morson BC. Primary malignant lymphoid tumors of the intestinal tract. Br J Surg. 1961;49:80.

Ebeling WW. Primary jejunal ulcer. Ann Surg. 1933;97:857.

Eisenman JI, Finck EJ, O'Loughlin BJ. Gallstone ileus: a review of the roentgenographic findings and report of a new roentgen sign. AJR. 1967;101: 361.

Elliott GM, Elliott KA. The roentgenologic pathology of so called pneumatosis cystoides intestinalis. AJR. 1963;89:720.

Falchuk ZM. Update on gluten-sensitive enteropathy. Am J Med. 1979;1085.

Farmer RG, Hawk WA. Metastatic tumors of the small bowel. Gastroenterology. 1964;47:496.

Fiegel LS, Fiegel St J. Ileocecal intussusception in the adult. AJR. 1957;78:662.

Fisher WW, Nice CM. Barium impaction as a cause of small bowel obstruction in an infant with cystic fibrosis. Ped Radiol. 1984;14:230.

Fisk JD, Schulman HM, Greening RR, McDonald GB, Sale GE, Thomas ED. Gastrointestinal radiographic features of human graft-vs-host disease. AJR. 1981;136:329.

Frazer AC, French JM, Thompson MD. Radiographic studies showing the induction of segmentation pattern in the small intestine in normal human subjects. Br J Radiol. 1949;22:123.

Gaisie G, Curnes JT, Scatliff JH, Coom RD, Vanderzalm T. Neonatal intestinal obstruction from omphalomesenteric duct remnants. AJR. 1985;144: 109.

Goldberg HJ, Sheft DJ. Abnormalities in small intestine contour and caliber. Radiol Clin North Am. 1976;14:461.

Golden R. Amyloidosis of small intestine. AJR. 1954;72:401.

Godwin JD. Carcinoid tumors. Cancer. 1975;36:560.

Good CA. Tumors of the small intestine. AJR. 1963;89:685.

Greenstein S, Jones B, Fishman EK, Cameron JL, Siegelman SS. Small bowel diverticulosis: CT findings. AJR. 1986;147:27.

Harbin WP, Andres J, Kim SH, Borden S. Internal hernia into Traves' field pouch. Radiology. 1979; 130:71.

Harris OD, Cooke WT, Thompson H, Waterhouse JAH. Malignancy in adult coeliac disease and idiopathic steatorrhea. Am J Med. 1967;42:899.

Herlinger H, Maglinte DDT. Jejunal fold separation in adult coeliac disease: relevance of enteroclysis. Radiology. 1986;158:605.

Hodgson JR, Hoffman NH, Huizenga KA. Roentgenologic features of lymphoid hyperplasia of the small intestine associated with dysgammaglobulinemia. Radiology. 1967;88:883.

Holmes WH, Starr PA. Nutritional disturbance in adults resembling coeliac disease and sprue. JAMA. 1929;92:975.

Hornsby AT, Baylin GH. Sprue vs. pancreatogenous steatorrhea. Radiology. 1954;63:491.

Ike BW, Rosenbusch G. Gastrointestinal malignant lymphoma; roentgenographic features and pathologic and morphologic correlations. Diagn Imag. 1981;50:66.

Jones B, Bayless TM, Fishman EK, Siegelman SS. Lymphadenopathy in coeliac disease, computed tomographic observations. AJR. 1984;142:1127.

Kantor JL. The roentgen diagnosis of idiopathic steatorrhea and allied conditions. Practical value of the moulage sign. AJR. 1939;41:758.

Kogutt MS. Necrotizing enterocolitis of infancy. Radiology. 1979;130:367.

Lerner HH, Gazin AJ. Pneumatosis intestinalis. Its roentgenologic diagnosis. AJR. 1946;56:464.

Lerner HH, Levinsin SS, Kateman AE. Meckel's diverticulum. AJR. 1953;69:268.

Levine MS, Drooz AT, Herlinger H. Annular malignancies of the small bowel. Gastrointest Radiol. 1987;12:53.

Lukes RJ, Collins RD. New approaches to the classification of the lymphomata. Br J Cancer. 1975; 31(Suppl 2):1.

Maglinte DDT, Miller RE, Lappas JC. Radiologic diagnosis of occult incisional hernias of the small intestine. AJR. 1984;142:931.

Maglinte DDT, Herlinger H. Small bowel radiography: an overview. Dig Dis Sci. 1984;29:1057.

Maglinte DDT, Chernish SM, De Weese R, Kelvin FM, Brunelle RL. Acquired jejunoileal diverticular disease: subject review. Radiology. 1986;158: 577.

Marshak RH, Wolf BS, Cohen N, Janowitz, HD. Protein-losing disorders of the gastrointestinal tract: roentgen features. Radiology. 1961;77:893.

Marshak RH, Linder AE, Maklansky D. Lymphoreticular disorders of the gastrointestinal tract. Roentgenographic features. Gastrointest Radiol. 1979;4:103.

Mast A, Elewaut A, Mortier G, Quatacker J, Defloor E, Roels H. Gastric xanthoma. Am J Gastroenterol. 1976;65:311.

McLeod AJ, Zornoza J, Shirkhoda A. Leiomyosarcoma—computed tomographic findings. Radiology. 1984;152:133.

Miller RE, Brahme F. Large amounts of orally administered barium for obstruction of small bowel. Surg Gynecol Obstet. 1969;129:1185.

Murphy SB. Classification, staging and end results of treatment of childhood non-Hodgkin's lymphomas: dissimilarities from lymphoma in adults. Sem Oncol. 1980;7:332.

Ormson MJ, Stephens DH, Carlson HC. CT recognition of intestinal lipomatosis. AJR. 1985;144:313.

Osborn AG, Friedland GW. Radiological approach to the diagnosis of small bowel disease. Clin Radiol. 1973;24:281.

Pansdorf H. Die fraktionierte Dundarmfullung und ihre klinische Bedeutung. Fortschr Rontgenstr. 1937;56:627.

Papandopulos VD, Nolan DJ. Carcinoma of the small intestine. Clin Radiol. 1985;36:403.

Pearce AE, Ivker M, Oller S. Fibroma of ileum and a review of benign small intestinal tumors. Surgery. 1954;36:299.

Pope TL, Shaffer H. Small bowel xanthomatosis: radiologic-pathologic correlation. AJR. 1985;144: 1215.

Quinn SF, Shaffer HA, Willard MR, Ross S. Bull's-eye lesions. a new gastrointestinal presentation of mastocytosis. Gastrointest Radiol. 1984;9:13.

Radin DR, Siskind BN, Alpert S, Bernstein RG. Small bowel varices due to mesenteric metastasis. Gastrointest Radiol. 1986;11:183.

Rambaud JL, Seligmann M. Alpha-chain disease. Clin Gastroenterol. 1976;5:341.

Ree HJ. Malignant lymphoma of Waldayer's ring following gastrointestinal lymphoma. Cancer. 1980; 46:1528.

River L, Silverstein J, Tope JW. Collective review: benign neoplasms of small intestine; critical comprehensive review with reports of 20 new cases. Surg Gynecol Obstet. 1956;102:1.

Sanders DE, Ho CS. The small bowel enema: experience with 150 examinations. AJR. 1976;127:743.

Seymour EQ, Griffin CN Jr, Kurtz SM. Carcinoid tumors of the duodenal cap presenting as multiple polypoid defects. Gastrointest Radiol. 1982;7:19.

Shapiro JH, Rubinstein B, Jacobson HG, Poppel MH. Enteroliths in small intestine. AJR. 1956; 75:343.

Shimkin PM, Waldman TA, Krugman RL. Intestinal lymphangiectasia. AJR. 1970;110:827.

Smith EEJ, Saunders JH, Bowley N. Pneumatosis intestinalis in the small bowel of an adult. A radiological sign of a serious post-operative complication. Br. J Radiol. 1981;54:266.

Starr GF, Dockerty MB. Leiomyomas and leiomyosarcomas of the small intestine. Cancer. 1955;8: 101.

Sussman JF, Chalck JI. Hepatodiaphragmatic interposition of the small intestine. Radiology. 1950;54: 726.

Tallrot K, Katevue K, Holsti L, Andersson M. Angiography and computed tomography in the diagnosis of primary lymphoma of the brain. Clin Radiol. 1981;32:383.

Wittich G, Salomonowitz E, Szepesi T, Szembirek H, Frenhwald F. Small bowel double-contrast enema in stage III ovarian cancer. AJR. 1984;142:299.

Wollaeger EE, Scudamore HH. Spectrum of diseases causing steatorrhea. Arch Intern Med. 1964;113: 819.

Zeitels J, Naunheim K, Kaplan EL, Strauss F. Carcinoid tumors. Arch Surg. 1982;117:732.

Chapter 11

Diseases That Affect Both Small and Large Bowel

INTESTINAL ISCHEMIA

The superior mesenteric artery provides the blood supply for the small and the large bowel as far as the splenic flexure of the colon. More distal segments are supplied by the inferior mesenteric artery. Signs of mesenteric artery occlusion depend on the rate of decrease in blood flow, as well as on the length of the affected segment and collateral vascular network. Circulatory disturbances of the superior mesenteric artery have a graver prognosis than those of the inferior mesenteric artery, since the entire small bowel and a major portion of the colon can be affected. Sudden and complete superior mesenteric arterial obstruction is a life-threatening condition (Fig. 11.1). Therefore, it is important to recognize the barium examination appearance of preceding partial or temporary mesenteric artery obstruction.

Acute occlusion of mesenteric arteries presents as an acute abdomen. The ischemic bowel is functionally obstructed. This results first in delayed transport of small bowel contents and is soon followed by symptoms of paralytic ileus. At the onset of clinical symptoms, the bowel appears gasless. An early specific sign of intestinal ischemia on plain roentgenograph of the abdomen is narrowing of the lumen of an affected segment and increasing separation between adjacent intestinal loops caused by thickening of the intestinal wall (Fig. 11.2). Edema of the intestinal wall is visible as swelling of Kerckring's folds in the small intestine, and vanishing haustra in the colon.

Distension of the colon and small bowel with collections of gas and liquid is a late nonspecific sign of intestinal ischemia, which accompanies considerable disturbance of blood flow. In mesenteric arterial occlusion, a plain roentgenograph of the abdomen recorded in a dependent position often reveals a functional obstruction (see chapter 5, page 153). Presence of gas in the intestinal wall and portal vein is a late but relatively specific sign of intestinal gangrene (Fig. 11.3). Occlusions of mesenteric arteries with consequent necrosis of the intestinal wall and gangrene are contraindications for oral or rectal contrast media examination of the alimentary tract.

The diagnosis may be confirmed by angiographic examination. However, in approximately half of all patients with nonocclusive intestinal ischemia, the arteriographic findings are normal. Routine angiography is not able to detect decreased blood flow in arteries but is valuable in estimating sufficient or insufficient collateral circulation. Arteriography and CT angiography are methods of choice for detection of occlusions in larger vessels.

A patient with nongangrenous ischemic intestinal disease should be radiologically examined in the beginning of the disease and three weeks later by oral administration of contrast medium or by barium enema. In this manner, information about the progression of the dis-

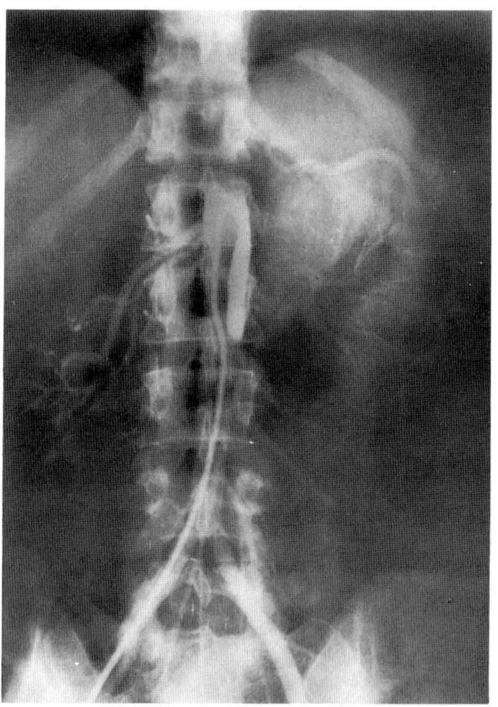

Figure 11.1. Thrombosis of the superior mesenteric artery. Selective arteriography.

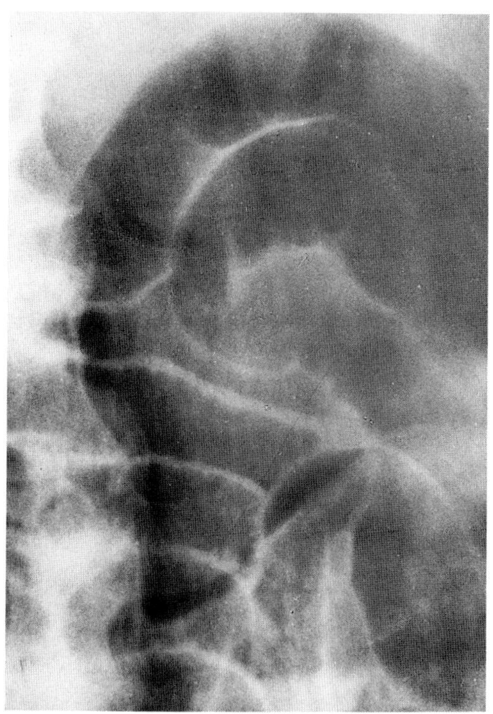

Figure 11.2. Ileus and thickened small bowel wall in ischemia.

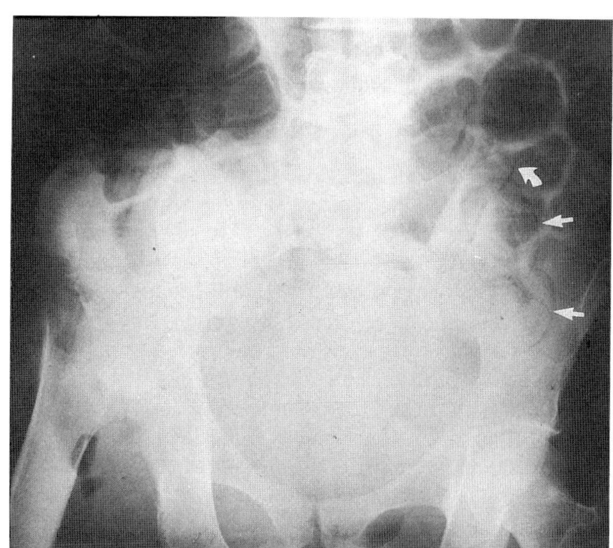

Figure 11.3. Linear pneumatosis intestinalis in bowel ischemia (arrows).

ease, such as the appearance of early strictures, can be obtained. The left colonic flexure, distal descending colon, and sigmoid colon are the most common sites of these pathologic entities. This is attributed to the poor anastomoses between upper and lower mesenteric arteries in this area. Location of an ischemic segment of bowel does not always correspond to the site of vascular occlusion or altered circulation. Perforation of the intestinal wall in an ischemic area can lead to pneumoperitoneum and peritonitis.

Anastomoses between the superior and inferior mesenteric arteries, as well as between the superior mesenteric artery and the celiac axis, and the inferior mesenteric artery and internal iliac artery, are sometimes very plentiful. In these instances, arterial occlusions may remain without clinical symptoms. The midgut is not supplied with a double circulation and is more likely to undergo necrosis.

Disturbances of circulation in mesenteric arteries are caused by atherosclerosis, vasculitis, coagulopathies, and compressions of the mesentery and gut, such as strangulated obstructions. Ischemic colitis may also be the consequence of sigmoid colon volvulus. Following volvulus reduction some patients develop postischemic stricture of the sigmoid colon, while others may later develop subacute colitis of the left hemicolon resembling chronic inflammatory diseases of the large intestine. Ischemic disease of the bowel may be a repercussion of microcirculatory disturbances where there are occlusions only of small arteries. There is evidence that digitalis may act as a provocative agent in developing intestinal ischemia, via constriction of splanchnic arteries. Ischemic lesions of the intestinal wall may also be caused by alterations in venous circulation.

Gangrenous ischemic enteritis and colitis result from occlusion of one of the major arteries that supply the bowel. Necrosis often affects all layers of the intestinal wall, although the mucosa and submucosa are the most vulnerable. This is followed by gangrenous necrosis, accompanied by putrefaction, and infection with colonic bacteria. In rare cases, only a portion of the intestinal wall will undergo necrosis. Gas in mesenteric veins, confirmed by computerized tomography, is an accurate sign of infarction. Sufficient collateral circulation can preserve the intestinal wall from complete necrosis. Infarctions of the large intestine are less frequent in those portions fixed to the posterior abdominal wall because of rich anastomoses.

Gangrene of the bowel mainly affects patients over 60 years of age with advanced atherosclerosis.

Nongangrenous ischemic enteritis and colitis are characterized by edema, submucosal bleeding, and ulceration. Radiologic findings in ischemic colitis are similar to those found in chronic inflammatory diseases of bowel (ulcerative colitis and Crohn's disease). In early stages, the mucosa is swollen and may bear ulcerations. Later, fibrosis leads to strictures with benign radiologic characteristics (Fig. 11.4).

Ischemic colitis is more common than enteritis. There are two possible variants. A *transitional form* is a consequence of temporary ischemia of the bowel supplied by atherosclerotic small arteries. Recovery of the mucosa is complete. In patients with a *stricturing form* of the disease, collateral circulation prevents the development of gangrene but is insufficient to permit complete recovery of the intestinal wall. Later, strictures and saccular widenings develop (Fig. 11.4C). Sac-like widenings of normal colon, pseudodiverticula, result from the fibrosis of adjacent affected segments. Combinations of transitional and stricturing ischemic colitis are also possible.

Radiographic signs of intestinal ischemia are:

1. Mural impressions (thumbprinting), asymmetric indentations of bowel contour caused by submucosal bleeding and edema (Figs. 4.74 and 11.5). They appear mainly (75%) in nongangrenous ischemic disease, follow early clinical symptoms, and can last for ten days. Thumbprinting appears in the stricturing form of the disease within nine days of the ischemic attack, and within six days of the attack in the transitional form.
2. Deep symmetric transverse indentations on the contour of the large intestine caused by muscle spasms which often accompany mural impressions.
3. Sawtooth ulcers distributed either symmetrically or asymmetrically along the bowel, where they may be found one to three weeks after initial symptoms (Fig. 11.6). Longitudinal ulcers are present in 60% of patients.

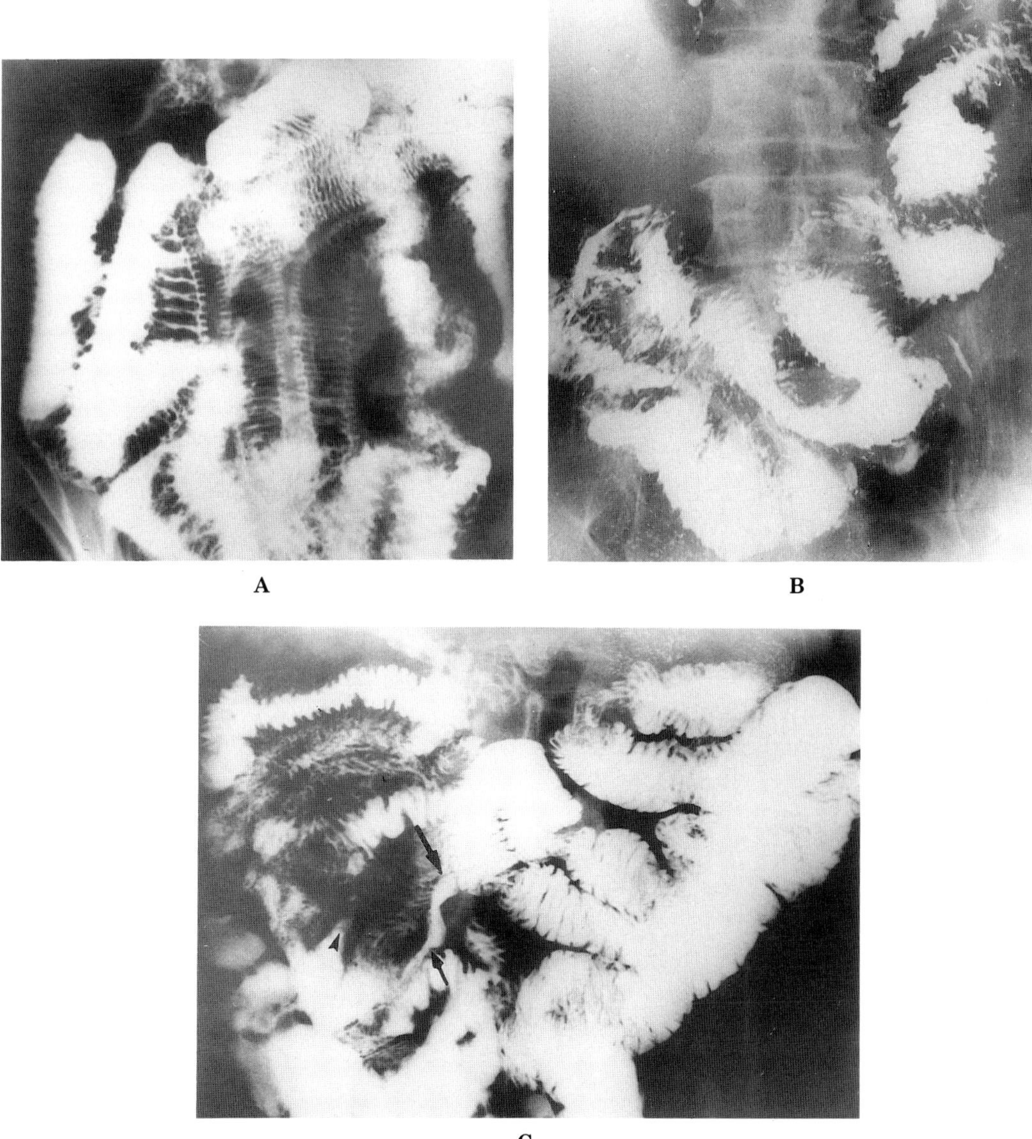

A

B

C

Figure 11.4. (A) Acute ischemic small bowel lesions. Edema and erosion of mucosa. (B) Subacute stage of small bowel ischemia. Distension of bowel lumen and thickening of folds. (C) Chronic small bowel changes. Strictures with benign characteristics (arrows and arrowhead).

They heal after 10 days in the transitional form and after 20 days in the stricturing form of the disease.

4. Presence of barium in the intestinal wall as a result of its penetration through deep ulcers.
5. Tubular strictures which appear at the beginning of the fourth week after the ischemic

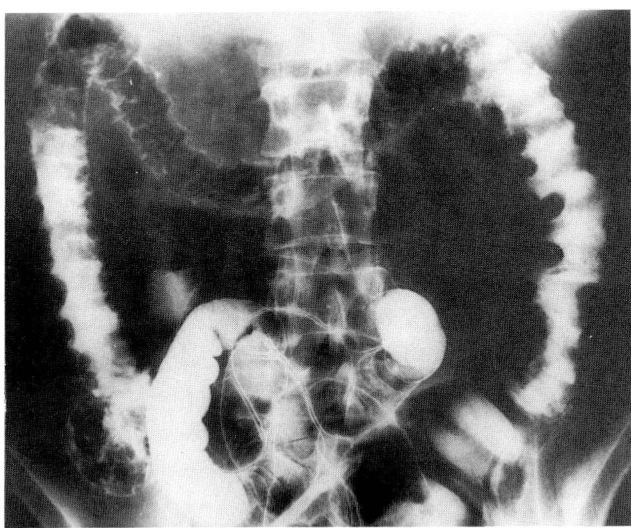

Figure 11.5. Ischemia of the colon. Thumbprinting, ulcers and symmetric spasm. (See Fig. 4.74.)

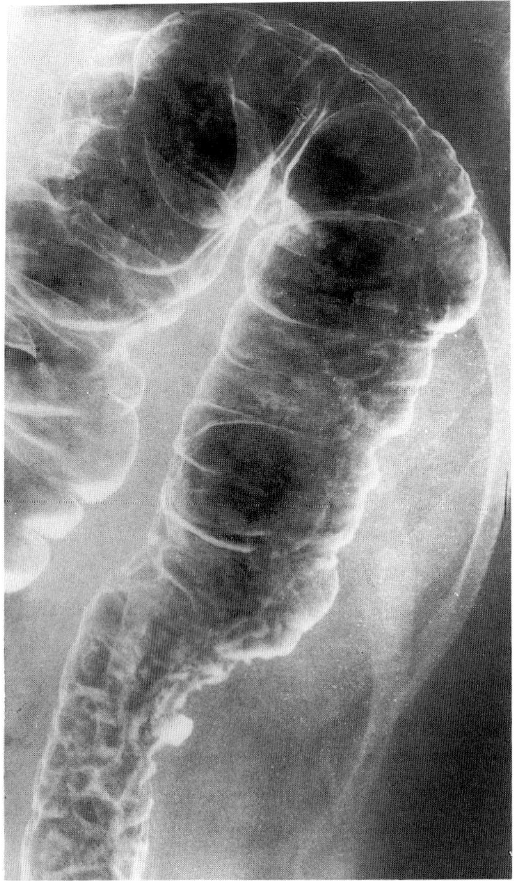

Figure 11.6. Postischemic lesions of the proximal descending colon. Ulcers and asymmetric narrowing. Anastomosis of the superior and inferior mesenteric arteries is not well developed in the splenic flexure region.

attack. They may affect the intestinal wall asymmetrically and are caused by fibrosis in the submucosa. These strictures have a benign radiographic appearance (Fig. 11.7). Sometimes, radiologically detectable lesions (ulcers, digital impressions) do not precede the strictures, which are then the first and only signs of ischemic bowel disease (Figs. 4C and 11.7). Eccentric strictures appear 48% of the time (Fig. 11.8).

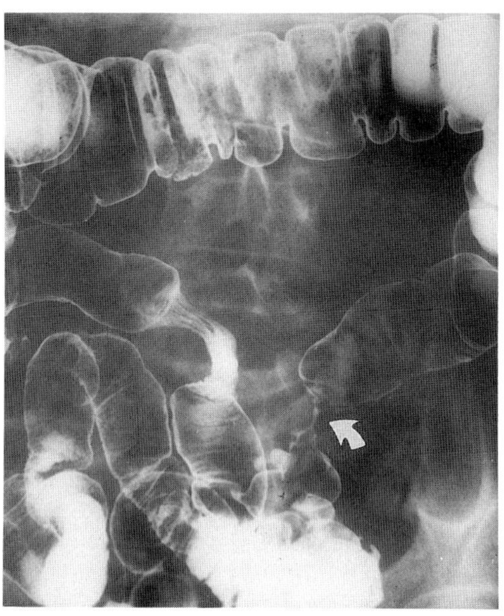

A

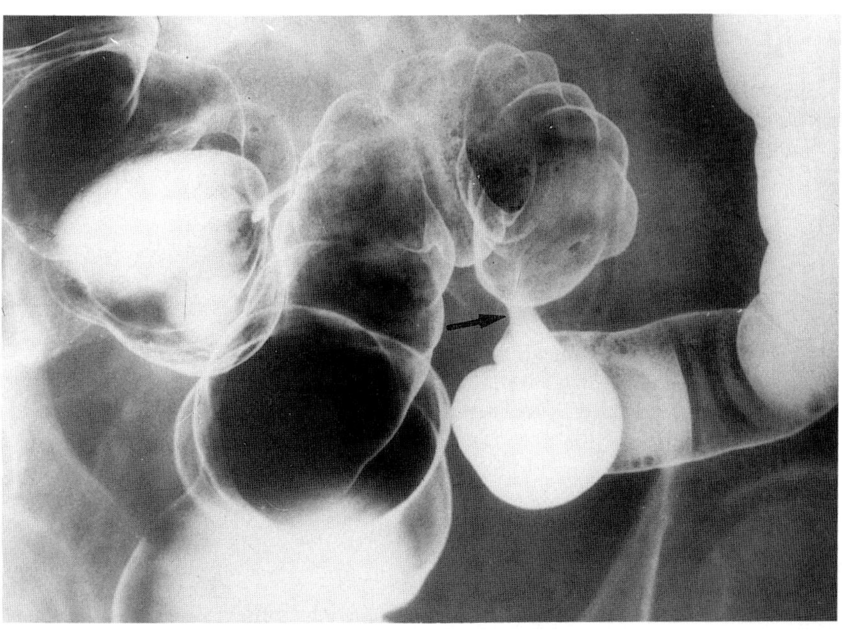

B

FIGURE 11.7. Ischemic stenosis. (A) At the transition from descending colon to sigmoid colon (arrow). (B) In mid-sigmoid colon (arrow). The sigmoid colon region, particularly the distal segment, is a location with less collateral arterial blood flow.

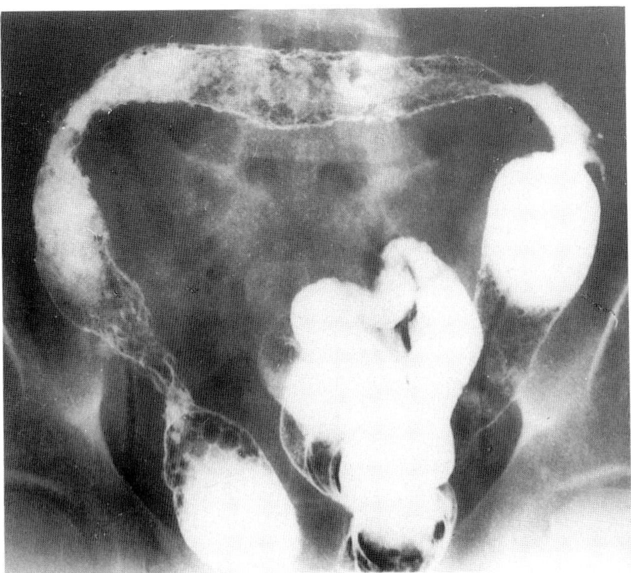

FIGURE 11.8. Microcolon with ulcers, pseudopolyps, and fibrosis. Repeated attacks of colonic ischemia with typical distribution of lesions. The colon is affected up to the left flexure.

6. Saccular widenings (pseudodiverticula) of normal intestinal wall are caused by fibrosis in adjacent diseased tissue. They may mimic those in Crohn's disease (Fig. 11.9), and are visible in 30% of patients.

Among radiographic signs of ischemic bowel disease, mural impressions and ulcers are the earliest to appear, and along with sac-like areas and strictures are the most frequent. Longitudinal ulcers and digital impressions are more specific for an ischemic etiology than are other signs.

Stricturing carcinoma distal to an ischemic lesion of the colon occurs in 1–5% of patients with ischemic colitis.

Thrombosis of mesenteric veins is not characterized by alarming symptoms in the majority of patients. On plain roentgenograph of the abdomen recorded in a dependent position, discrete collections of gas and fluid in the bowel are noted. The intestinal lumen is not significantly widened. Overall, radiologic signs on plain roentgenogram of the abdomen, or barium series are not sufficient for confirmation of the diagnoses. Computed tomography may demonstrate an occlusive thrombus in the superior mesenteric vein and associated mesenteric edema.

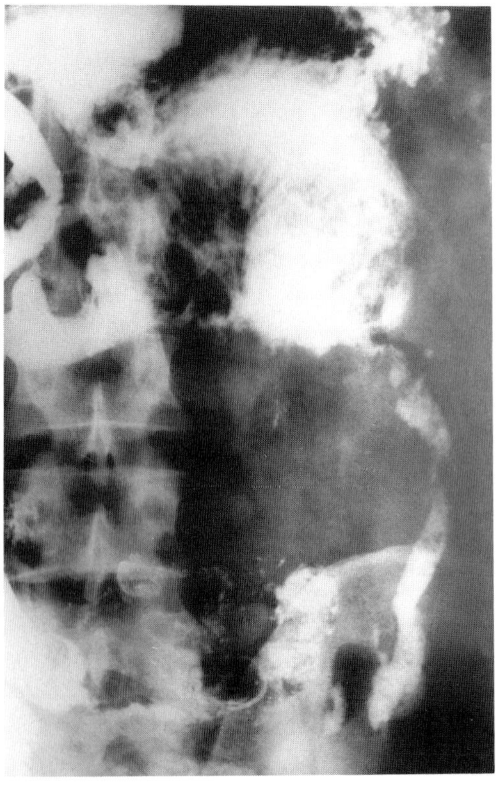

FIGURE 11.9. Long postischemic stricture of the small bowel with proximal distension.

INFECTIONS AND INFESTATIONS

Infections and infestations of the alimentary canal do not have pathognomonic radiographic characteristics. Stool culture and/or biopsy are often required for precise diagnosis. However, patients with bacterial, mycotic, or viral infections, and parasitic infestations of the digestive tube may undergo radiologic examination for a variety of clinical indications.

BACTERIAL INFECTIONS

Tuberculosis. Gastrointestinal tuberculosis is rare. Bacilli may infect the alimentary canal by ingestion or occasionally by hematogenous spread. Aphthoid ulcerations, defects of epithelium covering enlarged submucosal lymphoid follicles, may appear at the onset of the disease. The surrounding mucosa is commonly intact but aphthoid ulcerations may progress into deeper ulcers. Aphthoid ulcers are frequently found on colonic mucosa in Crohn's disease, enterocolitis caused by *Yersinia enterocolitica*, Behçet syndrome, candidiasis of the stomach and gut, amebic colitis, and shigellosis.

Tuberculous ulcers of the upper alimentary canal appear on a thickened wall. Radiologic findings in the stomach are consistent with the diagnosis of "hypertrophic gastritis." In the ileocecal region, the most common site for alimentary canal tuberculosis, lesions closely resemble those of Crohn's disease. Tuberculous colitis cannot be radiographically distinguished from other types of chronic colitis.

Other Bacterial Infections. *Bacillary dysentery* in its chronic form radiographically resembles ulcerative colitis.

Lesions caused by *Yersinia enterocolitica* or chronic lesions resulting from *Salmonella typhi* infection may mimic Crohn's disease of the ileocecal region.

SPIROCHETAL INFECTIONS

Treponema pallidum rarely invades the alimentary canal, but when it does the stomach is most often affected. Lues of the stomach resembles scirrhous carcinoma, and gummas appear as circumscript tumors. On occasion, the rectum may also be a site of involvement. When not treated, lues results in rectal ulcers, with progressive narrowing in the postulcerative phase.

MYCOTIC INFECTIONS

Candidiasis of the bowel is infrequent. The most common site of lesions caused by *Candida albicans* is the esophagus. However, the stomach may also be the site of alimentary canal candidiasis. Early lesions may take the form of aphthoid ulcerations. As a result of mucosal protrusions and colonies of fungi, the affected mucosa assumes a cobblestone pattern. In chronic disease, this is followed by ulcer formation and strictures.

Actinomycosis, as it affects the alimentary canal, is mainly a disease of the terminal ileum and cecum. Radiographic findings resemble other granulomatous and neoplastic diseases of this area.

Mucormycosis occurs almost exclusively in an immunosuppressed population. It is the least common among mycotic infections of the alimentary canal. This otherwise saprophytic microorganism invades blood vessels causing vasculitis, thrombosis, and ischemic necrosis. Tumor-like formation is a radiologic finding. Endoscopy reveals an ulcerated polypoid lesion covered with a black crust.

PROTOZOAL INFECTIONS

The colon is a primary location of chronic infection by *Entamoeba histolytica.* After ingestion of a cyst, the protozoon passes from an encysted into a vegetative form within the small intestine. The disease is characterized by ulcers affecting both mucosa and submucosa of the colon with a tendency to coalesce. Reactive proliferation of tissue leads to formation of pseudotumors called amebomas. Amebic abscesses and amebomas preferentially reside in the ileocecal area. Abscesses affecting the intestinal wall and the liver are readily demonstrated by ultrasound or CT.

VIRAL INFECTIONS

Patients with viral infections of the alimentary canal are seldom subject to radiologic examination. *Chlamydia trachomatis* infection may result in *Lymphogranuloma venereum* causing changes resembling Crohn's proctocolitis. Ulcerations, fistulas, and strictures are associated with diffuse inflammation in Douglas's cavity. The rectum and sigmoid colon are locations predisposed to these changes.

Rotavirus infections account for 75% of the gastroenteritis in children between six months and two years of age. Diarrhea is accompanied by hyperthermia and vomiting. The colonic mucosa is edematous as the result of infiltration of the lamina propria and swelling of the intestinal villi. Spasms and discrete rose-thorn ulcers resemble an ulcerative colitis. Differentiation is possible by detection of viremia.

Cytomegalovirus is transmitted by infected body fluids and stools. Parenchymatous organs and the alimentary canal of clinically asymptomatic patients may harbor the virus. The infection attacks newborns and subjects with decreased immunologic reactivity, such as patients under immunosuppressive therapy and those with neoplasms or AIDS. Cytomegalovirus infection may involve any portion of the gastrointestinal tract in AIDS patients. The colon is most commonly involved and either a diffuse pancolitis or segmental infection can result (Fig. 11.10). However, the cecum may be exclusively involved. Ulcers in the terminal ileum and cecum may bleed and even perforate. Vasculitis in the submucosa can result in focal ischemia. The colonic mucosa appears granular, with superficial erosions, aphthoid ulcers, and swollen folds. Spasms are quite common. Though in most cases colitis has a chronic clinical history, it may occasionally progress rapidly with profuse bleeding, perforation, and death. Computed tomography can demonstrate colonic wall thickenings and mucosal ulcerations.

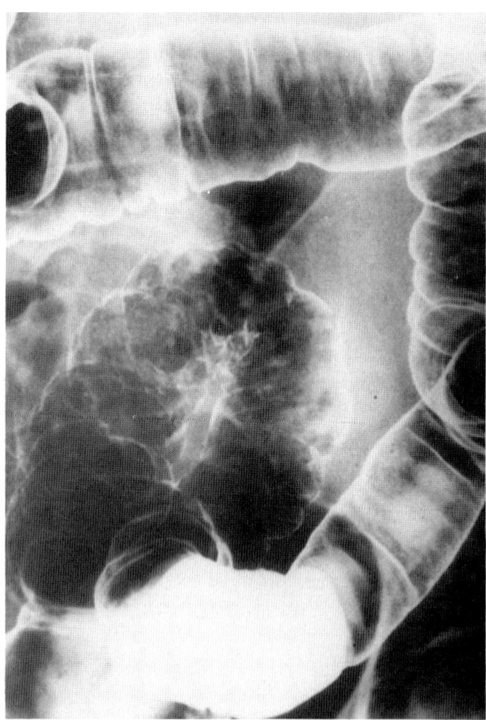

FIGURE 11.10. Cytomegalovirus colitis. Irregularities of the sigmoid colon.

Although the AIDS virus does not affect the alimentary canal directly, patients are placed at an increased risk from opportunistic infections with a high prevalence of *Cryptosporidium* and *Toxoplasma* (Coccidia parasites), cytomegalovirus infection and moniliasis of the esophagus. Alimentary canal carcinoma develops in 12% of patients with AIDS, and Kaposi's sarcoma in 8%.

Parasitic diseases are discussed in chapter 10, pages 379–380.

ULCERATIVE COLITIS AND CROHN'S DISEASE

Double-contrast enema is reliable and safe for examining patients with ulcerative colitis (UC) and Crohn's disease (CD). The sensitivity in adults exceeds 90%, whereas the sensitivity of a single-contrast barium enema in detecting CD lesions is 82%. The specificity of both methods in detecting UC and CD in children equals 100%. Lesions of both UC and CD, their natural histories, and the effect of therapy can be monitored by barium studies and CT. The natural history of UC and CD is unpredictable. They may both be accompanied by extraintestinal manifestations.

UC is a chronic inflammatory disease of unknown etiology. It usually affects the mucosa and submucosa of the large intestine, but may occupy all layers of the wall. In approximately 10% of patients, it also affects the terminal ileum, causing a backwash ileitis. When the process affects only a segment of the colon, the left hemicolon is more frequently involved.

Crohn's disease is chronic inflammation of unknown etiology. It may appear in any segment of the alimentary canal, from the oral cavity to the anus, as well as in extragastrointestinal organs. It originates at the terminal ileum in a majority of patients. Both small and large intestine are affected in 59% of patients, whereas the small or large intestine alone is affected in 30% and 11% of the cases respectively. Transmural, segmental, granulomatous lesions and ulcerations characterize CD. Considering the tendency for recurrence, surgical resections of the gut should be kept to a minimum. Therapy is mainly medical, and only high-grade obstructions, fistulae, or malignancies necessitate surgery.

Ulcerative colitis shows a predilection for young and middle-aged adults, but even newborns can be affected. In half of UC patients, symptoms begin before 30 years of age, females being affected twice as often as males. When the disease is severe at its onset, the mortality rate may be as high as 30%. When the disease begins more gradually, it has a better prognosis.

The incidence of UC and CD observed over

TABLE 11.1. PATHOLOGIC AND RADIOLOGIC FEATURES OF ULCERATIVE COLITIS AND CROHN'S DISEASE OF THE COLON

FEATURE	ULCERATIVE COLITIS	CROHN'S DISEASE
Extent	Entire large intestine	Rectum often intact
Wall involvement	Symmetrical	Asymmetrical
Early lesions	Edema, necrosis	Aphthoid ulcerations
Skip areas	Rare	50%
Granulomas	Exceptionally rare	Always
Early ulcers	Rose-thorn	Aphthoid
Mucosa	Diffuse ulcerations	Cobblestone pattern
Advanced ulcers	Circular and longitudinal	Longitudinal, deep
Ulcers	All mucosa inflamed	Inflamed and normal appearing mucosa
Intestinal wall	Not thickened	Thickened (lymphedema, granulomas)
Haustral markings	Disappear early	Preserved
Pseudopolyps	Often	Less often; smaller
Lymphatic follicles	Intact	Enlarged
Regional lymph nodes	Unaffected	Enlarged
Inflammation and fibrosis	Mucosa and submucosa only	Entire wall thickness
Wall deformation	Moderate	Severe
Appendices epiploicae	Intact	Affected
Adhesions	No	Yes
Fistulae	No	Yes
Mesentery and mesocolon	Unaffected	Affected
Terminal ileum disease	Seldom (backwash ileitis)	Often
Toxic dilatation	Yes	Yes
Carcinoma	Considerably increased risk	Increased risk

the past several decades has been almost constant. In countries of the West where it attacks one in approximately 3500 adults, the incidence of CD exceeds that of UC. The average age of CD onset is between 15 and 30 years and the proportion of diseased males and females is approximately 5:4. Crohn's disease is more common in some families than in the general population. It affects the colon less frequently than UC. Unlike UC, CD is not inclined to remissions and, despite therapy, almost 25% of diseased patients remain permanently disabled. Except for fibrosis, lesions of UC, in contrast to CD, are more likely to be reversible. In 14% of diseased individuals, the first attack of CD appears after the 50th year of age and, in this group, the colon is more frequently affected. However, the terminal ileum remains a favorable site for CD lesions.

In typical cases with a characteristic distribution of lesions, it is possible radiologically to distinguish UC from CD, as well as from other forms of chronic colitis and ileitis. Endoscopy with biopsy is diagnostic in approximately 90% of diseased patients (Table 11.1).

Cleansing enemas must be carefully administered in patients with UC and CD. Air insufflation for a double-contrast enema has to be performed with great care so as to not damage vulnerable intestinal wall. During a filling of the colon, barium advances faster than in normal persons due to spasms. Several phases may be identified in the natural history of UC and DC (Diagrams 11.1 and 11.2). Lesions characteristic of several phases are often simultaneously present in the same patient.

In brief, in *UC* the following phases may be observed.

1. A *congestive phase* is characterized by mucosal hyperemia along with edema, resulting in a granular mucosal appearance (Dia-

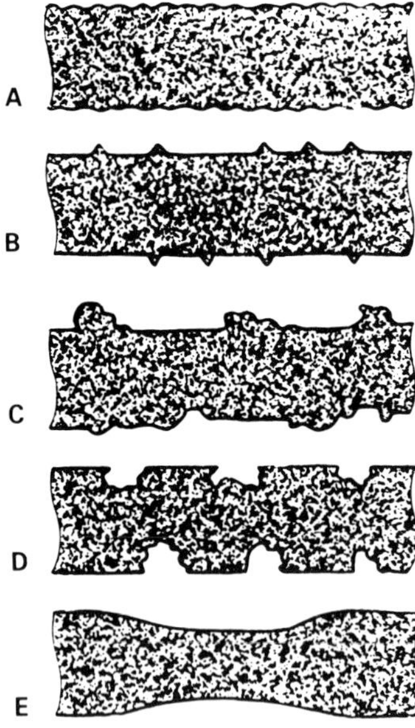

Diagram 11.1. Ulcerative colitis. (A) Congestive phase. Fine granularity of the mucosa. (B) Early ulcerative phase. Small rose-thorn ulcers. (C) Advanced ulcerative phase. (D) Chronic reparative and proliferative phase. Regeneratory formations "pseudopolyps" protrude into the lumen. (E) Fibrous-atrophic phase with shortening and stenoses. Lead-pipe appearance of the colon.

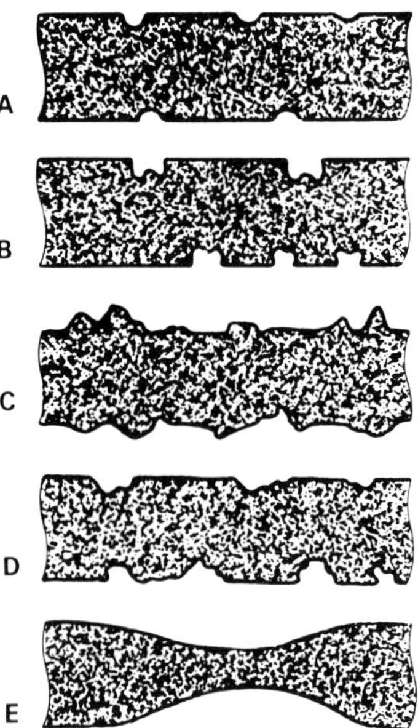

Diagram 11.2. Crohn's disease. (A) Enlarged lymphoid follicles. (B) Aphthoid ulcers. Defects of epithelium covering enlarged lymph follicles. (C) Granulomas, transverse and longitudinal ulcers resembling cobblestones. (D) Reparative and proliferative phase. Healing of ulcers and appearance of regenerating mucosal formations "pseudopolyps." (E) Stenotic phase.

gram 11.1 and Fig. 11.11A). Spasm of the colon or hypotonia with loss of haustral markings may be the first radiologic sign (Fig. 11.11B).

2. In the *early ulcerative phase* "rose-thorn" ulcers occur at various depths often at symmetric sites on the wall (Fig. 11.12A and B).
3. In the *advanced ulcerative phase*, ulcers penetrate deeper into the wall and become irregular. In severe forms ulcers may penetrate to the serosa. Confluent deep ulcers result in the longitudinal entrance of barium into the wall giving the appearance of a tramline (Fig. 11.13).
4. "Pseudopolyps" characterize a *reparative and proliferative phase*. These hyperplastic

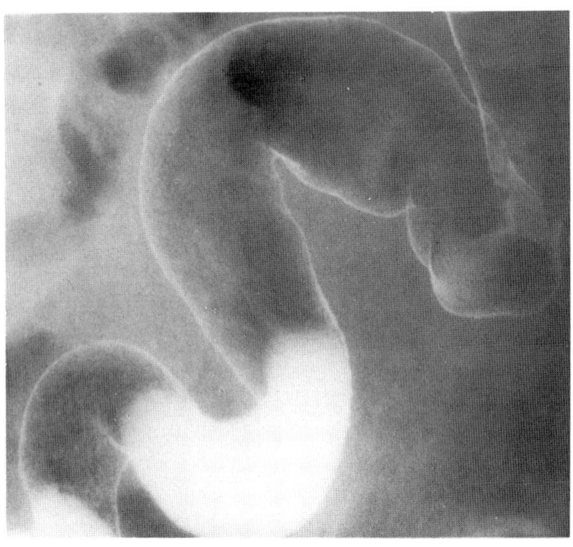

A

FIGURE 11.11. Ulcerative colitis. (A) The surface of the mucosa looks as if it is covered with powdered sugar. (B) Distal half of the transverse colon is without haustral markings. Loss of haustral markings proximal to the left flexure of the colon is a sign of pathology. Small pseudopolyps are present in the proximal transverse colon.

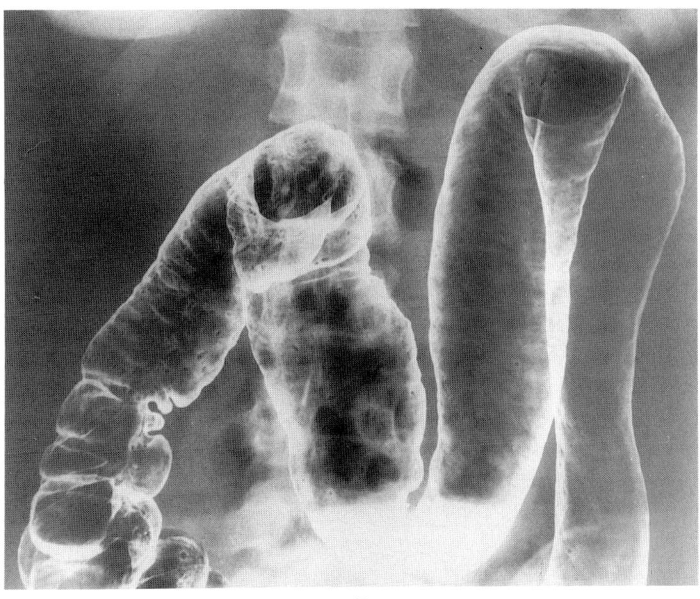

B

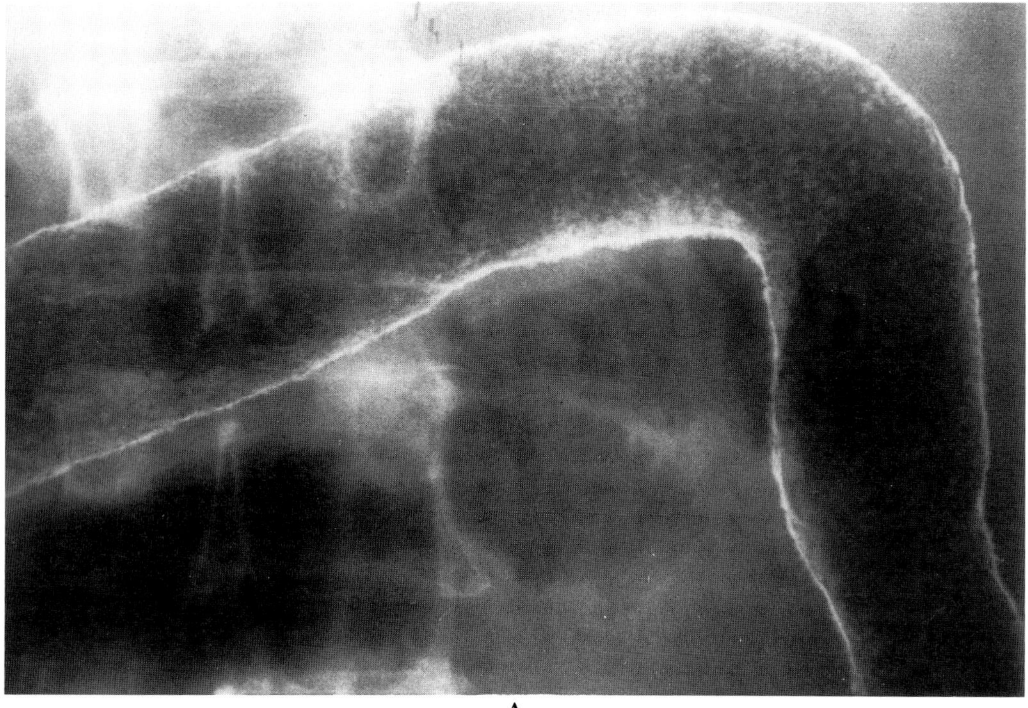

A

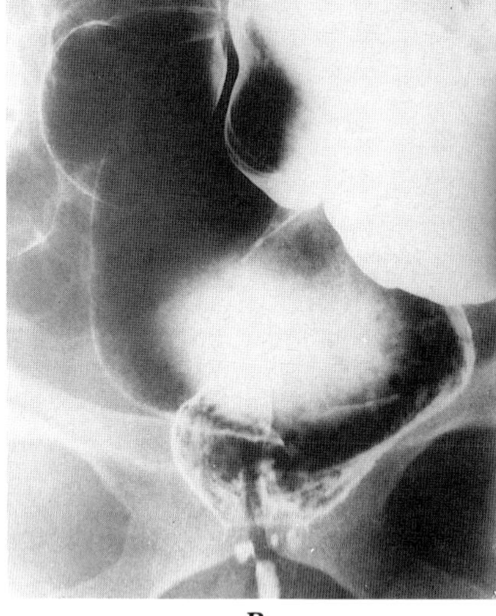

B

FIGURE 11.12. Ulcerative colitis. (A) Loss of haustral markings, granularity of mucosa and numerous shallow ulcers. (B) Edema and superficial ulcers in distal rectum.

growths of remaining mucosa appear in 64% of patients with UC (Figs. 11.14 and 11.15).

5. The *fibrous atrophic phase* begins with a dissolution of ulcerations and pseudopolyps. The intestinal wall is replaced with fibrosis and the lumen of a commonly shortened colon becomes narrow and its wall rigid. Haustral markings disappear throughout the entire colon as well as the rectal valves.

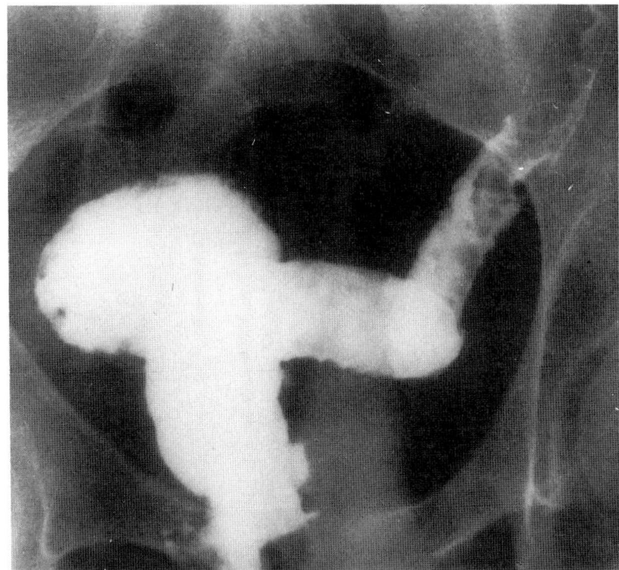

A

FIGURE 11.13. Advanced phase of ulcerative colitis. (A) Deep ulcerations, hyperplastic formations and mucosal edema. (B) Deep subserosal ulcerations. Barium appearances between layers of the colonic wall. Pseudopolyps of the sigmoid colon wall are evident. (*Figure continued on overleaf.*)

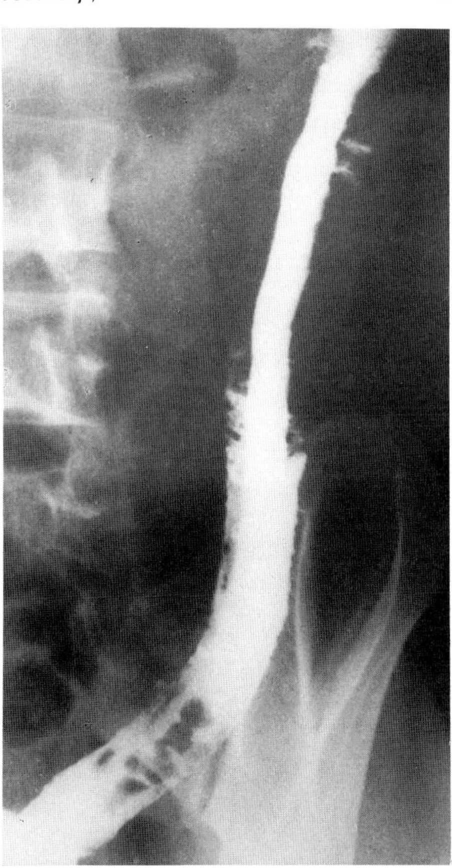

B

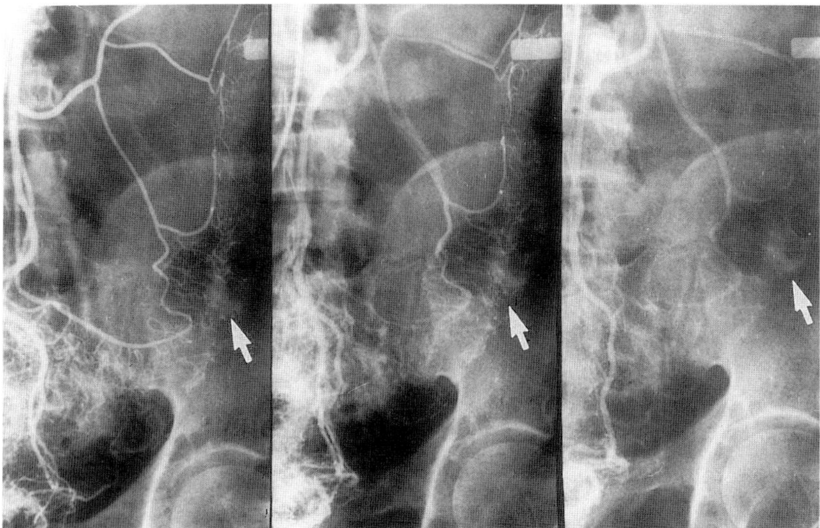

Figure 11.13 *continued.* Advanced phase of ulcerative colitis. (C) Bleeding from a deep ulcer. Selective inferior mesenteric arteriography (arrows).

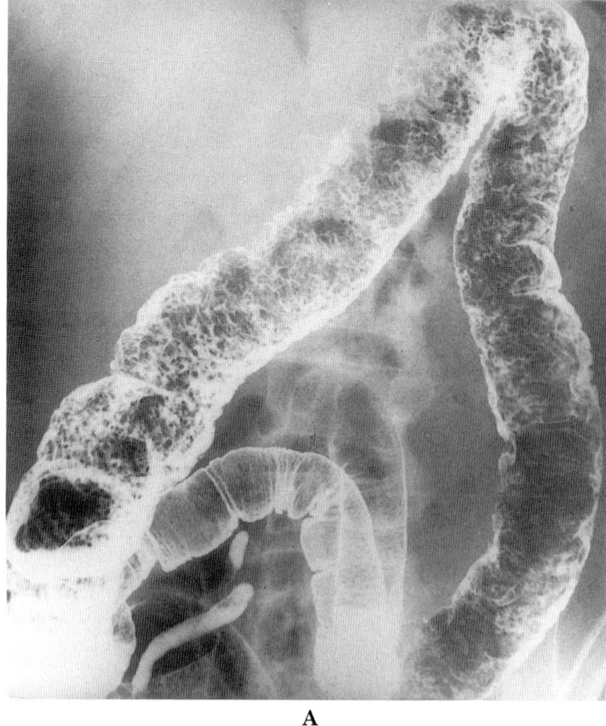

A

Figure 11.14. Chronic phase of ulcerative colitis. (A) Diffuse regenerating formations of colonic mucosa (pseudopolyps).

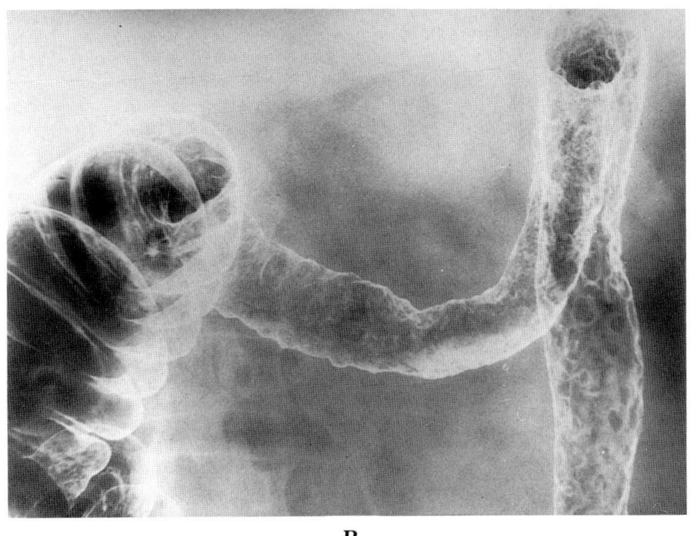

B

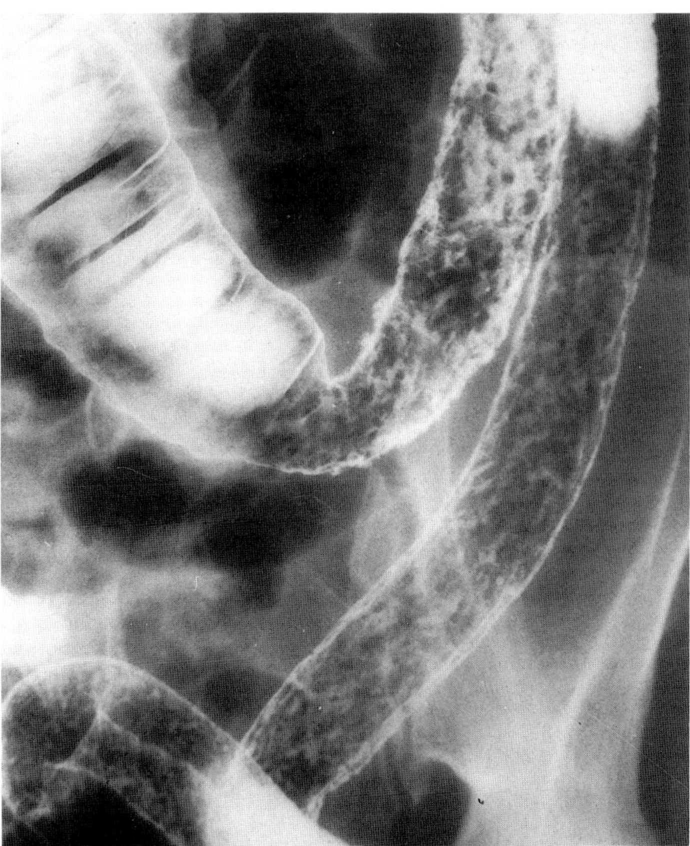

C

FIGURE 11.14 *continued.* Chronic phase of ulcerative colitis. (B) Pseudopolyps of various dimensions in the transverse and descending colon. (C) Pseudopolyps of the colon. Recurrence with ulcers in the transverse colon.

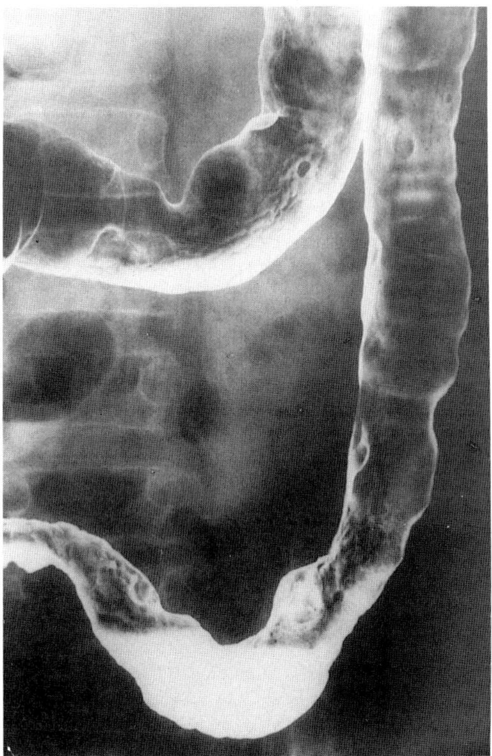

FIGURE 11.15. Late, chronic-reparative phase of ulcerative colitis. Mucosal atrophy and several pseudopolyps.

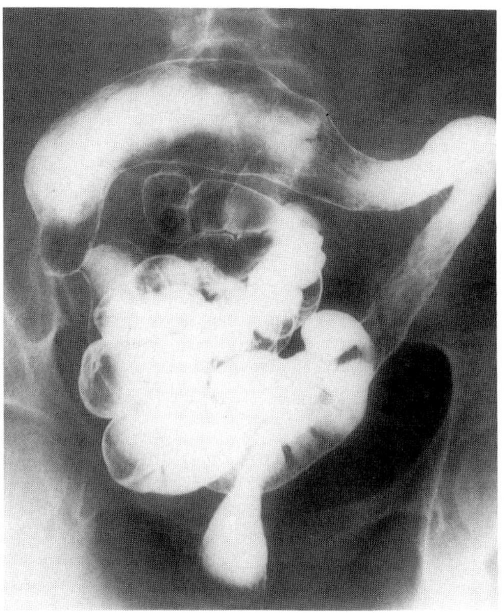

A

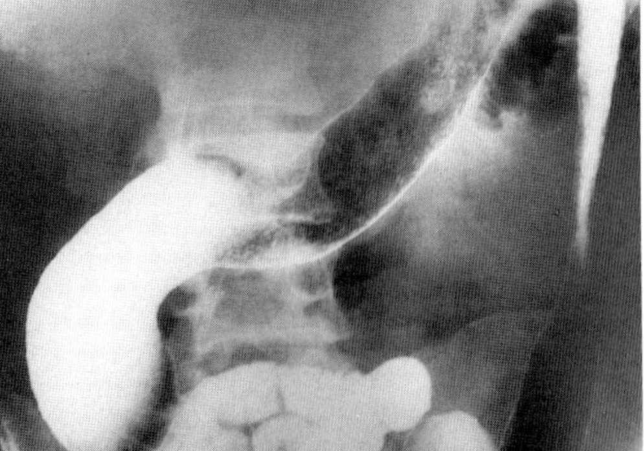

B

FIGURE 11.16. (A) Fibrotic and atrophic phase of ulcerative colitis. Shortened colon without haustral markings. "Secondary microcolon." "Colonization," widening of the ileum. (B) Stenosis of the descending colon.

Flexures are placed low and may be straightened. These findings refer to a "secondary microcolon," "burned-out colitis," or "leadpipe" appearance. As the result of the loss of the colon's reservoir function, the terminal ileum has a widened lumen (Fig. 11.16). Radiographic findings in this phase persist regardless of clinical remission. There are similar radiographic findings in cathartic colon (Fig. 11.17).

Crohn's disease is the most common disease affecting the small bowel. Gross pathologic lesions observed radiologically are poorly correlated with clinical symptoms in patients with CD. Statistically significant radiographic improvement can only be found in patients treated with prednisolone for six months or longer. Hence, repeated follow-up radiologic examinations of patients with CD are not usually indicated even though there is a high positive correlation between radiologic and pathologic findings of primary and recurrent CD affecting the small gut.

Crohn's disease most commonly begins in

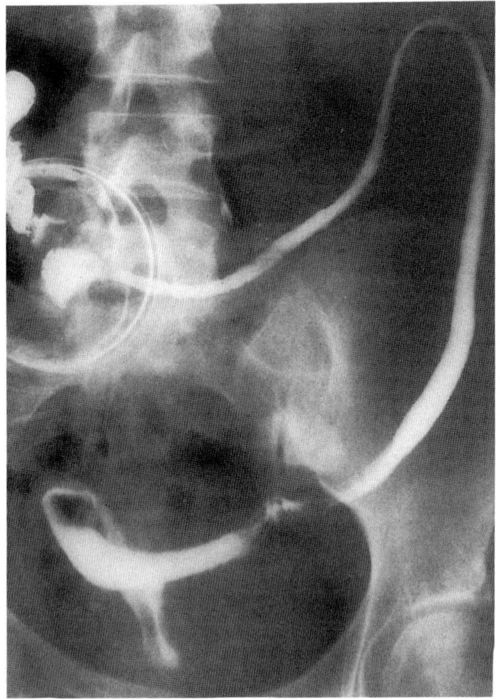

C

FIGURE 11.16. *continued.* (C) Lead-pipe appearance of the colon and colostomy.

the terminal ileum and is possibly related to distribution of lymphoid tissue. As a rule, CD affects the bowel segmentally. However, the distal 10–15 cm of ileum are always continuously affected. Alternating uninvolved segments are termed skip areas (Fig. 11.18). The *earliest* radiologic sign of CD is enlarged submucosal lymphoid follicles (Diagram 11.2 and Fig. 11.19. The next is an appearance of shallow aphthoid ulcers, defects of the epithelium covering enlarged lymphoid follicles, which are best revealed *en face* on double-contrast studies (Figs. 11.20 and 11.21). However, an earlier phase of CD can be seen exclusively in the small bowel. This is a diffuse granular mucosal pattern caused by the rounded tips of coalescent villi measuring 5–10 mm in diameter (Fig. 11.22). Inflammatory changes with atrophy and "pseudoatrophy" of villi are detected microscopically. Submucosal granulomas, a hallmark of CD,

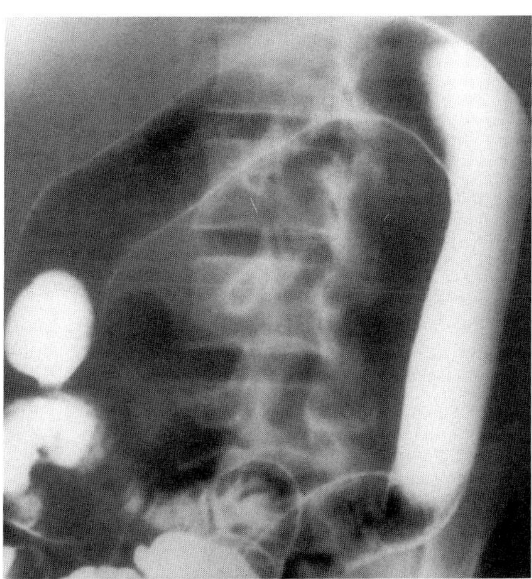

FIGURE 11.17. Cathartic colon. Colon is shortened and devoid of normal anatomical features.

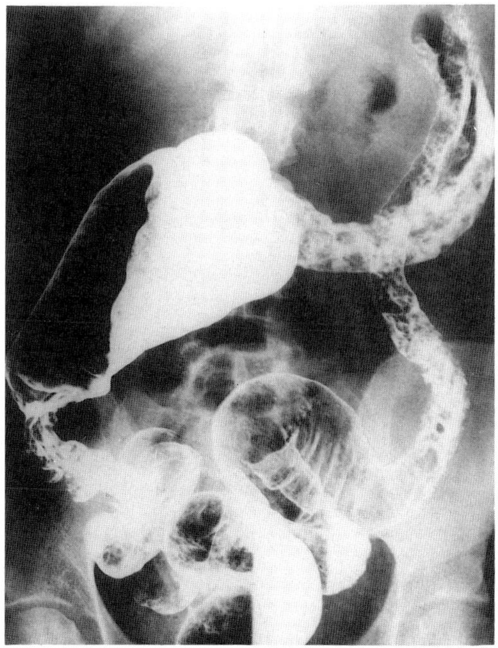

FIGURE 11.18. Crohn's disease affecting the colon and terminal ileum. Lesions are distributed segmentally. Ulcers result in cobblestone appearance with pseudopolyps. Pseudodiverticular changes of skip areas result from rigidity of adjacent wall.

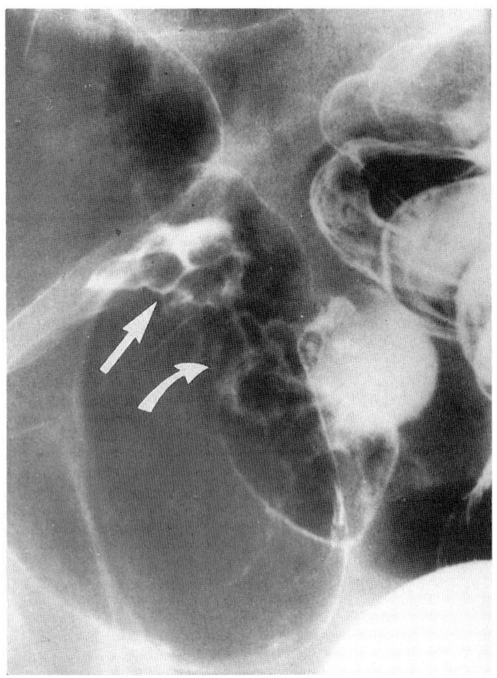

FIGURE 11.19. Crohn's disease. Enlarged lymphoid follicles of the terminal ileum without ulceration (arrows).

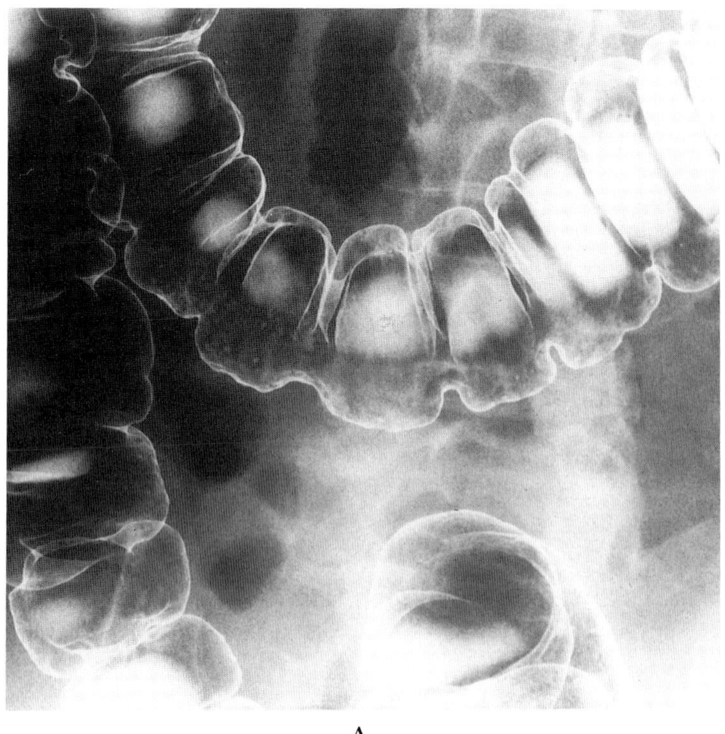

A

FIGURE 11.20. Aphthoid ulcers of Crohn's disease (A) in the colon.

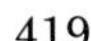

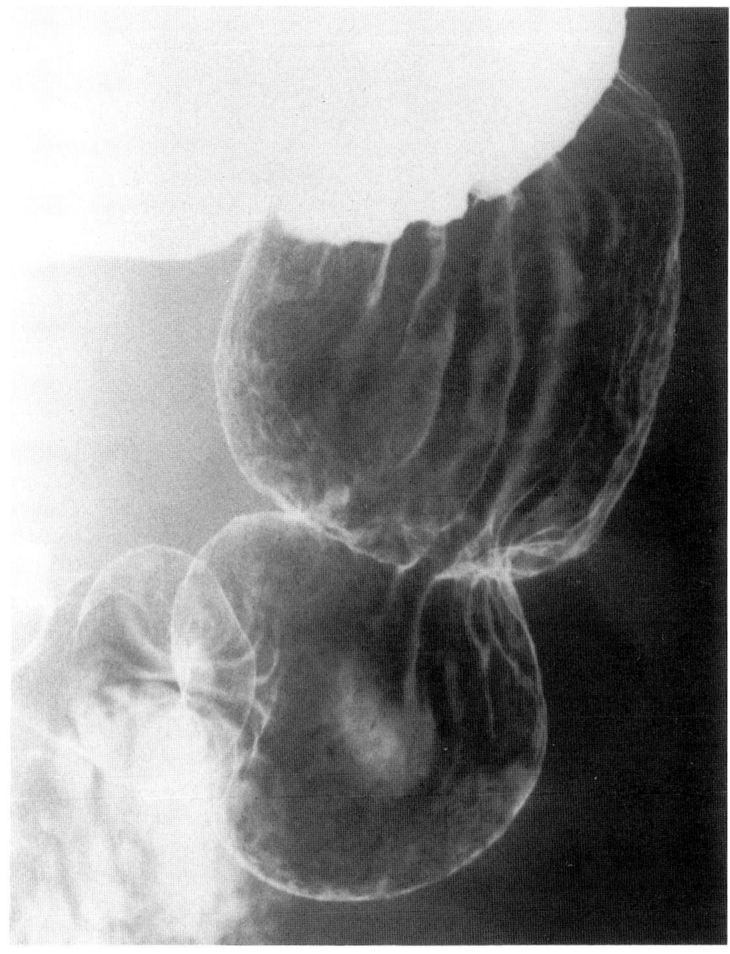

B

FIGURE 11.20. *continued.* Aphthoid ulcers of Crohn's disease (B) in the stomach.

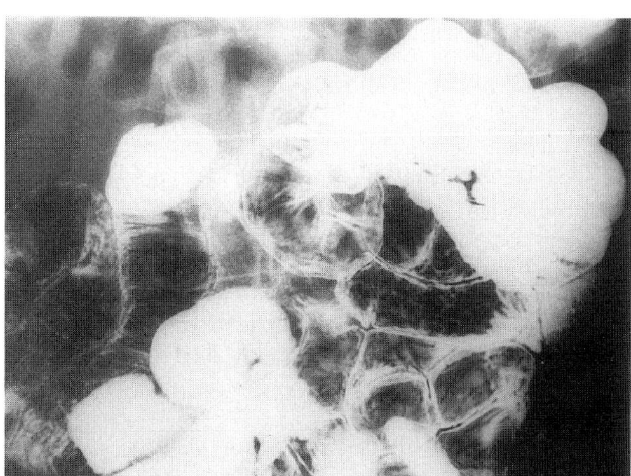

FIGURE 11.21. Aphthoid ulcers of Crohn's disease in the small bowel. Double-contrast follow-through study.

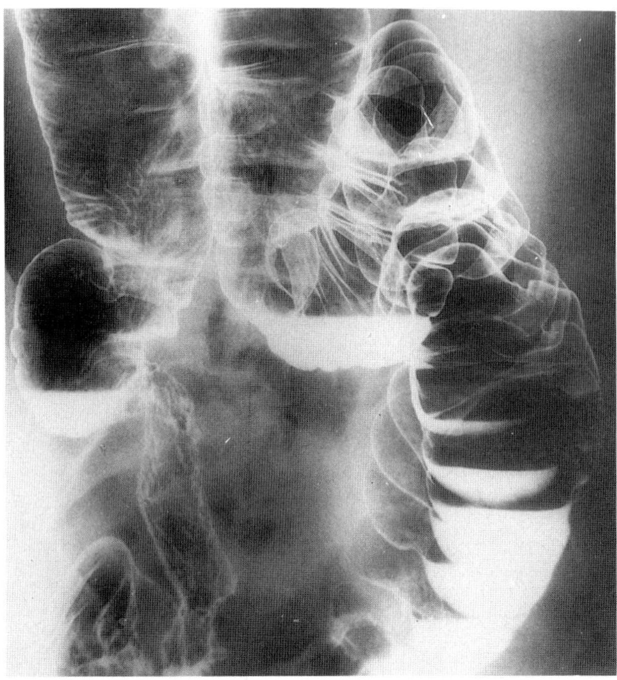

Figure 11.22. Granular mucosal pattern of the terminal ileum resulting from thickened coalescent villi. The earliest detectable phase of Crohn's disease involving the small bowel. Proximal ascending colon is also affected.

contain epithelioid cells and caseous necrosis. The plicae conniventes are edematous and lymphatic tissue is hyperplastic; impaired lymphatic circulation results in lymphedema (Fig. 11.23). In *advanced CD*, both longitudinal and transverse ulcers enlarge and coalesce, often resulting in a "cobblestone" appearance (Fig. 11.24). Stenoses may emerge (Fig. 11.25) as a narrowed featureless terminal ileum, the string sign, also referred as to Kantor's sign, which results from a combination of fibrosis and spasm (Fig. 11.26). Normal wall adjacent to fibrotic sections of the gut may undergo "pseudodiverticular" changes (Fig. 11.27). In CD affecting the ileocecal area, Stierlin's sign, described originally in patients with ileocecal tuberculosis, manifests as a failure of the cecum to fill with barium, due to spasm.

Transmural ulcerations can result in adhesions, and fistula formation with adjacent intestines, other organs, or the body surface. Fistulas are most common in the terminal ileum.

On occasion, only lymph nodes and vessels of the mesentery may be affected with inflammation with resultant fibrosis, obstruction of lymph circulation, and consequent thickening of the mesentery. The associated small intestine loop seems separated from adjacent bowel segments (Fig. 10.4), mimicking lymphoma of the mesentery.

Unlike UC, CD of the colon, *granulomatous colitis*, is characterized by more pronounced changes in the submucosa. The majority of lesions correspond to those in the small intestine. Hyperplastic lymph follicles along with aphthoid ulcers indicate an *early phase* (Fig. 11.28). Since aphthoid ulcers are not present in UC, this is an important differential diagnostic feature. Their fate is unpredictable as they may persist or disappear regardless of the evolution of CD lesions in other segments of the gut.

Deep ulcerations resulting in a cobblestone appearance of the inflammation spreading to the serosa, along with stenoses, characterize *advanced* CD (Fig. 11.29). Radiologic findings in the colon are often more impressive than in the small intestine. An altered lymphatic circu-

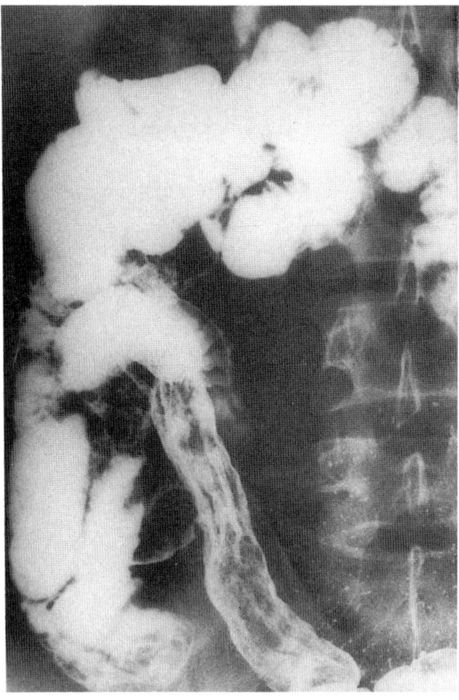

FIGURE 11.23. Crohn's disease. Widening of folds in the terminal ileum with granularity and ulcers.

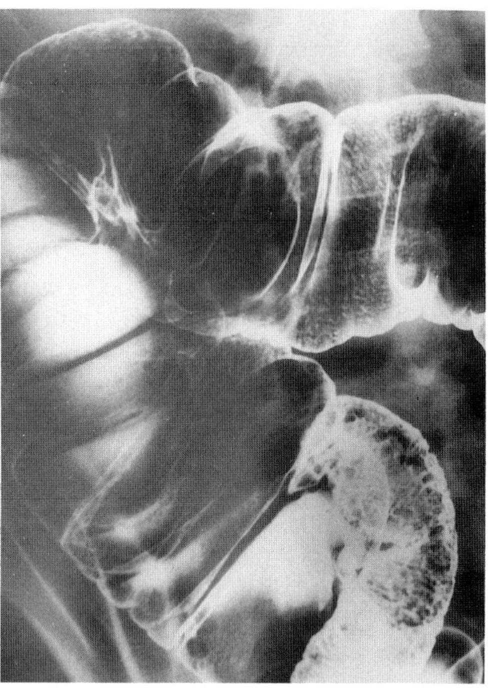

FIGURE 11.24. Crohn's disease. Cobblestone appearance of the terminal ileum. The transverse colon is also affected.

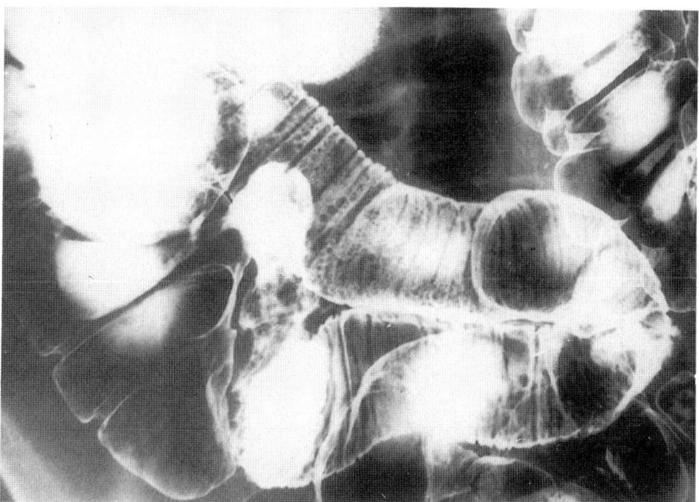

FIGURE 11.25. Crohn's disease. Stenoses, ulcers, and granulomas of the terminal ileum. Other portions of the bowel are without pathologic changes.

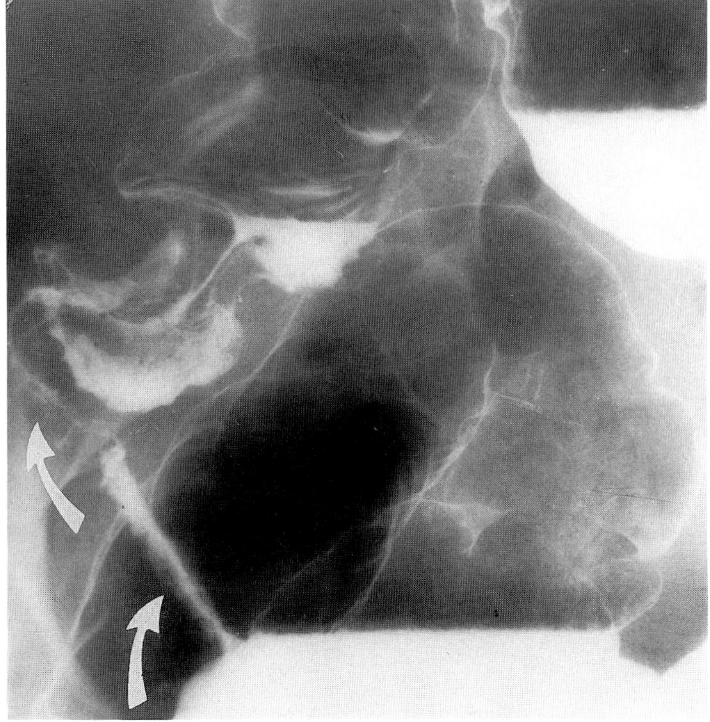

Figure 11.26. Crohn's disease. String sign in the terminal ileum (arrows).

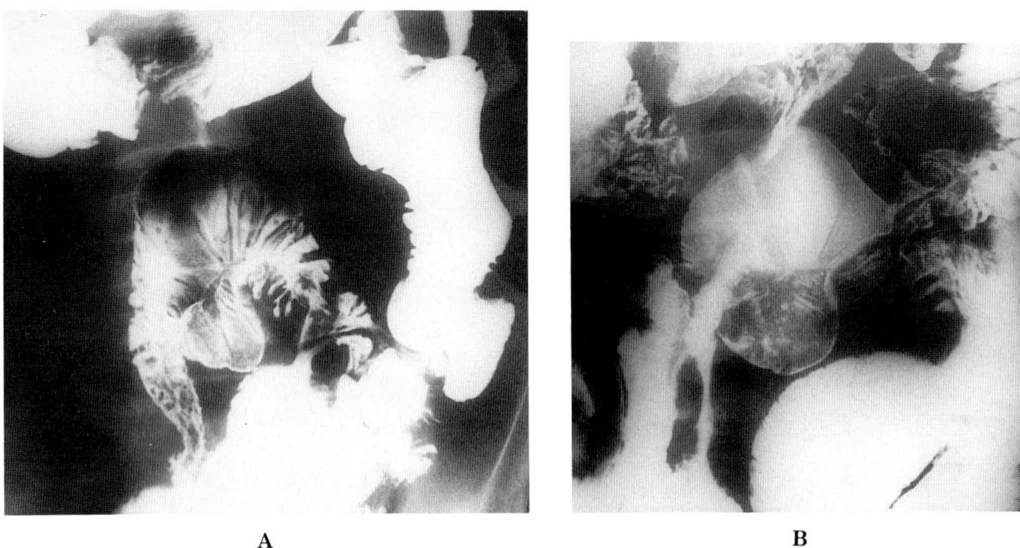

A B

Figure 11.27. Crohn's disease affecting small bowel. (A) Ulcers, granulomas, strictures, and pseudodiverticular distension of bowel wall. (B) Stenoses and pseudodiverticular distension of small bowel.

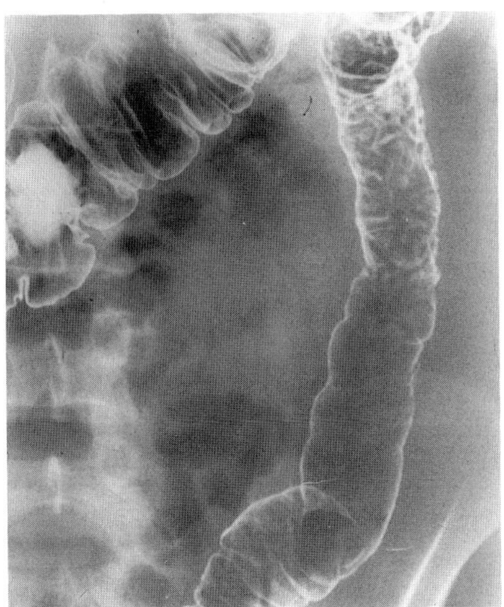

FIGURE 11.28. Crohn's disease. Aphthoid ulcers of the proximal descending colon.

lation can lead to "elephantiasis" of the colon. Haustral markings may be less pronounced, but tend to remain better preserved than in UC. "Pseudopolyps," not larger than 1–2 cm in diameter, appear in the *reparative and proliferative phases*, particularly on the edge of ulcers (Fig. 11.30).

Loss of compliance, with either symmetric or eccentric narrowing and shortening of the colon, characterize the *stenotic phase* (Figs. 11.31 and 11.32). Strictures arise no earlier than one year after the onset of CD symptoms. The strictures may vary in length and may cause obstruction. Nonelastic segments of the colon cause "pseudodiverticular" bulges of adjacent and opposite uninvolved intestinal wall (Figs. 11.31C–11.34). Intervening unaffected segments, skip areas, separate pathologically altered sections (Fig. 11.31). *The late phase* of CD is characterized by lack of haustral markings, and shortening and narrowing of the colon

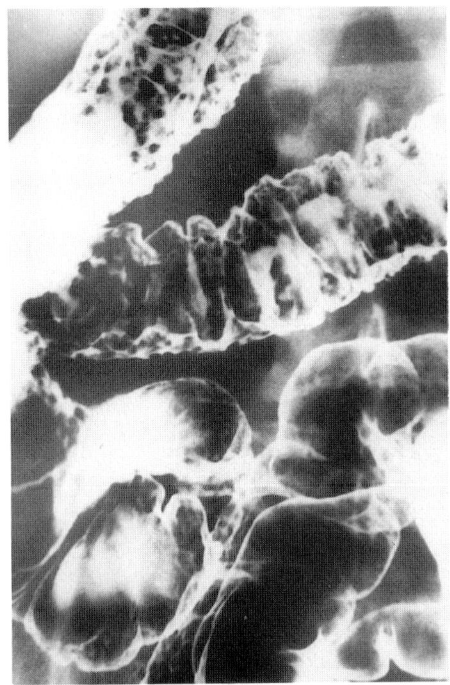

FIGURE 11.29. Crohn's disease. Cobblestone appearance of the ascending and transverse colon.

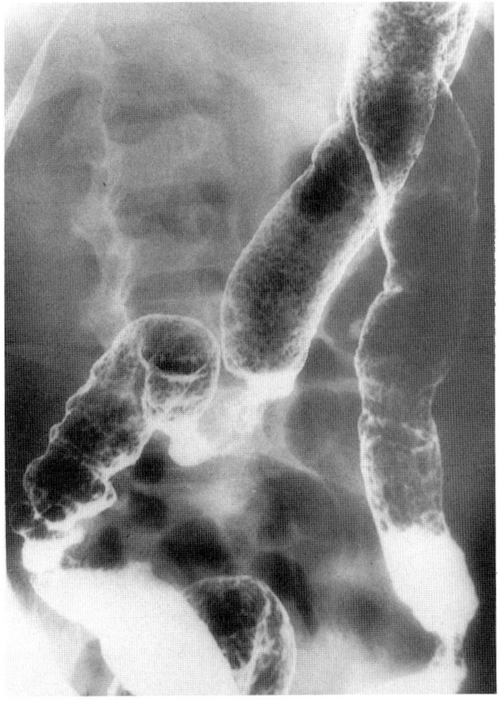

FIGURE 11.30. Crohn's disease. Alternating pseudopolyps and stenoses.

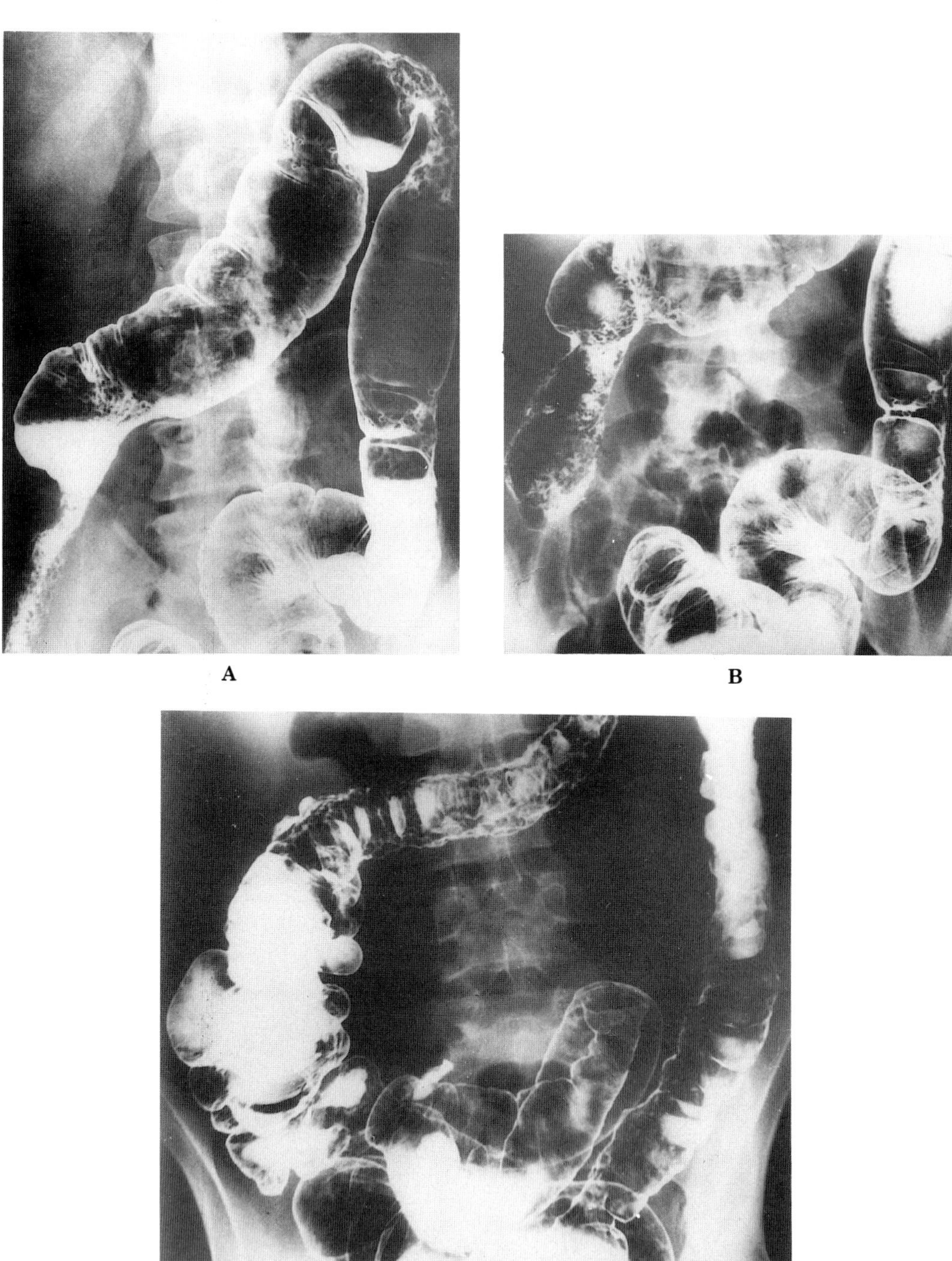

A B C

Figure 11.31. Crohn's disease. Double-contrast barium enema. (A) Involved segments alternate with skip areas. Spasm of the cecum and ascending colon. (B) Narrowed area became dilated during the course of the examination. (C) Lesions characteristic for all phases of Crohn's disease are seen: aphthoid ulcers of the descending colon, deep longitudinal and transverse ulcers resulting in "cobblestoning" and pseudopolyps in the transverse colon, and pseudodiverticular widenings of the proximal colon.

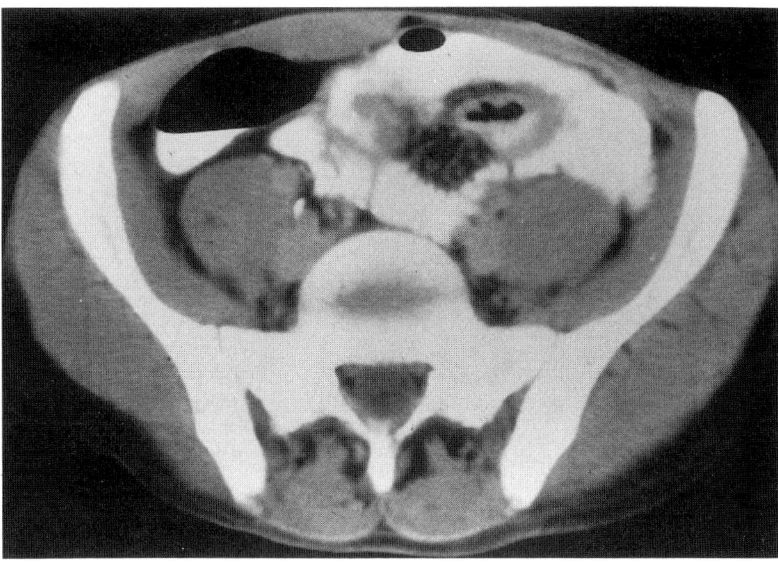

FIGURE 11.32. Crohn's disease affecting the small and large bowel. CT of intestinal lumen stenoses, with wall thickening.

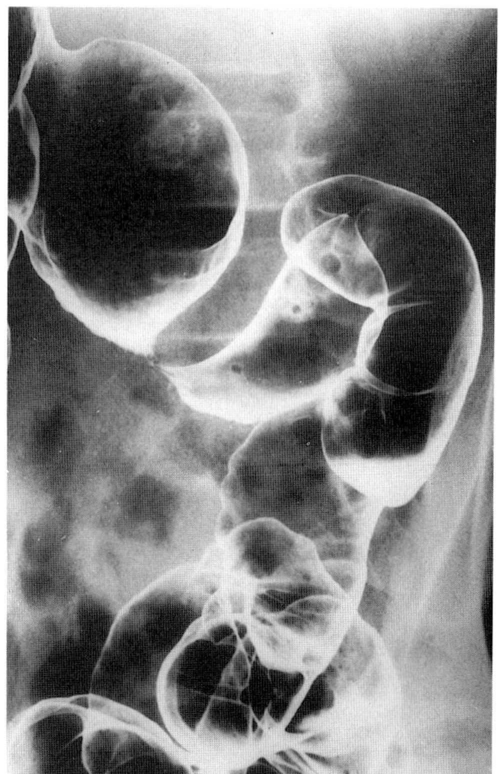

FIGURE 11.33. Stenotic phase of Crohn's disease. Severe stenosis of distal transverse colon.

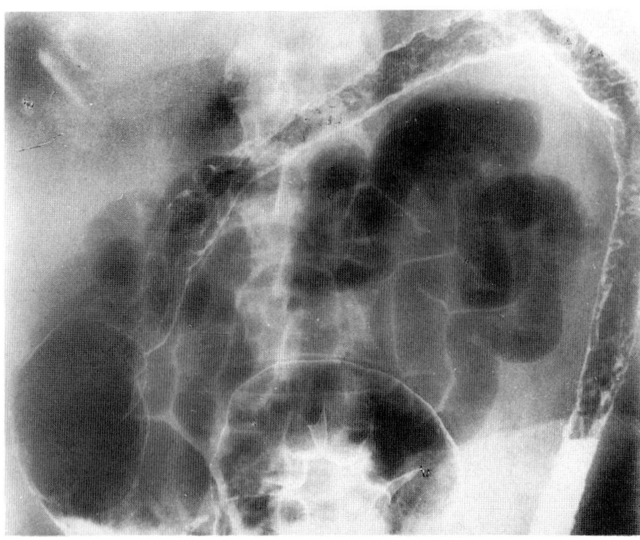

Figure 11.34. Stenotic and reparative-proliferative phase of Crohn's disease. Narrowing of the colon with numerous pseudopolyps. Pseudodiverticular distension of the cecum and proximal ascending colon. Normal sigmoid colon with distended lumen of air-filled small bowel.

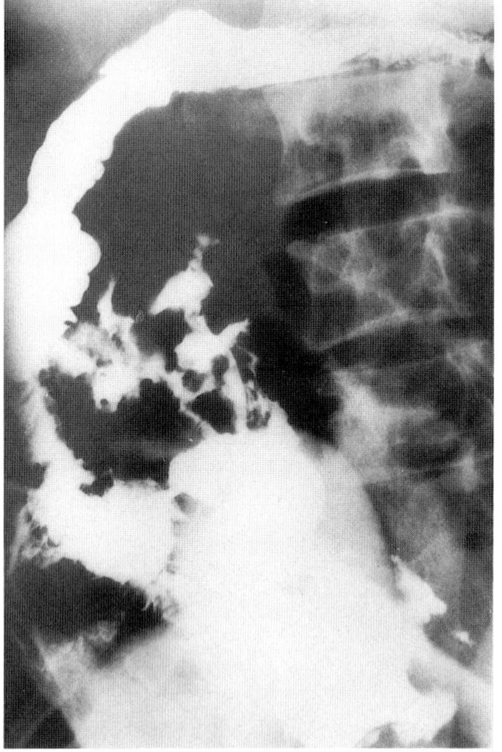

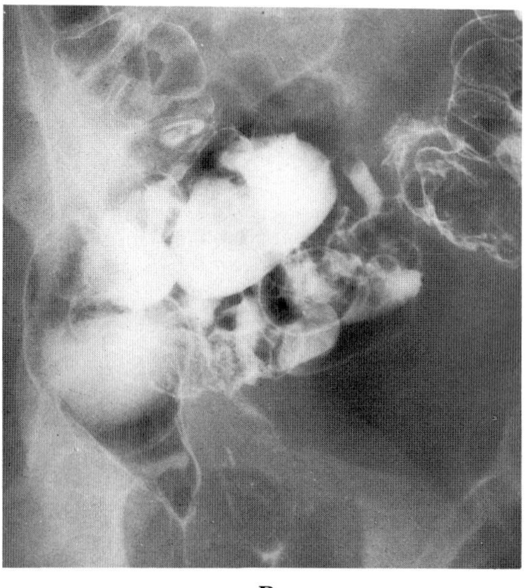

A B

Figure 11.35. Fistulas in Crohn's disease. (A) Multiple sinus tracts between the ileum, cecum, ascending colon, and mesentery. (B) Rectovaginal fistula. The major portion of the perineum and rectovaginal septum was destroyed.

(Figs. 11.33 and 11.34). Fistulas are common (Fig. 11.35).

Recurrences occur in 70% of patients after surgery for Crohn's disease. Recurrences of CD have the same morphology as the first attack (Fig. 11.36). They occur in 87% of patients with transmural lesions. Local recurrences without axial progression are most often seen and are most commonly located in the proximal intestinal segment near the site of resection in patients who have had surgery.

Complications of UC and CD may be either

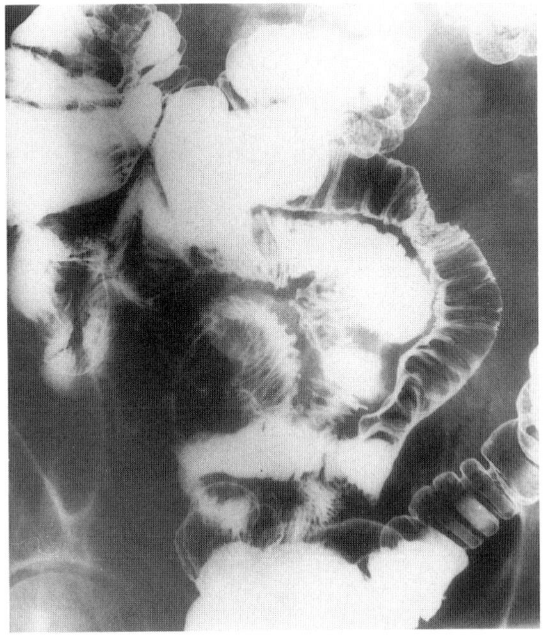

A

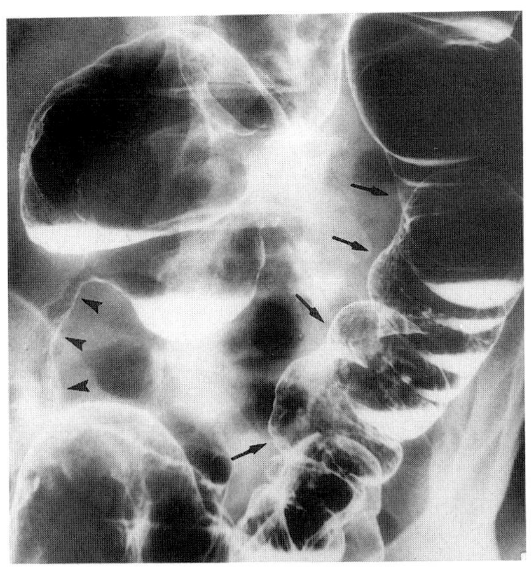

B

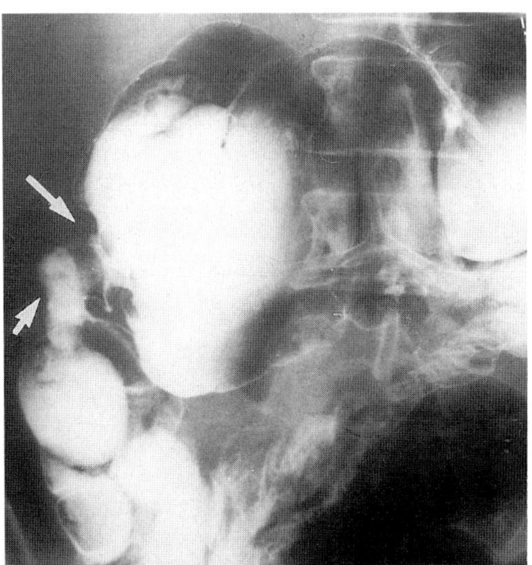

C

FIGURE 11.36. Recurrence of Crohn's disease. (A) Small bowel involvement after partial resection of the right hemicolon. (B) Right hemicolectomy for Crohn's disease. Stenosis of the anastomosed small bowel loop (arrowheads). Aphthoid ulcers of the distal descending colon (arrows). (C) Ileotransversostomy after right colectomy for Crohn's disease. Recurrence affects the site of anastomosis (arrows).

local or extraintestinal. Strictures, malignancies, and sinus tracts with abscesses are local complications. Hepatitis, pericholangitis, cholelithiasis, urolithiasis, arthritis, and uveitis are extraintestinal complications.

One of the most severe complications of UC and CD is *toxic megacolon* in which the diameter of the gas-distended transverse colon can exceed 5 cm in the supine position. Although toxic megacolon affects all sections of the large

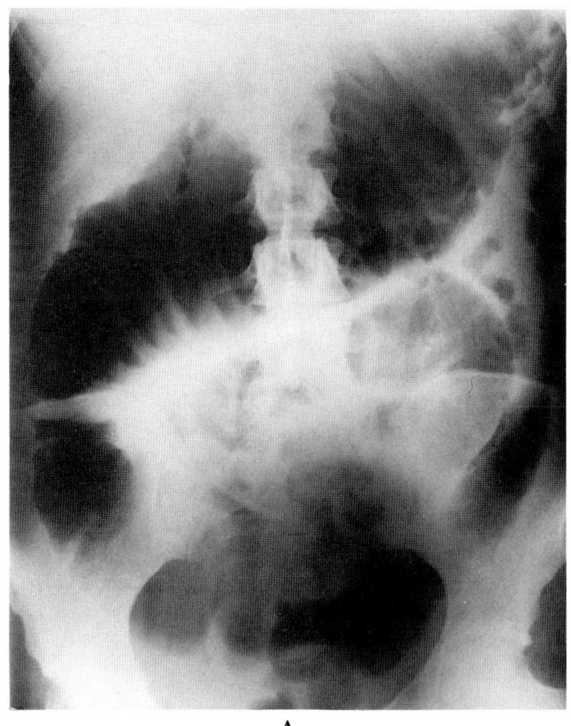

A

FIGURE 11.37. Toxic megacolon. Supine abdominal film. (A) In ulcerative colitis. (B) In Crohn's disease.

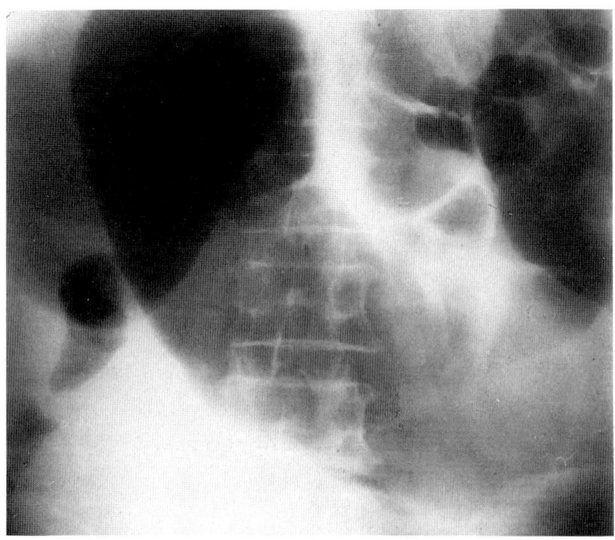

B

intestine, it is more readily demonstrated in the transverse colon. Haustral markings are absent or faintly visible (Figs. 4.5, 5.18, and 11.37). Enemas are contraindicated since the risk of perforation is high. Toxic megacolon may be well demonstrated by CT. Toxic megacolon occurs in about 4–6% of patients with CD and 1–3% of patients with UC.

Toxic dilatation may develop in any type of pancolitis, either ischemic, amebic or infectious, or even in nodular lymphoma affecting the entire colon. Performing barium enema does not predispose to toxic megacolon. Dilatation results from destruction of muscle and intramural neuronal plexuses. Necrosis of all layers of the wall results in rupture, often with fatal consequences. Gas within the wall is an ominous sign in toxic megacolon. The average mortality rate of toxic megacolon is 23%, taking into account both medically and surgically treated patients.

Colorectal carcinoma occurs in approximately 6% of patients with long-standing UC. Carcinoma is found in 1.6% of those diseased five years following onset of UC. Ulcerative colitis lasting more than eight years increases the risk of carcinoma by 20% for each succeeding decade.

Dysplasia of the mucosal epithelium is frequent in patients who subsequently develop carcinoma, and is considered a precursor of carcinoma. Supposed transformation of dysplasia to carcinoma is unpredictable. Since most dysplasia cannot be distinguished from surrounding normal epithelium macroscopically, the diagnosis is established histologically. Dysplasias have been verified by randomized biopsies in 15% of patients with long-standing UC. Endoscopic or double-contrast enema demonstration of macroscopically detectable dysplasia shows multiple mucosal nodules from several millimeters up to 1 cm in diameter, or villous or papillary areas of the mucosa (Fig. 11.38). Dysplastic nodules cannot be differentiated from hyperplastic growths. Nevertheless, collections of flattened nodules are associated with dysplasia in 50% of patients. Dysplasia detectable by the naked eye is more likely to become carcinoma.

There is a high incidence of carcinoma in both UC and CD. Carcinoma associated with UC (Fig. 11.39) is an adenocarcinoma distributed in the large intestine without site predilection. When originating from ulcerated mucosa, the carcinoma arises near the edge of the ulcerations, and multiple carcinomas may even develop. Annular, plaque-like and volcano-like adenocarcinomas are found more often than polypoid tumors. However, these cancers can assume morphologic characteristics of a benign stenosis. Early diagnosis of carcinoma can be achieved in 70% of UC patients.

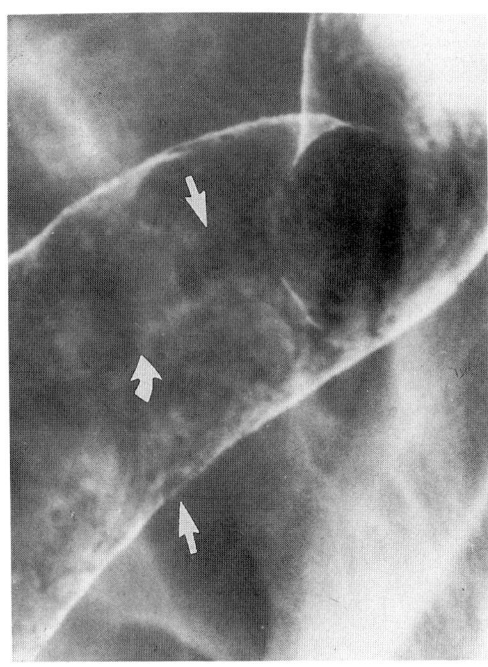

Figure 11.38. Chronic ulcerative colitis. Nodular lesions in the sigmoid colon (arrows). The bioptic diagnosis was dysplasia of colonic mucosa.

With CD, colorectal carcinoma is between 4 and 20 times more prevalent than in the general population. An average interval between diagnosis of CD and detection of intestinal carcinoma is 27 years, with a range from 13 to 39 years. Although carcinoma of the small intestine occurs earlier than in the general population, colorectal carcinoma attacks patients with CD at the same age as the general population. Carcinoma has the same distribution as CD and tends to appear in segments with more pronounced pathology. It may even occur within sinus tracts. Carcinomas in patients with CD have been poorly differentiated adenocarcinomas with poor prognoses (Fig. 11.40). In

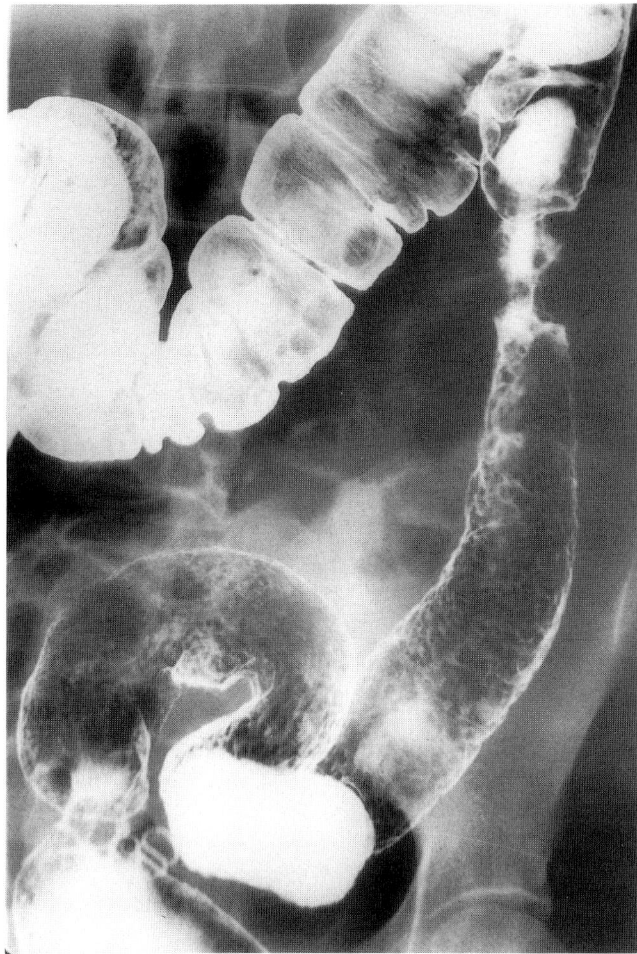

FIGURE 11.39. Carcinoma of the proximal descending colon in a patient with long-standing ulcerative colitis. Regenerating mucosal formations (pseudopolyps) of the descending and sigmoid colon.

more than half the patients, carcinomas associated with CD resemble benign strictures with prominent intramural growth. When intestinal obstruction occurs after a long silent period, carcinoma should be suspected.

Approximately 20% of patients with CD will, as a result of fistulas or transmural extension, develop an abdominal abscess which can be readily diagnosed by CT. The thickened wall of an abscess shows high attenuation in contrast to the inner portions, where attenuation values are between water and soft tissue. Many abscesses in CD can be percutaneously drained under US or CT guidance. The recurrence rate is much higher for an abdominal abscess in CD because of transmural extension.

Diagnosis of UC and CD is made by clinical symptoms, radiologic examination, and endoscopy with biopsy. Differentiation between UC and CD is presented in Table 11.1. Approximately 10–15% of patients with chronic colitis cannot be included in the classification of UC, CD, or other types of colitis using clinical, radiologic, and pathologic criteria. This type of colitis is referred to as *colitis of indeterminate type*. Computed tomography may give findings of both UC and CD. The intestinal wall is significantly thickened in CD, while it has been believed that this does not happen in UC. However, chronic UC is characterized by a *lamina muscularis mucosae* as much as 40 times thicker than normal. Computed tomography

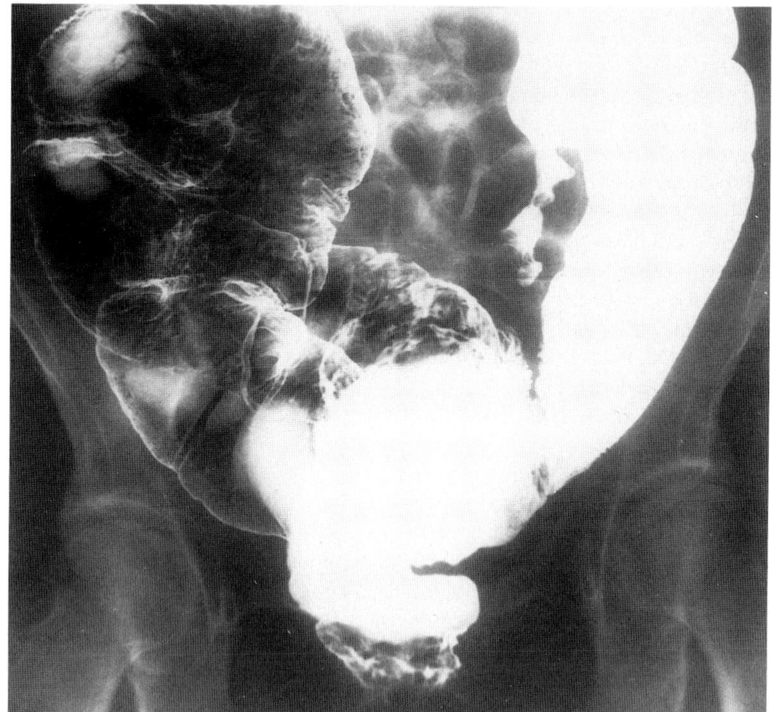

A

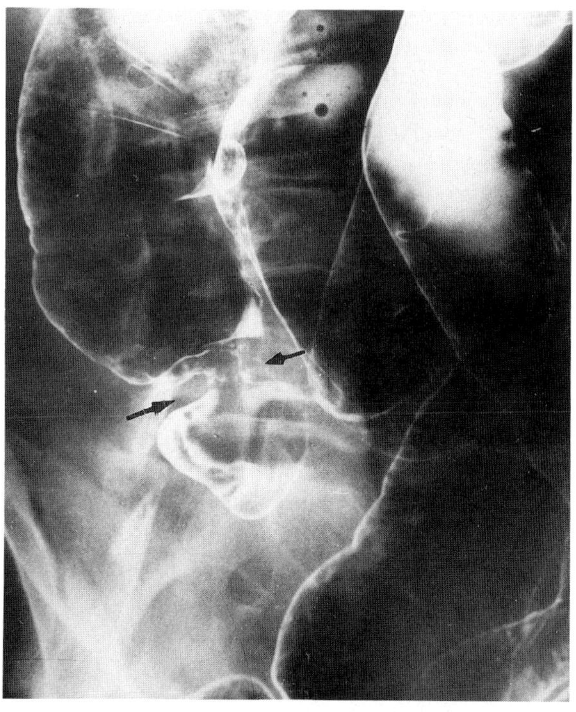

B

FIGURE 11.40. Carcinoma in Crohn's disease. (A) Involving very elongated sigmoid colon. The sigmoid colon and rectum are affected with Crohn's disease lesions. (B) At the transition from cecum to ascending colon (arrows).

shows a homogeneously increased attenuation in CD colitis, but an inhomogeneous appearance in patients with UC.

Normal anatomical elements such as *lineae innominatae* and mucous glands of the colon when filled with barium may resemble discrete ulcers. Aphthoid ulcers may be seen in amebic and tuberculous colitis, shigellosis, yersiniosis, Behçet's syndrome, and nodular lymphoma, as well as in CD. *Campylobacter* colitis is associated with aphthoid ulcers and hyperplastic lymphoid tissues both of which are segmentally distributed and show a predilection for the sigmoid colon and rectum.

An ischemic enteritis and colitis mainly affecting the elderly population may mimic UC and CD. Pseudomembranous enterocolitis, lesions caused by ionizing radiation, and tuberculosis can resemble UC and CD. In contrast to celiac disease, CD tends to result in focal areas of narrowing. Eosinophilic enteritis may be impossible to distinguish from CD radiologically. Long-term oral administration of antibiotics may also cause lesions of the colon resembling UC or CD (Fig. 11.41).

Hyperplastic pseudopolyps must not be mistaken for polyposis syndromes where haustral markings are preserved and other features of inflammation are lacking (Fig. 11.47). Distinguishing strictures caused by CD and UC from malignant tumors is also most important. A *cathartic colon* caused by damage to the mucosa and neuronal plexuses, as the result of laxative abuse, can resemble chronic UC (Fig. 11.17).

MISCELLANEOUS CHRONIC INFLAMMATORY DISEASES

In children, *allergic reactions* to cow's milk may result in mucosal ulceration and spasm leading to hemorrhagic diarrhea. Symptoms disappear when milk is excluded from the diet.

Although usually affecting the skin, *xanthomatosis*, resulting from proliferation of macrophages loaded with lipids (foam cells), may involve stomach, colon, and small bowel. Regular or irregular thickening of mucosal folds, and decreased pliability of the wall, results from macrophage infiltration of muscles and proliferation of connective tissue around vessels and nerves. The antrum is the most common portion of the stomach to be affected. Differential diagnosis includes processes which result in decreased pliability of the wall, moderate stenoses, and thickening of mucosal folds.

Graft-versus-host reaction occurs following allogeneic bone marrow transplantation and may affect the alimentary canal. Approxi-

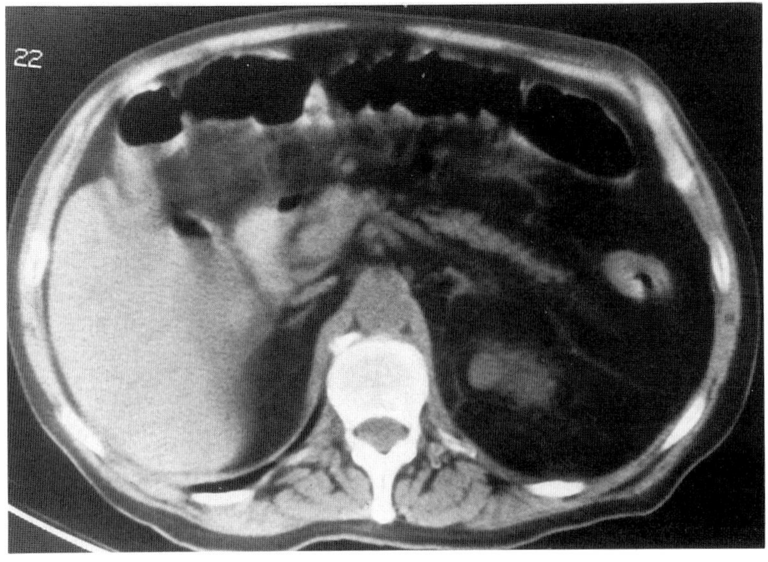

FIGURE 11.41. CT of colitis resulting from prolonged antibiotic therapy.

mately 5 to 15 days following clinical gastrointestinal symptoms, common radiologic findings include thickening of the wall and plicae conniventes with dilatation and the appearance of excess fluid in the lumen of the small intestine (Fig. 11.42). The small intestinal transit time may be shortened significantly. Late changes, in the resolutive phase, affect the terminal ileum, resulting in considerable thickening of the wall. Neither barium studies nor CT can differentiate between graft-versus-host reaction and viral enterocolitis.

Pseudomembranous colitis has associated involvement of the small bowel. The mucosa undergoes necrosis, and is covered with pseudomembranes containing an exudate with inflammatory cells, fibrin, and mucus (Fig. 11.43). Since perforation may result, contrast enema examination is contraindicated. Computed tomography reveals an intestinal wall thicker than 6 mm and a dilated lumen. Because segmental distribution also occurs, ischemic colitis and Crohn's disease should be considered in the differential diagnosis.

Bowel inflammation proximal to an obstruction occurs more often in the colon than in the small bowel. Lesions resembling ischemic or ulcerative colitis can be seen proximal to a site of chronic incomplete obstruction caused by neoplasm or benign stenosis. Mucosal relief elements are thickened and wall pliability is decreased (Fig. 11.44). Lesions, ranging from mucosal and submucosal edema to infarction and perforation, are attributed to dilatation proximal to the stenosis, resulting in ischemia of the intestinal wall. However, fecal stasis probably contributes to any inflammation. Bleeding into the intestinal wall and edema cre-

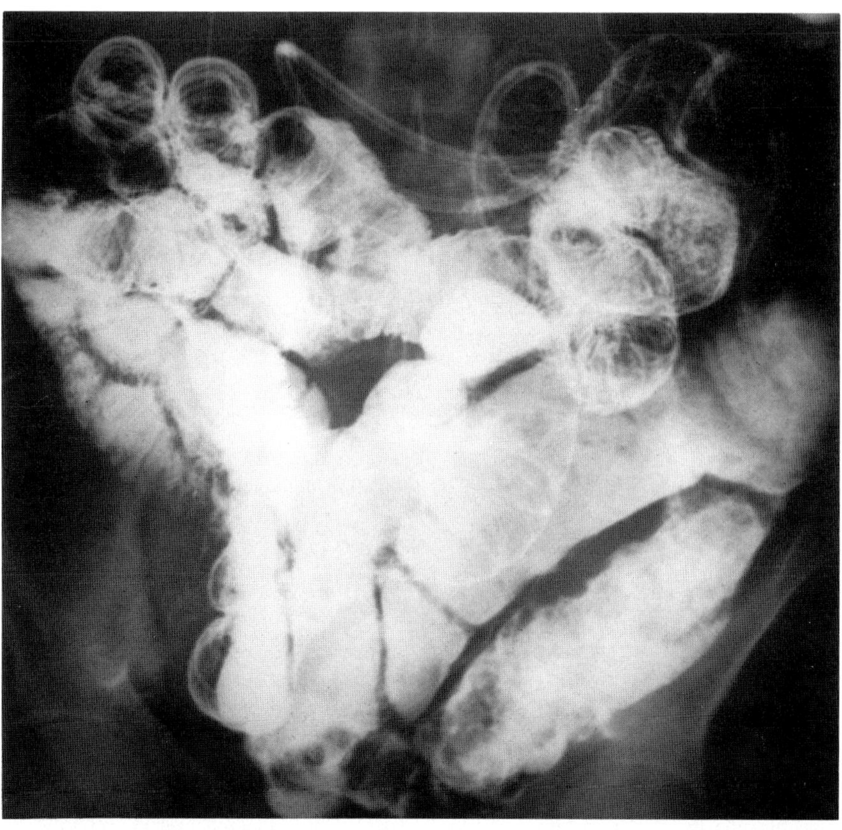

Figure 11.42. Enteroclysis in subacute phase of graft-versus-host reaction. Thickening of circular folds in the distal ileum with dilatation of the jejunum.

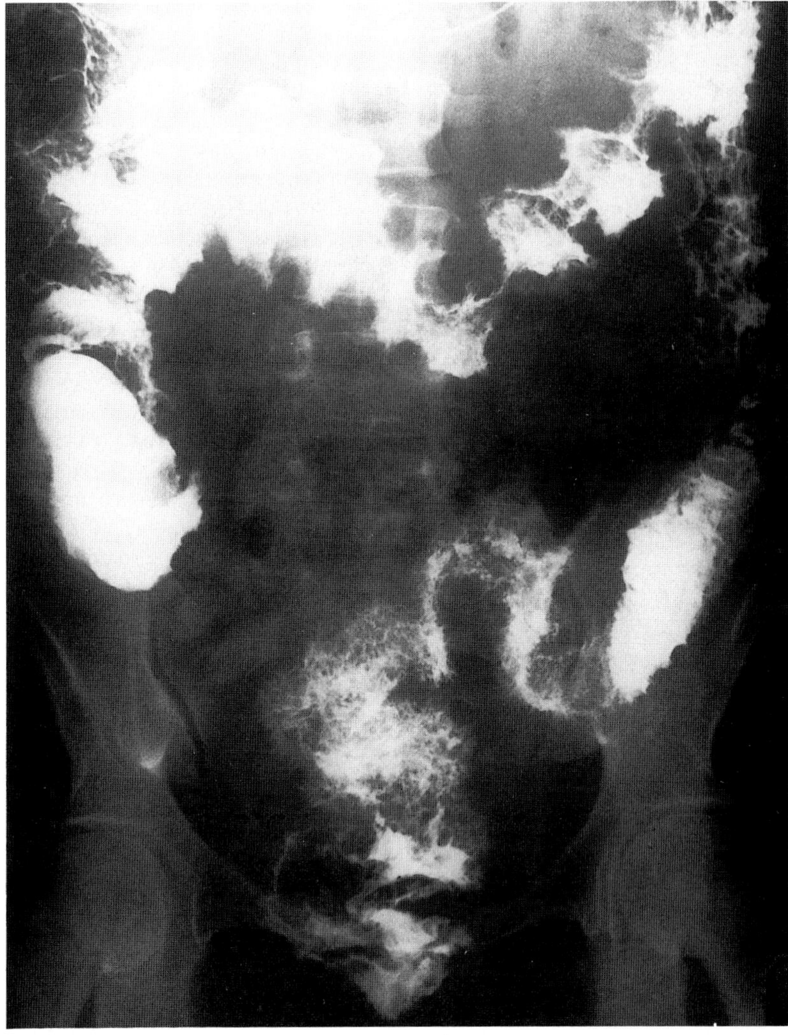

FIGURE 11.43. Pseudomembranous colitis. Irregular appearance resulting from pseudomembranes and mucosal ulcerations. Because contrast enemas are contraindicated, this figure is used only for purpose of illustration.

ate a characteristic thumbprinting pattern. These lesions may disappear as soon as the obstruction is relieved.

POLYPOSIS SYNDROMES

This group of syndromes, of dominant inheritance with varying gene expression, is featured by multiple polyps of the gastrointestinal tract. The majority of polyps are 5 mm in size or larger. Adenomas or hamartomas, polyps in hereditary polyposis syndromes, cannot be mutually differentiated on grounds of radiologic examinations.

An autosomal dominant mode of inheritance characterizes *familial polyposis*. These polyps may involve the entire gastrointestinal tract distal to the esophagus. However, the colon may be exclusively affected (Fig. 11.45). Histologically, these polyps are adenomatous or, in

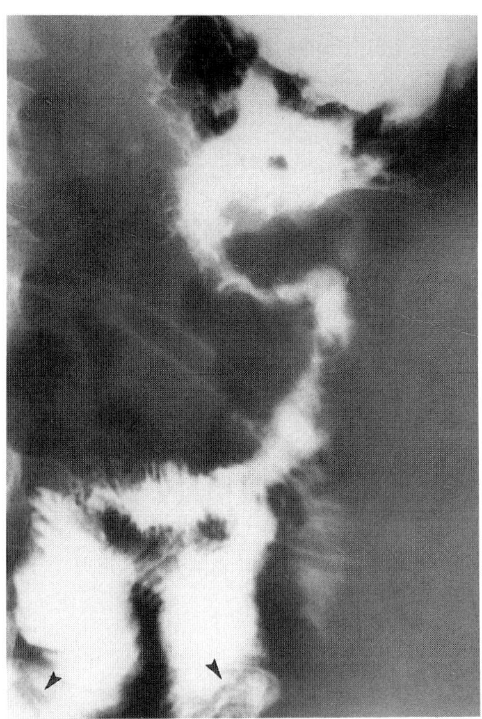

FIGURE 11.44. Enteritis proximal to adhesions (arrowheads). Gastric resection with jejunal anastomosis (Billroth II).

exceptional cases, adenomatous-hyperplastic. Advanced disease is characterized by 30 to 3000 polyps in the large intestine. The average number of polyps is 1000. Unlike multiple adenomas of the colon, an appearance independent of polyposis syndromes, familial polyposis consists of a density of 0.15–3 polyps per square centimeter of the large intestine, usually too numerous to count. Early forms that precede adenomas in familial polyposis are microscopic collections of tubules in the mucosa, which later grow into macroscopic polyps. The end of the second decade of life is the characteristic time for clinical symptoms to appear; however, some 10% of patients remain undiagnosed up to their 50s. On the other hand, manifestations have been observed as early as the newborn period. Both the number and size of polyps are greater in patients who exhibit clinical symptoms than in asymptomatic patients.

High-viscosity barium suspensions, such as those usually used for a double-contrast barium enema, tend to obscure mucosal details like innominate lines. Hence, they are unsuitable for the detection of very small polyps. In familial polyposis early diagnosis is essential because the risk of colorectal adenocarcinoma is 100%.

Besides alimentary canal adenomas, *Gard-*

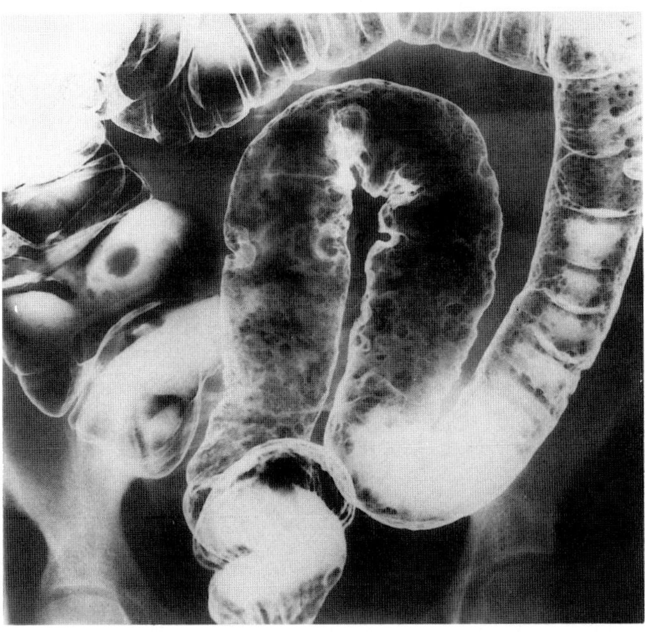

FIGURE 11.45. Familial polyposis of the large intestine.

ner's syndrome is featured by osteomas of the cranium and soft tissue neoplasms. *Turcot's syndrome* is characterized by alimentary canal adenomas and neoplasms of the central nervous system. In syndromes with gastrointestinal adenomas, it is mainly the colon that harbors polyps, which are rather uncommon in other sections of the alimentary canal.

Hamartomas, characteristic of another group of polyposis syndromes, do not undergo malignant transformation. In *Peutz-Jeghers syndrome*, hamartomas populate the gastrointestinal tract in association with mucocutaneous pigmentations of the mouth, nose, and anus. The small intestine is most affected with polyps (Fig. 11.46). *Juvenile polyposis* syndrome affects the colon predominantly with polypoid hamartomas (Fig. 11.47). It may be associated with alopecia and hyperpigmentation. The mode of inheritance is still obscure, but the disease seems to be hereditary in some cases. Polyps in *Cronkhite-Canada* syndrome

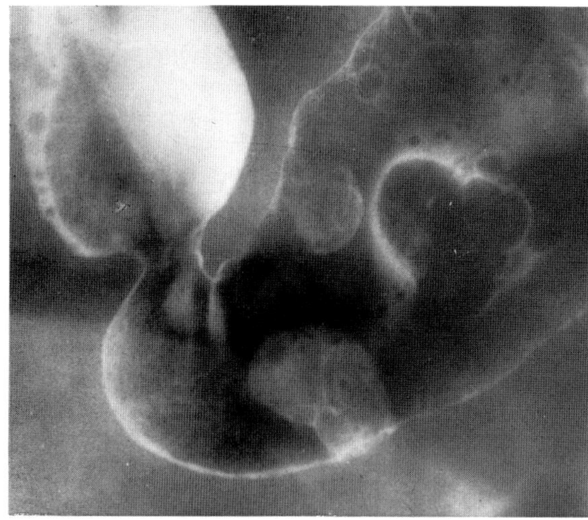

A

FIGURE 11.46. Peutz-Jeghers syndrome. (A) Gastric hamartomatous polyps. (B) Multiple hamartomas of the small bowel.

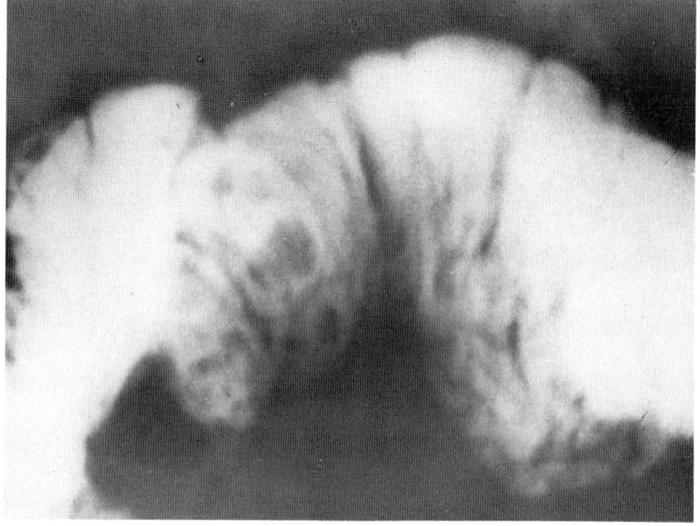

B

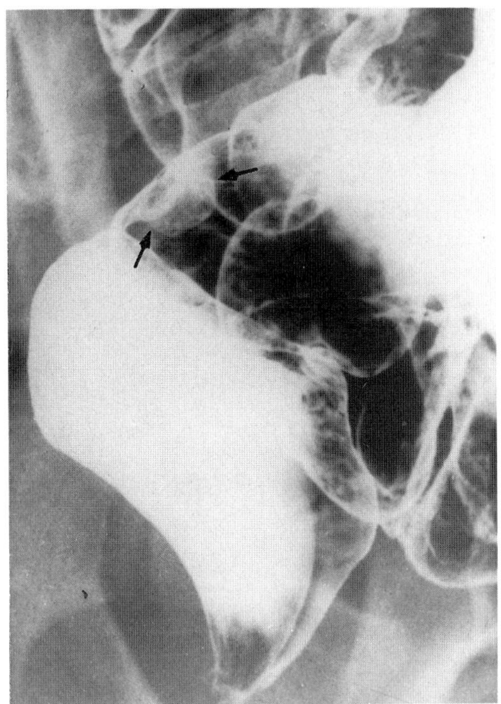

FIGURE 11.47. Juvenile polyp of the rectum—hamartoma (arrows) in a girl 5 years of age.

are also located in the colon. *Ruvalcaba-Myhre-Smith* syndrome is characterized by diffuse affection of the entire digestive tube with hamartomatous polyps. Radiologic findings are the same as in other polyposis syndromes. In *Cowden's* syndrome hamartomatous polyps occur in the gastrointestinal tract from the pharynx to the anus, with an average polyp size of 5 mm. Ectodermal dysplasias and tumors of the neck, breast, and bone may coexist coincidentally. The disease is inherited as an autosomal dominant trait.

Syndrome of the neural crest and colonic neoplasms are not hereditary. They develop later than familial polyposis and the number of tumors is low. Histologically these are malignant tubulovillous adenomas originating from neural crest remnants. This group also includes pheochromocytomas, carcinoids, and multiple endocrine neoplasias. Besides the colon, the small intestine and the stomach can be affected.

Nodular lymphoma of the colon can mimic polyposis syndromes (Fig. 11.48D). Polyposis affecting the colon should also be differentiated from follicular lymphoid hyperplasia, "pseudopolyps" in ulcerative colitis, and Crohn's disease. This should not be difficult since, in addition to

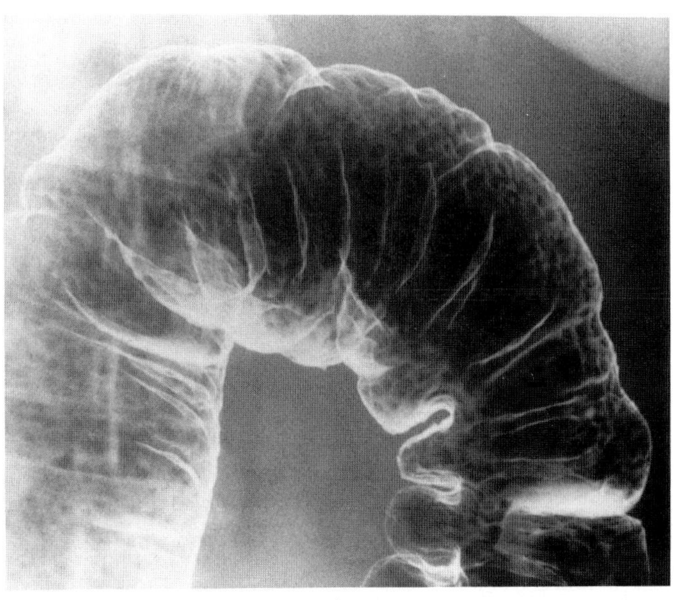

A

FIGURE 11.48. (A) Enlarged lymphoid follicles of the colon. (*Figure continued on the following two pages.*)

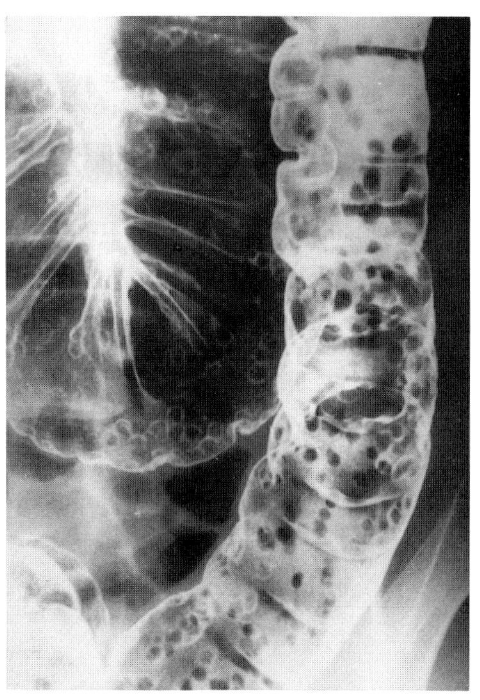

B

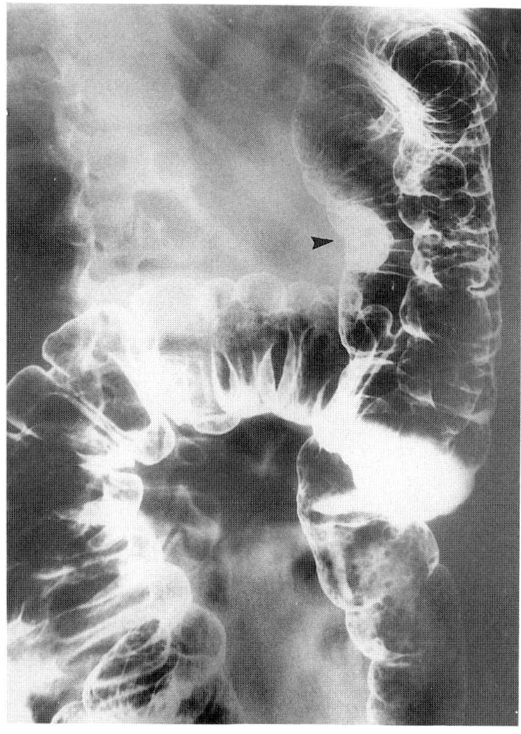

C

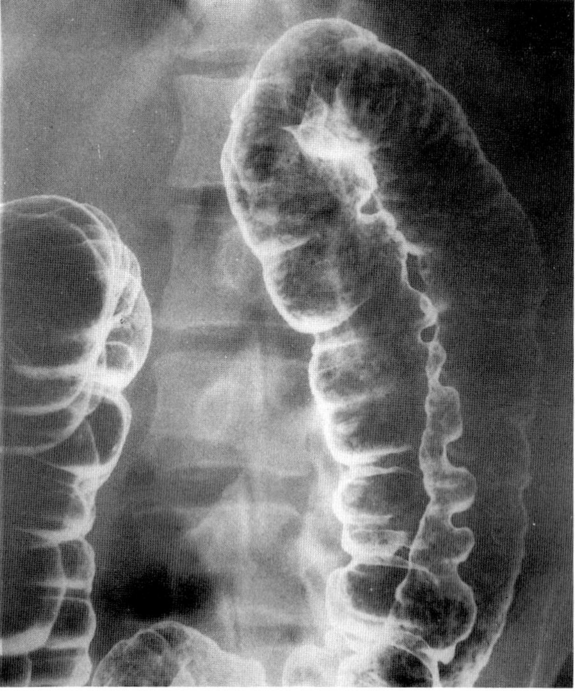

D

FIGURE 11.48 *continued.* (B) Familial polyposis. (C) Familial polyposis with large carcinoma (arrowhead) is evident. (D) Nodular lymphoma of the colon. Haustral markings are preserved from (A) to (D).

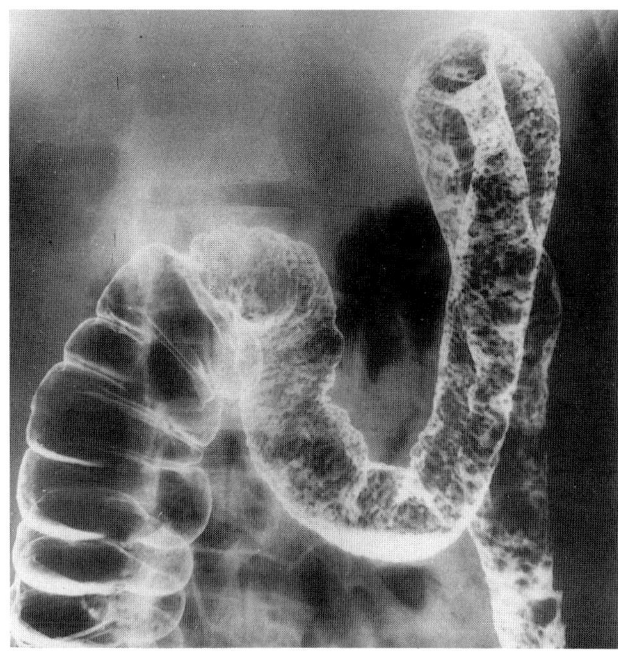

FIGURE 11.48 *continued.* (E) Regenerating mucosal formations, pseudopolyps, in ulcerative colitis. Loss of haustral markings.

loss of haustral markings, other lesions characteristic for chronic inflammation are also present (see text on ulcerative colitis and Crohn's disease, pages 408–432) (Figs. 11.14 and 11.48E).

FISTULAS

Sections of the alimentary canal may communicate with adjacent organs of the alimentary canal or with the body surface via fistulas. These are named according to the organs involved, for example, gastroenteric, gastrocolic (Fig. 11.49) or cholecystocolic. Fistulas may also occur with the urogenital system (Figs. 11.35B and 11.49D).

Fistulas can result from peptic ulcers, Crohn's disease, malignant neoplasms, diverticulitis, trauma, and surgery. Depending on the natural history of the disease, fistulas may tend to heal or may be permanently opened and progressive. Fistulas are revealed on barium examinations and those communicating with the body surface are successfully demonstrated at fistulography using water-soluble contrast media.

METASTASES OF THE ALIMENTARY CANAL AND PERITONEUM

Metastases may involve the intestine, mesentery, and mesocolon with equal frequency as a consequence of the mechanisms listed in Table 11.2. The modes of spread of malignant neoplasm may have recognizable radiologic features.

1. **Direct invasion from adjacent primary neoplasms.** Direct invasion of the bowel by contiguous primary tumors occurs with carcinoma

TABLE 11.2. SPREAD OF MALIGNANT TUMORS INTO THE BOWEL AND PERITONEAL FOLDS

A. Direct invasion
- I. From adjacent primary neoplasms
- II. From remote primary neoplasms
  1. Mesenteric spread
  2. Lymphatic spread

B. Intraperitoneal seeding

C. Embolic metastases

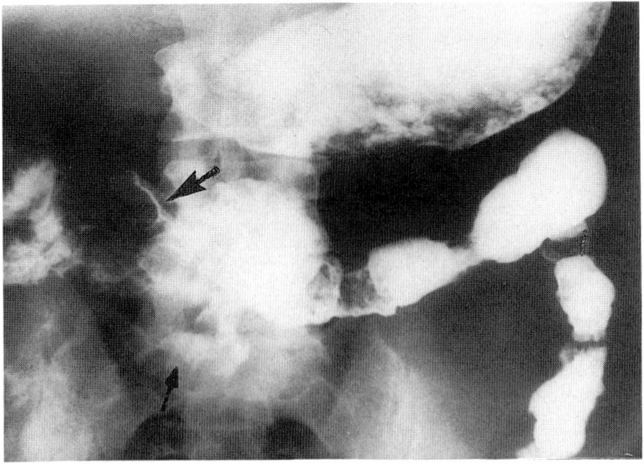

A

FIGURE 11.49. Colonic fistulas. (A) Multiple fistulas of the transverse colon in Crohn's disease (arrows). (B) Fistula between the gastric stump and transverse colon. (C) Carcinoma of hepatic fixture of the colon. Sinus tracts between the colon and duodenum (arrows).

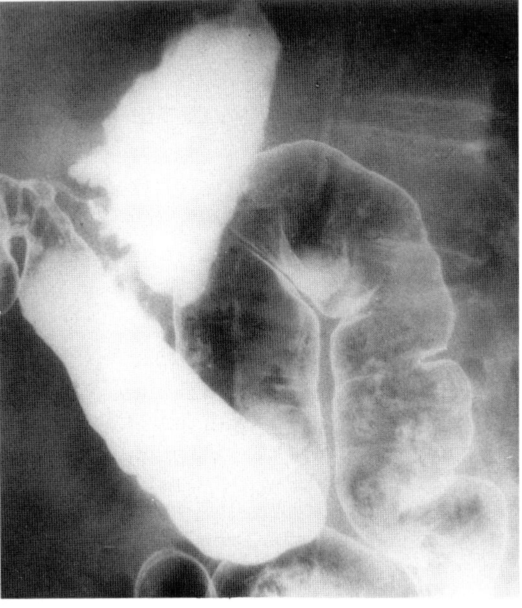

B

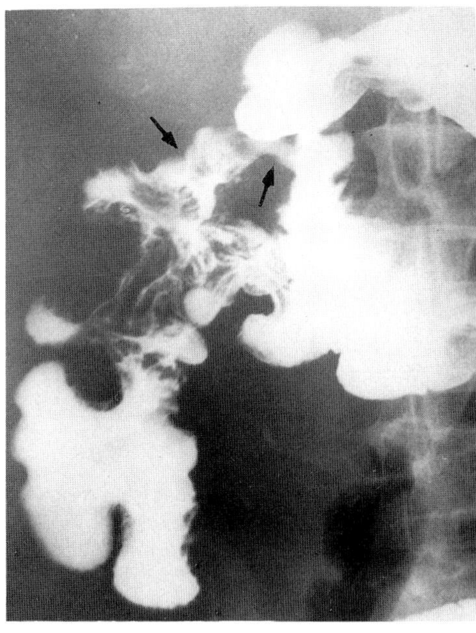

C

of the ovary, uterus (Fig. 11.50), prostate and kidney. Serrations of the mucosa and stenoses are more common signs than shouldering, which is more indicative of primary bowel neoplasia (Fig. 11.51).

2. **Direct invasion from remote primary neoplasms, with mesenteric spread.** The gastrocolic ligament and transverse mesocolon allow spread of gastric and pancreatic carcinoma into the transverse colon. Cells of *gastric carcinoma* extend down the gastrocolic ligament to the transverse colon which becomes involved along the superior aspect, between the tenia mesocolica and the tenia omentalis. Tumor masses infiltrate the colon, displacing it in a caudad direction. The desmoplastic reaction results in angulated and distorted mucosal folds. Although the mucosa is without ulcers it may produce a cobblestone appearance. Differentiation from Crohn's disease is possible since only the superior aspect of the colon is affected. The uninvolved inferior haustral contour re-

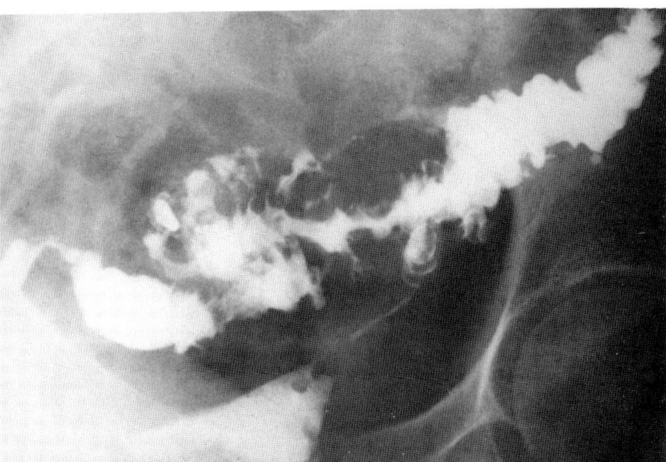

Figure 11.49 *continued.* Colonic fistulas. (D) Colo-vesical fistula in diverticulitis.

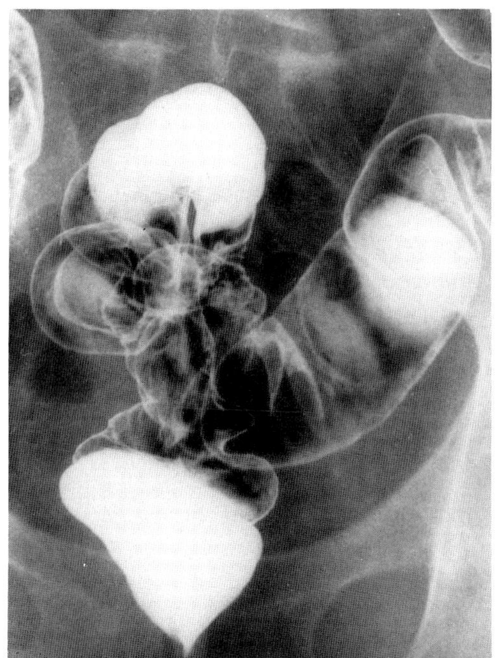

Figure 11.50. Carcinoma of the uterus infiltrates the rectum.

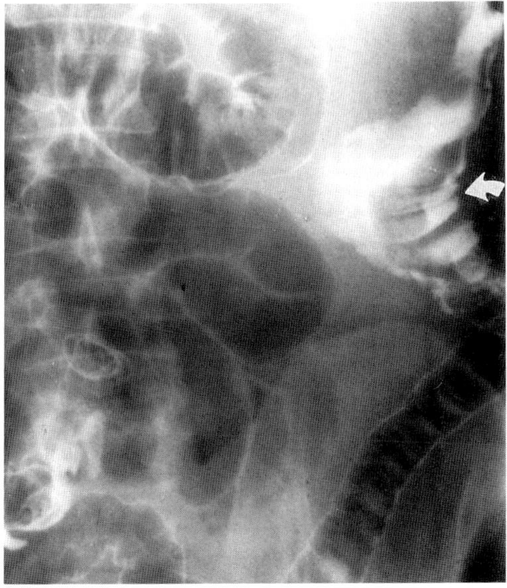

Figure 11.51. Carcinoma of the left suprarenal gland infiltrates the descending colon.

tains elasticity and undergoes saccular dilatation (Fig. 11.52). The spreading tumor may infiltrate the entire circumference of the colon, but does not usually infiltrate the extraperitoneally situated ascending and descending colon. Pelvic tumors such as carcinoma of the ovary and the urinary bladder can affect the transverse colon by spreading through the greater omentum to infiltrate the superior contour of the transverse colon (Fig. 11.53). The contour is serrated and the lumen narrowed.

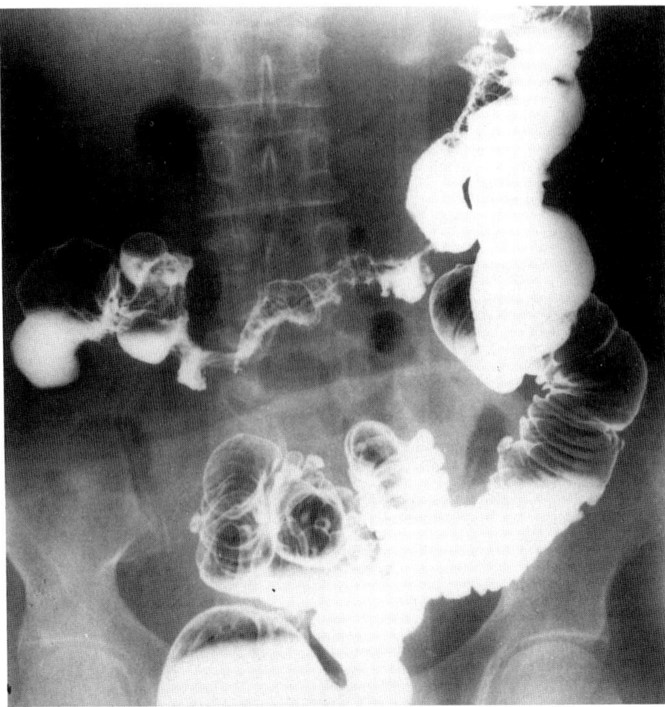

Figure 11.52. Carcinoma of the stomach spreading through the gastrocolic ligament infiltrates the transverse colon.

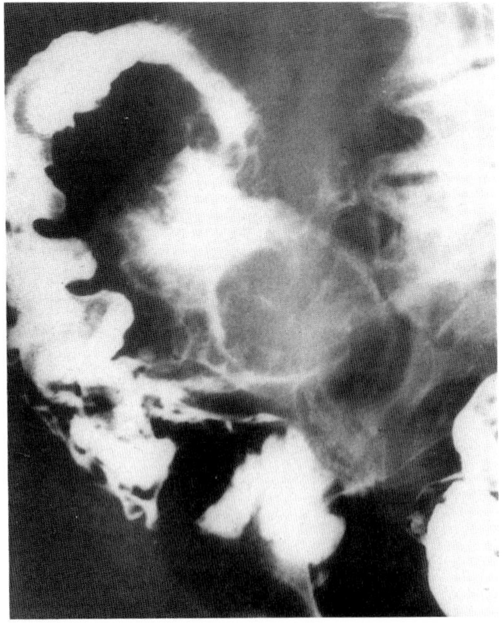

Figure 11.53. Ovarian carcinoma spreading through the greater omentum infiltrates the transverse mesocolon.

The tumor masses may protrude into the lumen to resemble invasion of gastric carcinoma through the gastrocolic ligament.

Carcinoma of the pancreas spreads directly along the transverse mesocolon and principally affects the inferior border of the transverse colon. Changes are identical to those with involvement by gastric carcinoma (Fig. 11.54).

Carcinoma of the hepatic flexure of the colon may infiltrate the second portion of the duodenum by spreading along the beginning of the transverse mesocolon (Fig. 11.49C). Spreading of transverse colon carcinoma along the gastrocolic ligament results in infiltration of the greater curvature of the stomach.

3. **Direct invasion from remote primary neoplasms, with lymphatic spread.** Dissemination of neoplasms by lymphatic permeation is not common. Blockage of distant lymph nodes may result from impaction of colon carcinoma cells with retrograde spread along lymph channels and subsequent involvement of adjacent intestinal segments.

4. **Intraperitoneal seeding.** Intraperitoneal seeding depends on the circulation of ascitic

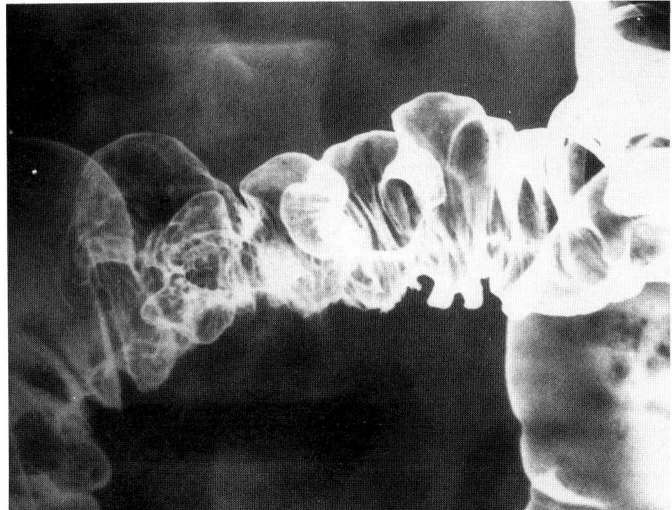

FIGURE 11.54. Carcinoma of the pancreas spreading through the transverse mesocolon infiltrates the inferior aspect of the transverse colon circumference.

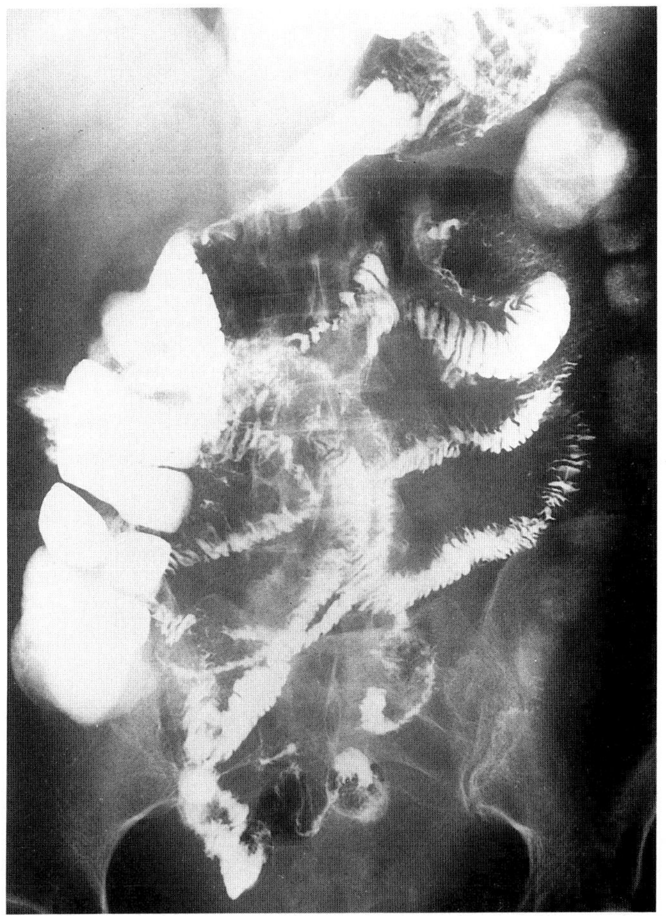

FIGURE 11.55. Carcinomatosis peritonei particularly affecting the mesentery. Follow-through barium study.

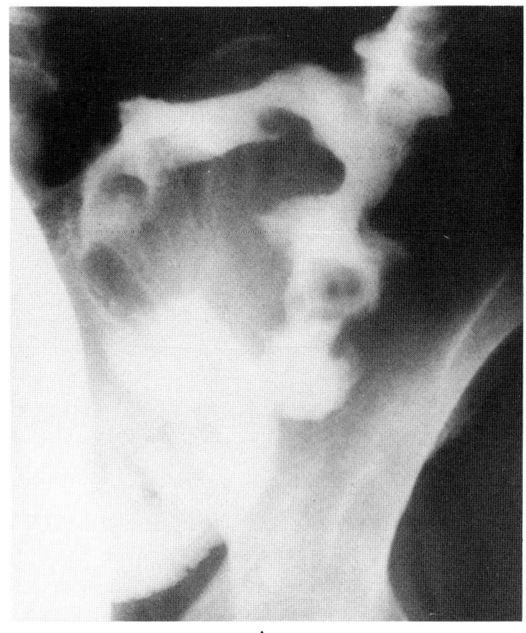

A

FIGURE 11.56. Hematogenous malignant melanoma metastases (A) to the jejunum and (B) to the terminal ileum.

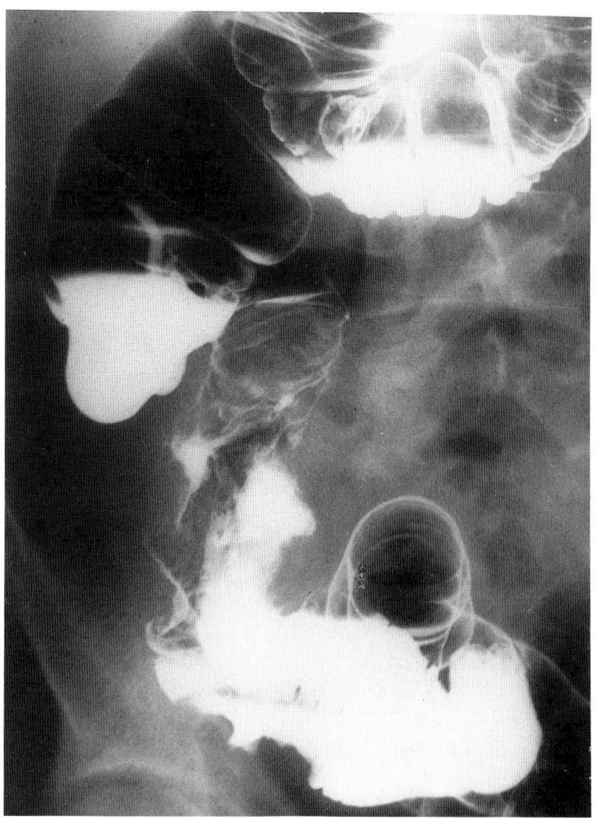

B

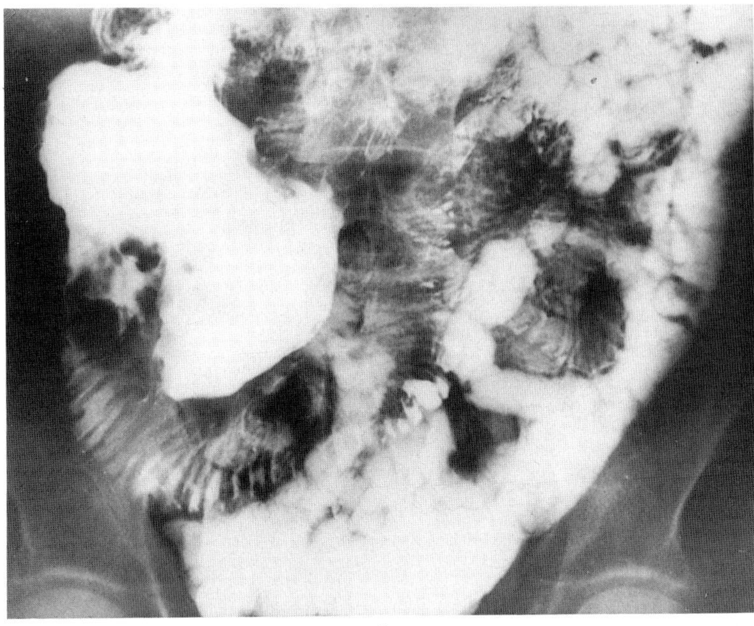

A

FIGURE 11.57. Malignant melanoma metastases. (A) Matted loops of ileum. Used by permission, Plavsic B, Robinson AE. Variations in gastrointestinal melanoma metastases. Acta Radiol Diagn. 1990; 31:493. *(Figure continued on overleaf.)*

fluid. Even a small amount of ascites can transport tumor cells. The principal barriers dividing the abdominal cavity and determining circulation of ascites are the transverse mesocolon, mesentery of the small intestine, and sigmoid mesocolon.

The distribution of ascites depends on several factors, such as gravity, patient position, or the presence of adhesions. Fluid from the inframesocolic compartment drains into the pelvis, the right lower quadrant, superior aspect of the sigmoid mesocolon, and right paracolic gutter. Stasis of ascites enhances the deposition and growth of malignant cells. Cells of pancreatic carcinoma and mucinous carcinoma of the stomach seed deposits along the mesentery of the small intestine and into the ileocecal region. The changes may mimic Crohn's disease. Metastases and desmoplastic reactions cause defects of the terminal ileum and the medial aspect of the cecum. However, the entire mesentery may be infiltrated with tumor masses (Fig. 11.55). Growth of secondary tumors on the superior aspect of the sigmoid colon results in tethering and nodular changes of the superior contour. Metastatic tumors in the right paracolic gutter result from seeding of secondary tumors by ascites which flows cranially from the pelvis. Growth of these tumors results in irregularities in the mucosal pattern of the ascending colon.

5. **Embolic metastases.** Embolic metastases to the gut are most commonly melanoma, or breast or lung carcinoma deposits. The most frequent symptom is partial obstruction. Hematogenous metastases grow in the submucosa as intramural formations protruding into the lumen. They are often ulcerated, resulting in a "bull's eye" appearance. A desmoplastic reaction is lacking. Malignant melanoma metastases to alimentary canal organs are most frequent in the small bowel (Figs. 11.56 and 11.57). The majority of these tumors are situated on the antimesenteric aspect.

The alimentary canal is affected in 8.2% of patients with far advanced carcinoma of the breast (Fig. 11.58). Hematogenous metastases to the colon are most frequent. Clinical and ra-

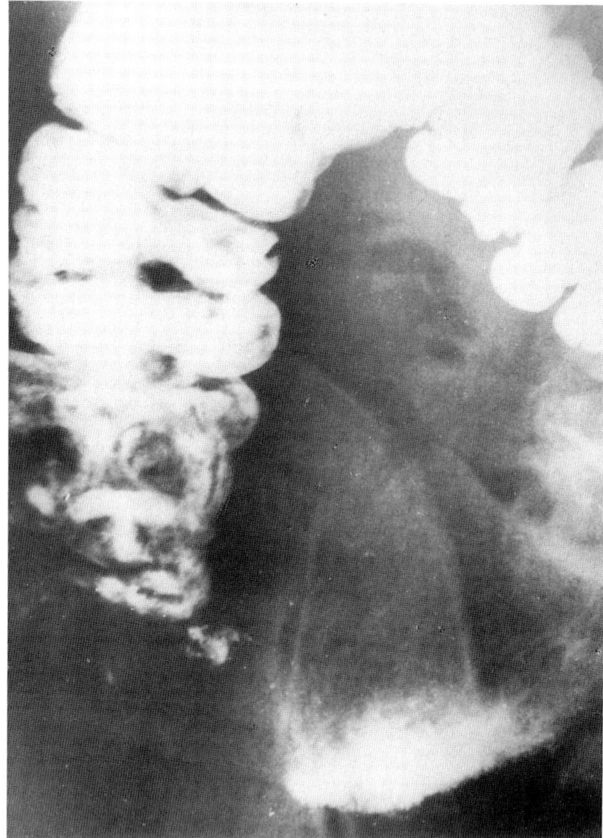

B

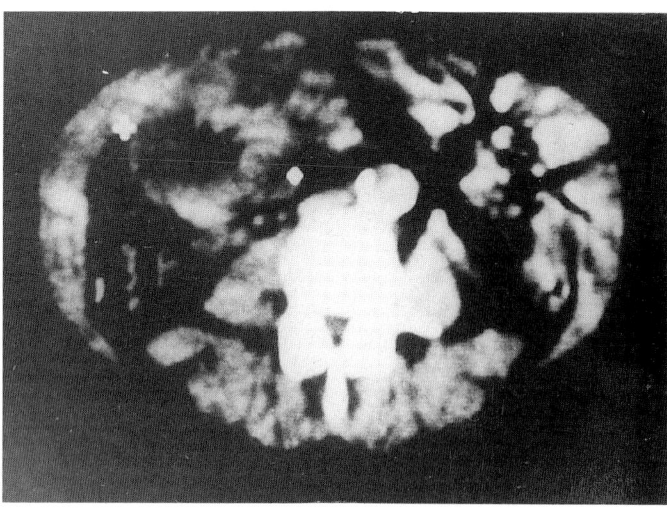

C

Figure 11.57 *continued.* Malignant melanoma metastases. (B) Barium empties from matted loops after several hours. (C) CT scan in the same patient.

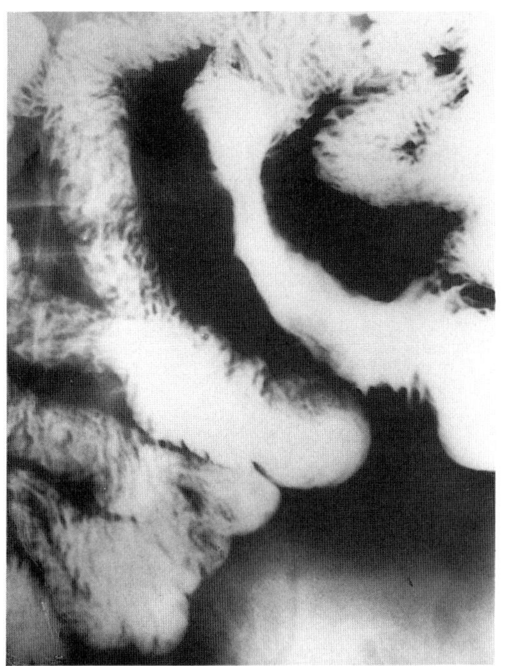

FIGURE 11.58. Hematogenous metastatic breast carcinoma in the small intestine.

diological symptomatology may simulate chronic inflammatory disease of the colon. Secondary gastric deposits of breast carcinoma frequently result in a linitis plastica appearance (Fig. 8.62).

Metastatases of bronchogenic carcinoma to the alimentary canal present as serosal deposits but may also affect inner layers of the wall.

BOWEL SURGERY AND POSTOPERATIVE APPEARANCE

Segments of the intestine may be *sutured*, for example, in case of bleeding. *Resected* portions may be short or long as in colectomy (Fig. 11.59). Moreover, sections of the bowel may be *anastomosed*, either with another section of the bowel or with other sections of the alimentary system, such as biliary or pancreatic ducts, or with the body surface. Anastomoses can be end-to-end, end-to-side, side-to-side, and side-to-end. Regarding peristalsis, there are isoperistaltic and anisoperistaltic anastomoses. In the latter, peristalsis in connected segments propagates in opposite directions.

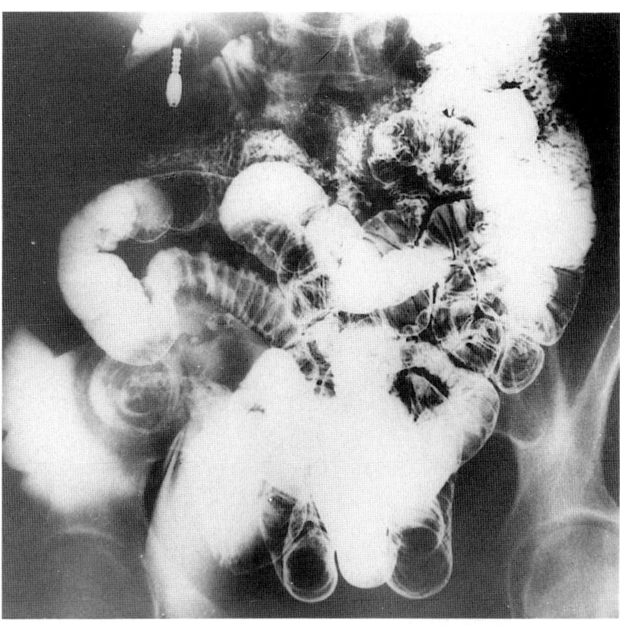

FIGURE 11.59. Colectomy. Air contrast enteroclysis with normal small bowel finding.

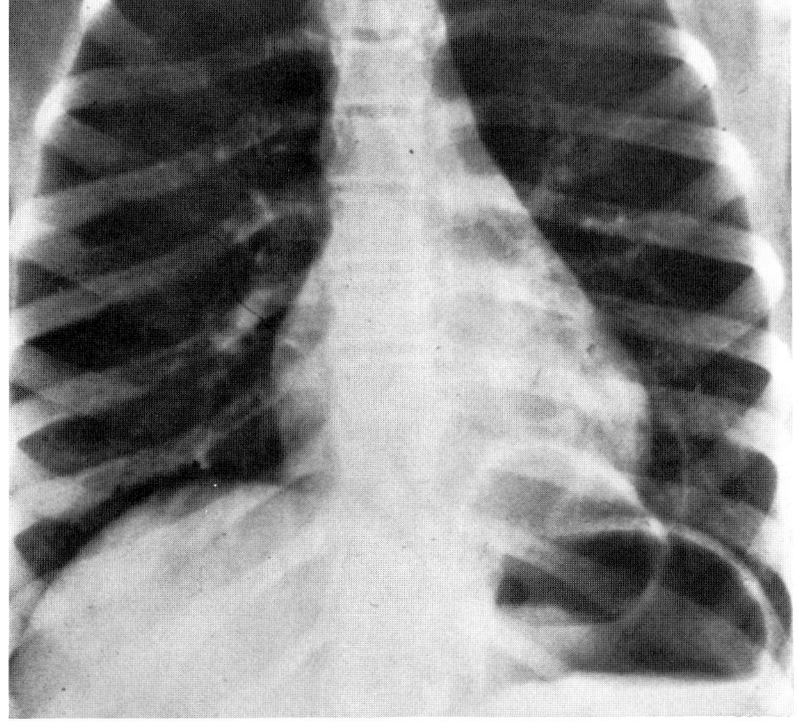

A

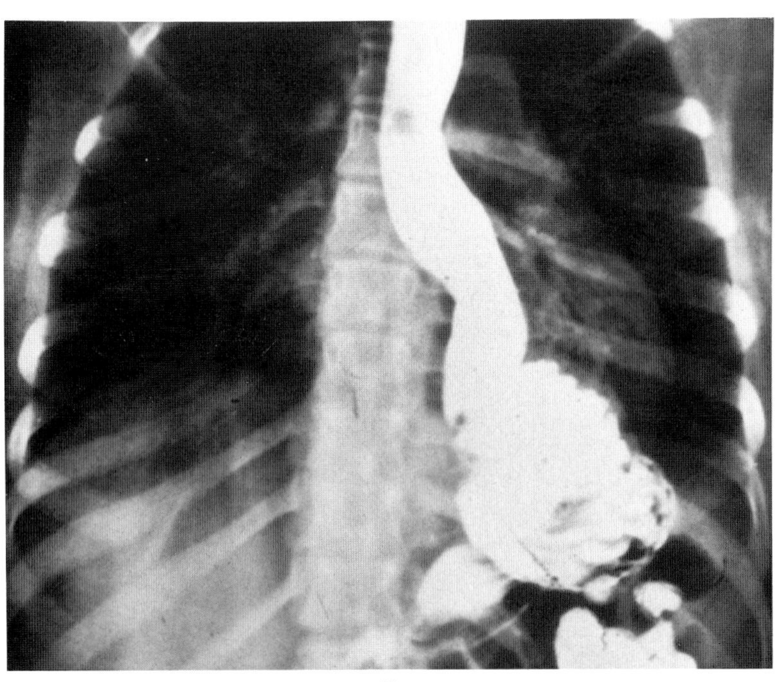

B

Figure 11.60. Hiatus hernia of the stomach. (A) Mimics a bullous lesion of the left lung base on chest film. (B) Barium study.

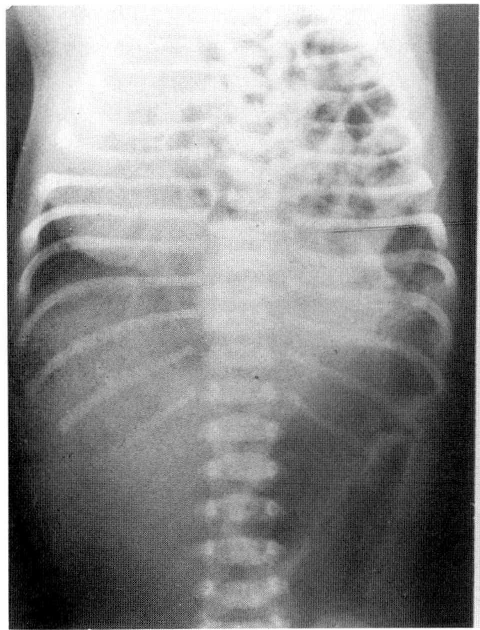
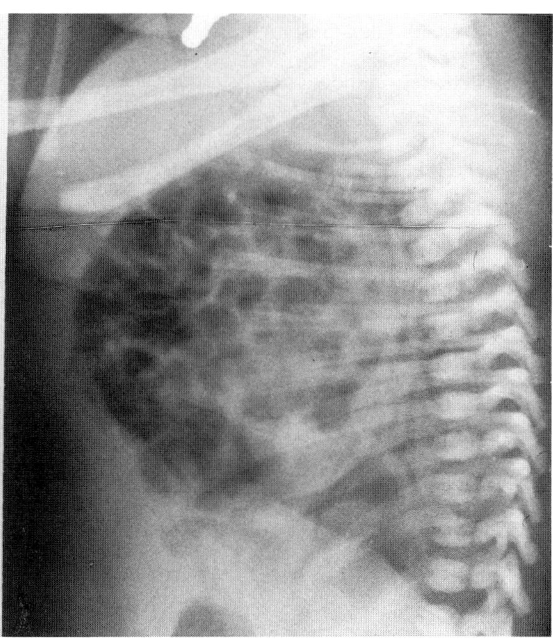

Figure 11.61. Hernia of small bowel through Bochdalek foramen.

Some anastomoses improve results of surgery performed on other organs, such as side-to-side anastomosis between afferent and efferent limbs in gastroenterostomies and Billroth II operations, which prevent recirculation without progression.

Segments of the intestine may be connected to artificial openings on the body surface, such as an ileostomy or colostomy.

Several days following surgery, or whenever a leak is suspected, examination can be performed with water-soluble contrast media.

DIAPHRAGMATIC HERNIA

Abdominal organs may be herniated into the chest through normal openings or through abnormal defects of the diaphragm (Fig. 11.60).

Hernias, other than hiatus hernia, through anatomical openings in the diaphragm are:

1. Bochdalek's hernia and pleuroperitoneal canal defects occurring on each side of the spine. The latter are not true hernias because herniated organs such as the stomach, spleen, or omentum do not contain a hernial sac (Fig. 11.61).
2. Anterior hernias passing through sternocostal triangular openings of the diaphragm. The left one is termed Larrey's space and the right one Morgagni's space. The transverse colon and the omentum may be contained within a sternocostal hernia.

THE EFFECTS OF DRUGS ON THE ALIMENTARY CANAL

Almost 25% of all drug reactions have associated gastrointestinal manifestations. The spectrum of alimentary canal reactions to drugs is limited and nonspecific.

Ulcerogenic medications provoke erosion and ulcer formation in the alimentary canal, particularly in the duodenum and stomach. Either novel ulcers occur or previously existing ulcers are reactivated. Aspirin, indomethacin, phenylbutazone, and corticosteroids have proved to be ulcerogenic. Corticosteroids contribute to the formation of antral gastric ulcers. Higher doses are more likely to provoke an ulcer, males are more commonly affected, and ulcers tend to occupy large areas. These ulcers are usually shallow. However, "silent" perforations can occur.

Stricture of the small intestine has been reported after administration of KCl tablets, which may also damage esophageal mucosa if not enteric-coated.

Immunosuppressive drugs and antibiotic therapy produce conditions favorable to the development of esophageal moniliasis and pseudomembranous colitis.

Anticoagulant drugs and medicamentous damage of the blood vessels may provoke hemorrhage into the intestinal wall. These changes can resemble ischemic intestinal disease. Digitalis may also provoke an ischemic intestinal attack due to arterial constriction.

Numerous drugs affect alimentary canal *motility*. Metoclopramide, acetylcholine, and serotonin increase intestinal motility. Neuroleptics, tranquilizers, anticholinergics, and antiparkinson drugs decrease alimentary canal tone and increase transit time.

Hypertonic water-soluble radiographic contrast media act as osmotic laxatives on the gastrointestinal tract. Accidental aspiration may be fatal in infants. These contrast media alter alimentary canal tone, reflected as changes in bowel caliber. Besides acting on tone, hypertonic contrast media accelerate bowel transit. This hyperperistalsis is mediated by serotonin and intramural cholinergic ganglionic cells.

Bibliography

Agha FP, Lee HH, Boland CR, Bradley SF. Mucormycoma of the colon: early diagnosis and successful management. AJR. 1985;145:739.

Balthazar EJ, Megibow AJ, Fazzini E, Opulencia JF, Engel I. Cytomegalovirus colitis in AIDS: radiographic findings in 11 patients. Radiology. 1985; 155:585.

Balthazar EJ, Gordon R, Hulnick D. Ileocecal tuberculosis: CT and radiologic evaluation. AJR. 1990; 154:499.

Bartram CI. Radiology in the current assessment of ulcerative colitis. Gastrointest Radiol. 1977;1:383.

Bartram CI, Thornton A. Colonic polyp patterns in familial polyposis. AJR. 1984;142:305.

Bar-Ziv J, Yagupski P, Karphus M, Mares A, Moor E: Congenital ulcerative colitis. Ann Radiol. 1982;25:59.

Bernstein WC, Bernstein EF. Ischemic ulcerative colitis following inferior mesenteric arterial ligation. Dis Colon Rectum. 1963;6:54.

Bienestock J, Befus AD. Mucosal immunology. A review. Immunology. 1980;41:249.

Binder SC, Pattersonn JF, Glotzer DJ. Toxic megacolon in ulcerative colitis. Gastroenterology. 1979; 66:909.

Braver JM. Drug reactions and the gastrointestinal tract. Postgrad Radiol. 1983;3:121.

Burney M, Farrar T, Sander RL. Gastrojejunocolic fistula. Am J Surg. 1950;24:709.

Choi SH, Sheehan FR, Pickren JW. Metastatic involvement of the stomach by breast cancer. Cancer. 1964;17:167.

Cockburn AG, Krolikowski J, Balogh K, Roth RN. Crohn's disease of penile and scrotal skin. Urology. 1980;15:596.

Collier PE, Turowski P, Diamond DL. Small intestinal adenocarcinoma complicating regional enteritis. Cancer. 1985;55:516.

Cronkhite LW, Canada WJ. Generalized gastrointestinal polyposis: an unusual syndrome of polyposis, pigmentation, alopecia and onychotrophia. N Engl J Med. 1955;252:1011.

Crooks DJM, Brown WR. The distribution of intestinal nodular lymphoid hyperplasia in immunoglobulin deficiency. Clin Radiol. 1980;31:701.

Davidson GP, Bishop RF, Townley RRW, Holmes IH, Ruch BJ. Importance of a new virus in acute sporadic enteritis in children. Lancet. 1975;1:242.

Dodds WJ. Clinical and roentgen features of the intestinal polyposis syndromes. Gastrointest Radiol. 1976;1:127.

Downey DB, Nakielny RA. Aphthoid ulcers in colonic tuberculosis. Br J Radiol. 1985;55:561.

Eisenberg RL, Montgomery CK, Margulis AR. Colitis in the elderly: ischemic colitis mimicking ulcerative and granulomatous colitis. AJR. 1979;133: 1113.

Ekberg O, Fork FT, Hildell J. Predictive value of small bowel radiography for recurrent Crohn's disease. AJR. 1980;135:1051.

Emeray CA, Jr. Regional enteritis and its oral manifestations. A case report. J Oral Med. 1979;34: 103.

Feczko PJ, Barbour J, Halpert RD, Ackerman LV. Crohn's disease in the elderly. Radiology. 1985; 157:303.

Fernbach SK, Lloyd-Still JD. The radiographic findings in severe rotavirus-induced colitis. J Can Assoc Radiol. 1984;35:192.

Frager DH, Frager JD, Brandt JL, Wolf EL, Rand LG, Klein RS, Beneventano TC. Gastrointestinal complications of AIDS: radiologic features. Radiology. 1986;158:597.

Framer RG, Hawk WA, Turnbull RB Jr. Clinical patterns in Crohn's disease: a statistical analysis of 615 cases. Gastroenterology. 1975;68:627.

Francis RS, Berk RN. Typhoid fever. Radiology. 1974;112:583.

Frank PH, Riddell RH, Feczko PJ, Levin B. Radiological detection of colonic dysplasia (precarcinoma) in chronic ulcerative colitis. Gastrointest Radiol. 1978;3:209.

Frank D, Raiicht RF. Intestinal perforation associated with cytomegalovirus infection in patients with acquired immune deficiency syndrome. Am J Gastroenterol. 1984;79:201.

Franken EA, Bixler D, Fitzgerald JF, Gamet DJ, Russ MA. Juvenile polyposis of the colon. Ann Radiol. 1975;18:499.

Fraudsen PJ, Jarnum S, Malstrom J. Crohn's disease of the duodenum. Scand J Gastroenterol. 1980;15: 683.

Gardiner R, Stevenson GW. The colitides. Radiol Clin North Am. 1982;20:797.

Gardner EJ, Richards RC. Multiple cutaneous lesions occurring simultaneously with hereditary polyposis and osteomas. Am J Genet. 1953;5:139.

Glick SN, Teplick SK. Crohn's disease of the small intestine: diffuse mucosal granularity. Radiology. 1985;154:313.

Goldberg HJ. The barium enema and toxic megacolon: cause-effect relationship? Gastroenterology. 1975;68:617.

Goldberg HJ, Caruthers SB, Nelson JA, Singleton JW. Radiographic findings of the national cooperative Crohn's disease study. Gastroenterology. 1979;77:925.

Goldberg HJ, Gore RM, Margulis AR, Moss AA, Baker EL: Computed tomography in the evaluation of Crohn's disease. AJR. 1983;140:277.

Goldstein SJ, Crooks DJM. Colitis in Behçet's syndrome. Radiology. 1978;128:321.

Gore RM, Marn CS, Kirby DF, Vogelzang RL, Neiman HL. CT findings in ulcerative, granulomatous and indeterminate colitis. AJR. 1984;143:279.

Gricco MB, Bordan DL, Geiss AC, Beil AR. Toxic megacolon complicating Crohn's colitis. Ann Surg. 1980;191:75.

Halpert RD. Toxic dilatation of the colon. Radiol Clin North Am. 1987;25:147.

Hamilton SR. Colorectal carcinoma in patients with Crohn's disease. Gastroenterology. 1985;89:389.

Hildell J, Lindstrom C, Wenckert A. Radiographic appearances in Crohn's disease, I: accuracy of radiographic methods. Acta Radiol Diagn. 1979;20: 669.

Hildell J, Lindstrom C, Wenckert A. Radiological appearances in Crohn's disease, II: the course as reflected at repeat radiography. Acta Radiol Diagn. 1979;20:933.

Hooyman JR, MacCarthy RL, Caroenter HA, Schroeder KW, Carlson HC. Radiographic appearance of mucosal dysplasia associated with ulcerative colitis. AJR. 1987;149:47.

Hyams IS, Goldman H, Katz AJ. Differentiating small bowel Crohn's disease from lymphoma. Role of rectal biopsy. Gastroenterology. 1980;79:340.

Hyson EA, Burrell M, Toffler R. Drug-induced gastrointestinal disease. Gastrointest Radiol. 1977;2: 183.

Iida M, Matsui T, Fuchigami T, Iwashita A, Yao T, Fujishima M. Ischemic colitis: serial changes in double-contrast barium enema examination. Radiology. 1986;159:377.

James EM, Carlson HC. Chronic ulcerative colitis and colon cancer: can radiographic appearance predict survival patterns? AJR. 1978;130:825.

Johnson MM, Vosburgh JW, Wiens AT, Walsh GC. Gastrointestinal polyposis associated with alopecia, pigmentation and atrophy of fingernails and toenails. Intern Med. 1962;56:935.

Jones B, Fishman EK, Kramer SS, Siegelman SS, Saral R, Beschorner WE, Yeater AU, Lake AM, Yolken RH, Tutschka P, Santos GW. Computed tomography of gastrointestinal inflammation after bone marrow transplantation. AJR. 1986;146: 691.

Kantor JL. Regional (terminal) ileitis. Its roentgen diagnosis. JAMA. 1934;103:2016.

Kattan KR, King AY. Presacral space revisited. AJR. 1979;132:437.

Kelvin FM, Woodward BH, McLeod ME, Fetter BF, Scott-Jones R. Prospective diagnosis of dysplasia (precancer) in chronic ulcerative colitis. AJR. 1982;138:347.

Kerber GW, Frank PH. Carcinoma of the small intestine and colon as a complication of Crohn's disease. Radiologic manifestations. Radiology. 1984; 150:639.

Kerber GW, Greenberg M, Rubin JM. Computed tomography evaluation of local and extraintestinal complications of Crohn's disease. Gastrointest Radiol. 1984;9:143.

Kilcheski T, Kressel HY, Laufer I, Rogers D. The radiographic appearance of the stomach in Cronkhite-Canada syndrome. Radiology. 1981;141:57.

Kilpatrick ZM, Silverman JF, Belancourt E, Forman J, Lawson JP. Vascular occlusion of the colon and oral contraceptives. N Engl J Med. 1968;278:438.

Koetel G, Schmiedl U, Majer MC, Weber P, Jenss H, Kauper K, Hess CF. Diagnosis of fistulae and sinus tracts in patients with Crohn's disease: value of MR imaging. AJR. 1989;152:999.

Kullnig P, Steiner H, Porsch G, Smolle J. Gastrointestinal Polypose bei Coeden-Syndrom. Radiologe. 1987;27:232.

Laufer I, Mullens JE, Hamilton J. Correlation of endoscopy and double-contrast radiography in early stages of ulcerative and granulomatous colitis. Radiology. 1976;118:1.

Laufer I, Costopoulos L. Early lesions of Crohn's disease. AJR. 1978;130:307.

Ledesma-Medina J, Reid BS, Girdany BR. Colitis cystica profunda. AJR. 1978;131:529.

Marston A, Pheils MT, Thomas ML, Marson BC. Ischaemic colitis. Gut. 1966;7:1.

Mathis JM, Zelenik ME, Staab EV. CT detection of bowel infarction. Comput Radiol. 1985;9:177.

Max RJ, Kelvin FM. Nonspecificity of discrete colonic ulceration on double-contrast barium enema study. AJR. 1980;134:1265.

McGovern VJ, Goulston SJM. Ischemic enterocolitis. Gut. 1965;6:213.

McKusick VA. Genetic factors in intestinal polyposis. JAMA. 1962;182:277.

Meyers MA. Distribution of intra-abdominal malignant seeding: dependence on dynamics of flow of ascitic fluid. AJR. 1973;119:198.

Meyers MA. Intraperitoneal spread of malignancies and its effect on the bowel. Clin Radiol. 1981; 32:129.

Meyers MA, Whalen JP. Roentgen significance of the duodenocolic relationships: an anatomic approach. AJR. 1973;117:263.

Miller TL, Skucas J, Gudex D, Listinsky C. Bowel cancer characteristics in patients with regional enteritis. Gastrointest Radiol. 1987;12:45.

Morson BC, Konishi F. Contribution of the pathologist to the radiology management of the colorectal polyps. Gastrointest Radiol. 1982;7:257.

Ni XY, Goldberg HI. Aphthoid ulcers in Crohn's disease: relationship to bowel appearance. Radiology. 1986;158:589.

Nolan DJ, Gourtsoviannis NC. Crohn's disease of the small intestine: a review of the radiological appearances in 100 consecutive patients examined by barium infusion technique. Clin Radiol. 1980; 31:597.

Nolan DJ, Piris J. Crohn's disease of the small intestine: a comparative study of the radiological and pathological appearances. Clin Radiol. 1980;31: 591.

Ott DJ, Chen YM, Gelfand DW, Swearingen FV, Munitz HA. Detailed per-oral small bowel examination vs. enteroclysis. Radiology. 1985;155:29.

Ottinger LW. Mesenteric ischemia (current concepts). N Engl J Med. 1982;307:535.

Pope TL, Shaffer H. Small bowel xanthomatosis: radiologic-pathologic correlation. AJR. 1985;144: 1215.

Quioque T, Glick SN, Teplick SK. Inflammatory changes proximal to obstructing lesions in the small intestine. Gastrointest Radiol. 1985;10:157.

Reeders JWAJ, Rosenbusch G, Tytgat GNJ. Radiological aspects of ischaemic colitis. Diagn Imag. 1981;50:4.

Rutledge RH. Pseudoulcerative colitis proximal to obstructing colon carcinoma. Am J Surg. 1969; 35:384.

Sacher DB. New concepts of cancer. Mt Sinai J Med. 1983;50:133.

Sartoris DJ, Harell GS, Anderson MF, Zboralske MF. Small bowel lymphoma and regional enteritis: radiographic similarities. Radiology. 1984;152: 291.

Sasson L. Entrance of barium into intestinal glands during barium enema. JAMA. 1960;173:343.

Shapir J, Frank P. Radiologic manifestations of the syndrome of neurocrest and colonic tumors. Gastrointest Radiol. 1985;10:383.

Simpkins KC. Aphthoid ulcers in Crohn's colitis. Clin Radiol. 1977;28:601.

Siskind BN, Burrell MI, Klein ML, Princethal RA. Toxic dilatation in Crohn's disease with CT correlation. J Comput Assist Tomogr. 1985;9:193.

Smerud MJ, Johnson CD, Stephens DH. The diagnosis of bowel infarction: a comparison of plain films and CT scans in 23 cases. AJR. 1990;154:99.

Smit JN, Winship DH. Complications and extraintestinal problems in inflammatory bowel disease. Med Clin North Am. 1980:64:1161.

Sommers SC. Ulcerative and granulomatous colitis. AJR. 1978;130:817.

Stevenson GW, Goodacre R, Jackson R, Ragbeer M, Rowland R. Dysplasia to carcinoma transformation in ulcerative colitis. AJR. 1984;143:108.

Tielbeek AV, Rosenbush G, Muytjens HL, Yap SH, Strijk SP, Boetes C. Roentgenologic changes of the colon in Campylobacter infection. Gastrointest Radiol. 1985;10:358.

Traube J, Simpson S, Riddell RH, Levin B, Kirsner JB. Crohn's disease and adenocarcinoma of the bowel. Dig Dis Sci. 1980;25:939.

Tumen HJ. Toxic megacolon in fulminating disease. JAMA. 1965;191:838.

Turcot J, Despres JP, St Pierre F. Malignant tumors of the central nervous system associated with familial polyposis of the colon. Dis Colon Rectum. 1959;2:465.

Virus of infantile gastroenteritis. Br Med J. 1975;3: 555. Editorial.

Whelan G. Cancer risk in ulcerative colitis: why are results in literature so varied? Clin Gastroenterol. 1980;9:469.

Whittaker LD, Pemberton JD. Mesenteric vascular occlusion. JAMA. 1938;111:21.

Williams L. Innominate grooves in the surface of the mucosa. Radiology. 1965;84:877.

Winthrop JD, Balfe DM, Shackelford GD, McAlister WH. Ulcerative and granulomatous colitis in children—comparison of double-contrast and single-contrast studies. Radiology. 1985;154:657.

Wolf BS, Marshak RH. "Toxic" segmental dilatation of the colon during the course of fulminating ulcerative colitis. Roentgen findings. AJR. 1959;82: 985.

Chapter **12**

Radiology of the Colon, Ileocecal Area, and the Rectum

Barium enema examination should identify the position and length of the colon, presence of haustral markings, width of the lumen, and mucosal relief features. The normal mucosa of the large intestine, as seen on roentgenographs, has a smooth surface resulting in a regular contour (Fig. 12.1). An elongated colon may, by its foldings, create saccular formations which fill and empty during the course of a barium enema (Fig. 12.2). This should not be considered pathologic. Fluoroscopy with spot filming allows detection of lesions not visible in standard positions (Fig. 12.3).

Compared to a double-contrast barium enema examination, colonoscopy can more accurately detect small lesions such as polyps. However, it is associated with more complications and is usually three times more expensive than a double-contrast barium enema.

FUNCTIONAL SPHINCTERS OF THE COLON

Barium enema examination may demonstrate areas of narrowing of the colon at relatively constant sites, where the mucosal surface remains completely intact. These result from spasm of functional "sphincters." Their locations are on the inferior lateral wall of the cecum, at the transition of the cecum into the ascending colon, in the mid-transverse and mid-descending colon, at the transition of the descending into the sigmoid colon, in the mid-sigmoid colon and at the junction of sigmoid colon and rectum (Fig. 12.4). Functional stenoses can be easily distinguished from organic lesions by the use of a spasmolytic agent and distension of the bowel by air or barium.

IRREGULARITY OF THE NORMAL COLON CONTOUR

Irregularities in the normal colon contour result from the presence of barium in haustreolae, mucoid glands, and innominate lines. *Haustreolae* (Figs. 12.5 and 12.6) are transient irregularities of the mucosal surface resulting from contractions of the lamina muscularis mucosae. They may encompass the entire circumference of the colon, or may merely occupy a portion of it. As peristaltic impulses cause contractions of the muscular coat of the mucosa, haustreolae change their position, migrating through adjacent segments. These are physiologic movements which mix intestinal contents. Cholinergic stimulation, such as vagus predominance innervation or administration of pilocarpine, enhance the appearance of haustreolae. Their changes in position and dimension make it easy to distinguish them from other, anatomical structures.

Penetration of barium into *mucoid glands* (Lieberkühn's crypts) may create an impression of discrete rose-thorn ulcers of the colonic mucosa (Diagram 12.1A and Fig. 12.7). *Innominate lines* may mimic tiny ulcers or mucoid

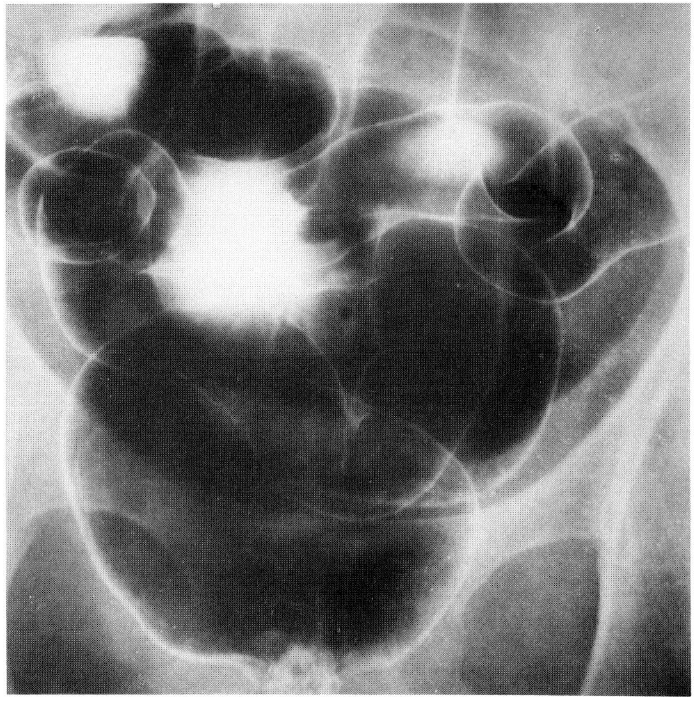

A

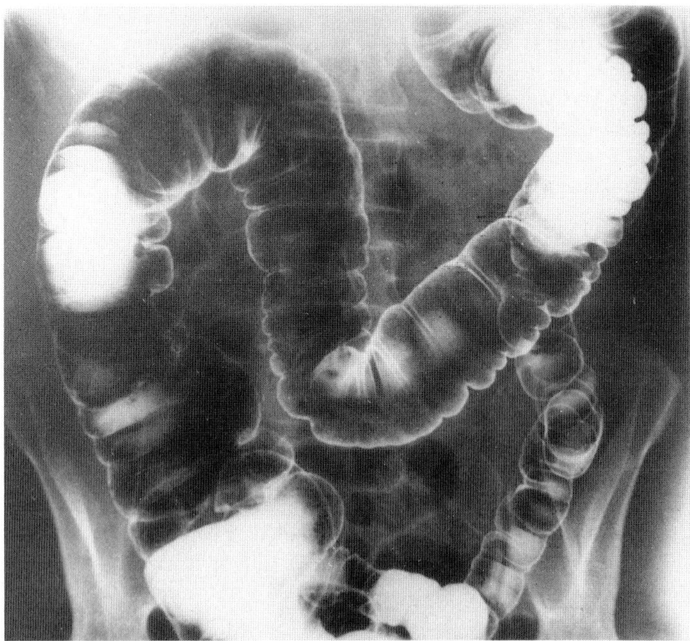

B

Figure 12.1. (A) Normal rectum and sigmoid colon in supine Trendelenburg position. (B) Normal colon. Double-contrast barium enema examination.

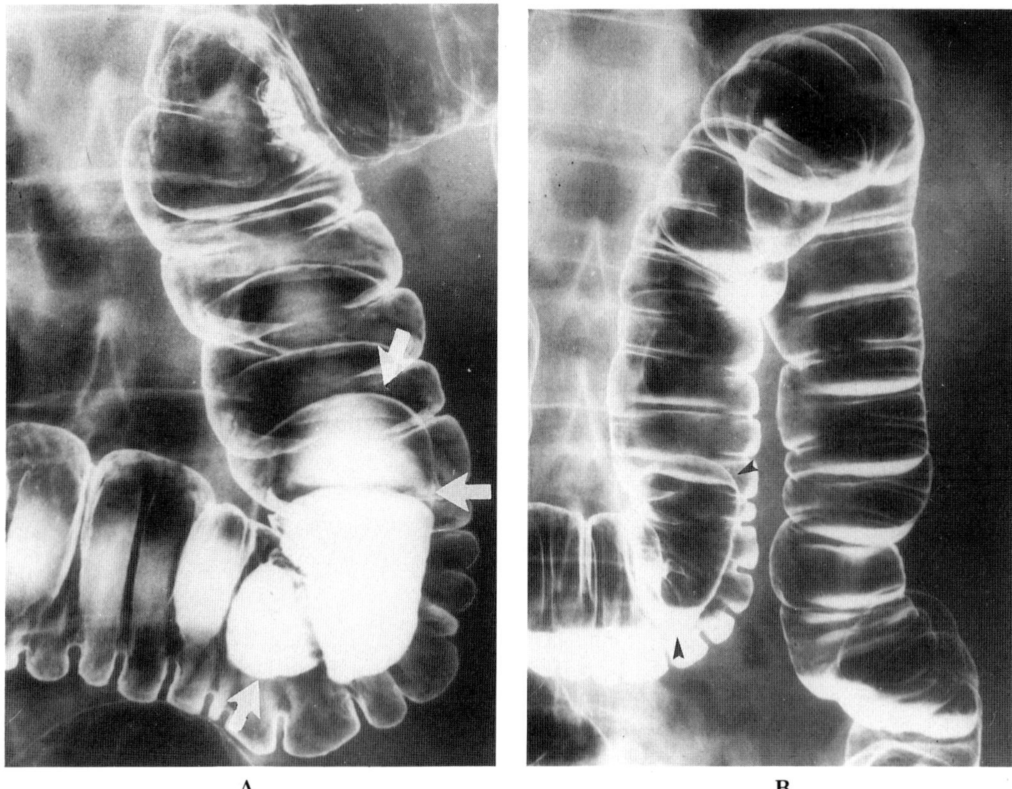

FIGURE 12.2. Sacculations form in colon curves which seemingly (A) fill with barium (arrows) and (B) empty (arrowheads).

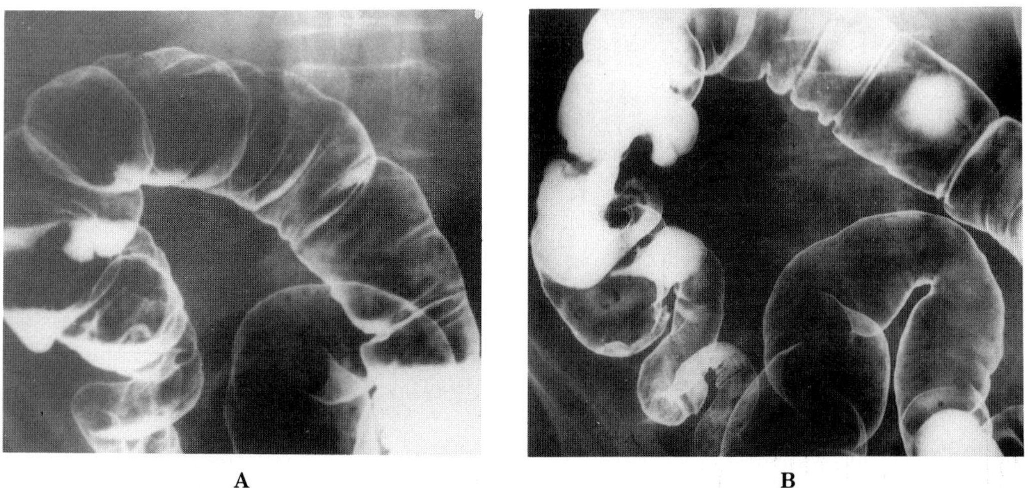

FIGURE 12.3. Carcinoma of the ascending colon. (A) Not seen in erect position but (B) seen in supine position.

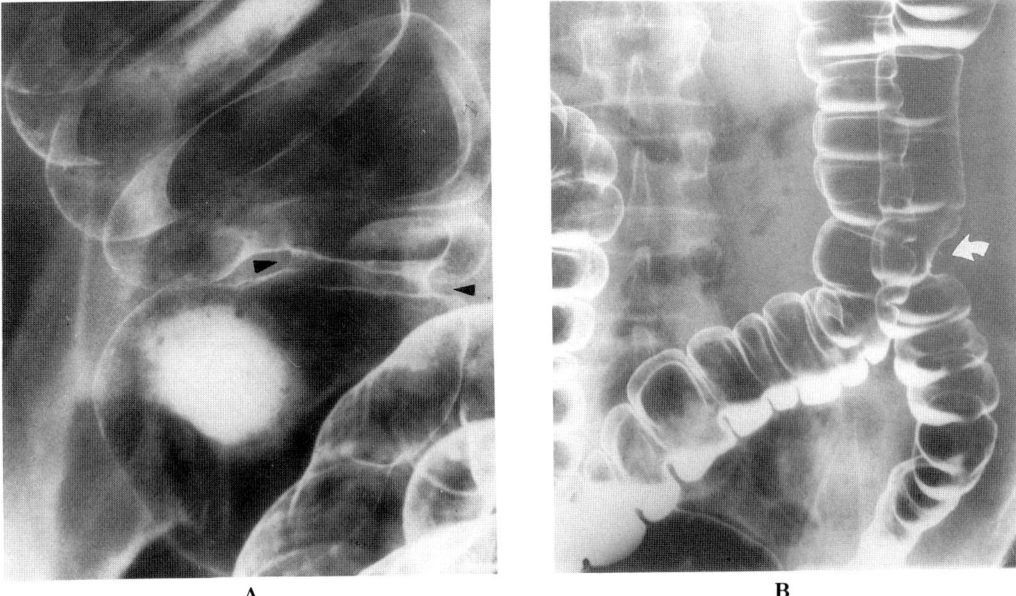

Figure 12.4. Functional sphincters of the colon. (A) At the transition from cecum to ascending colon (arrowheads). (B) In the middle of the descending colon (arrow).

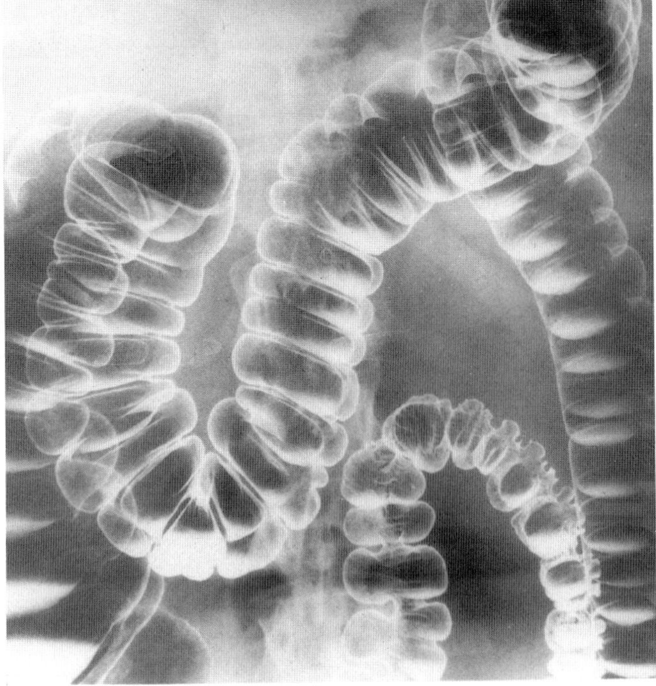

Figure 12.5. Contractions of the lamina muscularis mucosae, in the sigmoid colon.

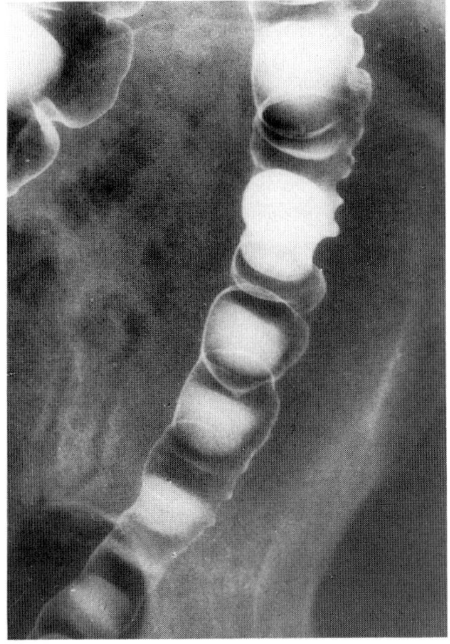

A

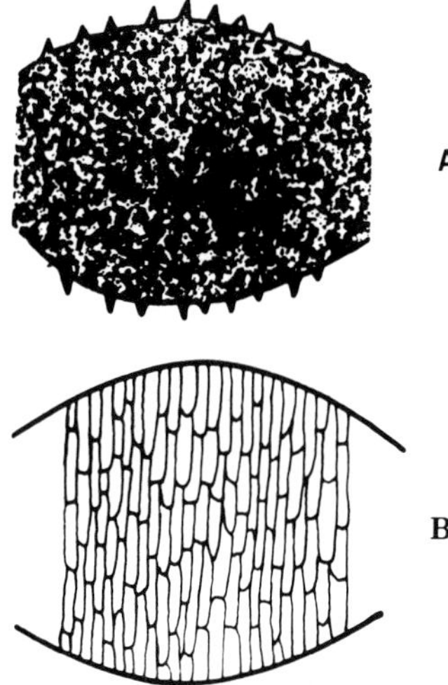

Diagram 12.1. (A) Mucosal glands of the colon filled with barium. (B) Innominate lines, normal elements of mucosal relief of the colon.

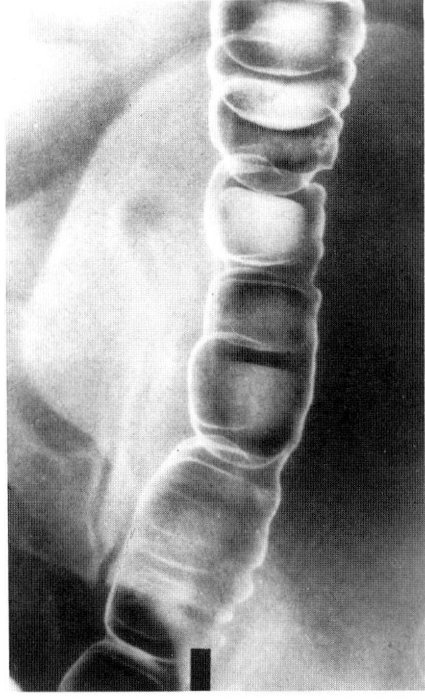

B

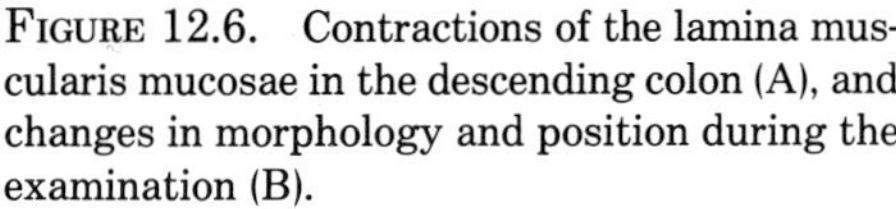

Figure 12.6. Contractions of the lamina muscularis mucosae in the descending colon (A), and changes in morphology and position during the examination (B).

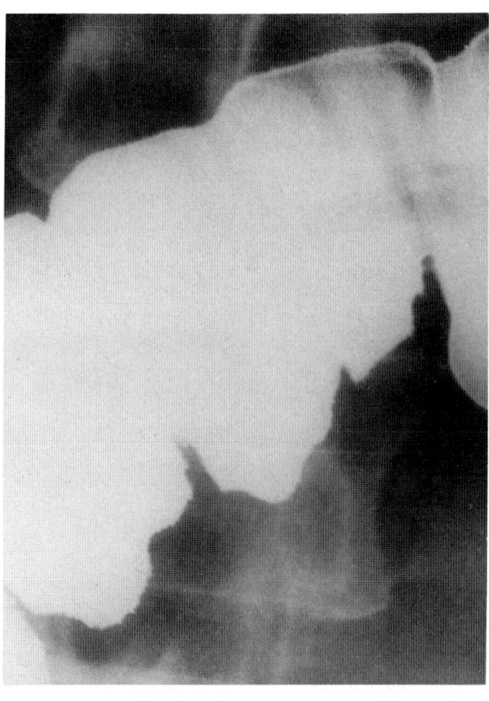

Figure 12.7. Irregularities of colon contour resulting from entrance of barium into mucosal glands.

glands filled with barium when seen on the contour of the colon during single-contrast studies. However, a double-contrast enema examination reveals discrete grooves perpendicular to the longitudinal axis of the colon (Diagram 12.1B and Fig. 12.8). These are normal surface elements of the colonic mucosa, and can be effaced by overdistension of the colon by air.

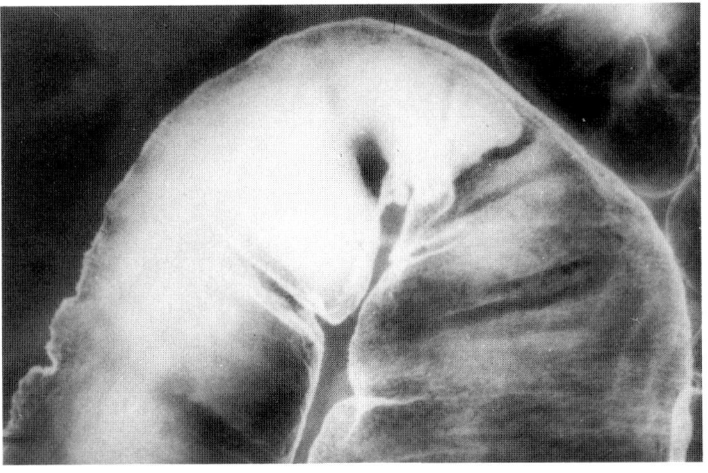

A

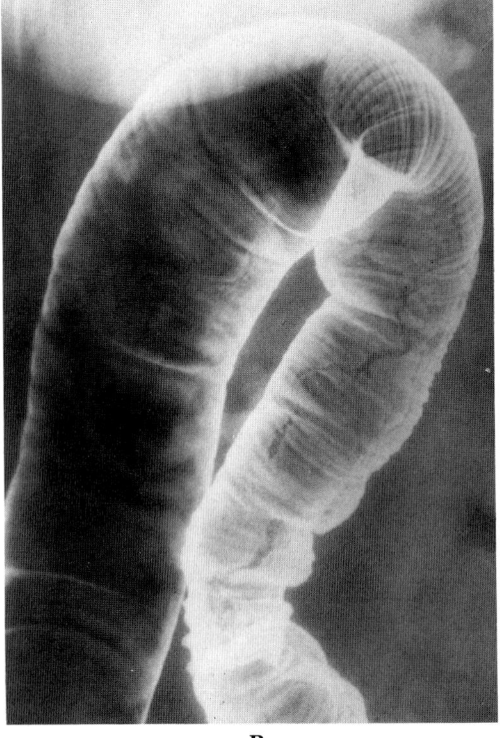

B

Figure 12.8. (A) and (B) Innominate lines of the colon. (B) Stripes of mucus in the descending colon.

FUNCTIONAL DISORDERS

IRRITABLE COLON SYNDROME

Also referred to as spastic colon, mucoid colitis, or neurosis of the colon, the irritable colon syndrome is diagnosed on the basis of clinical symptoms. Irritable colon accounts for more than one third of gastroenterological clinical examinations. Dysfunction of the autonomic nervous system appears to be related to anxiety states and possibly to dietetic factors and is likely to result in irritable colon. However, no pathologic substrate can be histologically detected. Clinical presentation includes pain, and diarrhea or obstipation, with large amounts of mucus secretion. Barium enema is needed to exclude any pathologic lesion. The findings may be normal, but hypertonia and hypermotility of the affected segment, most commonly the sigmoid colon, cause haustral markings to be prominent (Fig. 12.9). The lumen of the colon is narrowed and easily filled with barium, while evacuation is complete. Irritable colon with pronounced spasms can be an etiologic factor for diverticulosis of the distal colon.

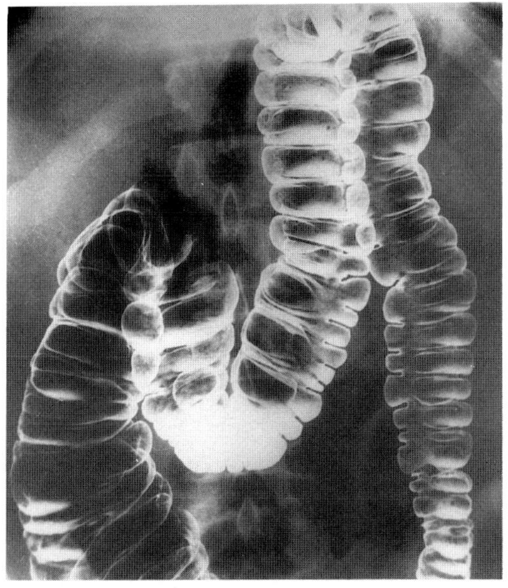

FIGURE 12.9. Hyperhaustration and contractions of the lamina muscularis mucosae of the colon in a patient with irritable colon syndrome.

ABNORMAL ANATOMICAL LOCATION OF THE COLON

CONGENITALLY ABNORMAL ANATOMICAL LOCATION

Malrotation of the intestine may be either partial (Fig. 12.10) or complete (Fig. 3.6). Sections of the colon and cecum can be fixed atypically during embryonic migration, or the pathway of the migration may differ from normal. *Ptosis* is characterized by low fixation of flexures (Fig. 12.10H). All segments of the colon may be elongated creating a *dolichocolon* (Fig. 12.10H and I). Only a double-contrast enema allows analysis of a very elongated, tortuous colon, that results in overlapping. An elongated colon and mesocolon predispose toward pathology such as volvulus.

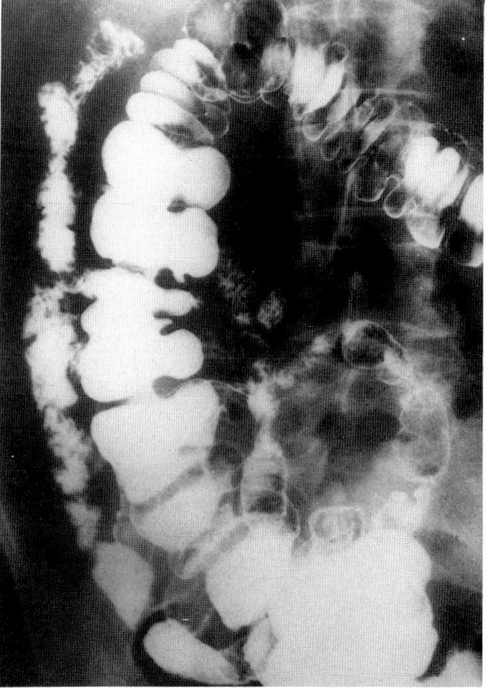

A

FIGURE 12.10. Congenital positional anomalies of the colon. (A) Distal sections of small bowel are lateral to the cecum and ascending colon. (*Figure continued on following three pages.*)

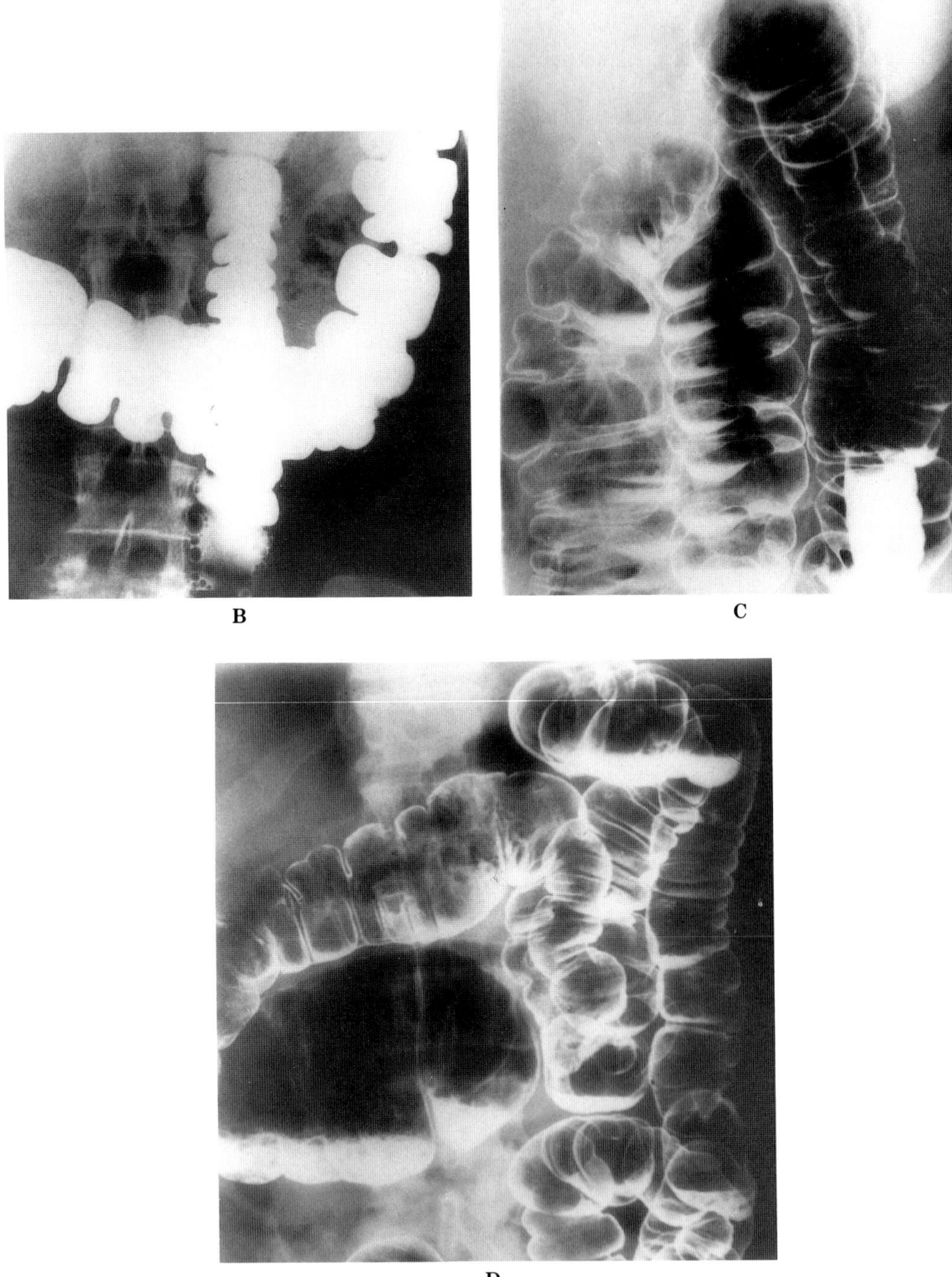

B

C

D

FIGURE 12.10 *continued.* Congenital positional anomalies of the colon. (B) Atypical course of the left colic flexure with medial fixation of the descending colon. (C) Both ascending and descending colon are almost in the mid-line. (D) The cecum is horizontally positioned with the tip directed medially.

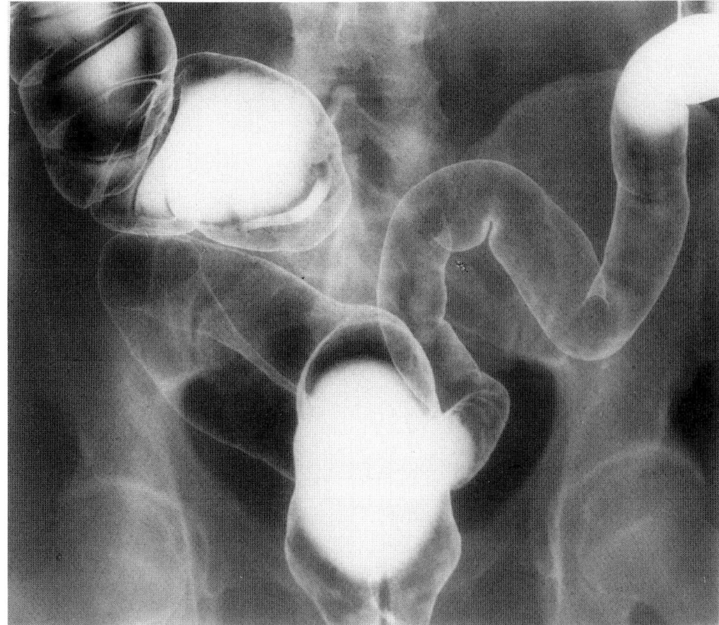

E

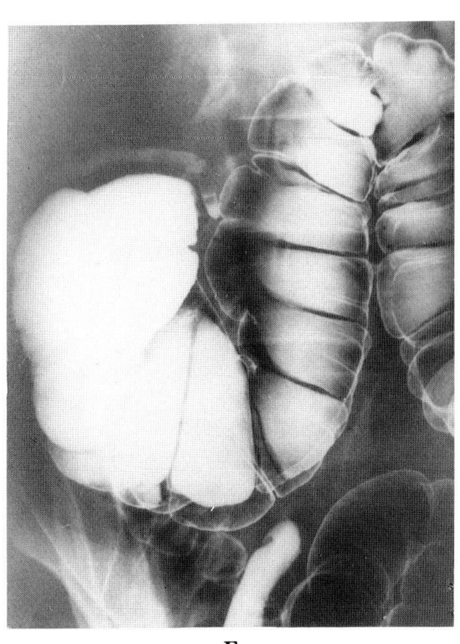

F

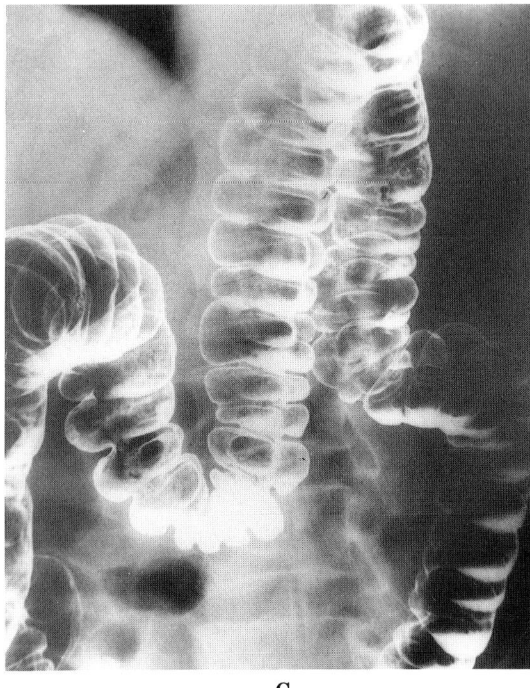

G

FIGURE 12.10 *continued.* Congenital positional anomalies of the colon. (E) Elongated and somewhat atypical course of the sigmoid colon with medial position of the cecum. (F) Medial position of the ascending colon with the tip of the cecum directed cranially. (G) Anomalous course of the transverse colon. Similar appearance may result from herniation of greater omentum into the chest.

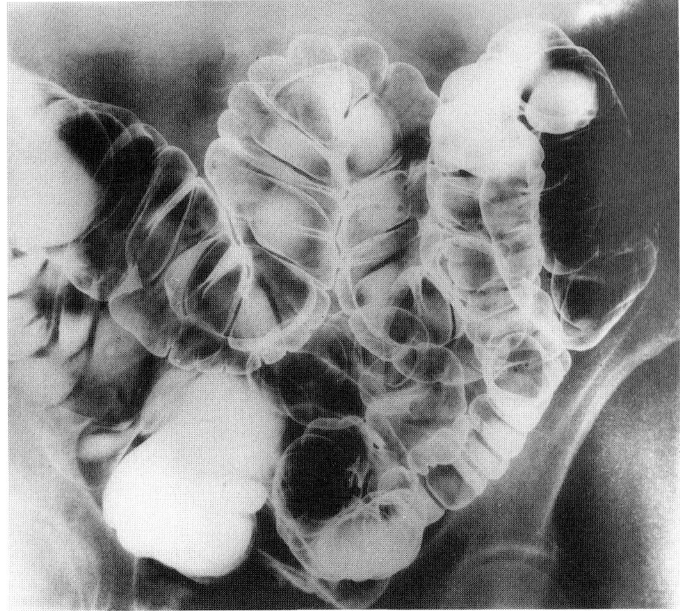

H

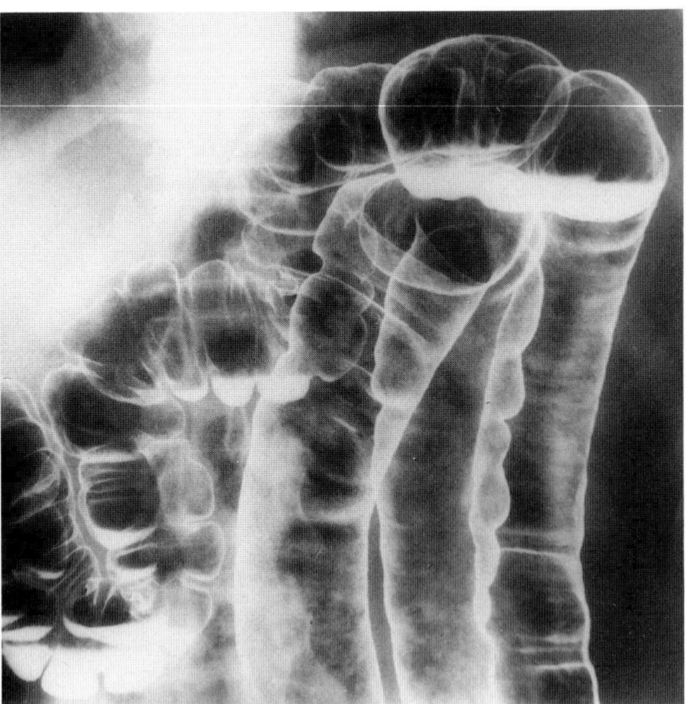

I

Figure 12.10 *continued.* Congenital positional anomalies of the colon. (H) Elongated, tortuous colon with low fixation of flexures (coloptosis). (I) Very elongated sigmoid colon reaching the splenic flexure of the colon.

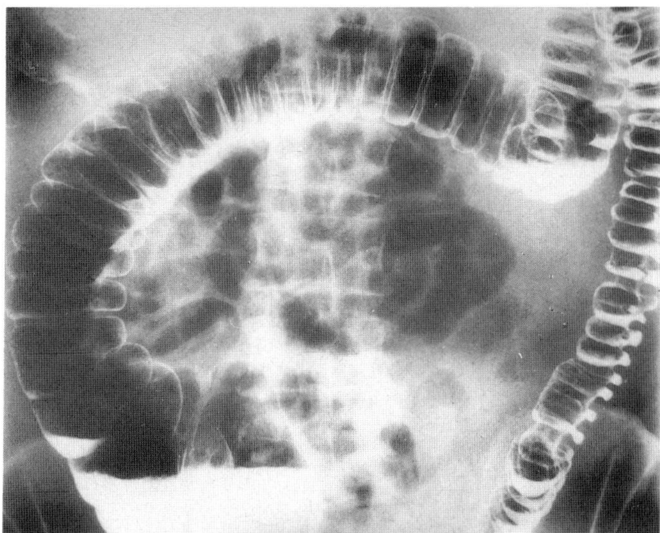

Figure 12.11. Air-filled small bowel dislocates the colon toward the periphery of the abdomen. Reversible diverticula of the descending colon.

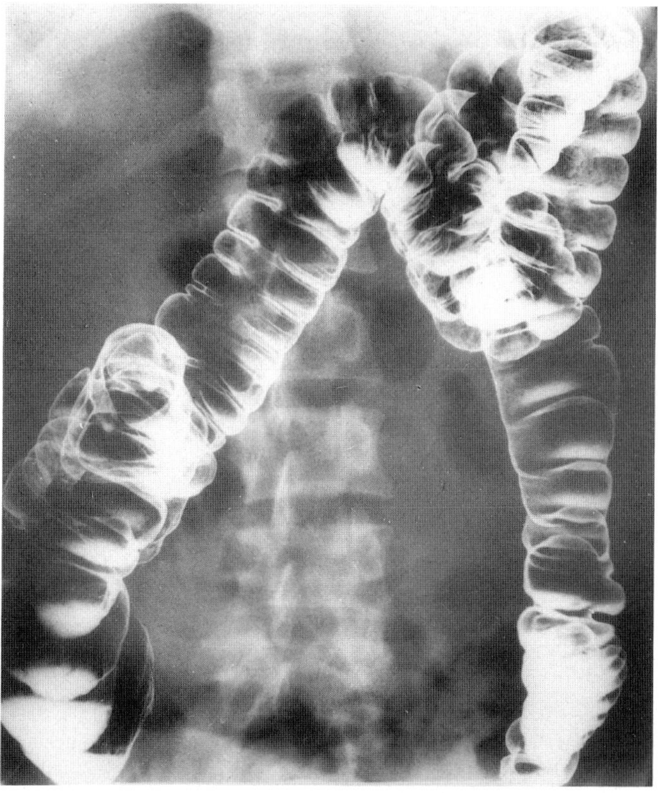

Figure 12.12. Enlarged liver displaces hepatic flexure of the colon caudally.

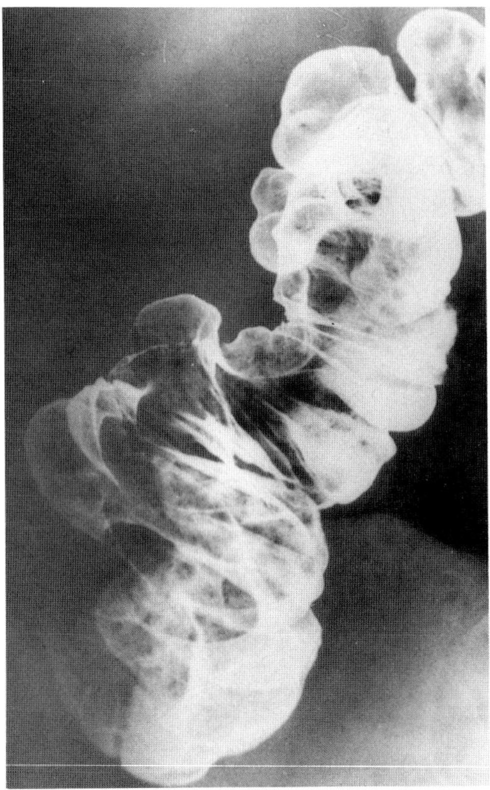

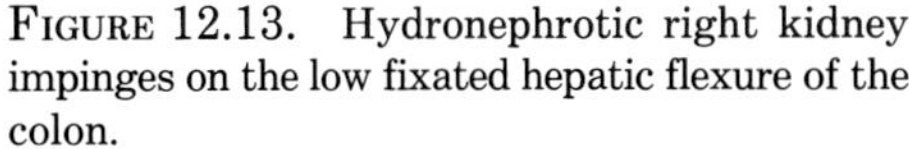

Figure 12.13. Hydronephrotic right kidney impinges on the low fixated hepatic flexure of the colon.

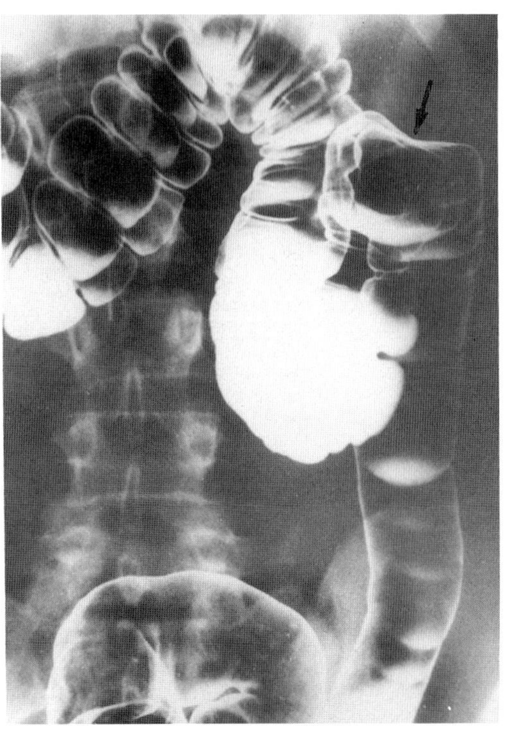

A

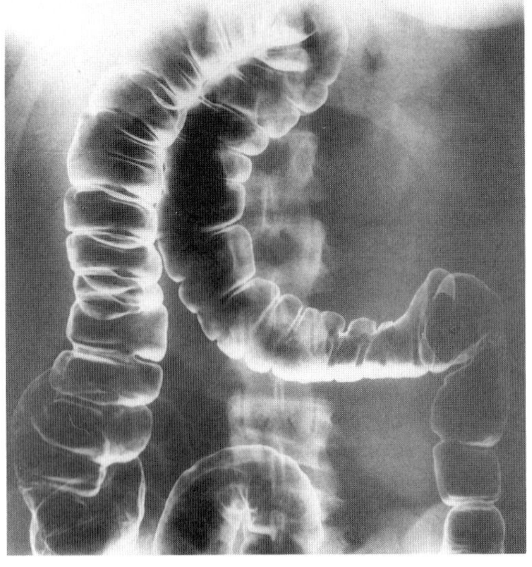

B

Figure 12.14. Impingement of splenic flexure of the colon by spleen enlarged (A) slightly, (B) greatly.

Chilaiditi's syndrome results from interposition of the right colic flexure between the liver and the diaphragm (Figs. 4.8 and 5.26). Insufficient development of the falciform ligament of the liver may result in this anomaly. The presence of haustral markings provides a basis for differentiation from pneumoperitoneum and subphrenic abscess. Contrast enema is diagnostic when plain film fails to demonstrate haustral markings.

Acquired Abnormal Positioning

An enlarged liver and spleen displace the right and left colonic flexures respectively, in a caudad direction. The sigmoid colon may be displaced by masses in the pouch of Douglas.

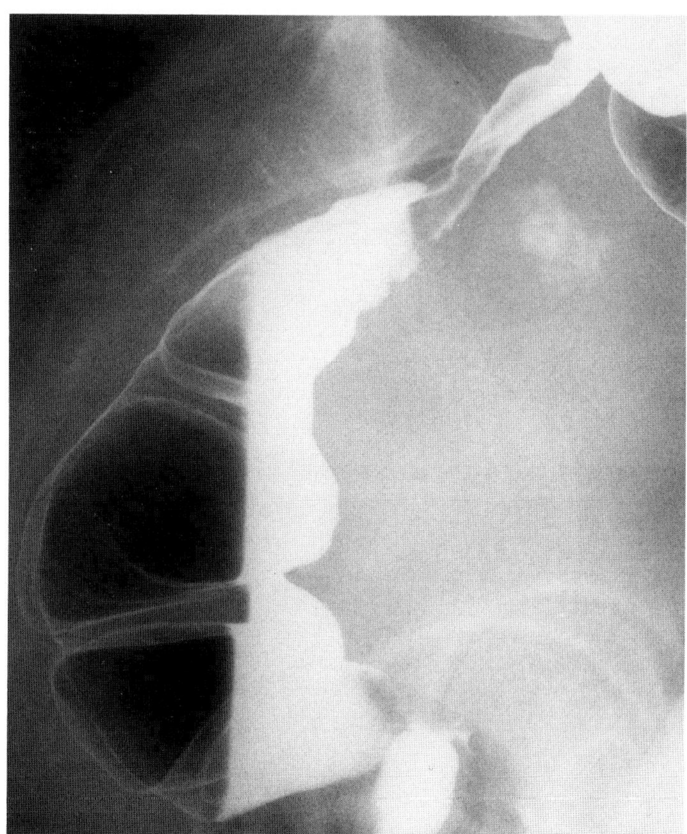

FIGURE 12.15. Narrowing of the distal sigmoid colon by a large calcified fibromyoma of the uterus.

A mass in the presacral space may impinge on the posterior aspect of the rectum. Figures 12.11 to 12.15 demonstrate acquired changes of position of the colon.

Hernias of the colon may be either internal or external (Fig. 12.16). Internal hernias are omental, paraduodenal, pericecal and intersigmoid. Sections of the colon may enter the chest either through anatomical openings of the diaphragm or through ruptures. Diaphragmatic hernia may resemble an infiltrative process of the lung. The presence of gas and haustral markings within a herniated segment, usually the transverse colon, are a diagnostic sign. If haustral markings are not readily demonstrated on plain film, barium enema can be diagnostic. Sternocostal openings (Larrey and Morgagni) and lumbocostal defects (Bochdalek) (Fig. 11.61) also allow herniation into the chest.

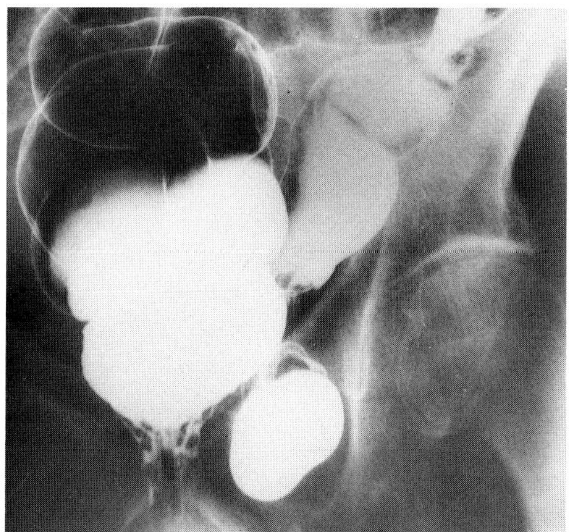

FIGURE 12.16. Sigmoid colon within inguinal hernia.

Freely movable sections of the colon may be herniated through the abdominal wall.

CONGENITAL ANOMALIES OF THE COLON

A membrane covers the anus in patients with anal *atresia*. Obstruction of the distal rectal segment characterizes rectal atresia. These are both detectable on plain films taken at least 10 hours after birth, when the rectum is filled by gas. Although it has been considered that the child should be in an upside-down position, with a radiopaque marker placed at the anal dimple, similar definition can be obtained by prone positioning and horizontal beam imaging (Fig. 12.17). However, a careful search for a fistula opening is often more rewarding.

In stenosis or atresia of the rectum, the anus is normally patent. Occasionally, other sections of the large bowel may harbor atresias.

Duplications of the large bowel are anomalies affecting only a short section of the whole organ. When duplications communicate with the intestinal lumen, they may fill and empty with barium during a contrast examination. If communication with the main lumen does not exist, they appear as elongated or oval negative defects of the contrast column.

Congenital fistulas of the large intestine, often associated with imperforate anus, communicate with the urinary tract, vagina, or per-

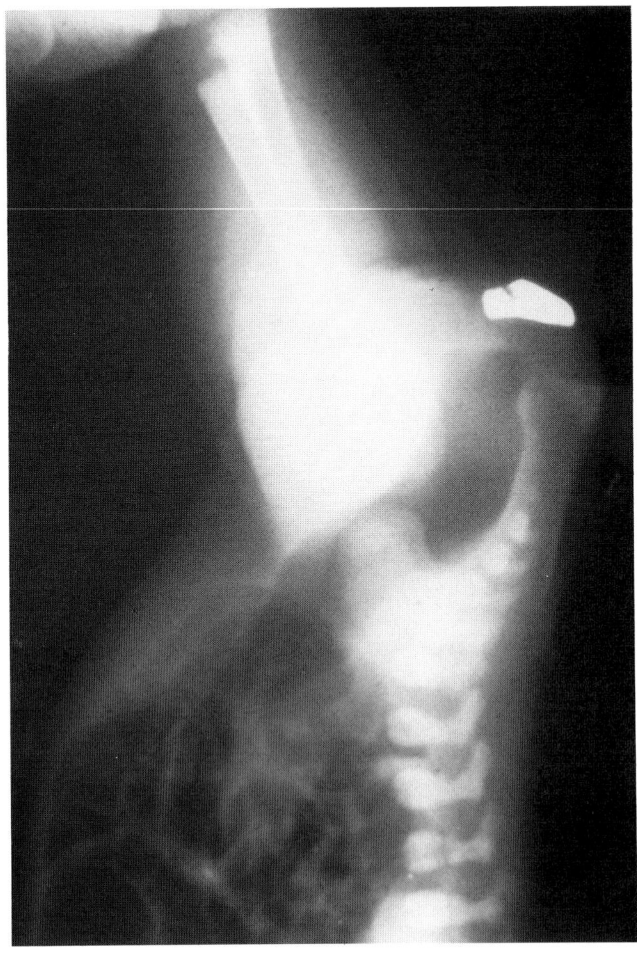

FIGURE 12.17. Atresia of the rectum. Opaque marker is placed on the anal dimple. Plain films demonstrate gas accumulating at the distal end of the colon and rectum. (A) Upside-down position.

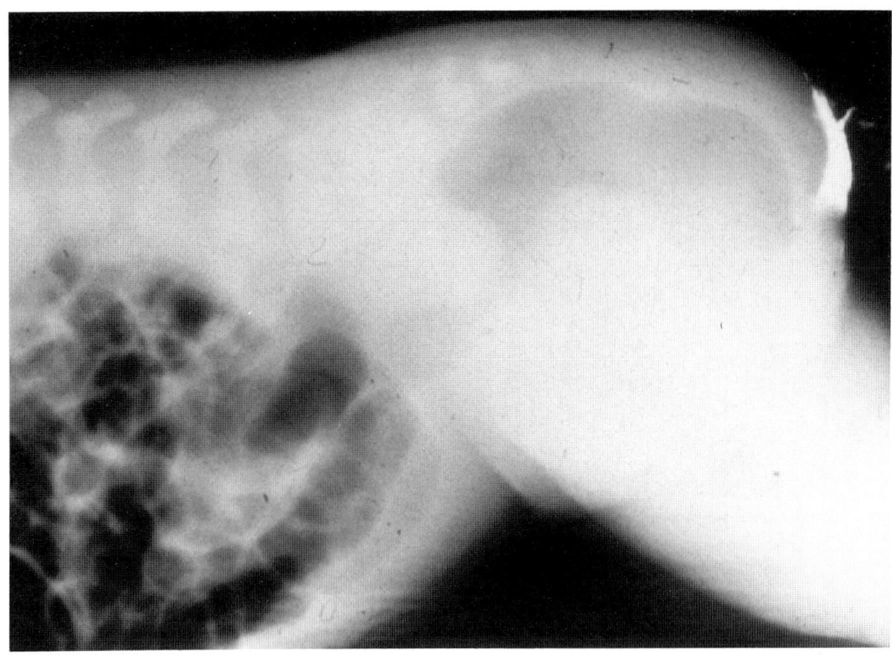

FIGURE 12.17 *continued.* (B) Prone lateral projection demonstrates the atresia equally well and is easier to perform.

ineum. Communications with other organs are exceptional.

Microcolon may result from various causes. The most common segment affected is the sigmoid colon (Fig. 12.18).

Chronic inflammation may result in narrowing of the colon. Since it is accompanied by other symptoms of inflammatory disease, it should not be confused with a congenital anomaly. A narrow left hemicolon in newborns may result from immature or absent intramural ganglion cells, proximal meconium impaction, or small left colon syndrome.

MEGACOLON

HIRSCHPRUNG'S DISEASE

Also known as congenital or aganglionic megacolon, Hirschprung's disease exhibits symptoms during the first year of life, and only exceptionally after 10 years of age. Its incidence is 1/5000 newborn children. A partial or total lack in ganglionic cells of the myenteric plexus and possibly also of the submucous plexus, in a segment of the bowel, results in congenital megacolon. Defective migration of ganglion cell precursors into the hindgut may be a causative factor. Adrenergic fibers in affected segments are also morphologically abnormal. The inability of an aganglionic area to propagate bowel contents results in the dilatation of proximal segments. Dilated segments are, however, normally supplied by ganglionic cells, while the narrowed segment is aganglionic (Figs. 12.19). Hyperplasia of extramural parasympathetic and postganglionic sympathetic fibers results in muscular contraction. Since the internal anal sphincter fails to relax, the normal defecation reflex is weakened. Preferential sites for aganglionic segments are the rectum and sigmoid colon which are best demonstrated in both lateral and oblique projections on a single-contrast study (Fig. 12.19A). Aganglionic segments are usually between 5 and 10 cm long, although the aganglionic segment may be as short as 10 mm. However, the entire large intestine may be involved, result-

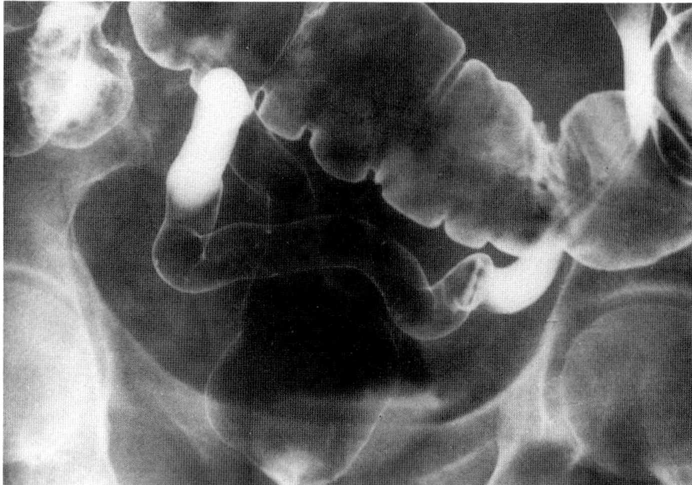

FIGURE 12.18. Congenital sigmoid microcolon.

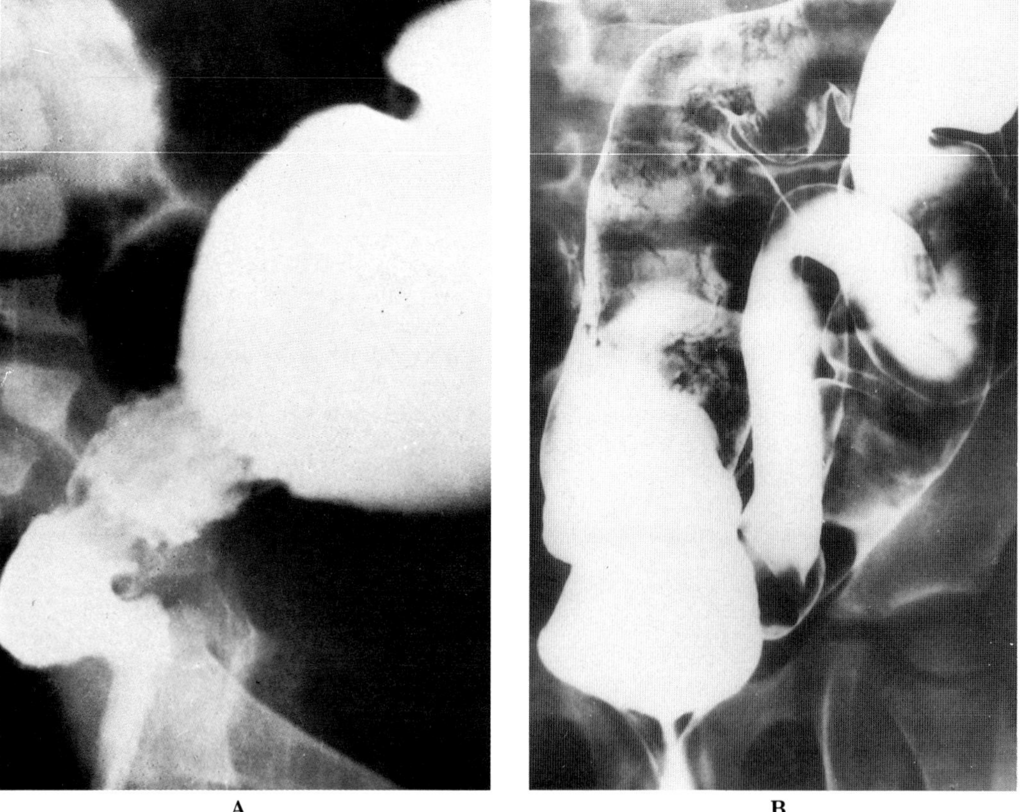

A B

FIGURE 12.19. Congenital megacolon, Hirschprung's disease. (A) Aganglionic zone in the rectum. (B) Aganglionosis of the sigmoid colon. (*Figure continued on the following two pages.*)

ing in distension of the small intestine and shortening of the colon. Skip areas are most unusual. Occasionally, congenital megacolon may be associated with the megacystic megaureter syndrome.

Unless treated surgically, a completely aganglionic colon, which affects 5–8% of patients with Hirschprung's disease, can be lethal (Fig. 12.19C). Complete absence of ganglionic cells in the large intestine and terminal ileum results in prolonged retention of barium in the colon. A moderately shortened colon harbors acquired diverticula which tend to enlarge. These are the sequelae of spasm in the aganglionic colon. Diverticula in infants with symptoms of obstruction should lead to consideration of Hirschprung's disease.

Dilute barium enema suspension should be administered carefully so as to not damage the intestinal wall, since fecal stasis may cause inflammation and injury (Fig. 12.19D). Barium is usually retained in the colon proximal to the transitional zone for 24 hours or longer in patients with congenital megacolon. The diffi-

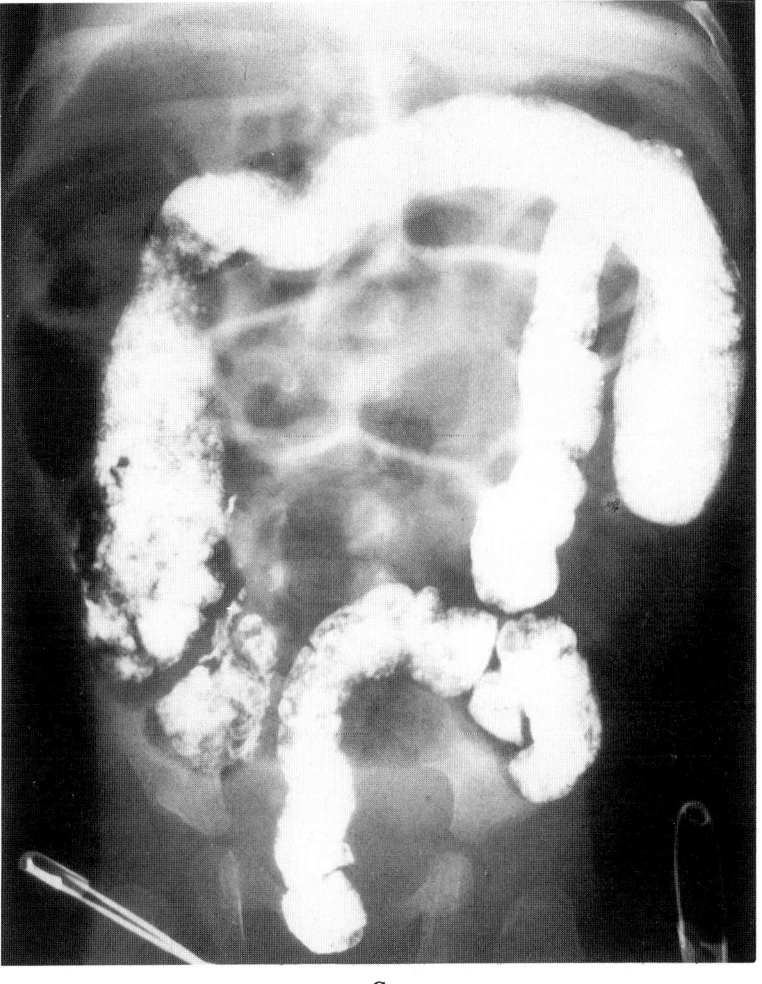

C

Figure 12.19 *continued.* Congenital megacolon, Hirschprung's disease. (C) Complete aganglionosis of the large bowel. Film taken 24 hours after barium enema with stagnation of barium in the colon and gaseous distension of the small bowel.

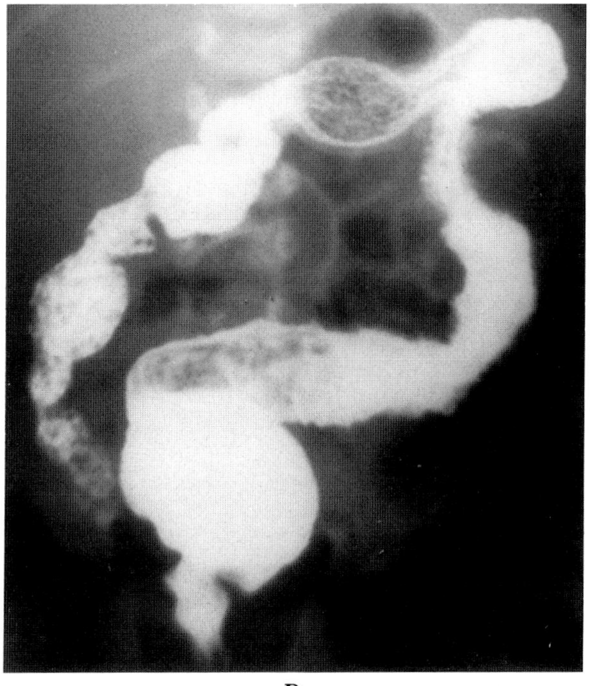

D

Figure 12.19 *continued.* Congenital megacolon, Hirschprung's disease. (D) Colitis resulting from stasis of feces. Aganglionic segment is in the rectum.

culty in evacuation of barium from the dilated more proximal bowel is sufficient reason to stop the barium flow once the narrow, aganglionic segment is demonstrated. Use of water-soluble radiographic contrast medium does not carry the risk of further impaction.

Opening of the anal canal is a normal response to dilatation of the rectum by a balloon in normal subjects and in patients with idiopathic obstipation. This rectosphyncteric reflex is absent in patients with a congenital megacolon. A combination of contrast enema examination and manometry can replace biopsy of the rectum in patients with a characteristic aganglionic segment. However, a very short segment of involvement can escape radiologic detection.

Hirschprung's disease is rarely diagnosed in adulthood. When seen, a proximal segment of the colon adjacent to the transitional zone is dilated and filled with feces, and the aganglionic segment is a funnel-shaped narrowing. Differential diagnosis in adults includes: psychogenic megacolon, Chagas' disease, strictures resulting from inflammation or radiotherapy, mural and extramural neoplasms, phenothiazine and anticholinergic therapy, neurogenic disorders, and idiopathic megacolon (Table 12.1).

Table 12.1. Causes of Colon Dilatation

Causes
Hirschprung's disease
Scleroderma
Toxic megacolon
Cathartic abuse
Neuromuscular disease
Some medication (for example, glucagon, Buscopan, tranquilizers, etc.)
Hypothyroidism
Sprue
Psychogenic disorders
Idiopathic megacolon

Idiopathic Megacolon

Idiopathic megacolon refers to markedly dilated segments of the large bowel of unknown etiology. The most often affected segment is the rectal ampulla, which is packed with solid feces. Occasionally the dilatation may be enormous (Fig. 12.20). No stenosis, either organic or functional, can be demonstrated distal to the dilated segment. Symptoms occur at middle age or even later. Stagnation of large amounts of the feces may result in damage to the mucosa. Similar megacolon is sometimes a result of long-term laxative abuse. Also contributing to the development of megacolon are psychological disorders. However, an underlying causative factor has not yet been revealed. Idiopathic megacolon must be distinguished from congenital megacolon and ileus of the colon.

DIVERTICULA

Congenital Diverticula

Analogous to acquired diverticula, congenital diverticula are found in the colon and cecum, but not in the rectum. These are true diverticula, consisting of all layers of the intestinal wall. They are rare and cannot be radiographically distinguished from acquired diverticula.

Acquired Diverticula

Outpouchings of mucosa and submucosa through the main muscular coating are referred to as "false" or acquired diverticula of the large intestine. They may be either solitary or multiple (Fig. 12.21). The presence of multiple di-

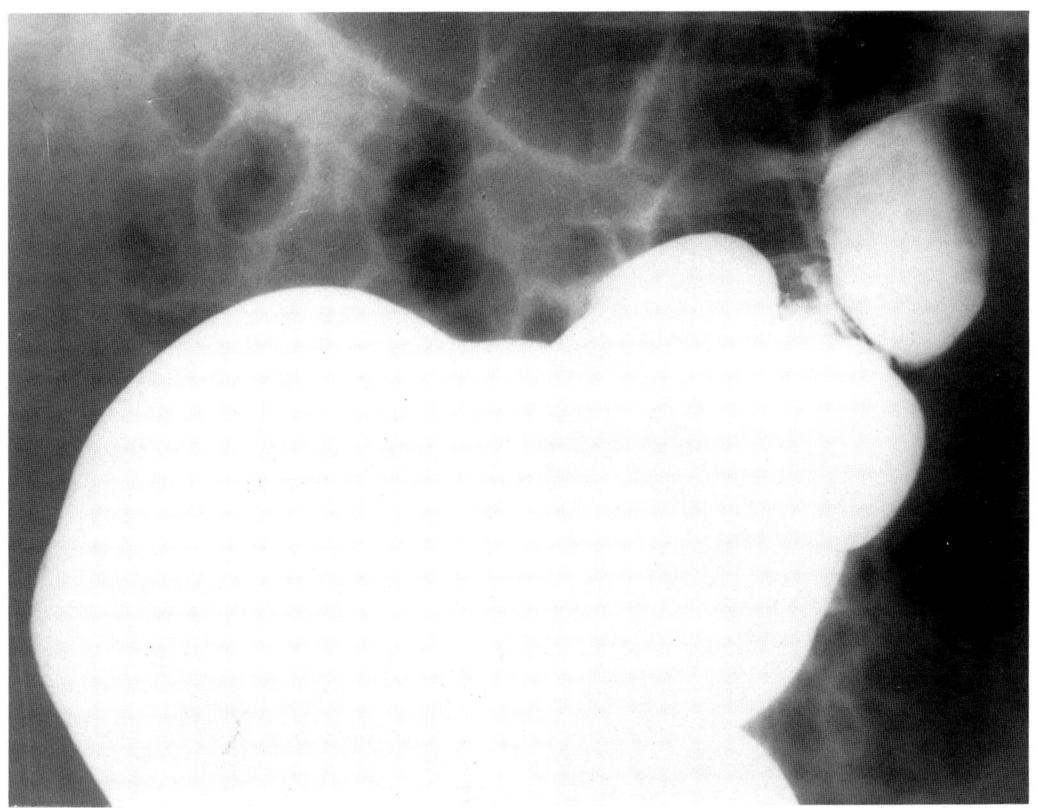

Figure 12.20. Idiopathic megacolon.

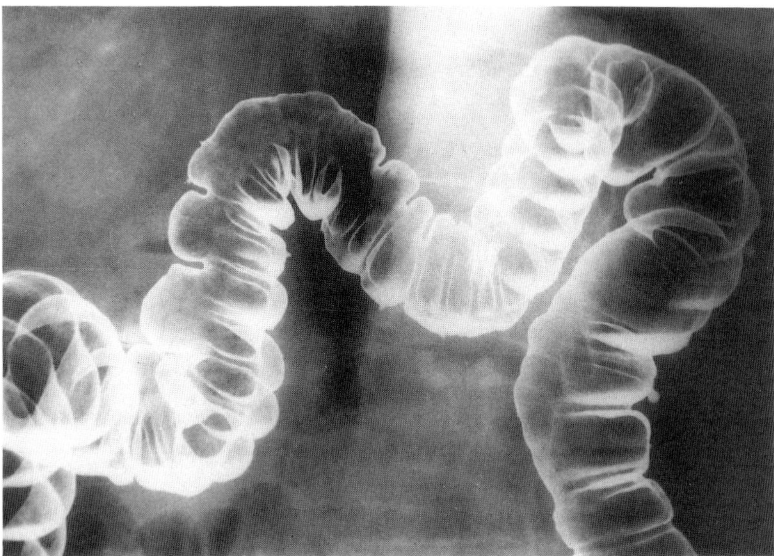

Figure 12.21. Diverticula of the colon.

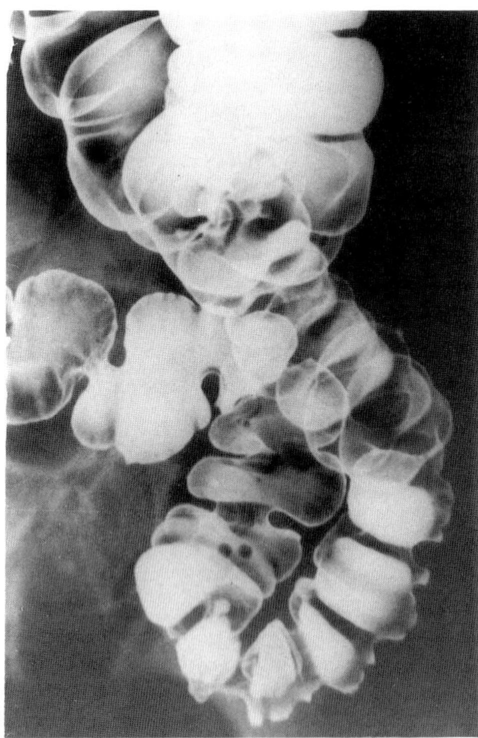

Figure 12.22. Reversible intramural diverticula of the colon.

verticula is termed diverticulosis. In an early phase, mucosal prolapses through the muscular coating may be reversible. This is particularly true for small intramural diverticula confined to the intestinal wall (Fig. 12.22). As a diverticulum enlarges, prolapse becomes irreversible and assumes either an intramural or extramural position (Fig. 12.23).

Diverticula are readily demonstrated by either double-contrast or single-contrast enema examination. However, nonvisualization may result from feces or viscous mucus filling the diverticular lumen. Barium residues may persist in diverticula even weeks after a barium examination (Fig. 4.18).

Diverticula may be small in size, merely a few millimeters in diameter. However, diverticula larger than 15 mm are rare. Giant diverticula of the colon are a separate pathologic entity. Diverticula often occur in places where small arteries penetrate muscle layers of the intestinal wall, thus they are found near the mesocolon.

In Western countries, either solitary or multiple diverticula of the large bowel are found in approximately 10% of the population over the age of 40, and 20% of patients over the age of 50. In time diverticulitis occurs in 20% of pa-

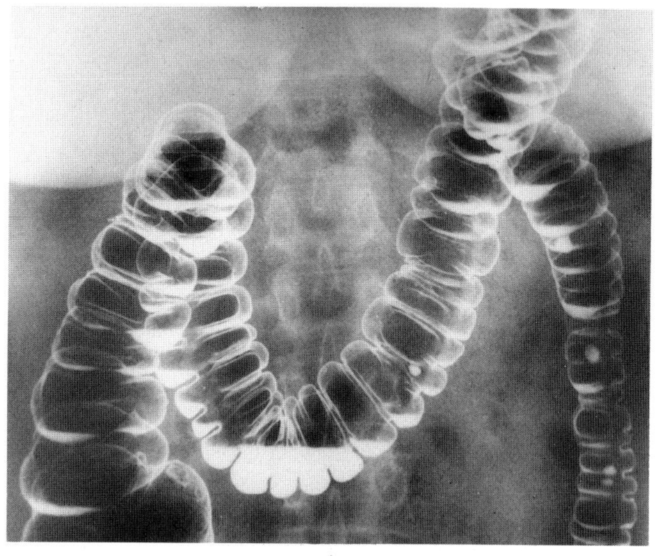

A

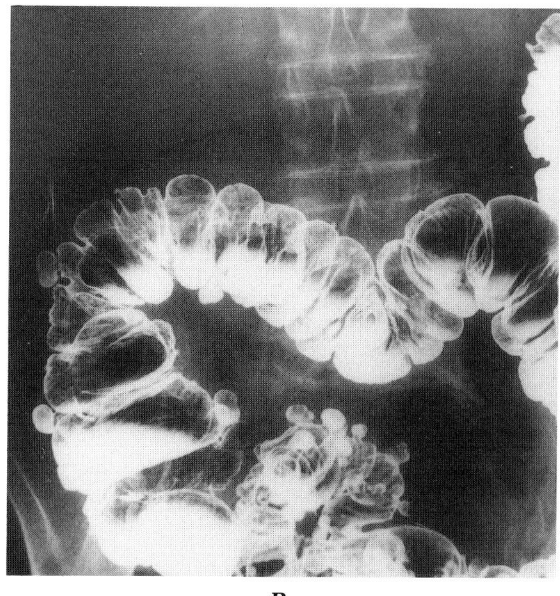

B

Figure 12.23. Diverticulosis of the colon. (A) Early phase. (B) Advanced phase.

tients with pronounced diverticulosis. The prevalence of colonic diverticula is lower in countries where a high-residue diet prevails. Unless complicated, diverticula do not cause clinical symptoms. The sigmoid colon and distal segments of the descending colon are the most common sites of diverticulitis.

Unlike the colon, the rectum has a complete longitudinal muscular layer and is not associated with diverticula. In a simplified approach to changes in the muscular coat of the colon, diverticula may be divided into two groups which are described below.

Diverticulosis without muscular hypertro-

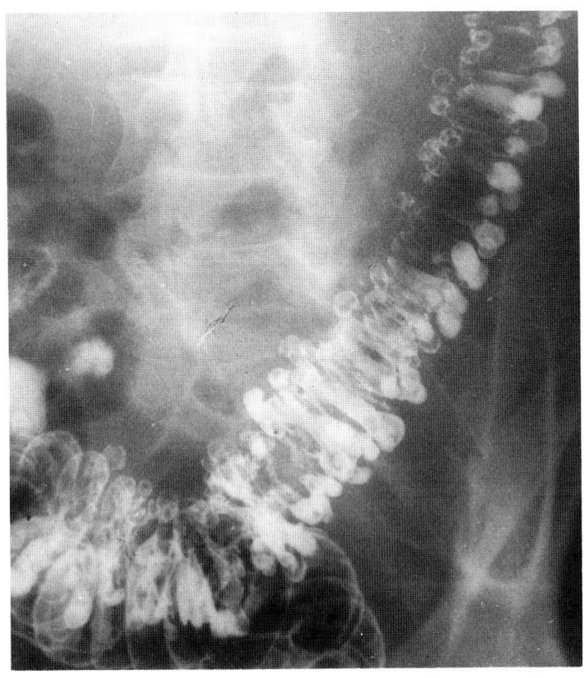

A

Figure 12.24. Diverticulosis with muscle hypertrophy. (A) Affecting the descending and sigmoid colon. (B) Sigmoid colon involvement.

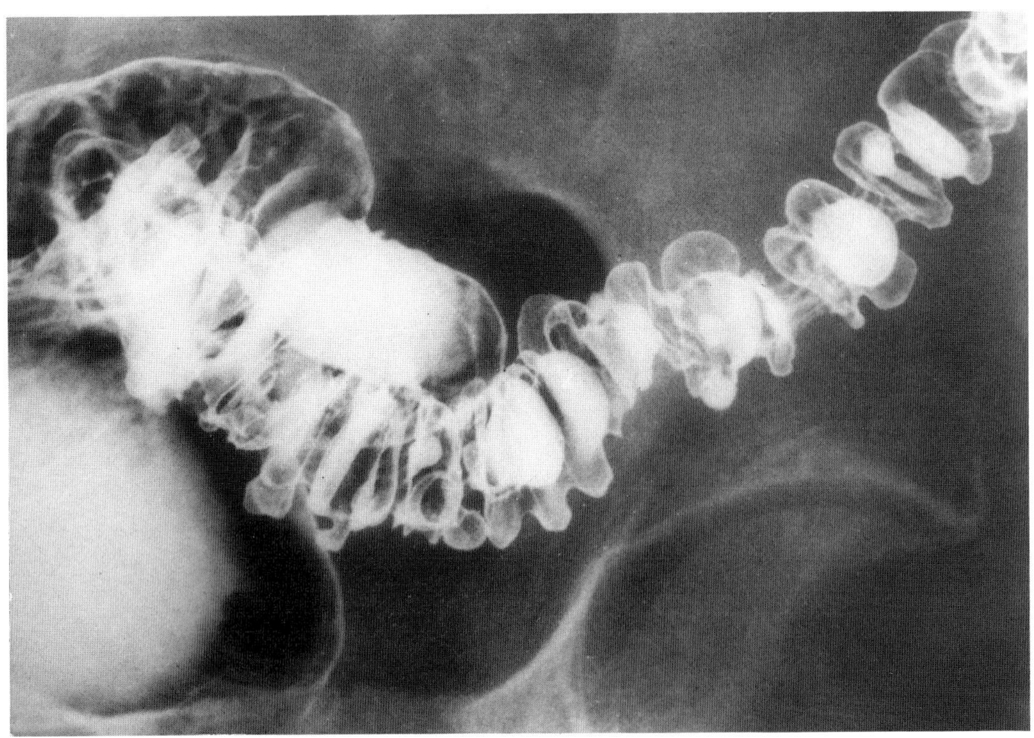

B

phy, also referred to as simple diverticulosis, is characterized by multiple diverticula without significant changes in the adjacent wall. However, as a result of the reduction in mucosal surface due to multiple mucosal prolapses, shortening and narrowing of the affected colonic segment may occur (Figs. 12.21 and 12.23A). Increased intraluminal pressure, such as in irritable colon syndrome, may contribute to the formation of simple diverticulosis.

Diverticulosis with muscular hypertrophy is confined to the sigmoid colon and the distal section of the descending colon (Fig. 12.24). It most probably results from long-standing spasm that accompanies irritable colon syndrome. Affected segments are short and narrow and are populated by numerous diverticula. The walls intervening between the diverticula have deeply indented margins as a result of the hypertrophy of circular muscle, and to a lesser degree, from muscular spasm. Muscles hypertrophy as a sequela of prolonged spasms, forming a sort of muscle bundle lattice through which mucosa and submucosa prolapse due to increased intraluminal pressure. Muscular changes result in diverticulosis and are not its consequence. Therefore, spasmolytics do not significantly change radiologic features in this form of diverticulosis.

Differentiation of diverticula from polyps is described in the section on colonic polyps (see pages 491-492).

COMPLICATIONS

Diverticulitis, inflammation of a diverticulum, occurs most often in the sigmoid and descending colon. Clinical "diverticulitis" is actually a peridiverticular inflammatory response, often with formation of a peridiverticular abscess resulting from perforation of a diverticulum. Inflammation is confined to a small area immediately adjacent to the perforation (Fig. 12.25). Barium outside the wall, in

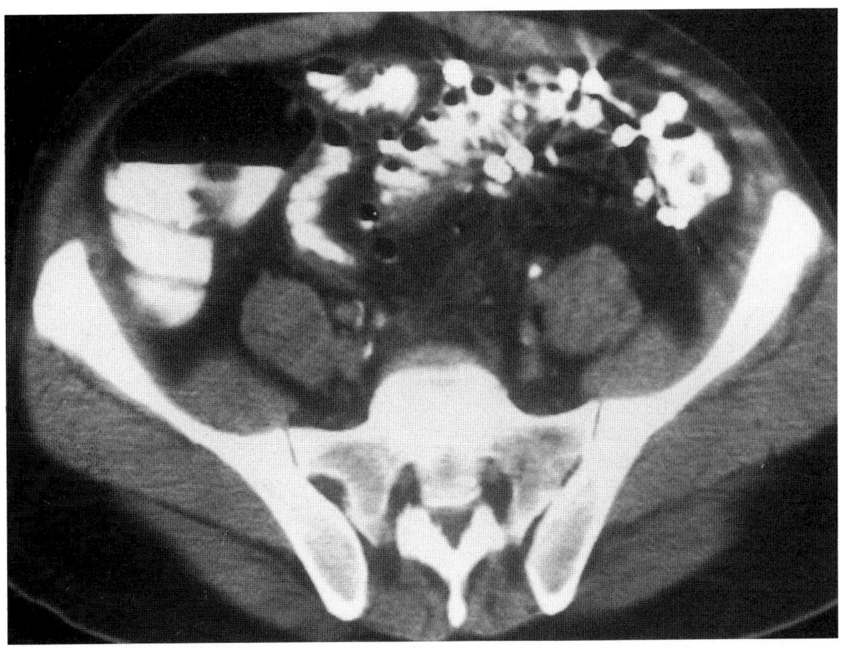

C

FIGURE 12.24 *continued.* Diverticulosis with muscle hypertrophy. (C) CT examination of diverticulosis of the sigmoid colon with muscular hypertrophy.

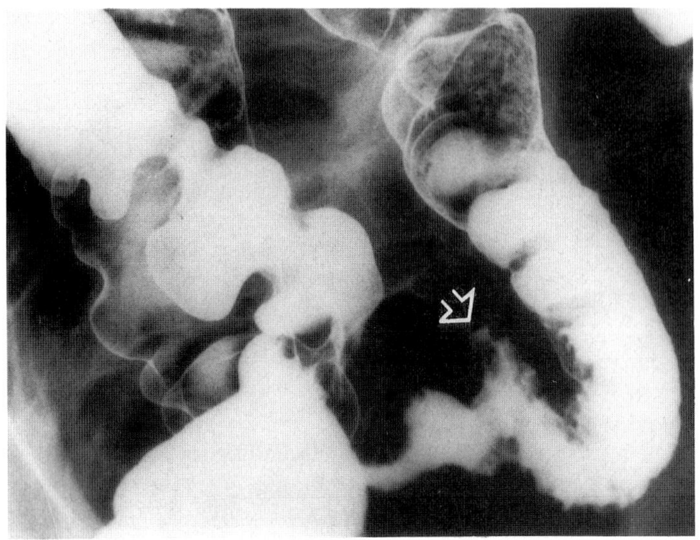

Figure 12.25. Diverticulitis. Perforation localized by adhesions (arrow).

general, does not refer to free perforation, but rather to penetration of barium into the peridiverticular abscess. It has not been proved that stagnation of luminal contents within diverticula leads to diverticulitis.

A single-contrast enema, using either water-soluble contrast medium or barium, should be used in patients with suspected diverticulitis, since colonoscopy is contraindicated. However, in most instances diagnosis of diverticulitis is based more on clinical findings than on radiologic abnormalities.

A sharp contour demarcates an intramural diverticular *abscess* (Fig. 12.26A) resulting from fusion of inflamed intramural diverticula. A pericolic abscess, commonly situated in pericolic adipose tissue or in the mesocolon, creates a poorly demarcated impression and may have serrated contours (Fig. 12.26B and C).

The following are roentgenographic and CT (Fig. 12.26D) signs of a pericolic or paracolic abscess:

1. Displacement of the colonic wall.
2. Sinus tract between the abscess and colon lumen.
3. Narrowing of the colon .
4. Altered mucosal relief.
5. A gas-fluid level.

The intestinal wall is thickened in the inflamed area. Computed tomography can readily separate an abscess from a phlegmon and can show gas in the retroperitoneal space. Wall thickening of the colon can result from other causes such as carcinoma, lymphoma, Crohn's disease, ulcerative colitis, and ischemic colitis. Gas in the retroperitoneal space and mesenteric abscess are readily demonstrated by CT.

Computed tomography criteria for diagnosing diverticulitis are:

1. Presence of diverticula in the sigmoid colon.
2. Thickening of the colon wall to more than 4 mm.
3. Inflammation of pericolonic fat.
4. Intramural sinus tract and/or abscess.
5. Pericolonic or paracolonic abscesses associated with sigmoid diverticula.
6. Fistulous tract originating from the sigmoid colon.

Stage 0 diverticulitis is confined to the sigmoid wall. In stage I, an abscess or phlegmon, not larger than 3 cm, is limited to the mesocolon. Stage II sigmoid diverticulitis is inflammation unrestricted by the mesocolon. It may affect structures of the pelvis such as the colon, small intestine, omentum, or female internal

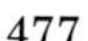

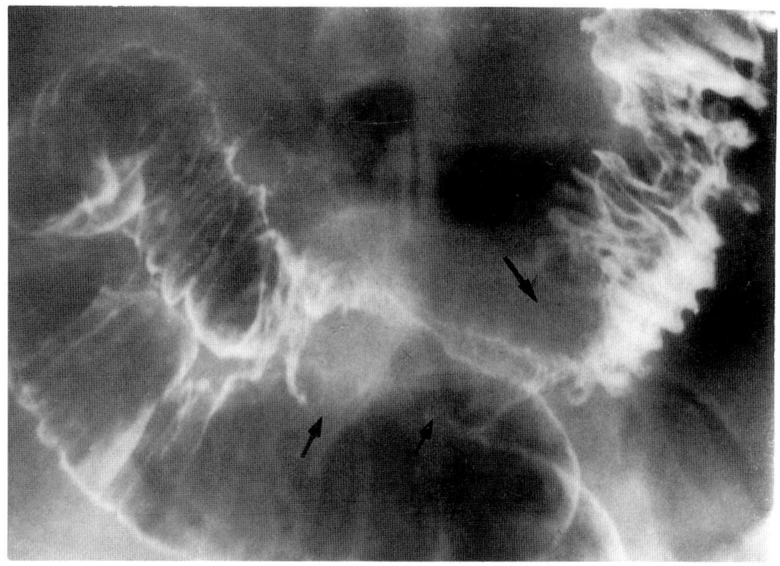

A

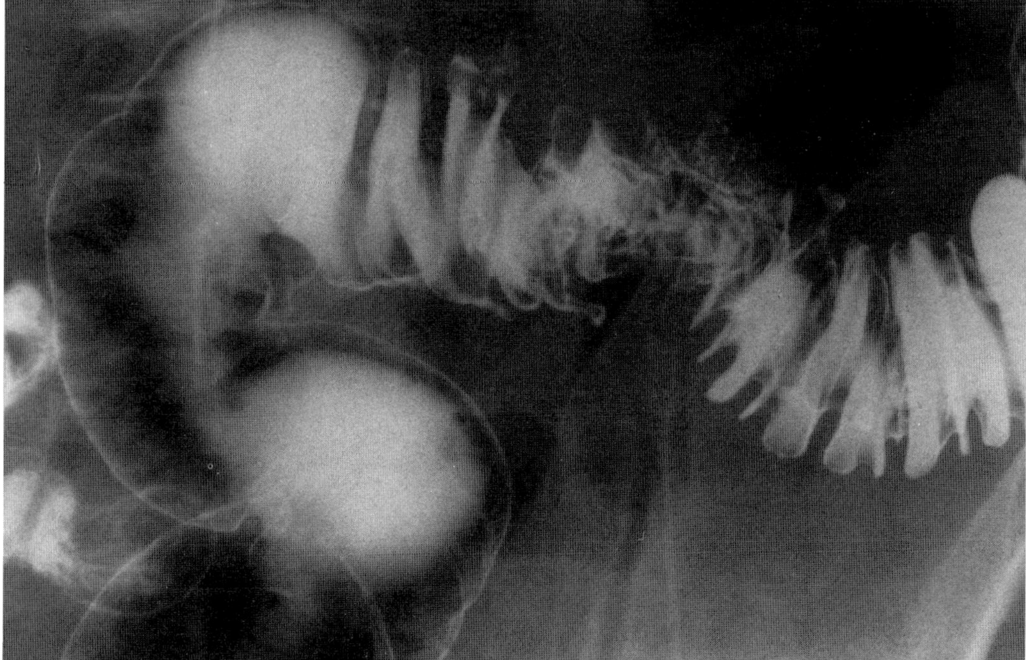

B

Figure 12.26. Diverticular abscess. (A) Intramural (arrows). (B) Small extramural. (*Figure continued on overleaf.*)

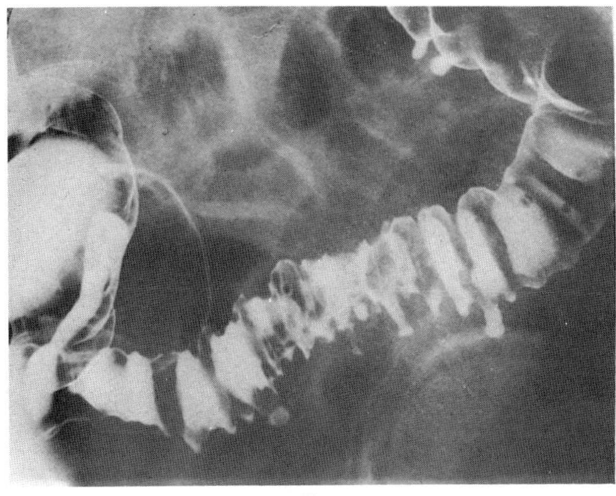

C

FIGURE 12.26 *continued.* Diverticular abscess. (C) Large extramural abscess. (D) CT of sigmoid diverticulitis with formation of an abscess.

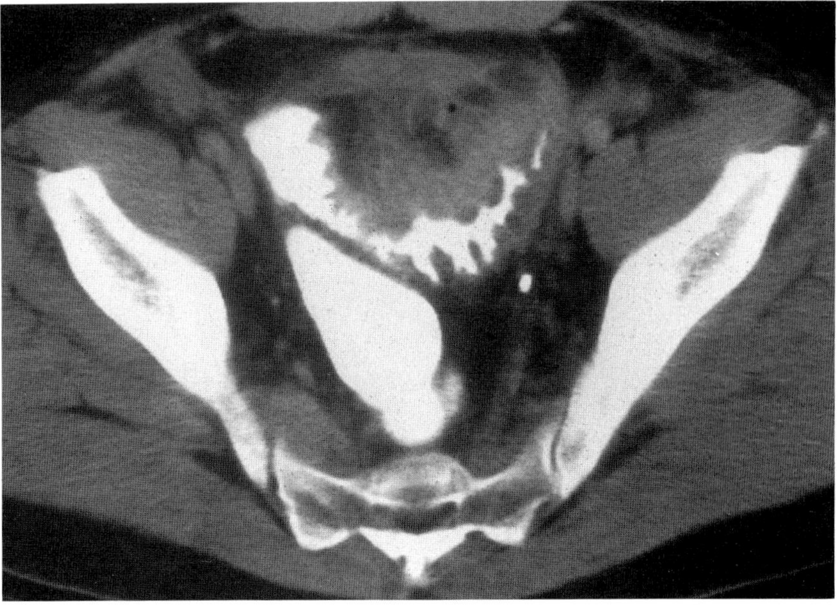

D

genital organs. Stage III is defined by extension into other sections of the peritoneal cavity and retroperitoneum. When generalized peritonitis with sepsis results, this is considered stage IV diverticulitis. Computed tomography results in defining diverticulitis are equal or even superior to those obtained from a contrast enema and can be followed by CT-guided percutaneous drainage if necessary.

Fibrosis can result from diverticulitis. Narrowing and decreased pliability of the wall follows, and may interfere with the patency of the intestine (Fig. 12.27). *Fistulae* may connect a colonic diverticulum with the urinary bladder or, less frequently, with small bowel or vagina. Perforation of a purulent sigmoid diverticulum may result in a suppurative process in the mesentery followed by a spread upward to the posterior perirenal space. *Free perforation* into the peritoneal cavity is unusual and is accompa-

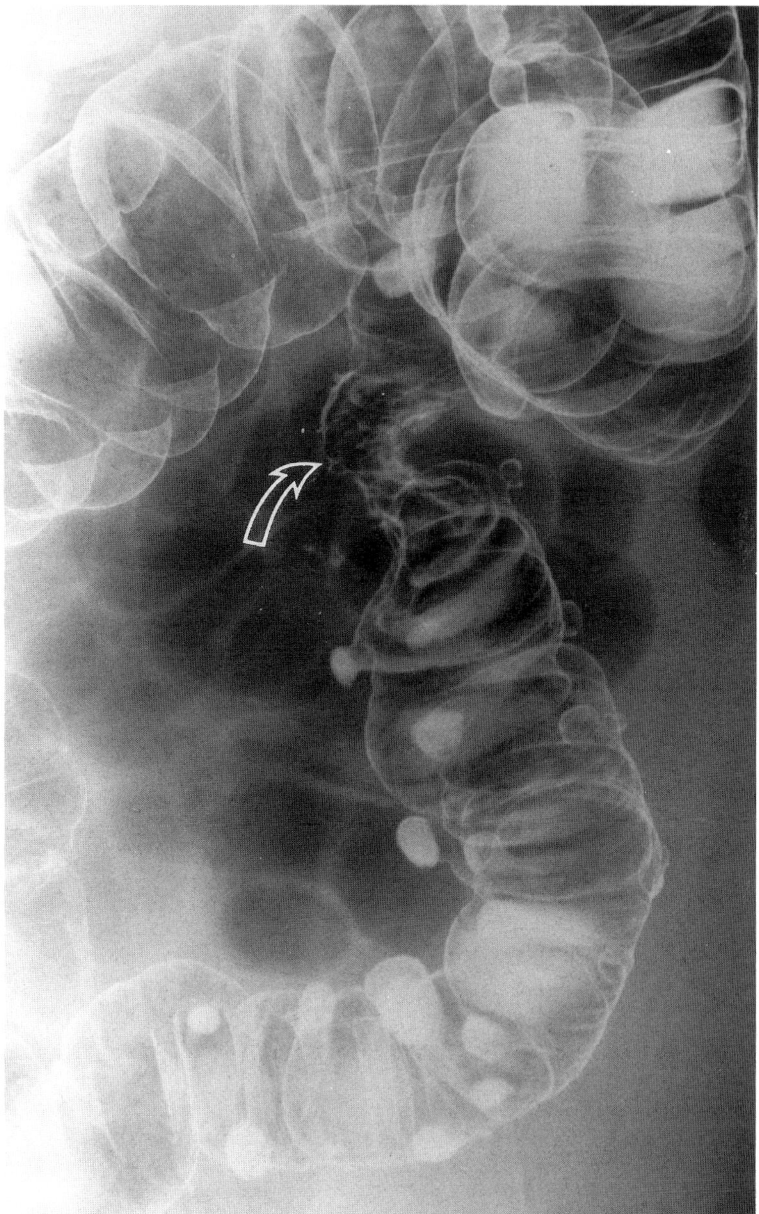

FIGURE 12.27. Post-diverticulitis stricture in the descending colon (arrow).

nied by pneumoperitoneum and peritonitis, either limited or generalized. Any enema is contraindicated under these circumstances.

Bleeding may occur from diverticula affected by inflammation, as well as from diverticula without signs of inflammation. Diverticula of the right hemicolon tend to bleed more frequently.

Both diverticula and carcinoma occur frequently in the sigmoid colon. However, it is not easy to determine if diverticulosis is a *predisposing factor* in the development of carcinoma.

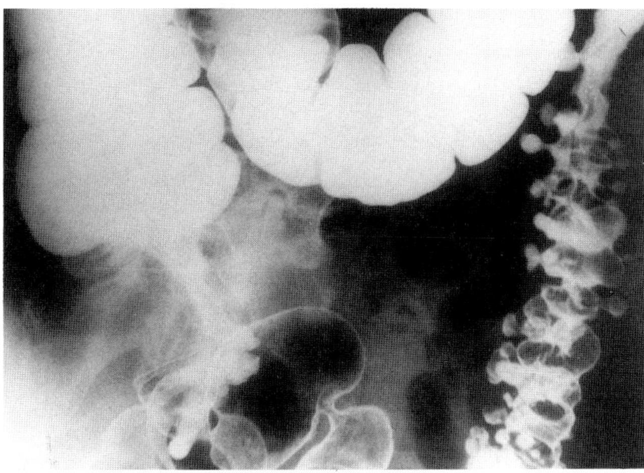

Figure 12.28. Descending colon diverticulosis. Large ascending colon carcinoma with functional, poststenotic dilatation due to destruction of intramural neuronal network.

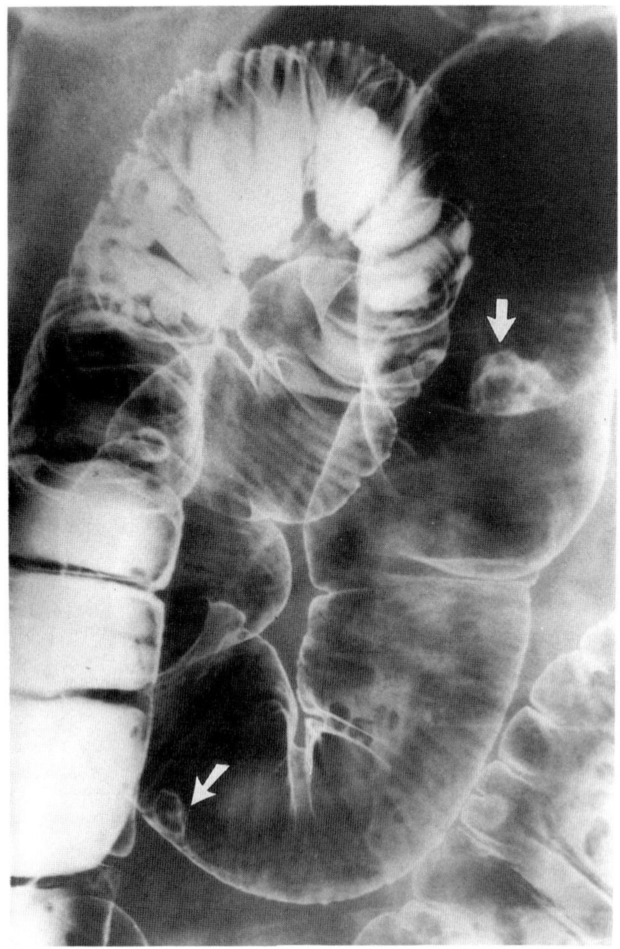

Figure 12.29. Polyps (arrows) and diverticulosis of the sigmoid colon.

Carcinoma occurring in an area populated with diverticula results in the following radiographic signs: destruction of mucosal relief, tumor mass, and abrupt transition with the adjacent unaffected wall. The signs of a malignant neoplasm are usually altered by diverticulosis and, for this reason, the tumor is often not detected before an advanced stage. When there are up to 15 diverticula in the sigmoid colon, 3.1% of carcinomas remain undetected, whereas when there are more than 15 diverticula, 20% of carcinomas remain undetected. Simultaneous occurrence of diverticula and carcinoma in other segments of the large intestine is also quite common (Fig. 12.28). Diverticula need to be differentiated from polyps (Fig. 12.29).

GIANT DIVERTICULA OF THE COLON

Diverticula exceeding 5 cm in diameter are referred to as giant and result from gaseous distension in the presence of a check valve mechanism. This mechanism results from narrowing of the diverticular neck, due to infection and inflammation. This appearance may also result from perforation of a diverticulum or, rarely, from perforation of a bowel duplication. Inflation of the resulting pseudocyst eventually results in a giant diverticulum appearance.

Giant diverticula are located in the sigmoid colon and are visible on a plain abdominal film as a gas collection. During contrast enema examination only 50% of giant diverticula will be filled. Torsion or perforation occurs in 10% of patients with giant diverticula. Differential diagnosis includes sigmoid and cecal volvulus, mesenteric cyst, and abscess. However, CT can readily establish the diagnosis.

OBSTRUCTIONS

Obstruction of the large intestine may be either mechanical or functional. Mechanical obstruction can be partial or complete. In children, particularly males up to five years of age, obstruction is mostly caused by an *ileocolic intussusception*. This may result in partial or complete obstruction. A characteristic pattern forms when the ileum is intussuscepted into the colon (Fig. 10.14). In ileocecal intussusception the appendix may be inverted and directed horizontally. Although uncommon, this may be seen on plain film—the appendix appears as a tubular structure filled with gas. As with other intussusceptions, the barium which fills the space between the intussusceptum and the intussuscipiens creates a coiled-spring appearance (Fig. 12.30). In adults, intussusception is commonly related to a polypoid neoplasm.

Neoplasms are the most common cause of mechanical obstruction of the large intestine in elderly patients.

Only freely movable sections of the colon, with a long mesocolon, are subject to torsion. The sigmoid colon most frequently undergoes *volvulus*. The second most frequent location of volvulus is the cecum. A greatly distended sigmoid colon filled with gas, sometimes reaching up to the diaphragm, is the hallmark of a sigmoid volvulus. The site of torsion may be shown by barium enema (Fig. 5.16). In contrast to a transverse colon distended by gas, where the bowel assumes a "U" shape, the sigmoid co-

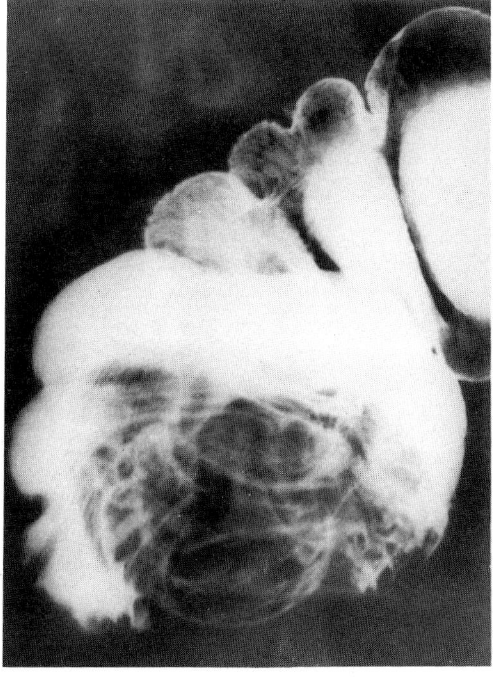

A

FIGURE 12.30. Intussusception. (A) Colocolic. Coiled spring appearance. (*Figure continued on overleaf.*)

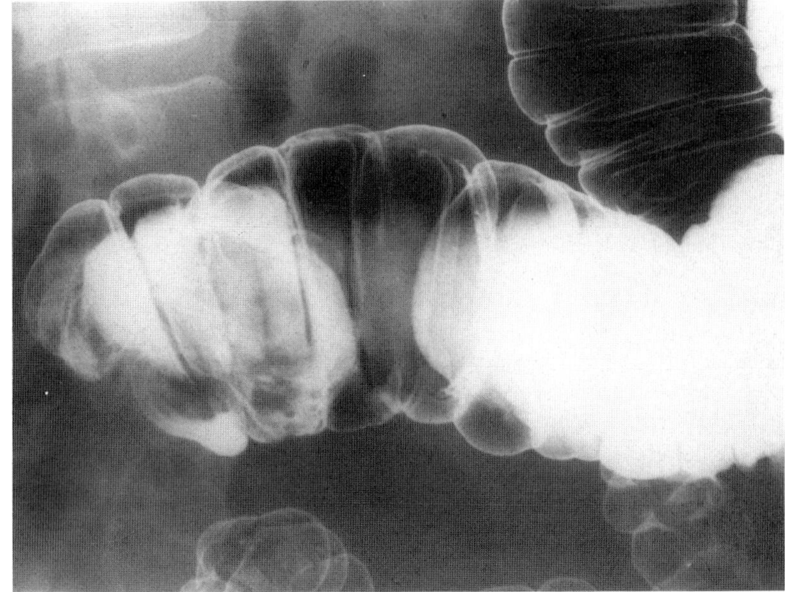

B

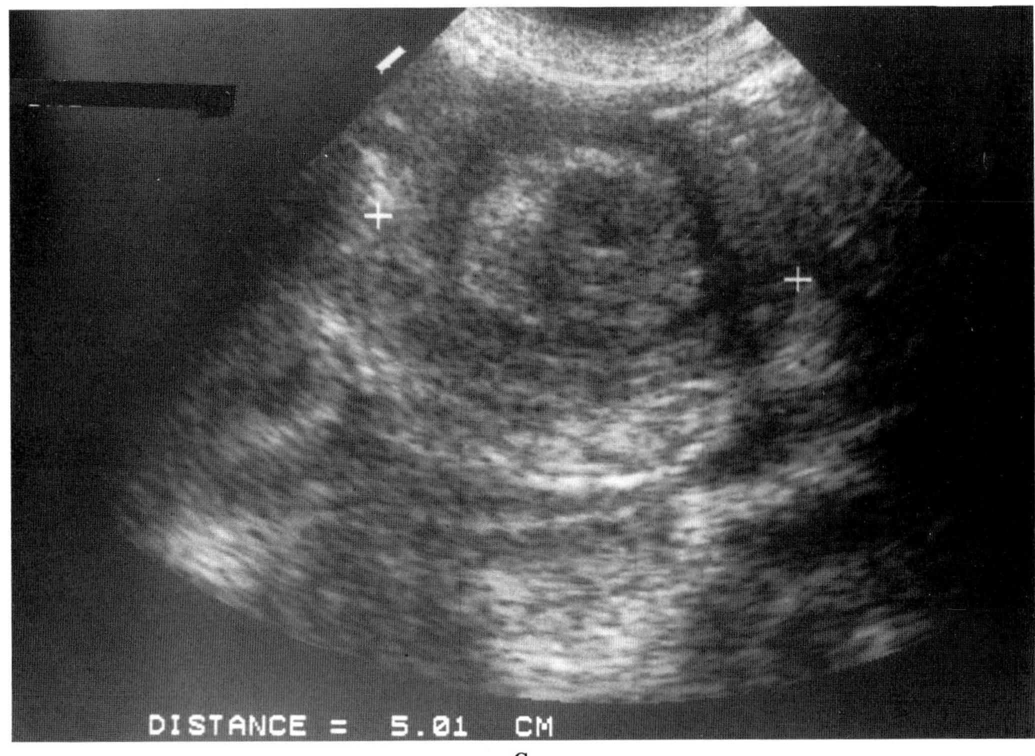

C

Figure 12.30 *continued.* Intussusception. (B) In the transverse colon resulting from polypoid carcinoma. (C) Ultrasound presentation of (B). Concentric ring appearance of intussusception (between cursors). (Courtesy of W.L. Wells, MD, Louisiana State University, New Orleans.)

lon with volvulus has been described as resembling an inverted "U" or "coffee bean." Cecal volvulus occurs in patients with a long mesocecum. The cecum is dilated with gas and the volvulus is often accompanied by mechanical obstruction of the small bowel (Figs. 12.84 to 12.86). Besides volvulus, *adhesions and incarcerated hernias* may lead to obstruction.

An *ileosigmoid knot*, caused by twisting of ileum around the root on the sigmoid mesocolon, results in obstruction, and resembles a sigmoid volvulus on barium enema.

The site of any mechanical large bowel obstruction is revealed by a contrast enema examination. It has been proved that oral application of barium does not convert a partial large bowel obstruction into a complete one.

LYMPHOID FOLLICLES OF THE COLON

Lymphoid follicles are commonly demonstrated, especially in the distal half of the colon of a healthy population up to 30 years of age. In children, enlarged lymphoid follicles are mostly without pathologic significance. They present as regular, spherical or oval, submucosal protrusions up to 3 mm in diameter, without a meniscoid ring of barium around the base (Fig. 12.31). Adenomatous polyps of the same dimensions have similar appearances. Endoscopy seldom identifies enlarged lymphatic follicles. When larger than 4 mm in diameter, lymphatic follicles of the colon may refer either to colitis, such as Crohn's disease, or to dysgammaglobulinemia, hypogammaglobulinemia, or the initial phase of lymphoma.

The colon, as well as other sections of the alimentary canal, may be involved in hypersensitivity reactions. The lymphatic follicles are not enlarged, but "urticaria" of the colon is radiologically indistinguishable from prominent lymphatic follicles, eosinophilic enteritis, and herpes zoster of the colon. *Colitis cystica profunda*, characterized by cysts coated with columnar epithelium and filled with mucus, exhibits a radiographic pattern similar to that of enlarged lymphatic follicles. The former results

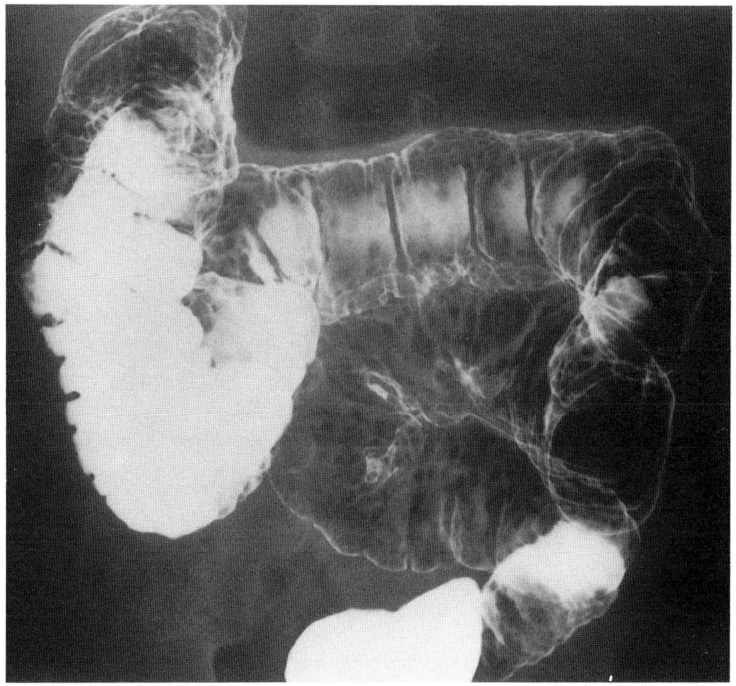

FIGURE 12.31. Lymphoid hyperplasia of the colon. Atypically positioned cecum.

from epithelial implantation following bowel surgery.

GRANULOMATOUS DISEASES OF THE LARGE BOWEL

Crohn's colitis is described in chapter 11.

Radiologically, collagenous colitis has an appearance similar to that of enlarged lymphatic follicles or of an early phase of Crohn's colitis.

Chronic granulomatous disease in childhood, a hereditary disorder, affects the colon with granulomas of unknown etiopathogenesis. The entire colon, or sections of it, may be affected with granulomas of different sizes; however, the majority are less than 10 mm in diameter.

PNEUMATOSIS COLI

Also referred to as pneumatosis intestinalis, pneumatosis coli may assume either a cystic or linear form. Intramural, mainly subserosal, spherical gas collections that change their shape under compression characterize cystic pneumatosis of the colon (Fig. 12.32). Plain films may sometimes reveal cysts, but CT is diagnostic. Mechanical injury to the mucosa may be related to cystic pneumatosis of the colon, since affected patients are those with frequent cough attacks, long-lasting intestinal obstruction, or recent endoscopy. Infectious etiologies have also not been excluded. Liberation of gas from the cysts can lead to pneumoperitoneum.

Pneumatosis coli cystica is usually asymptomatic. Endoscopy reveals spherical pliable

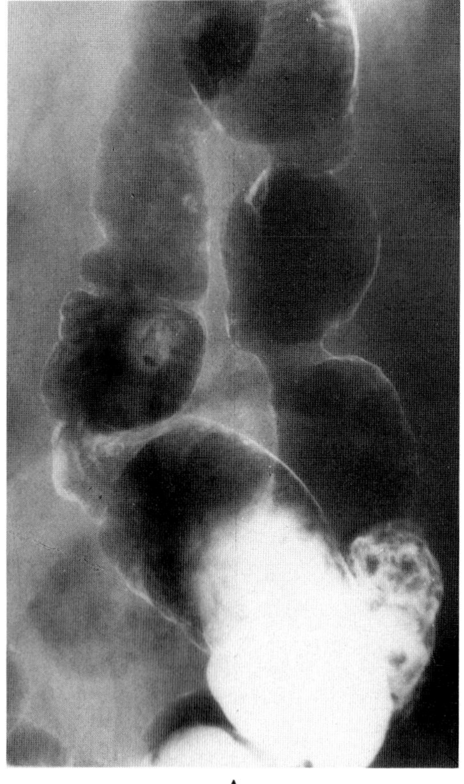

A

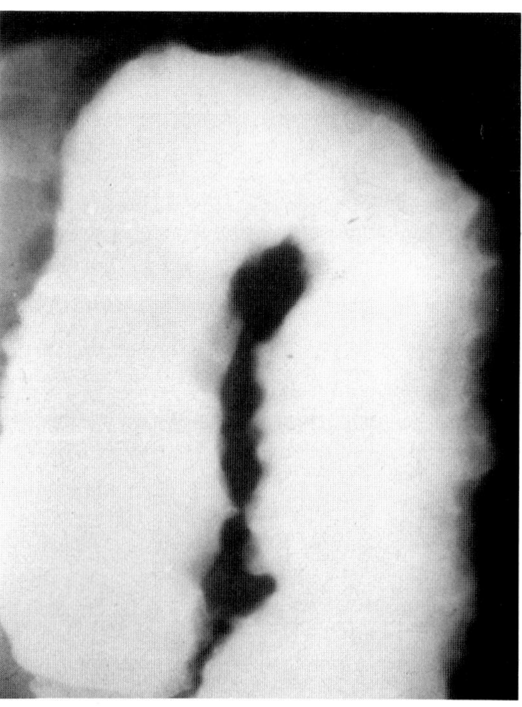

B

Figure 12.32. Cystic pneumatosis of the colon. (A) Several cysts seen on a double-contrast enema. (B) Multiple cysts seen on a single-contrast enema.

submucosal cysts. Linear intramural gas collections are an ominous sign of impending perforation, particularly in patients with intestinal ischemia (Fig. 11.3). Differential diagnosis of intramural cysts includes granulomas and benign neoplasms.

AMYLOIDOSIS

Among portions of the alimentary canal, the colon is the least frequently affected by amyloidosis. Either a primary or secondary form may affect the colon. Amyloid is deposited between the basement membrane and the endothelium of capillaries and arterioles.

Less pronounced haustral markings without mucosal irregularities are more characteristic of an early phase. Alternating stenoses and dilatations of the colon appear later. Amyloidosis should be distinguished from other chronic inflammatory diseases.

SCLERODERMA

The colon is not usually affected by scleroderma. Radiographic findings are characterized by saccular dilatations and intervening areas of relative stenosis of the bowel; these are attributed to degenerative changes of smooth muscles. Large wide-mouthed colonic diverticula are often situated on the antimesocolic aspect of the wall. These are formed by the coalescence of two or more adjacent haustral compartments due to loss of the intervening folds.

RADIATION PROCTOCOLITIS

Radiotherapy for malignant neoplasms in the pouch of Douglas, especially cervical carcinoma in females, may cause injury to the large intestine. As in other sections of the gastrointestinal tract, the mucosa is the tissue layer most sensitive to radiation because of rapid cell division. In approximately 10% of patients, a dose of 4500 Gy results in lesions both of the adjacent rectum and of the sigmoid colon. As a result of its considerable mobility, the small bowel is less commonly damaged. The mucosal surface shows irregularities in an acute phase. Small ulcerations may follow the hyperemia end edema caused by radiation. Chronic lesions, characterized by progressive narrowing of affected segments, develop 6–24 months after radiotherapy (Fig. 12.33). The lumen of the

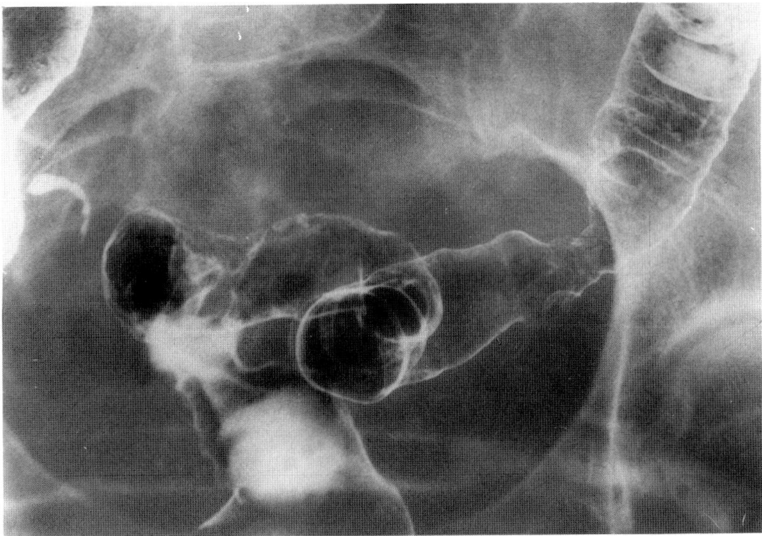

FIGURE 12.33. Radiation injury to the sigmoid colon. (A) Subacute phase with multiple stenoses. (*Figure continued on overleaf.*)

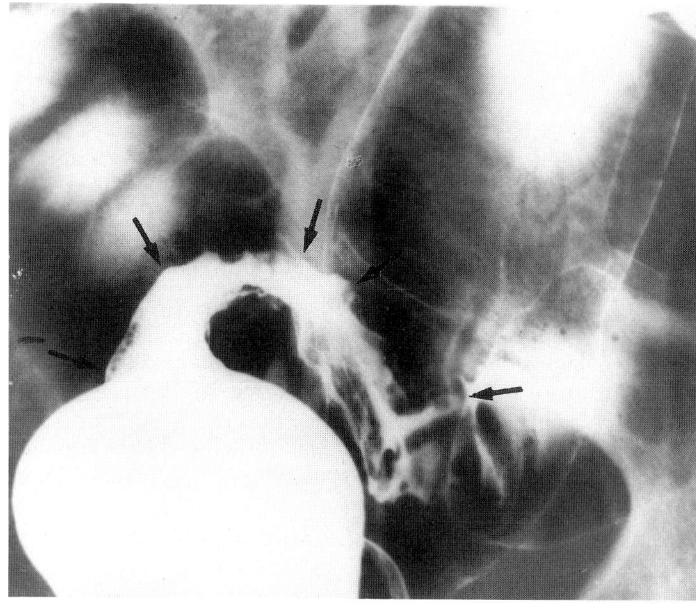

Figure 12.33 *continued.* Radiation injury to the sigmoid colon. (B) Chronic phase. Single, long stenosis (arrows).

rectum is reduced and fistulas with adjacent organs may be formed in the chronic phase.

GRAFT-VERSUS-HOST REACTION

Following allogeneic bone marrow transplantation, graft-versus-host disease occurs; after several weeks this affects the alimentary canal. Haustral markings disappear, the mucosa is swollen and ulcerated, and, in rare cases, completely destroyed. In the chronic phases, the intestinal wall is thickened.

NEOPLASMS OF THE LARGE BOWEL

Benign Neoplasms

Polyps of the Large Intestine. Detection of large bowel polyps is of the utmost importance since it is believed that the majority of large bowel carcinomas develop from adenomatous polyps (Fig. 12.34). Several facts substantiate this opinion:

1. Invasive carcinoma foci exist in adenomas of benign appearance.
2. Carcinomas smaller than 5 mm do not occur, while polyps of such dimensions are often found.
3. Carcinomas develop in all patients with untreated familial polyposis.
4. An 80% decrease in incidence of rectosigmoid carcinoma is found in patients who have undergone annual endoscopy with polypectomy.

Polyps are present at autopsy in the large bowel in one-third of all adults. Such a high prevalence of large bowel polyps illustrates their importance. Colonoscopy is an accurate technique for detection and removal of polyps, but it is expensive and bears risks. This procedure carries a mortality of 0.05%. Double-contrast barium enema is consequently the procedure of choice for detecting colonic polyps.

Polyps are mucosal outgrowths that protrude into the alimentary canal lumen (Figs. 12.35). Although the term "polyp" denotes a benign excrescence, benign polyps are indistinguishable from malignant tumors of similar morphology without microscopic analysis. Use of the term "pseudopolyp" is even less accurate since it re-

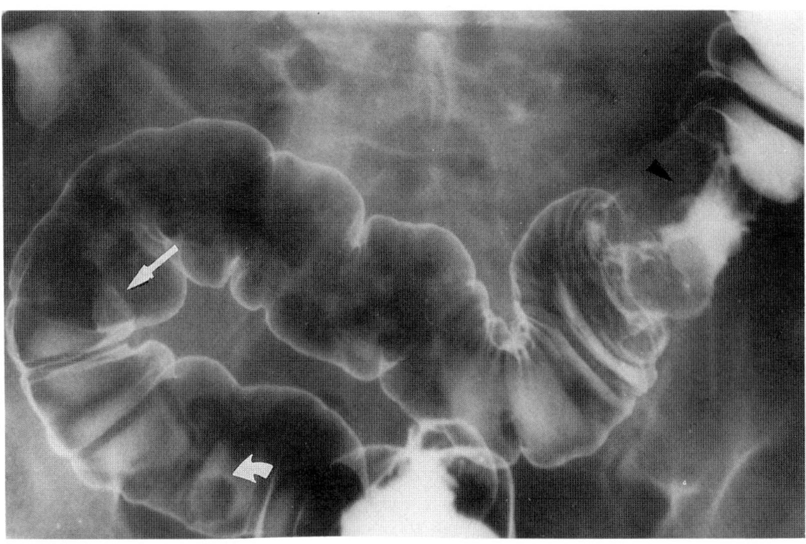

Figure 12.34. Carcinoma (arrowhead) and adenomatous polyps (arrows) of the sigmoid colon.

fers to a postinflammatory hyperplastic outgrowth of mucosa. Polyps can be adenomatous, hyperplastic, villous, tubulovillous, or hamartomatous (Table 12.2). Almost 90% of large bowel polyps are adenomas with high malignant potential. Adenomatous polyps are the most frequent tumors of the large intestine, and are most commonly found in men over 50 years of age.

The majority of polyps (65%) discovered by double-contrast enema are less than 1 cm in diameter. At least 80% of these polyps are ade-

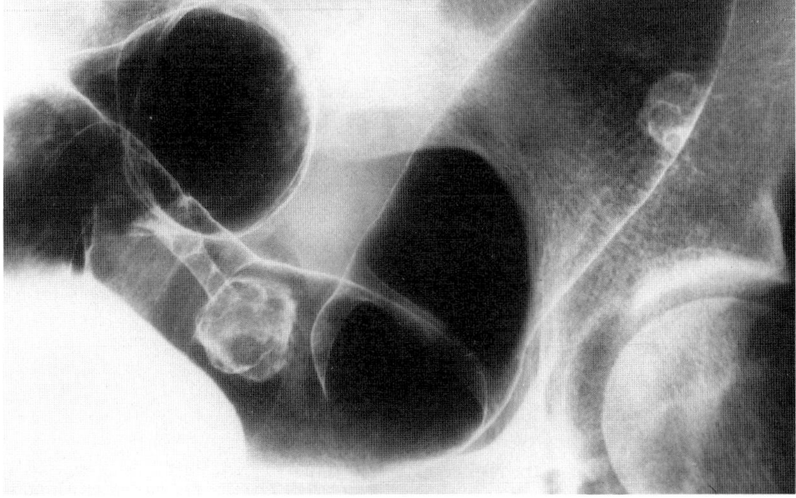

Figure 12.35. (A) Sessile and pedunculated polyp of the sigmoid colon. (*Figure continued on overleaf.*)

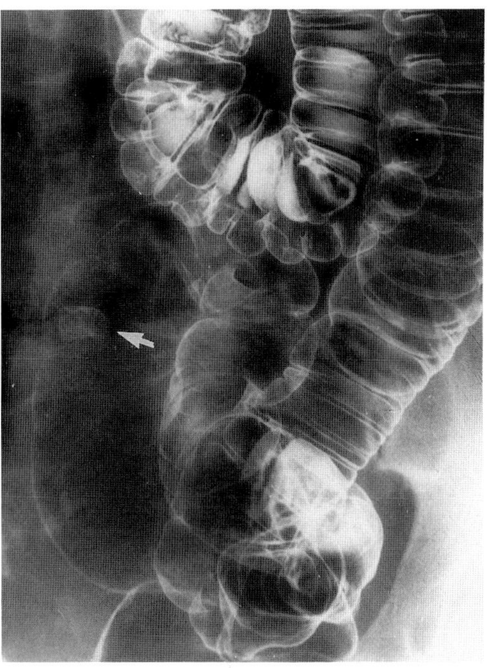

Figure 12.35 *continued.* (B) Adenomatous polyp of the sigmoid colon (arrow).

Table 12.2. Polyps of the Large Intestine

Solitary
Adenoma
Hamartoma
Hyperplastic
Villous adenoma
Endometriosis
Carcinoma
Carcinoid
Multiple
Adenoma
Hamartoma
Hyperplastic
Polyposis syndromes

nomas. In fact, 83% of polyps between 6 and 10 mm in diameter are adenomas, 6% villous adenomas, and 1% carcinomas. The remainder are hyperplastic polyps.

Polyps measuring 1–5 mm are often adenomatous and may be endoscopically removed. However, a lower incidence of polyps, with malignant alteration in only 2% of adenomatous polyps, has also been reported. Colonoscopic investigations have demonstrated that 70% of patients with multiple adenomatous polyps develop new adenomas within 2.5 years while, in the same time period, patients with only one polyp develop them in 35% of cases. The majority of polyps smaller than 3 mm are hyperplastic. Indeed, the percentage of adenomas dramatically increases among polyps larger than 3 mm in size. Dysplasia and carcinoma can be found in polyps 6–10 mm in size. Polyps smaller than 3 mm are rarely demonstrated by double-contrast techniques. However, dysplasia and carcinoma do not occur in this group of small polyps.

There is no accurate gross pathologic, and therefore no radiologic, distinction between benign and malignant polyps. Differentiating an advanced carcinoma from a benign outgrowth is much easier. The properties of polyps listed in Table 12.3 can sometimes be correlated with their behavior. Clinically the most important feature of a polyp is its size, since polyps larger than 10 mm in diameter undergo malignant alteration in 70% of patients. It cannot be determined by radiologic means whether the rate of polyp growth is linear or exponential. Apparent increase of polyp size is an absolute indication for endoscopic or operative polypectomy.

The presence of a stalk is not a reliable sign of a benign polyp since some carcinomas will have a stalk. The majority of polyps are sessile. It is believed that contact with alimentary canal contents in motion creates the stalk (Diagram 12.2) and that the indentation of the wall at the insertion of the stalk is a consequence of traction. Sessile polyps can be confused with

Table 12.3. Benign versus Malignant Polyps of the Large Bowel

	Polyp	
	Benign	Malignant
Size	<1 cm	>1 cm
Growth	Slow	Fast
Surface	Commonly smooth	Commonly irregular

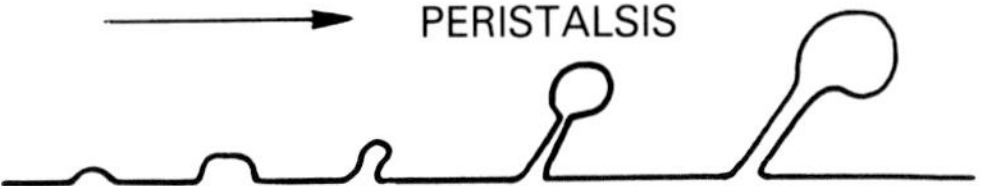

DIAGRAM 12.2. Formation of a polyp stalk.

air bubbles. Fecal residue adherent to the bowel wall can also resemble polyps. However, barium will not coat a fecal surface as well as a polyp. The "base" of adherent feces is indistinct and blurred (Fig. 12.39).

The distribution of polyps is very similar to that for carcinomas of the large bowel (Diagrams 12.3 and 12.4), and multiple polyps may occur in patients without polyposis syndromes. A polyp adjacent to a carcinoma (a "sentinel polyp") is a common finding in patients with colorectal carcinoma. Approximately 40% of large bowel carcinomas are located in the rectosigmoid region. In elderly people, a higher number of polyps are found in the right colon and fewer are found in the rectosigmoid region (Diagram 12.3). The same is true for carcinomas. Large polyps are found more frequently in the right colon.

More than 95% of colonic polyps can be visualized by double-contrast enema. Combining this method with colonoscopy, 99% of large intestinal polyps can be detected. If the results of the two methods differ significantly, one or both examinations should be repeated. This will reduce the number of false-positive and false-negative results to a minimum. On double-contrast roentgenography, polyps appear as mucosal outgrowths that protrude into the lumen (see the section on interpretation of double-contrast studies, pages 98–113). A double-contrast examination enables visualization of polyps as small as 1 mm in size. However, when searching for polyps of such minute dimensions the number of false-positive findings increases and the specificity of the examination decreases.

A single-contrast study is inferior to double-contrast examination in detection of polyps smaller than 10 mm (Fig. 12.36). However, a single-contrast examination is more suitable for elderly and incontinent patients. It is easier

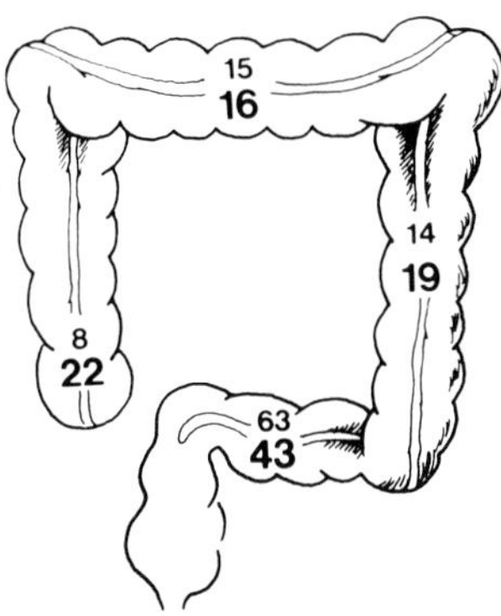

DIAGRAM 12.3. Distribution of large intestinal polyps in patients under 60 years of age (fine) and over the age of 60 (bold). (Used by permission, Bernstein MA, Feczko PJ, Halpert RD, et al. Distribution of colonic polyps: Increased incidence of proximal lesions in older patients. Radiology. 1985;144:35.)

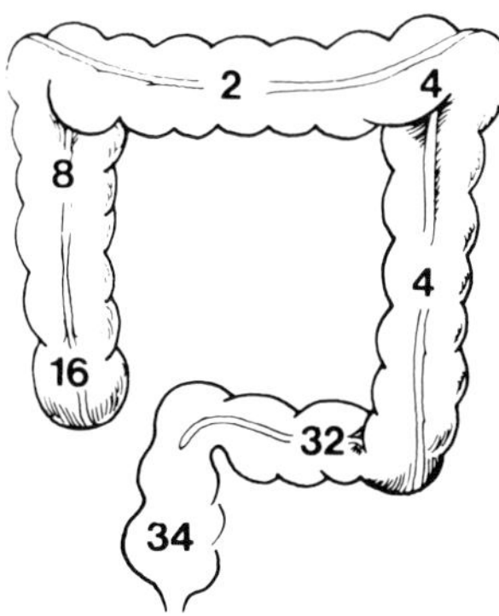

DIAGRAM 12.4. Distribution of large bowel carcinoma. (Numbers used by permission, Fork FT, Lindstrom C, Eklund G. Double contrast examination in the carcinoma of the colon and rectum. A prospective clinical series. Acta Radiol Diagn. 1983;24:177.)

and quicker to perform. Polyps appear as negative filling defects within the solid column of contrast medium. The sensitivity of single-contrast enema can approximate the sensitivity of double-contrast enema when modifications are applied. For such examinations a remote con-

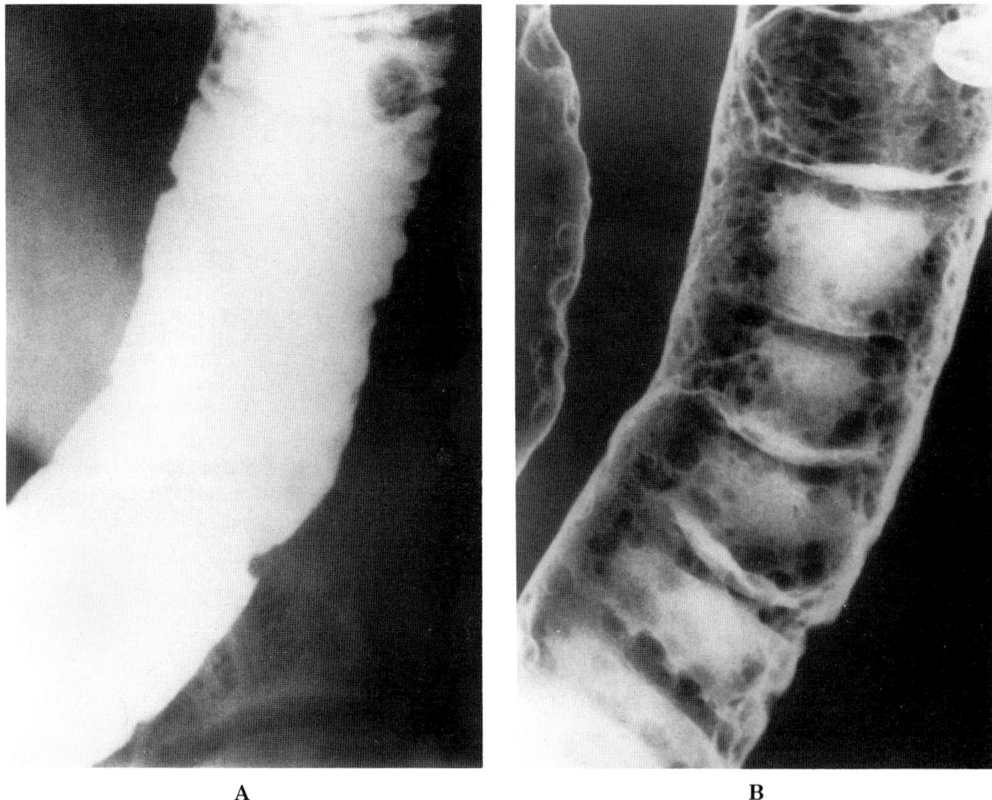

Figure 12.36. Familial polyposis of the colon. (A) Single-contrast barium enema. Only the very large polyps are seen. (B) Double-contrast enema demonstrates a greater number of polyps.

trol fluoroscopic apparatus with capabilities for X-ray tube angulation is most suitable. A rare-earth screen-film combination should also be used. This technique reduces scatter and results in high radiographic contrast, with use of high kilovoltages of up to 120 kilovolt (peak) (kVp). All areas of the colon except the distal sigmoid should be gradually compressed with a cone and manually palpated during fluoroscopy. A highly stable diluted barium suspension (18% w/v) is most suitable. Using these modifications 66% of polyps 5–9 mm in size can be detected; this approximates the 71% sensitivity obtained by double-contrast studies. The sensitivity of both methods in detection of polyps larger than 10 mm is identical and equals 95%. A single-contrast examination does not increase the number of false-positive results. It is a safe method for the detection of polyps in elderly patients and is an accurate technique for the detection of carcinoma.

Villous Adenoma. Also referred to as papillary adenoma, villous adenoma is a pliable, polypoid, broad-based neoplasm with an irregular villous surface. However, villous adenoma may on occasion have a stalk. The presence of viscous mucus between villi and liquid mucoid contents makes a villous adenoma easily compressible. Lace-like collections of barium among the villi are characteristic for a villous adenoma (Figs. 12.37 and 12.38). A homogeneous spherical component, eccentrically situated and attached near the intestinal wall, can be diagnosed by CT, even with an attenuation less than 10 Hounsfield units (HU). In contrast to villous adenoma, neoplasms with necrosis contain a liquid component that is less homogeneous and

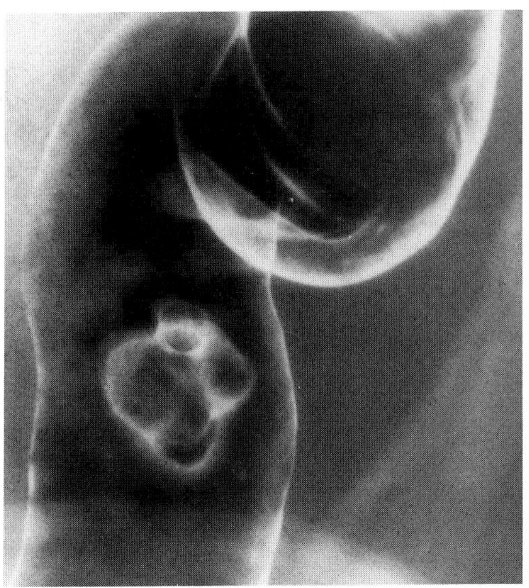

FIGURE 12.37. Polyp. Villous adenoma of the descending colon.

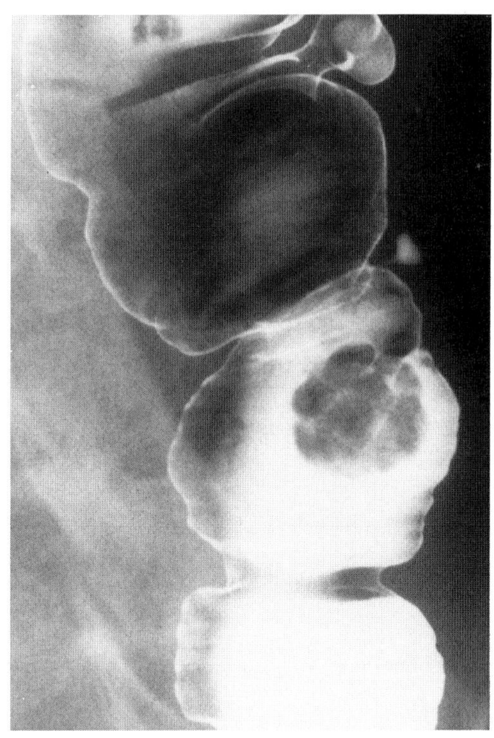

FIGURE 12.38. Villous adenoma of the colon. Diverticula proximally.

more centrally located, with attenuation values less than 3.9 HU. Attenuation in *colitis cystica profunda* equals that of water.

With tumors smaller than 2 cm in diameter, air insufflation in the large intestine may improve CT demonstration of a villous adenoma. Villous adenomas are most common in the rectum, but may be found in any section of the large intestine. The diameter of a villous adenoma may vary from 1–8 cm. Much attention has been paid to indentation of the intestinal wall at the base of a villous adenoma. However, this is not a sign of malignancy and, as in other polyps, is a result of traction due to moving intestinal contents. Malignant transformation occurs in 30% of villous adenomas.

Polyps of the large bowel, including villous adenomas, must be differentiated from residual fecal material adherent to the intestinal wall. This residue may resemble a sessile polyp but its irregular, rugged surface tends to be poorly coated by barium (Fig. 12.39). Air bubbles are mobile (Fig. 12.40). A diverticulum that does not project outside the intestinal contour can still be differentiated from a polyp. Seen *en face*, the base of a polyp is more transparent than a diverticulum filled with barium. The contrast ring surrounding the base of a polyp has a sharp inner and vague outer margin, these relations being reversed with a diverticulum (Fig. 12.41). An inverted diverticulum cannot be distinguished from a polyp by radiologic means.

The following are radiographic features of colon polyps:

1. There is a negative defect in a barium pool.
2. In oblique projections a sessile polyp may resemble a bowler hat, with a brim and dome. In contrast to a diverticulum, the dome of a polyp always protrudes into the lumen.
3. The barium meniscus surrounding the stalk of a polyp is encircled by a barium ring around the head of the polyp so as to give the appearance of a Mexican hat or target (Fig. 12.41A).
4. A ribbon-like transparency of the stalk appears, connecting the point of insertion to the head of the polyp (Fig. 12.46). The ap-

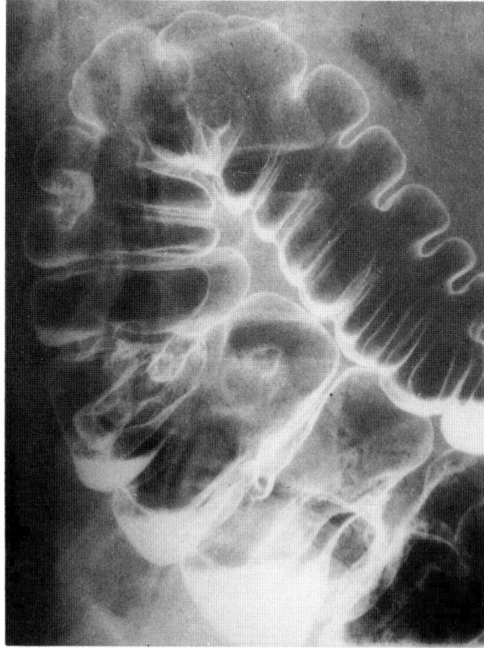

A

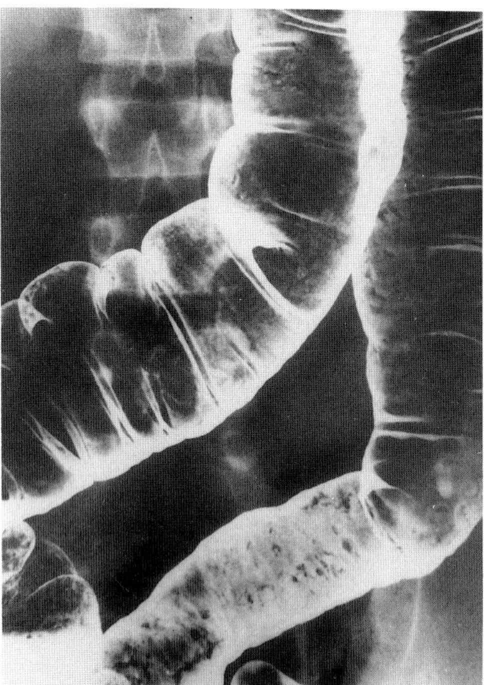

B

Figure 12.39. Insufficient colon cleansing. (A) In contrast to polyps, feces are not thoroughly coated with barium. (B) Discrete fecal remnants.

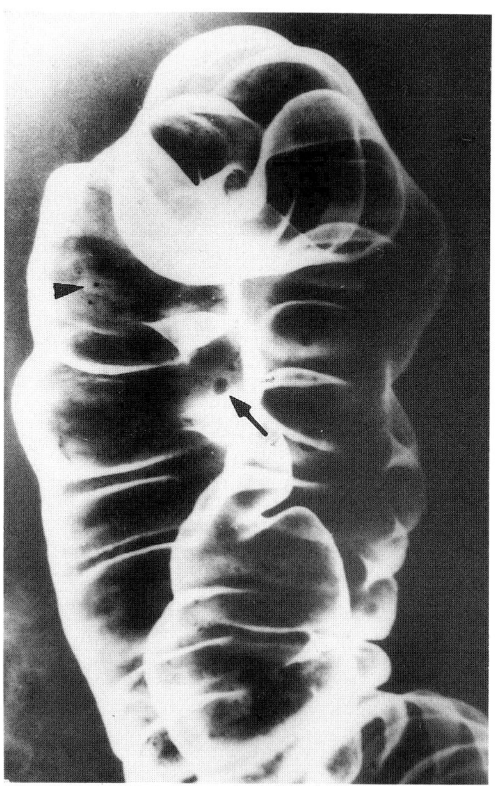

Figure 12.40. Air bubbles may resemble sessible polyps on double-contrast studies (arrow and arrowhead).

pearance of a polyp on double-contrast studies depends on whether it occurs on the dependent or the nondependent wall.

In contrast, the following are signs of a diverticulum:

1. When coated with a thin layer of barium, or filled with barium, a diverticulum may be seen projecting out of the intestinal contour (Fig. 12.42).
2. Seen *en face*, the diverticulum is a ring-shaped opacity with a neck projecting in the center (Fig. 12.41B).
3. A gas-fluid level is seen within a diverticulum partly filled with barium.

Polyps 5 mm in diameter or larger should be detected by a double-contrast enema examination. In the elderly, polyps smaller than 3 mm in diameter may be ignored, but in young and

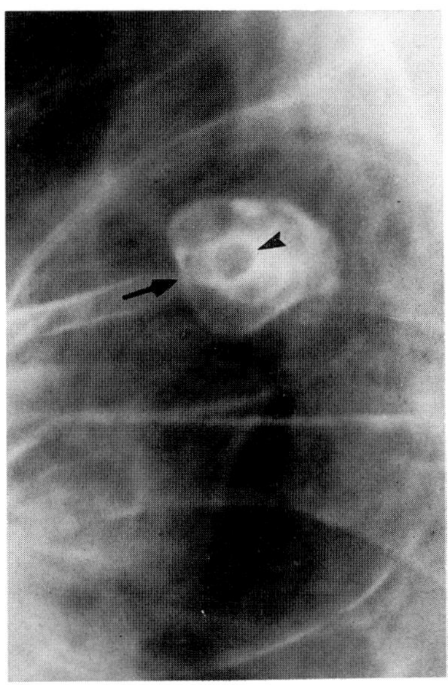

A

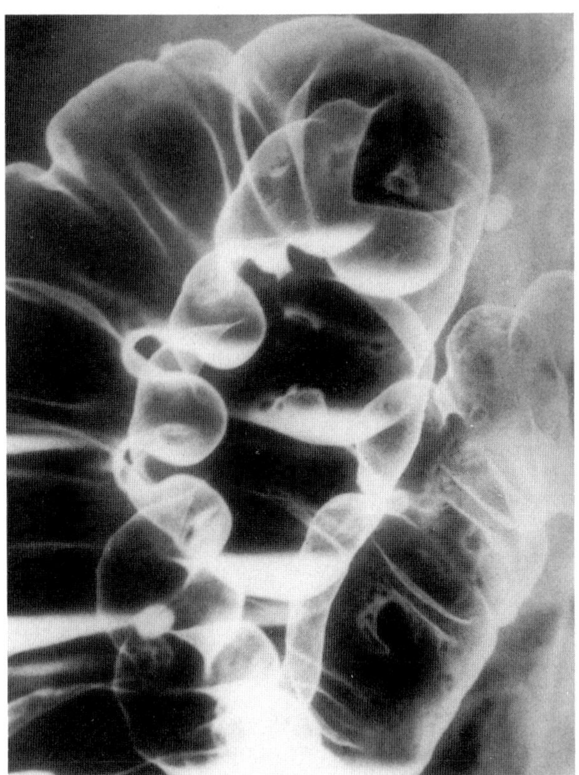

B

Figure 12.41. (A) Polyp on a stalk seen *en face*. Small circle (arrowhead) is created by the stalk and large circle (arrow) by the polyp head. (B) Diverticulosis of the colon. Diverticula seen in profile and *en face*. The latter exhibits the orifice.

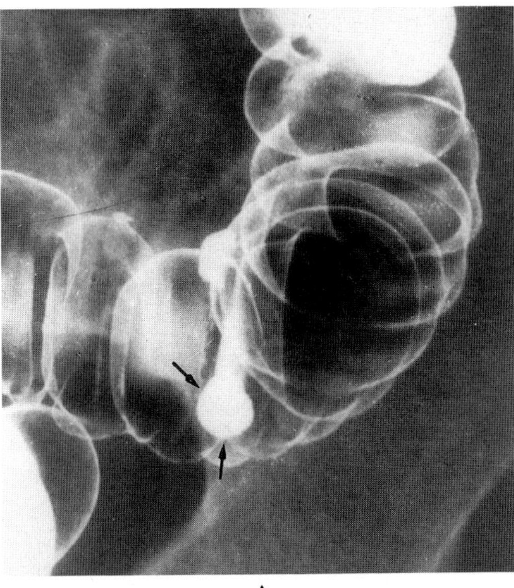

A

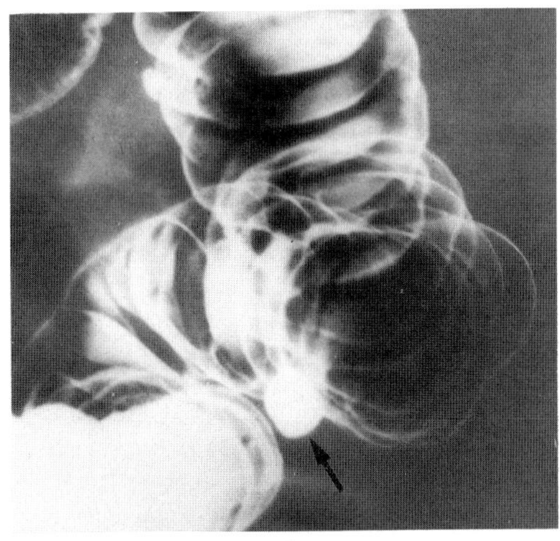

B

Figure 12.42. (A) Diverticulum filled with barium presents as a more radiopaque formation than a polyp (arrows). (B) However, profile projection is more diagnostic (arrow).

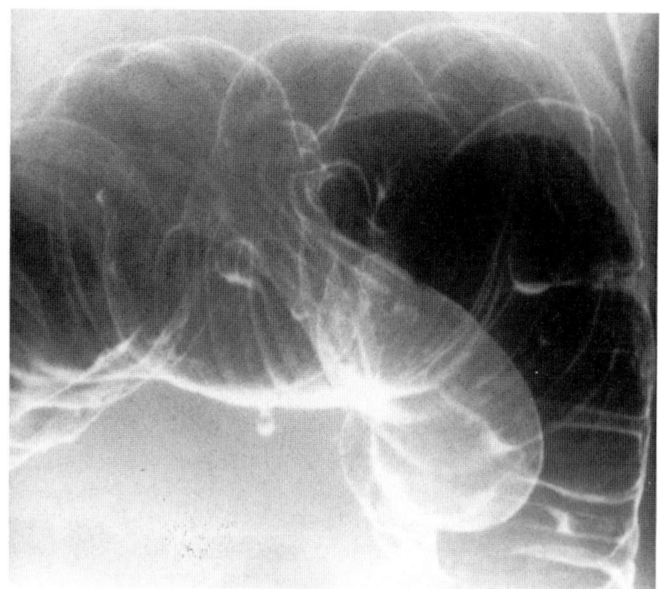

Figure 12.43. Lipoma of the transverse colon. Several diverticula.

middle-aged people, diagnostic and therapeutic endoscopy is indicated. Although all polyps larger than 10 mm have to be detected by a double-contrast enema examination, even large polyps can be missed, as the result of perception errors, unawareness of double-contrast study interpretation, or a very redundant colon.

Polyps in children are morphologically similar to polyps in adults but differ microscopically since they are often hamartomatous or hyperplastic. Solitary polyps appear most frequently up to the fifth year of age and sometimes disappear spontaneously.

Mesenchymal benign tumors of the large intestine are not common. *Leiomyoma*, a neoplasm of hard consistency, resembles other benign colonic tumors, but tends to be larger. Necrosis of tumor tissue results in ulceration which may then simulate a malignant neoplasm. *Lipoma* is a submucosal, oval or spherical, sharply demarcated tumor, sometimes pedunculated (Fig. 12.43). Since lipomas have a liquid consistency intra-abdominally, they tend to change shape on compression. Barium and water enemas may reveal lipomas, but CT is diagnostic. *Angiomas* are oval, compressible tumors which seemingly diminish, or even vanish, with

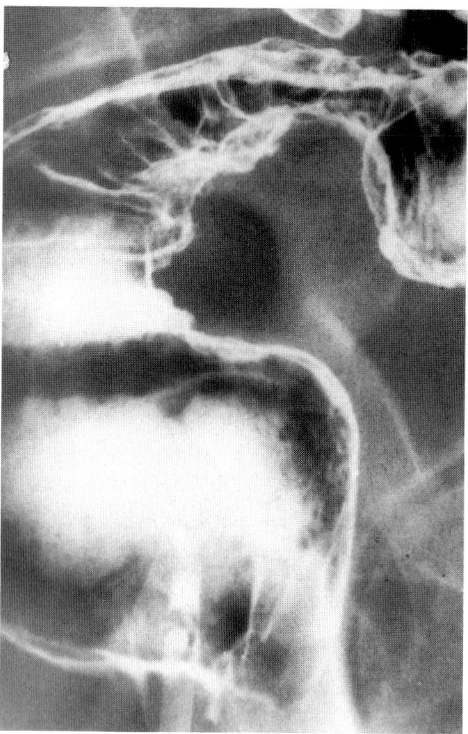

Figure 12.44. Endometriosis of the sigmoid colon and rectum.

air distension of the colon. *Endometriosis* refers to serosal endometrial implants which leave the mucosal relief completely preserved. Endometrial implants are frequently situated in the sigmoid colon and rectum, and tend to cause reactive fibrosis (Fig. 12.44). During the menstrual cycle, formations of endometrium change their dimensions. Differentiating endometriosis from other extramucosal growths is not always accurate by a barium enema.

MALIGNANT TUMORS OF THE LARGE INTESTINE

Carcinoma. Colorectal carcinoma is second in incidence only to lung carcinoma, among malignant neoplasms of internal organs in the developed world. Residents of highly developed industrial countries are more often affected, especially elderly patients. In spite of advances in diagnostic and surgical techniques, the 5-year survival rate is still 50%, or even less. Both sexes are equally affected with the exception of multiple primary carcinomas which are more frequent in females (Fig. 12.45).

Risk factors include a tendency to develop colonic adenomas and a familial history of colorectal carcinoma. If not treated, all patients with familial polyposis develop adenocarcinoma. Extensive ulcerative and Crohn's colitis place patients at increased risk. Chronic irritation from other causes, such as ureterosigmoidostomy, has also been implicated. Nutritional factors also seem to be important in induction of colorectal carcinoma.

It is widely believed that colorectal carcinoma arises from adenomatous polyps (Fig. 12.46). Consequently, polypectomy lowers the mortality rate from colorectal carcinoma. Some colorectal carcinomas probably start growing as conglomerates of malignant mucosal cells.

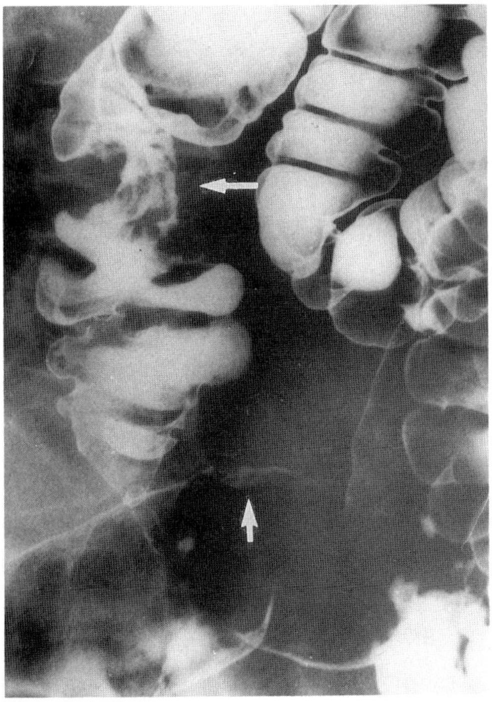

FIGURE 12.45. Two carcinomas (arrows) in the sigmoid and ascending colon.

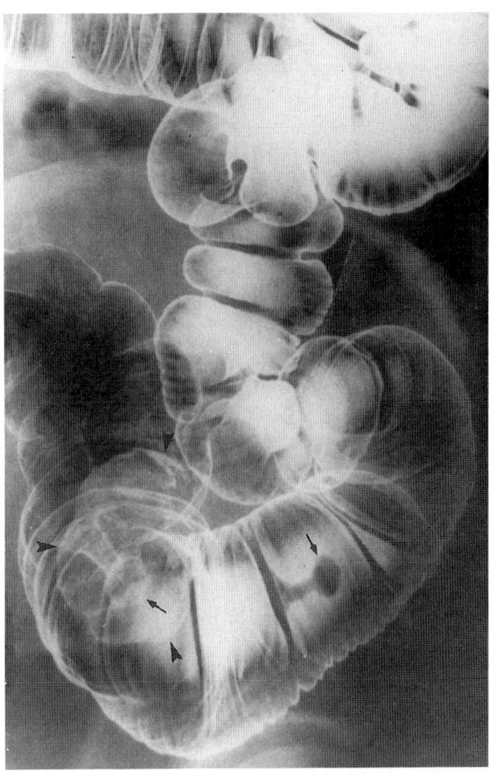

FIGURE 12.46. Two polyps on a stalk (arrows). A large carcinoma in the same region (arrowheads).

Approximately 5% of adenomas removed endoscopically contain invasive carcinoma. However, biopsy of a polyp is not an accurate procedure unless careful histology of the entire polyp is carried out after polypectomy, since malignant transformation can be focal. The risk of malignancy within an adenoma depends on its size and histologic type, and the presence of epithelial dysplasia. Size is the simplest and most practical predictor of malignancy. Because of X-ray divergence at roentgenography, polyps may appear larger than actual size. To best estimate the actual size, correction for magnification is required. This is approximately 30% for conventional roentgenography and 45% for spot-films. Filming an adjacent object, such as a catheter, under the same radiographic conditions readily allows calculation of the correction factor.

A risk of invasive carcinoma does not exist, for practical purposes, in polyps smaller than 5 mm in diameter. The risk of carcinoma is 1%, 5%, and 10% for adenomas whose size is 6–10 mm, 10–20 mm, and larger than 20 mm, respectively. Dysplasia is more frequent and more prominent in large rather than in small adenomas. Colorectal carcinoma is found in 10% of patients over 40 years of age who have occult blood in the stool. It was thought that 50% of colorectal carcinomas could be detected by digitorectal examination and almost 70% by sigmoidoscopy. However, over the past two decades the incidence of carcinoma has increased in the right hemicolon by 8% and has decreased in the left hemicolon. The use of double-contrast barium enema detection, colonoscopy, and endoscopic polypectomy may be responsible for an apparent increased incidence of right-sided carcinoma of the colon (Diagram 12.4).

Early carcinoma does not penetrate deeper in the intestinal wall than the submucosa, and is commonly polypoid. It has a better prognosis than the advanced form.

Approximately 5% of patients with colorectal carcinoma harbor multiple synchronous colorectal carcinomas (Fig. 12.45). As a rule, simultaneously occurring carcinomas are found in different segments of the large intestine. At least one-third of patients with colorectal carcinoma bear coincidentally occurring adenomatous polyps (Fig. 12.46). Thus the entire large intestine must be examined.

Liver metastases are present in 15–20% of patients at the moment when the large bowel carcinoma is detected. Two years after surgery for colorectal carcinoma, liver metastases occur in an additional 29% of patients.

Three macroscopic types of carcinoma may be found: annular, polypoid, and ulcerative. Almost 95% of these are histologically adenocarcinomas. In the right hemicolon, they grow mainly as polypoid lesions. Annular lesions are more frequent in the left hemicolon, and lead to obstruction. Despite different morphology and clinical symptoms, prognoses for both left-sided and right-sided carcinomas are equal. Some carcinomas may possess combined gross pathologic properties. A saddle carcinoma may transform into a circumferential carcinoma. When they are necrotic, polypoid and circumferential carcinomas may ulcerate.

Annular carcinoma, the most frequent gross pathologic type of colorectal carcinoma, causes a short, circumferential stenosis. It is believed

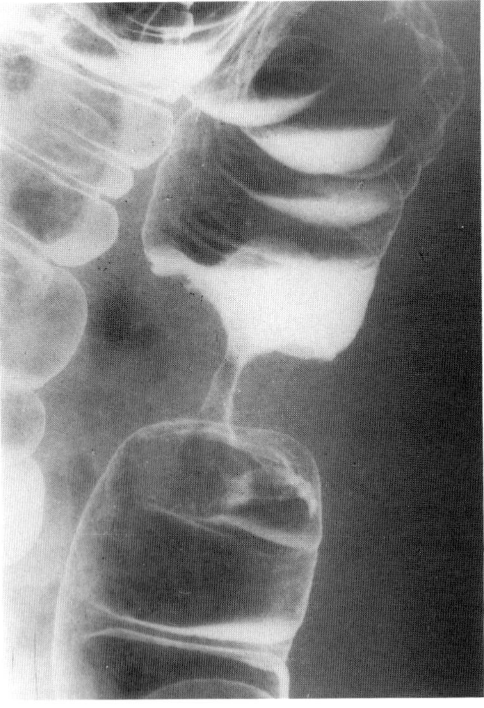

Figure 12.47. Annular adenocarcinoma of the colon. (A) Barium study.

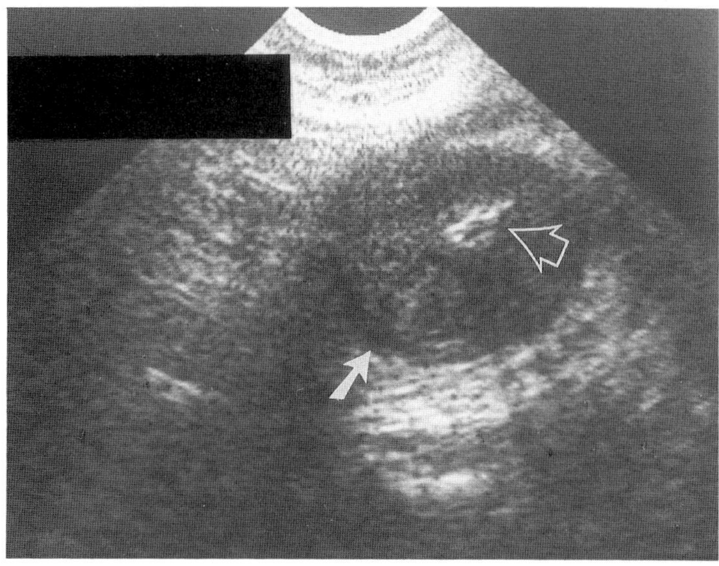

FIGURE 12.47 *continued.* Annular adenocarcinoma of the colon. (B) Ultrasound examination. Thick wall of the descending colon carcinoma (closed arrow) and small residual lumen (open arrow).

that the progression of polypoid carcinoma results in an annular appearance. On barium enema examination there is induration of the intestinal wall, destruction of mucosal surface, and abrupt demarcation from adjacent normal segments, sometimes with overhanging margins (Figs. 12.47–12.51). Obstruction and fistula formation are common complications.

Polypoid carcinoma often bleeds with necrosis developing because of an insufficient blood

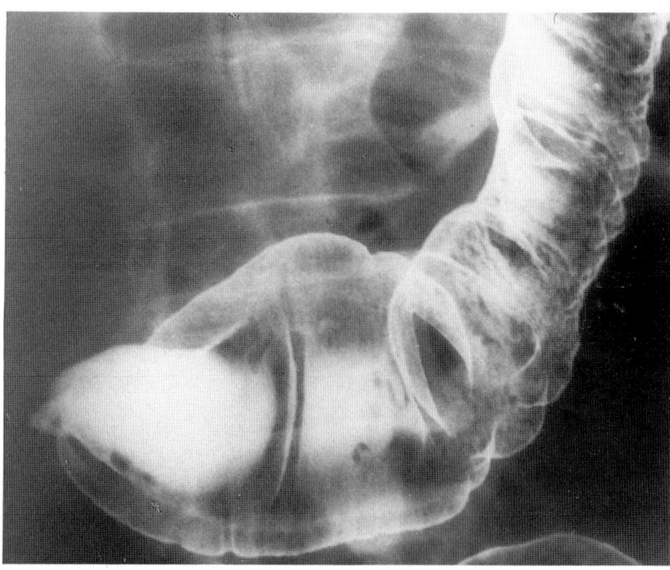

FIGURE 12.48. Annular carcinoma of the transverse colon.

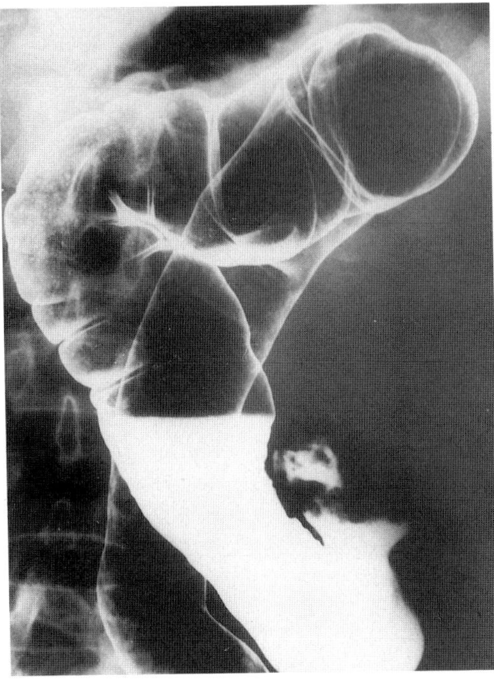

FIGURE 12.49. Annular carcinoma of the distal descending colon.

supply. Masses protruding into the lumen are a characteristic finding (Figs. 12.52 and 12.53). When situated on the nondependent wall, polypoid carcinoma may present, on double-contrast studies, as a thin white line (Figs. 12.94 and 12.96). A negative defect results when there is accumulation of barium on the dependent wall. Polypoid carcinomas and polyps may both cause intussusception. Large masses can obstruct the lumen. When intussusception presents in an adult, a careful search for underlying carcinoma is appropriate (Fig. 12.30B).

When *ulcerated carcinoma* is situated on the dependent wall, barium accumulates in the crater and resembles a volcano (Fig. 12.54).

The gross pathologic appearance of carcinoma does not depend on microscopic structure.

Carcinomas in patients with long-standing ulcerative colitis are adenocarcinomas, and may be multiple. The incidence of colorectal carcinoma is also increased in patients with Crohn's disease. In both instances the carcinomas usually assume characteristics of malignant growths, but may sometimes appear as long smooth strictures.

Colorectal carcinomas spread via lymph and

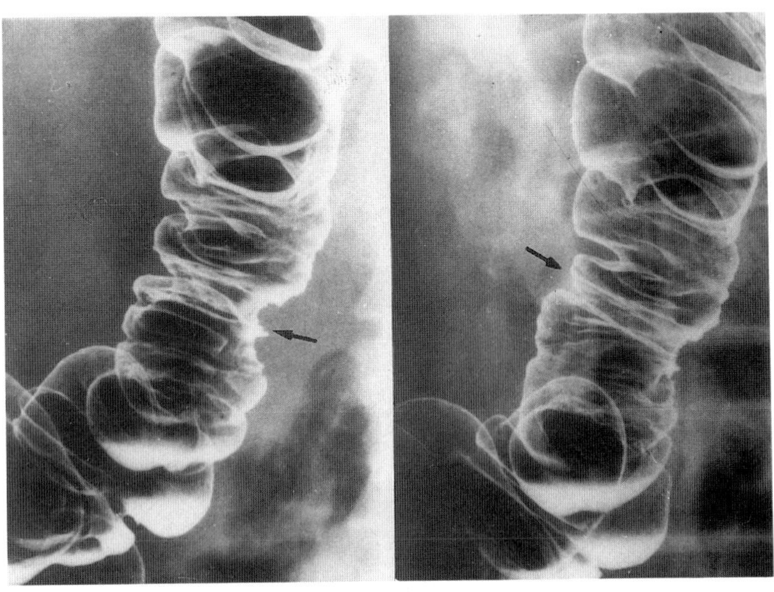

FIGURE 12.50. Spastic changes simulated an annular carcinoma on colonoscopy. Double-contrast enema study demonstrates changes in morphology during examination (arrows).

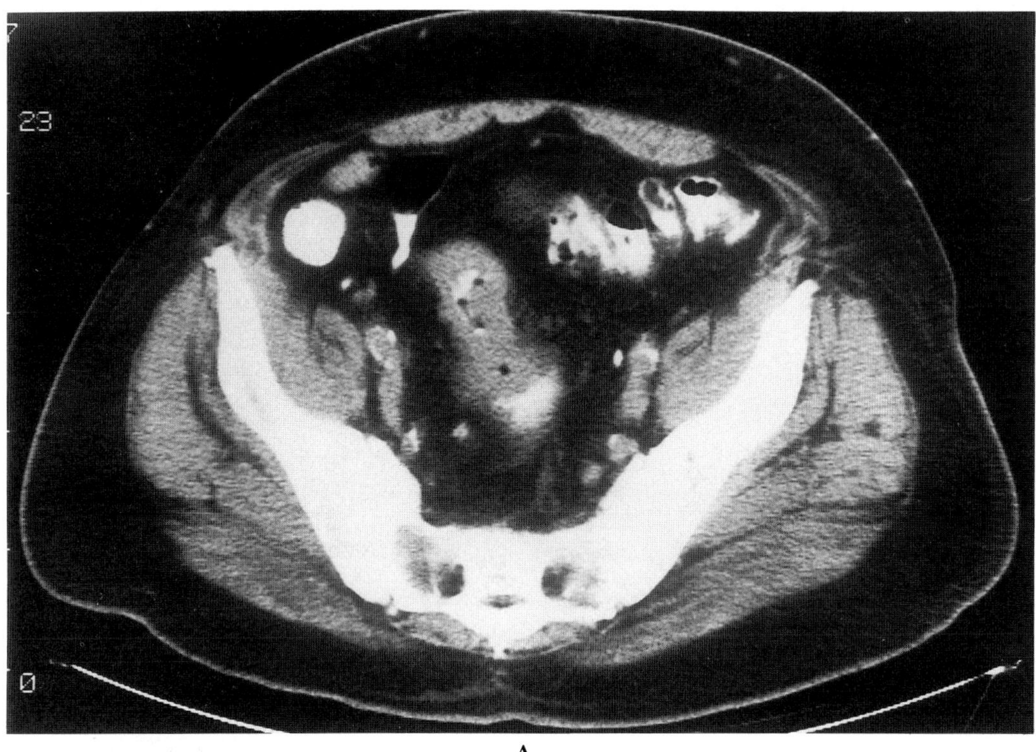

A

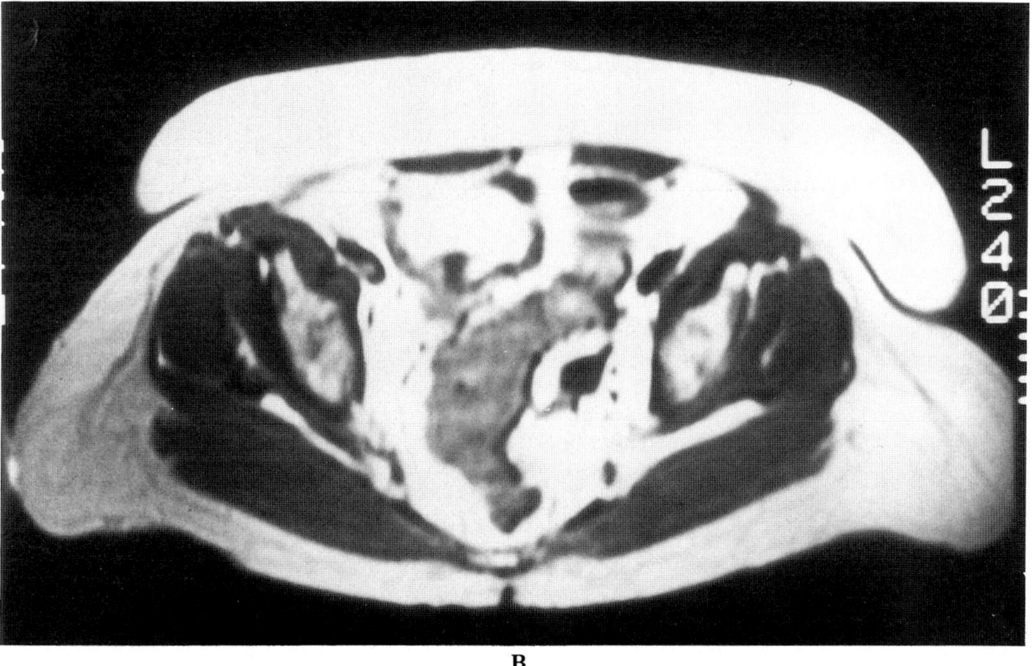

B

FIGURE 12.51. Annular sigmoid colon carcinoma. (A) CT presentation. (B) MRI presentation of proton density image.

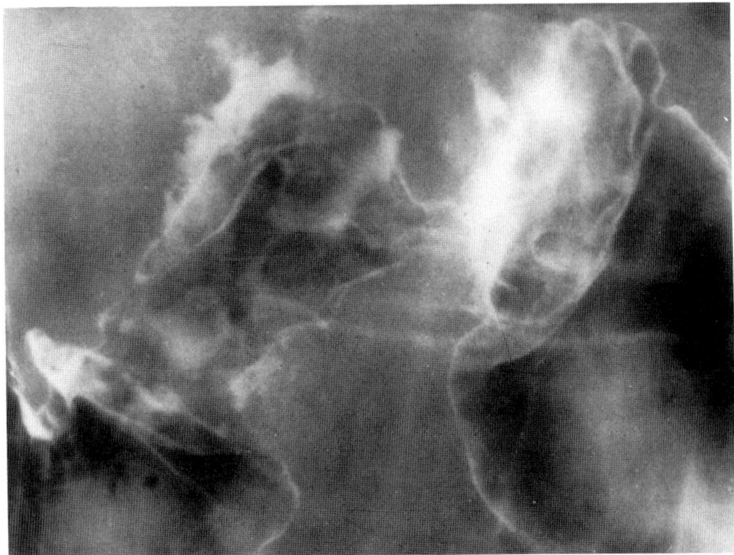

Figure 12.52. Apple-core appearance of colon carcinoma.

blood, and by direct invasion of adjacent structures. They may infiltrate the mesocolon, causing a serrated appearance of the colonic wall. Invasion into the gastrocolic ligament leads to affection of the greater curvature of the stomach. Impression on the intestinal wall by expansile growths does not cause tethering of the contour.

Duke's classification defines the depth of carcinoma infiltration of the intestinal wall and the presence of metastases. In the A-stage, carcinoma is confined to the intestinal wall. The B-stage is characterized by affection of adipose tissue of the serosa. In the C-stage, carcinoma cells also involve regional lymph nodes. Distant metastases characterize the D-stage. Colorectal carcinoma can also be classified according to the TNM classification. Computed tomography can detect primary and secondary carcinoma of the colon, and can identify involvement of adjacent vessels, lymph nodes, liver, adrenals, and bone. The main sign of a colonic carcinoma is thickening of the wall, which normally measures no more than 3 mm. Any thickening to 6 mm or more is considered definitively abnormal. The extent of carcinoma spread, especially from the rectum, can be demonstrated by CT. Several factors may make it difficult to detect

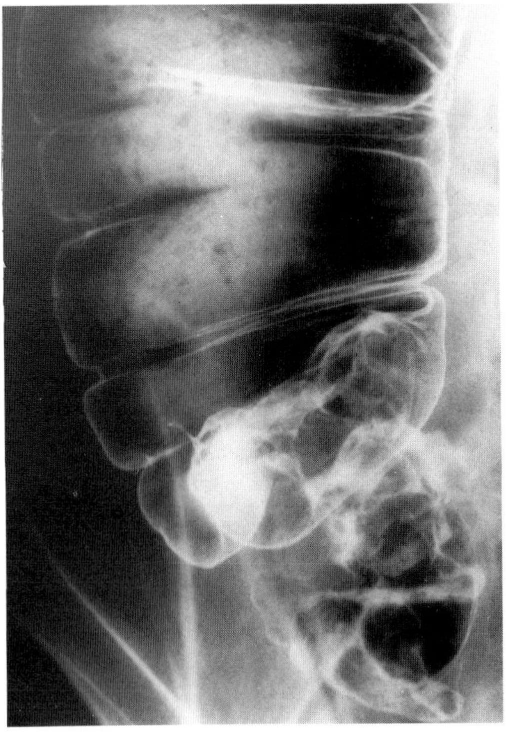

Figure 12.53. Polypoid carcinoma of the cecum. (A) Barium study.

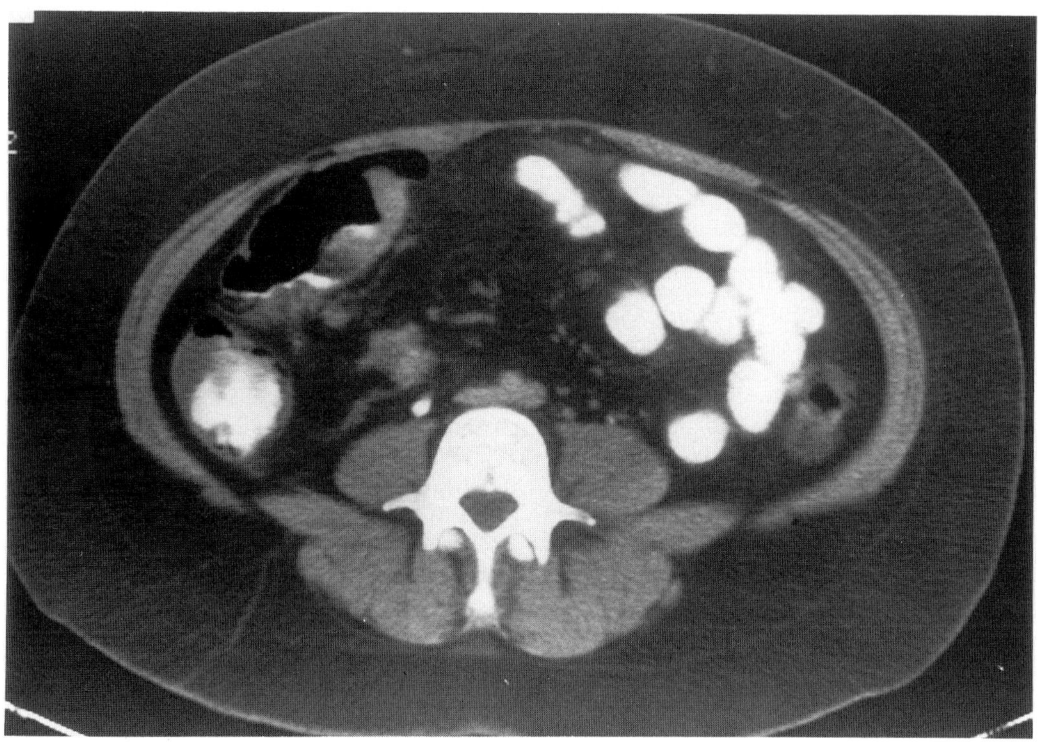

FIGURE 12.53 *continued.* Polypoid carcinoma of the cecum. (B) CT study.

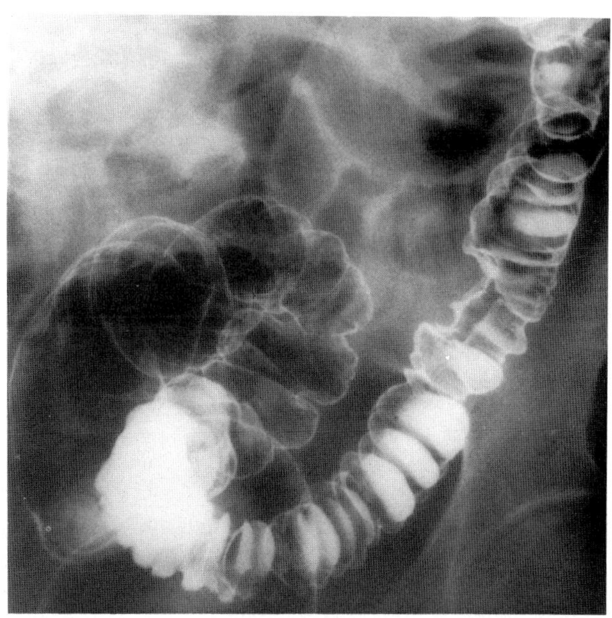

FIGURE 12.54. Ulcerated carcinoma of the distal descending colon.

direct invasion of the rectum on CT, including a normal lack of fat planes between the levator ani muscles, and obscuration by the lower segment of the prostate and by the posterior aspect of the urinary bladder. Colonic carcinoma can be staged by CT according to the following classification: stage I is characterized by intraluminal polypoid mass without change in the wall; in stage II, the wall of the colon is thicker than 16 mm and no invasion is seen; stage III includes invasion of adjacent organs and muscles; stage IV shows distant metastatic disease.

Preoperative staging of local distribution of the colorectal carcinoma by MR imaging can be as precise as with CT. Thickening of the intestinal wall may also be demonstrated by US, with transrectal echosonography demonstrating the depth of tumor penetration.

After apparently successful resection for colorectal carcinoma, diagnostic efforts are directed toward detection of metachronous and/or undetected synchronous adenomas and carcinomas. In patients with large tumors, complete evacuation of barium may not be successful and small lesions will remain invisible. Recurrent disease attacks approximately half the patients within two years of surgery for colorectal carcinoma. Local recurrences account for nearly one-third of recurrences. Anastomotic recurrences are most frequent after an anterior resection, where a residual tumor grows into the suture line (Fig. 12.55). Abdominoperineal resection results in local recurrences in 30–50% of patients. Presacral masses found after such operations are not all recurrent tumors, however; 75% of solid masses are recurrent carcinomas and the rest are either abscesses or necrotic tissue.

Distant metastases occur in 45% of patients with colorectal carcinoma and are the most difficult therapeutic problem. Magnetic resonance imaging is the most sensitive method for demonstrating liver metastases and distinguishing recurrent disease from scars. Recurrent disease shows medium to high signal intensity on T2-weighted images. In contrast, fibrous tissue demonstrates low signal intensity on T2-weighted images. When recurrent disease is found, the average survival rate is less than a year.

Annular colorectal carcinoma must be distinguished radiographically from postinflamma-

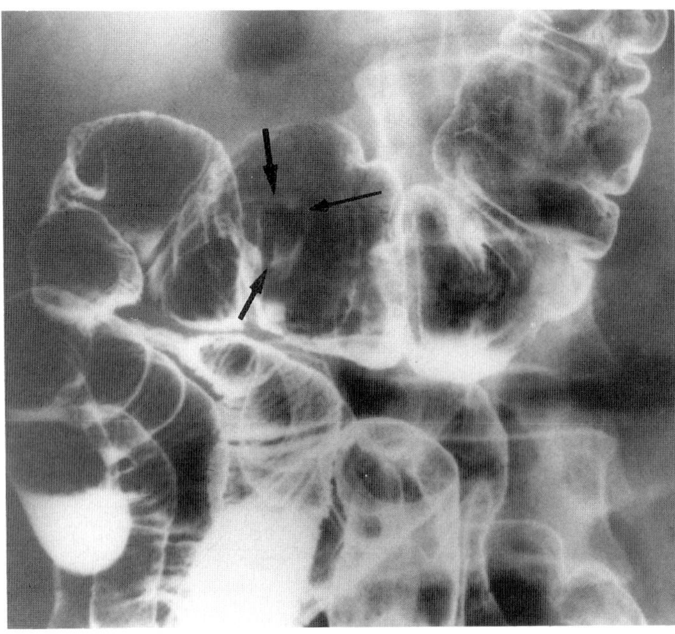

Figure 12.55. Recurrent polypoid carcinoma at the ileotransversostomy site (arrows).

TABLE 12.4. STENOSES OF THE LARGE BOWEL

Benign
Inflammatory
Crohn's disease
Ulcerative colitis
Colonic or pericolonic diverticular abscess
Bowel ischemia
Radiation injury
Neoplasms
Malignant
Carcinoma
Lymphoma
Carcinoid
Metastases

tory strictures and other stenoses (Table 12.4). Polypoid carcinomas may resemble polyps, granulomas, or sarcomas. Hypertrophic intestinal tuberculosis may be indistinguishable from carcinoma. Very rare idiopathic ulcers of the large intestine may mimic an ulcerated carcinoma.

Ischemic intestinal changes proximal to a circumferential carcinoma are very rare. These most probably result from increased intraluminal pressure, and have characteristics of ischemic colitis. Poststenotic dilatation of the intestine results from tumor destruction of nerve plexuses (Figs. 3.15B, 12.28, and 12.48).

A double-contrast enema can detect carcinoma in any segment of the large bowel with an accuracy rate of almost 95%. False-positive and false-negative rates are below 5% when double-contrast enema examination is combined with colonoscopy. Undetected carcinomas, most commonly located in the sigmoid colon or in the flexures, are usually visible on films, but are missed as a result of perceptional errors. Colonoscopy is highly accurate, but has more complications, and adequate visualization of the cecum is possible in only 65% of patients. Despite "blind spots," colonoscopy yields a smaller number of false-negative results than double-contrast barium enema examination.

Recurrent Local Colorectal Carcinoma. Recurrent carcinoma results in the early appearance of focal mucosal mural irregularities at the anastomotic site. Later, a neoplasm may assume considerable dimensions, corresponding morphologically to a primary carcinoma (Figs. 12.55 and 12.65).

The accuracy of a double-contrast enema examination in detecting primary and recurrent carcinoma is high, provided that all sections of the intestine are demonstrated and that an overabundance of barium, or flocculation from any cause, such as excessive mucus or improper cleansing of the colon, does not interfere with the quality of the study (Fig. 12.56).

Carcinoid. One half of the total number of gastrointestinal carcinoids grow in the ileocecal region. The incidence is higher in the rectum than in the colon. Argentaffinomas are spherical or oval, smooth-surfaced tumors readily discovered by a double-contrast enema. When large enough, they can be demonstrated by CT (Fig. 12.97). If smaller than 2 cm in diameter, they neither affect the muscular coat of the bowel, nor metastasize. The probability of metastases in regional lymph nodes and the liver increases with increasing tumor size. The prognosis is better with carcinoid than with colorectal carcinoma.

Lymphoma. The large bowel may be subjected to both primary and secondary lymphomas. According to Dawson's criteria a primary lymphoma should be considered when:

1. Lymph nodes on the body surfaces are not enlarged.
2. Mediastinal lymph nodes are not enlarged.
3. Only regional lymph nodes may be enlarged without affection of the spleen and liver.
4. The total number of white blood cells and the differential count are normal.

Lymphomas affecting the alimentary canal are non-Hodgkin's. Lymphoma is not commonly found in the large bowel; involvement usually occurs in the ileocecal area and the rectum. The large intestine is eventually affected in almost 25% of patients who die from a non-Hodgkin's lymphoma.

In the early phases, lymphoid follicles are enlarged. Polypoid tumors resembling a carcinoma are common later. Pliability of the wall may be preserved in part, but the intestine does not readily collapse as in normal subjects. Lymphoma may affect the colon diffusely, re-

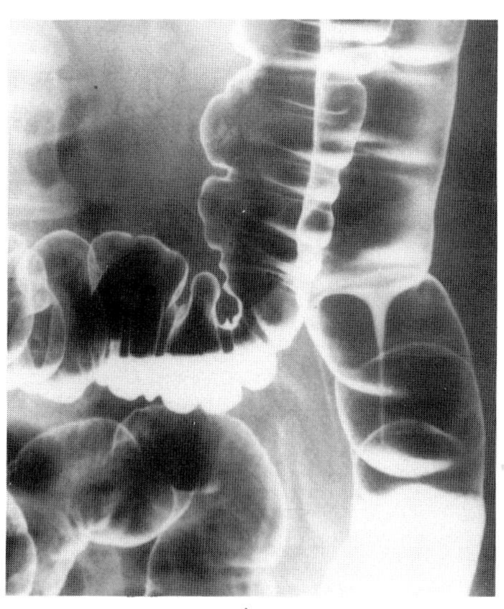
A

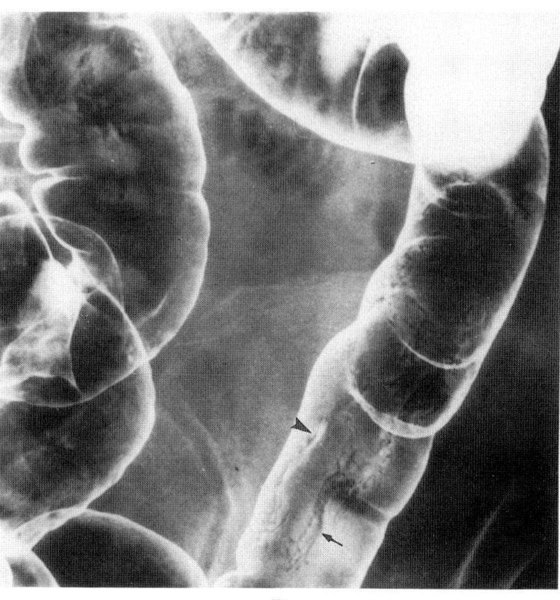
B

Figure 12.56. Colonic mucus. (A) Thin stream in the descending colon. (B) Stripes of mucus in the descending colon (arrows and arrowhead).

sembling a polyposis syndrome. In contrast to regenerating inflammatory pseudopolyps, lymphoma and polyposis syndromes tend to spare haustral markings.

Approximately 30–50% of lymphomas involving the colon are *multinodular* in appearance. Morphological properties are:

1. Sessile nodules of different sizes with an average diameter of 7 mm.
2. Cecal tumors that tend to be larger than lymphomas from other locations.
3. Preservation of haustral markings.
4. Incomplete emptying of barium from the colon frequently occurs. Simultaneous affection of the stomach, small bowel, and spleen is quite common.

Less common forms of nodular lymphoma are irregular polypoid filiform nodules with a central excavation (Fig. 12.57). Early lesions of nodular lymphoma may mimic aphthoid ulcers. In contrast to the lesions of Crohn's disease, similar lesions in lymphoma tend to be more

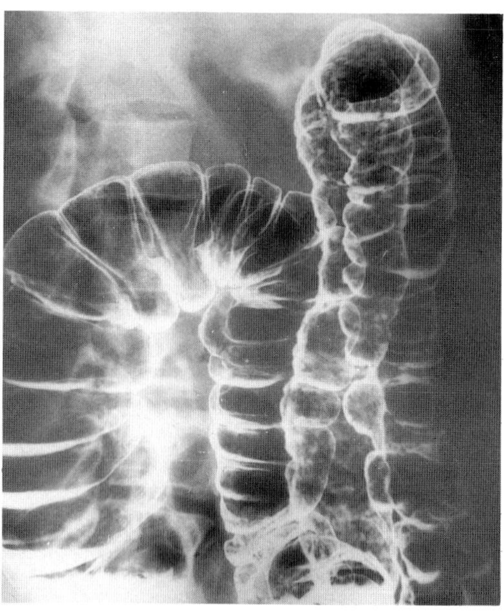

Figure 12.57. Nodular lymphoma affecting the left colon. Haustral markings are preserved.

numerous and somewhat less well demarcated. Acute toxic dilatation of the colon may result from a diffuse multinodular lymphoma.

Differential diagnosis of a nodular lymphoma includes multiple nodular lesions that affect the large intestine. Hyperplastic lymphoid follicles are usually smaller, and tend to be less aggregated. However, endoscopy with biopsy is diagnostic.

Leiomyosarcoma. Often ulcerated, the polypoid hard mass of a leiomyosarcoma is hardly distinguishable from other neoplasms originating from deep layers of the intestinal wall. Leiomyosarcomas tend to be larger than benign counterparts.

Liposarcomas of the large intestine are very rare (Fig. 12.58). The fat density of the neoplasm allows a relatively specific diagnosis with CT.

Metastatic Malignancies. Metastases to the colon have a variable appearance depending on whether there is direct invasion from either ad-

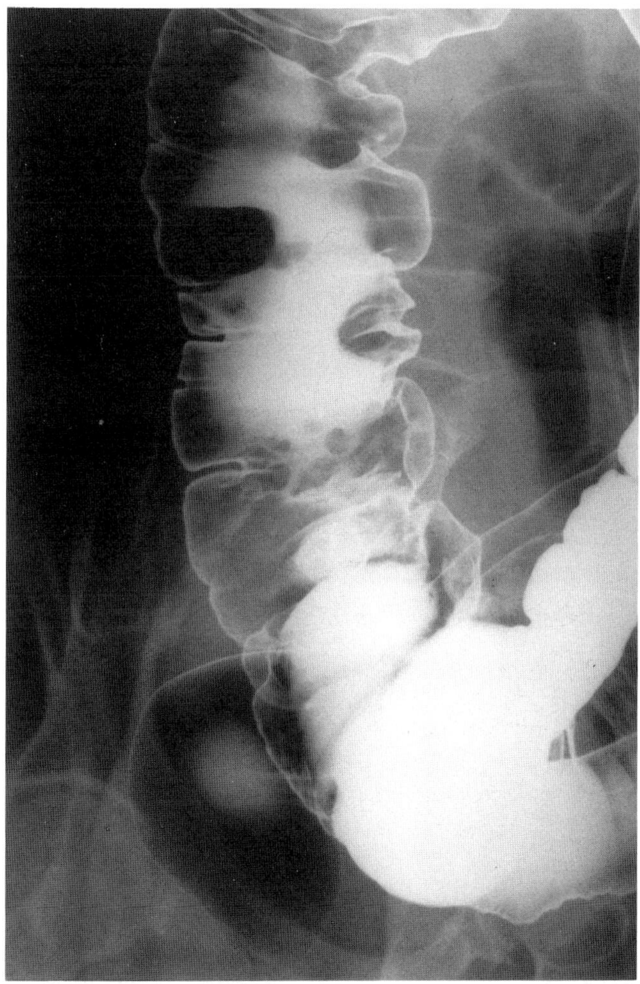

Figure 12.58. Primitive mesenchymal tumor of the right colon. Liposarcoma. (Courtesy R.F. Thoeni, MD, University of California, San Francisco.)

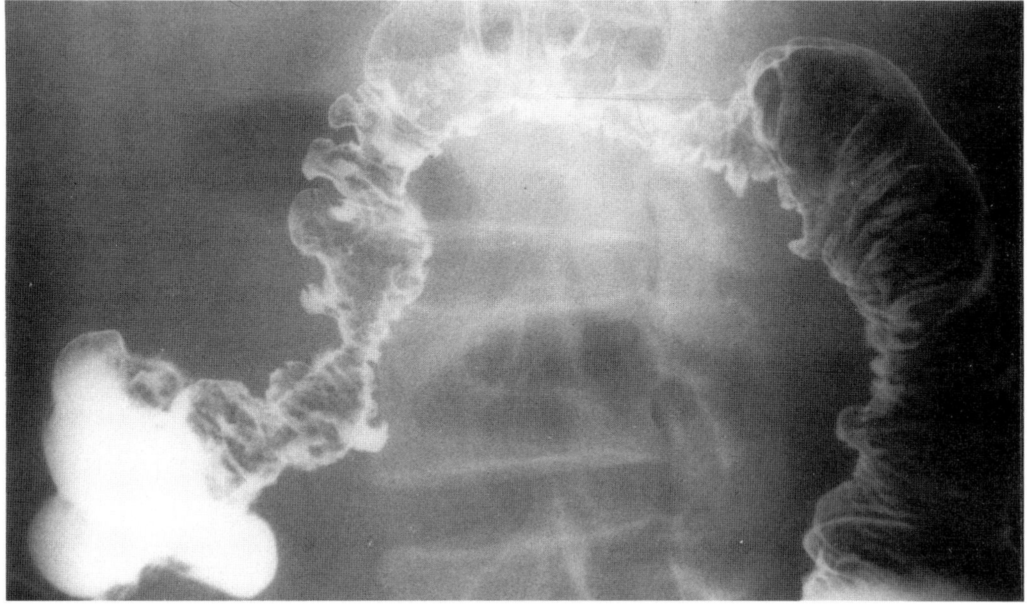

Figure 12.59. Carcinoma of the pancreas, spreading through the transverse mesocolon, primarily infiltrates the inferior aspect of the colon.

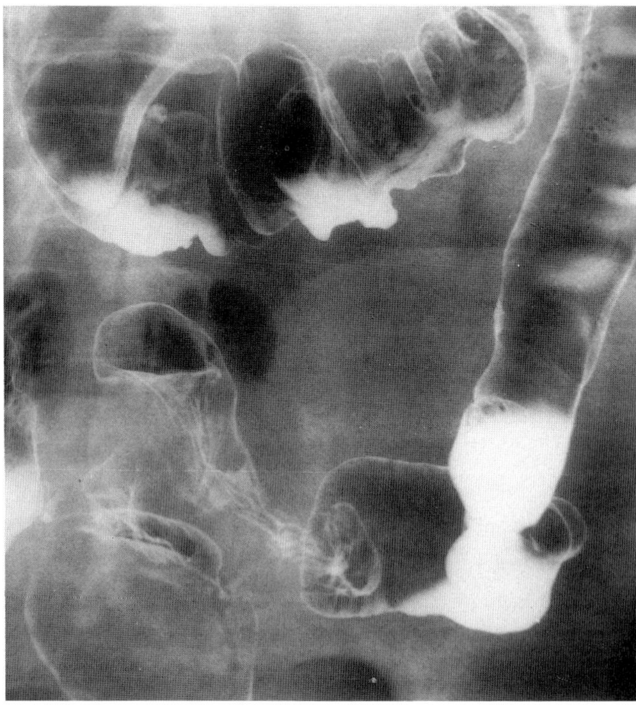

Figure 12.60. Carcinoma of the left ovary infiltrates the sigmoid mesocolon and sigmoid colon.

jacent or distant structures, peritoneal seeding, or lymphatic or hematogenous emboli (see chapter 11). Neoplasms of the kidney, duodenum, suprarenal glands, biliary tract, and genitourinary tract may penetrate into the large bowel *per continuitatem*. The morphology of secondary tumors depends on the route of affection (Figs. 12.59–12.61).

Angiodysplasia. By definition, angiodysplasia is an acquired dilatation of blood vessels of the submucosa and mucosa of the large bowel. On double-contrast studies, the mucosal surface may resemble a piece of coral. Angiodysplasias are often subject to bleeding. The angiographic pattern is not characteristic and may resemble the blood vessels of a lipoma (Fig. 4.89).

Injuries. Blunt abdominal trauma infrequently results in large intestinal injury. In order of decreasing frequency, the transverse colon, sigmoid colon, and cecum are affected. Blood and lymph collect at the site of injury. Subserosal collections create thickening of the bowel wall, decreased pliability, and narrowing of the lumen (Fig. 12.62).

Perforations often result in pneumoperitoneum and ileus. Any enema is contraindicated, since the increase in pressure can propel intestinal contents into the peritoneal cavity.

Perforations of the Colon in Patients Bearing a Renal Allograft. Immunosuppressed patients with a renal allograft are prone to gastrointestinal complications such as bleeding, perforations of peptic ulcers, acute pancreatitis, ischemic colitis, and perforation of the colon. Immunosuppressive therapy, often as a side effect, obscures the usual symptoms of underlying complications. Spontaneous perforation of the colon occurs in 2.3% of patients with renal transplants. The majority of perforations result from a nonocclusive intestinal ischemia, defined as mucosal necrosis with patent arteries

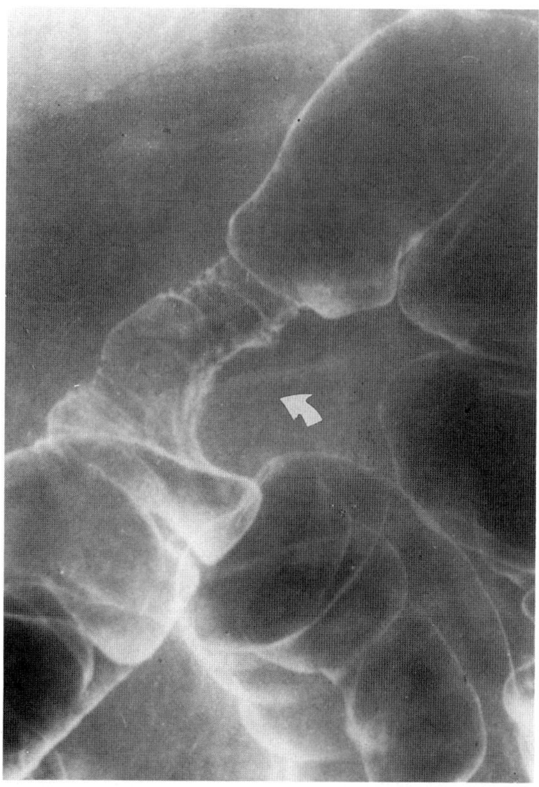

Figure 12.61. Hematogenous deposit of bronchial carcinoma in the transverse colon (arrow).

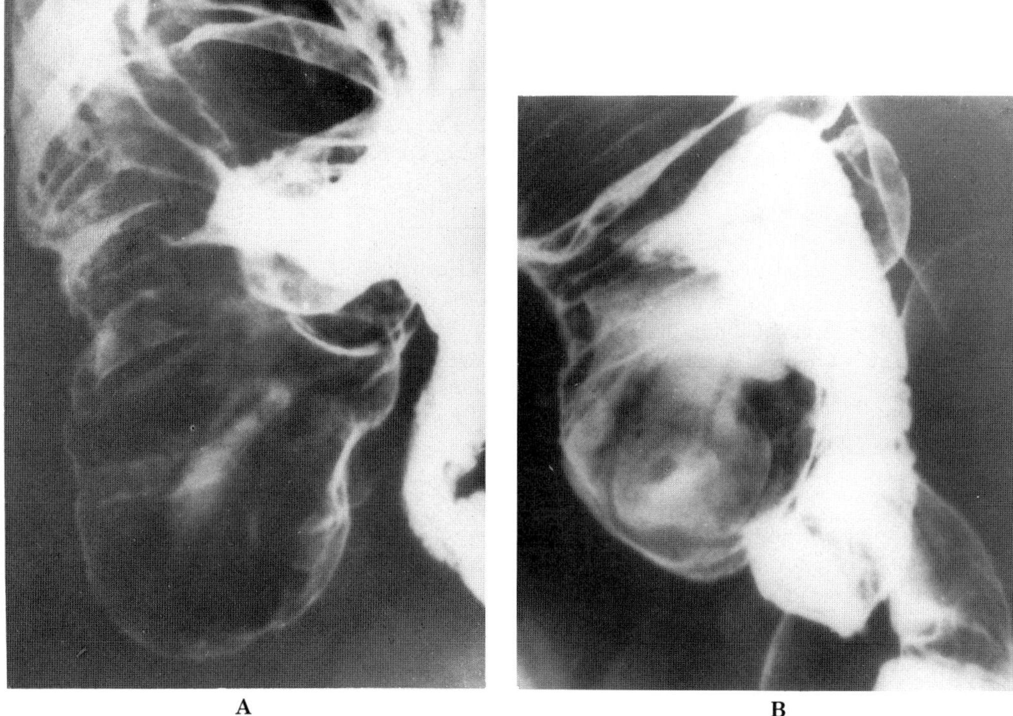

FIGURE 12.62. Subserosal hematoma of the cecum. Both (A) and (B) show rigidity of the wall.

and veins. This may result from transplantation surgery, uremia, infection, and immunosuppressive agents. Twenty-four percent of perforations related to a renal transplant are due to a ruptured diverticulum. Perforation may occur at any time—one day after surgery, or years later. An early diagnosis of such a perforation is essential since the mortality rate is 41–71%.

PATHOLOGY OF THE APPENDICES EPIPLOICAE

Normal appendices epiploicae are not seen on barium studies. However, when they are enlarged, such as in patients with Crohn's disease or any other etiology, they may exhibit symptoms of colon compression from an extrinsic mass (Fig. 12.63). Stenosis may be accompanied by muscle spasm. Gangrenous appendices epiploicae may lead to stenosis of the colon secondary to torsion.

THE POSTOPERATIVE LARGE INTESTINE

Water-soluble contrast media should be used for enemas performed soon after colonic surgery. However, when free perforation into the peritoneal cavity is suspected, both enema and colonoscopy are contraindicated and the diagnosis should be established by plain abdominal radiography. Barium in the peritoneal cavity contributes to granulomas. These may produce adhesions resulting in intestinal obstruction. A double-contrast barium enema can reveal the postoperative recurrence of carcinoma and metachronous polyps and carcinomas. Recurrences of Crohn's disease in postoperative patients are also demonstrated.

Colectomy is performed prophylactically to prevent a colorectal carcinoma in patients with familial polyposis or Gardner's syndrome. Instead of an ileostomy, the ileum may be connected to the anus or to the rectum (Fig. 12.64).

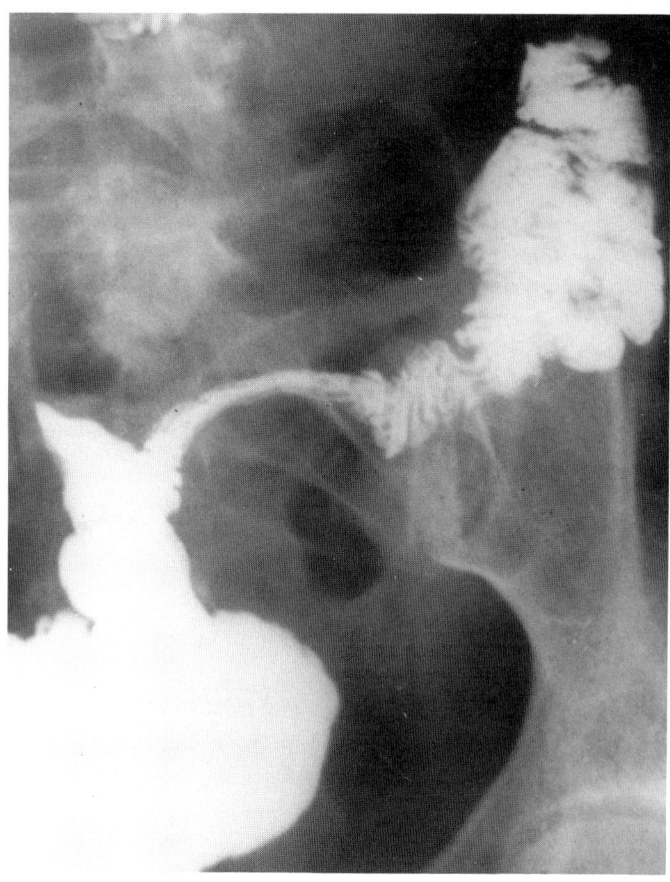

FIGURE 12.63. Necrosis of appendices epiploicae. Displacement of the sigmoid colon.

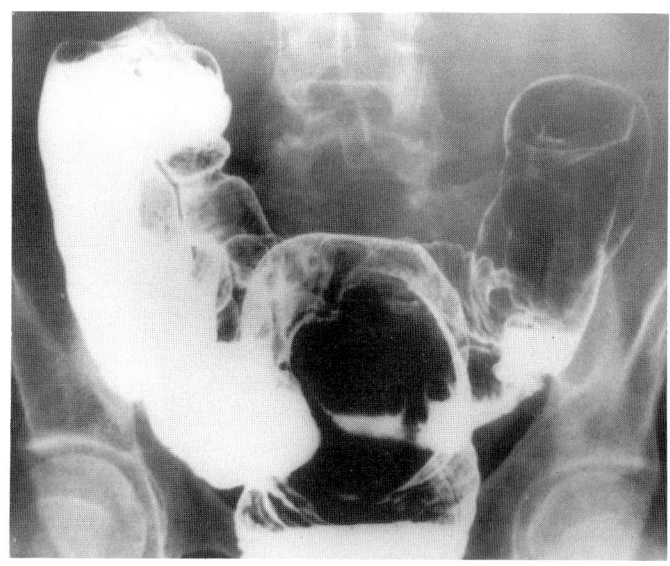

FIGURE 12.64. Colectomy. Ileum anastomosed to the rectum has assumed morphologic characteristics of the colon.

After colectomy and mucosal proctectomy (removal of rectal mucosa only) an endorectal or ileoanal anastomosis is formed. Proximal to the anastomosis, a reservoir may be formed with a 50 cm long ileal loop, either "S" or "J" shaped. The latter is smaller in volume. Such an operation requires a temporary ileostomy, until proximal sutures heal. This type of surgery preserves continuity of the bowel; permanent ileostomy is avoided and sphincteric function is preserved. A contrast enema, CT, or scintigraphy can be used in examining these patients.

After resection, the proximal segment of the colon can be anastomosed to the distal segment or with a loop of the small intestine (Fig. 12.65). Both proximal and distal segments often have to be examined in patients with a temporary or definitive colostomy (Fig. 12.66).

RADIOLOGY OF THE ILEOCECAL AREA

The ileocecal area, particularly the terminal ileum, has a predilection for certain pathologies, such as intussusception, chronic inflammations (Crohn's disease, tuberculosis, and actinomycosis), lymphoma, and carcinoid tumors. Due to its anatomical relationships, radiologic analysis is more complex than in other sections of the large intestine. The mucosal folds of the terminal ileum are often longitudinal and can be demonstrated by controlled compression during follow-through barium studies, enteroclysis, retrograde ileography, or oral pneumocolon. The cecum is normally fixed to the posterior abdominal wall, but may be mobile if a mesocecum is present. Double-con-

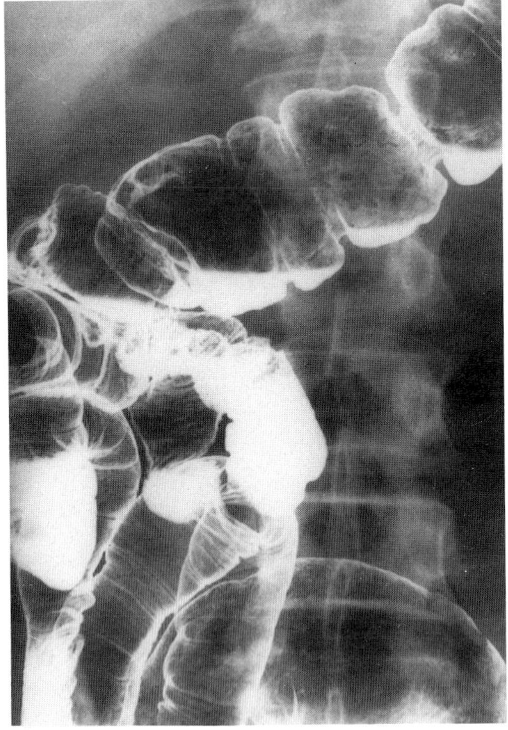

A

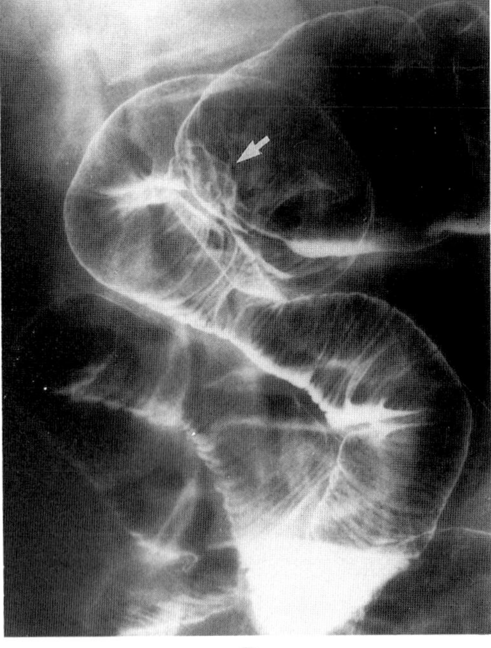

B

FIGURE 12.65. Right colectomy with ileotransversostomy for carcinoma of the colon. (A) Normal appearance one year following surgery. (B) Recurrence of carcinoma two years following surgery (arrow).

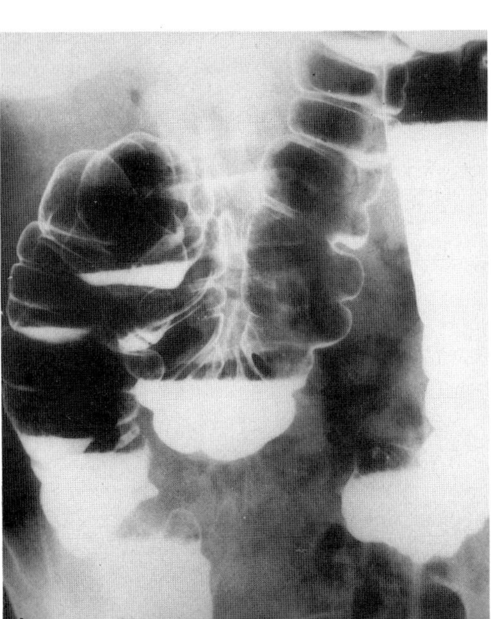

A

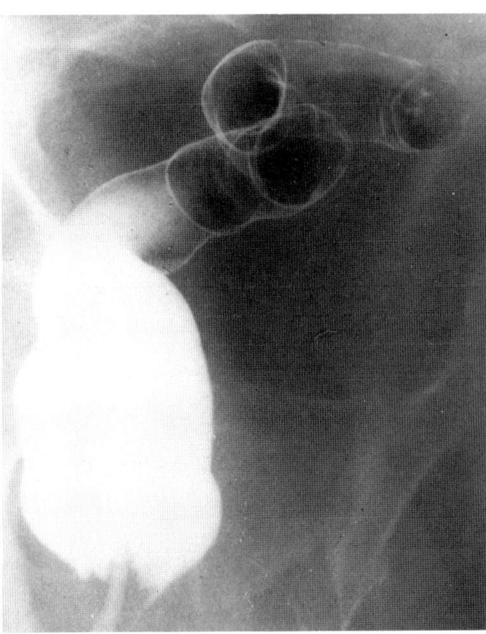

B

FIGURE 12.66. Colostomy. (A) Barium administered via the colostomy with edema of the ileocecal valve. (B) Administration of barium via the anus shows blind distal arm of the colon.

trast studies can show details of an ileocecal valve.

The *ileocecal valve* varies in its location and thickness, measuring 3–5 mm. In 7% of patients, the ileocecal valve is situated on the posterior wall of the cecum. The shape of the valve may be protruding, stellate, or oval (Fig. 12.67). When the cecum is either intentionally or unintentionally filled with only barium, differentiating the ileocecal valve from a neoplasm is still possible, since the terminal ileum enters the cecum symmetrically, in the center of a negative defect created by the valve (Fig. 12.68). The lips of the valve may be enlarged due to hypertrophy, edema, fat deposi-

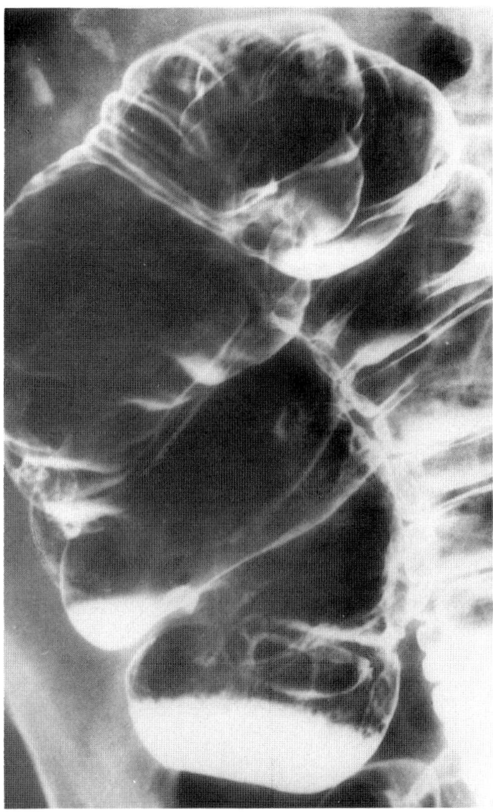

A

FIGURE 12.67. Ileocecal valve. (A) Stellate form. (*Figure continued on the following two pages.*)

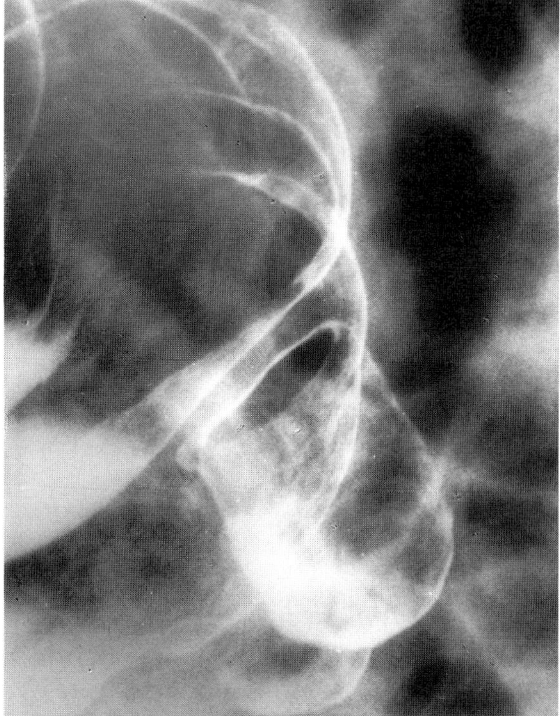

B

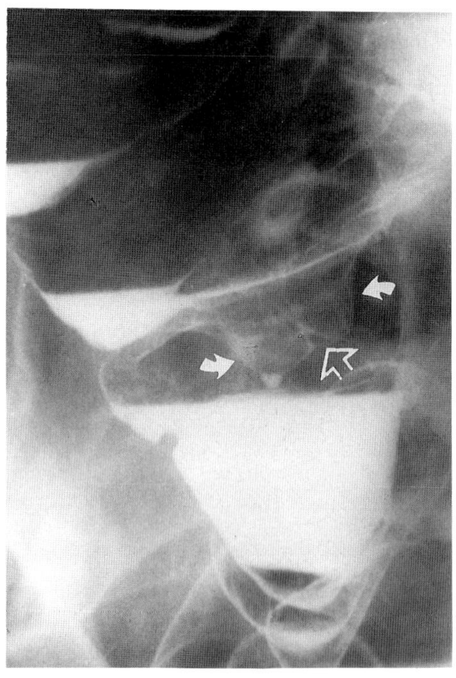

C

Figure 12.67 *continued.* Ileocecal valve. (B) Oval form. (C) Protruding form (arrows).

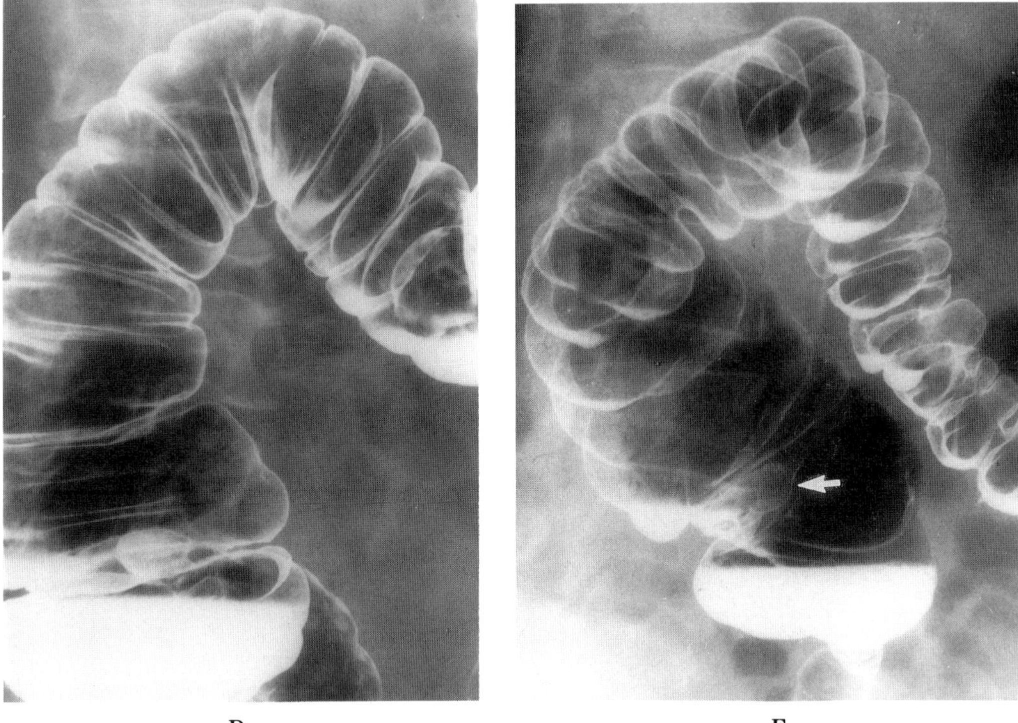

FIGURE 12.67 *continued.* Ileocecal valve. (D) Typical, most common form. (E) On the posterior lateral aspect of the large bowel (arrow).

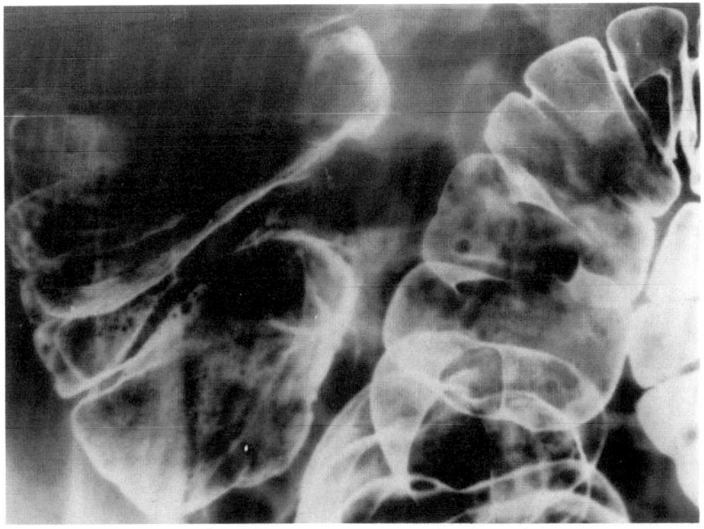

FIGURE 12.68. Normal ileocecal valve. Regular, symmetric, wedge-shaped defect. Terminal ileum demonstrated with air on double-contrast enema.

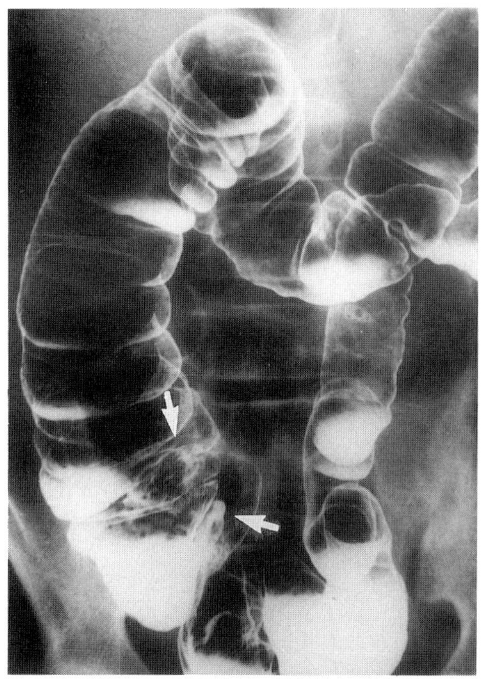
A

Figure 12.69. Carcinoma of the ileocecal valve. (A) Barium studies (arrows). (B) CT examination.

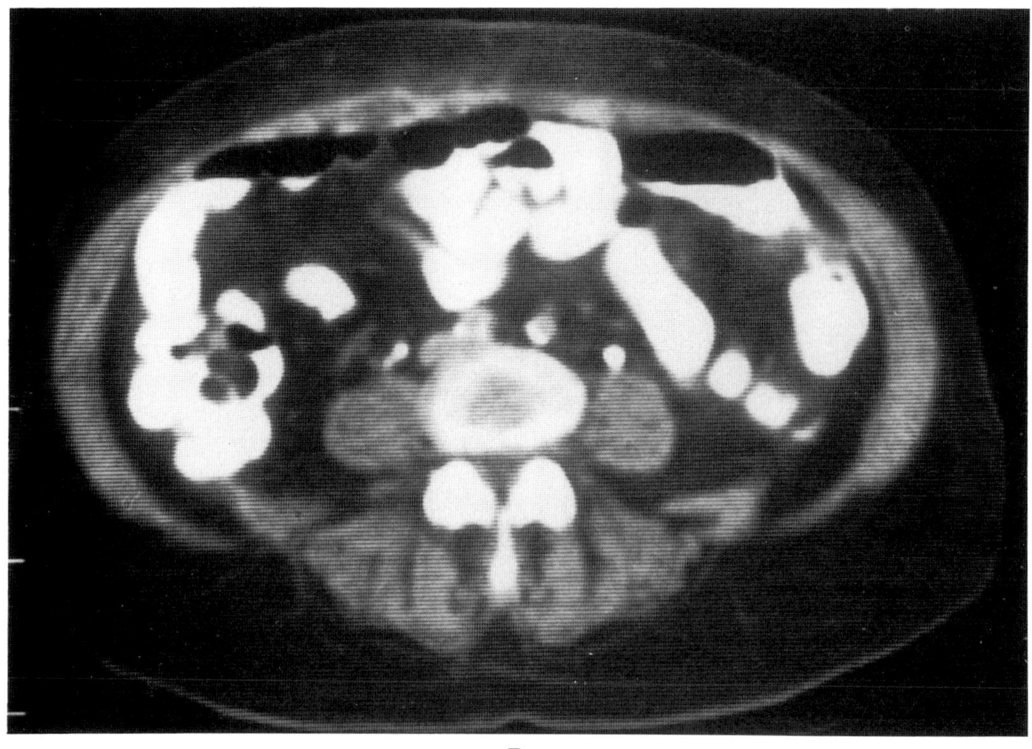
B

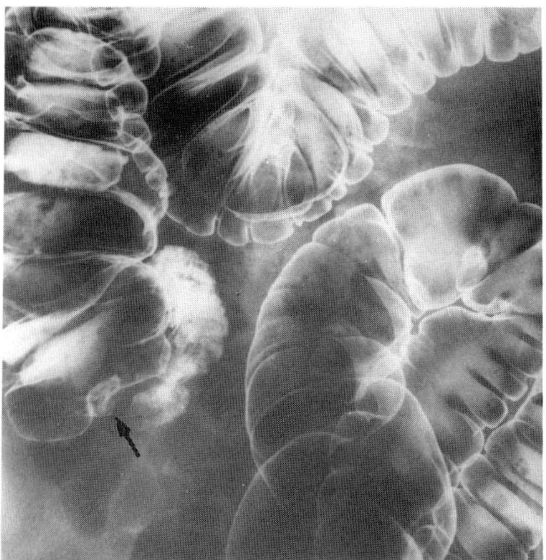

FIGURE 12.70. The cecum after appendectomy (arrow).

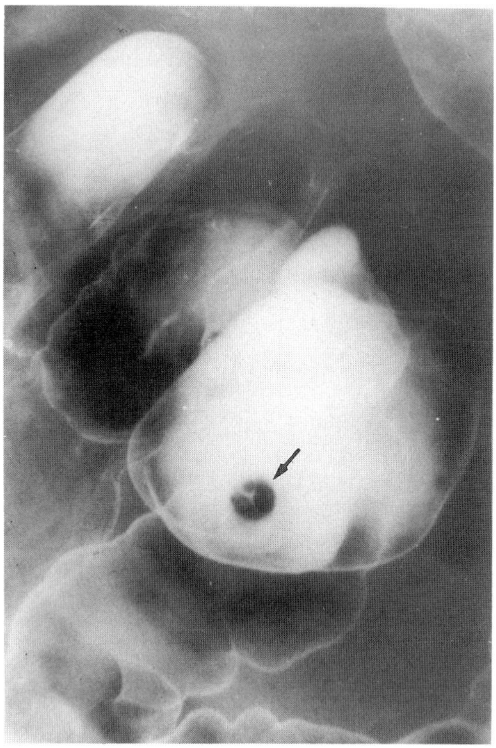

FIGURE 12.72. Ostium of the appendix (arrow).

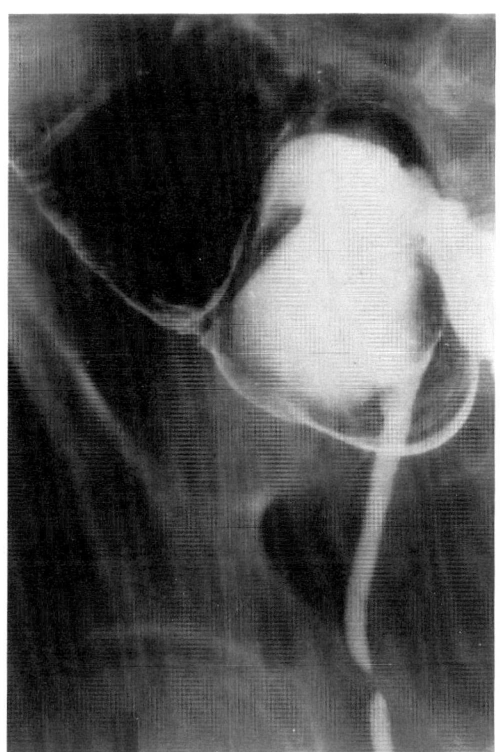

FIGURE 12.71. Very elongated appendix.

tion, or inflammation. *Lipomatosis* of the ileocecal valve is characterized by lobulated protrusions. Differentiation from neoplasm can be difficult, and similar changes may result from prolapse of the mucosa of the terminal ileum into the cecum. Approximately 2% of *adenocarcinomas* of the large bowel originate from the ileocecal valve, and are commonly polypoid in appearance (Fig. 12.69). *Carcinoid* of the valve may appear as an oval protrusion, or may be lobulated, assuming the morphology of a malignant lesion. A postappendectomy scar may appear as a neoplasm of the cecal floor (Fig. 12.70).

Failure of the *appendix* to fill with barium has no pathologic significance. The length of the appendix may vary considerably (Fig. 12.71). The direction of its course is important to note in case of perforation (Figs. 12.72–12.74). The normal appendix is commonly freely movable on palpation.

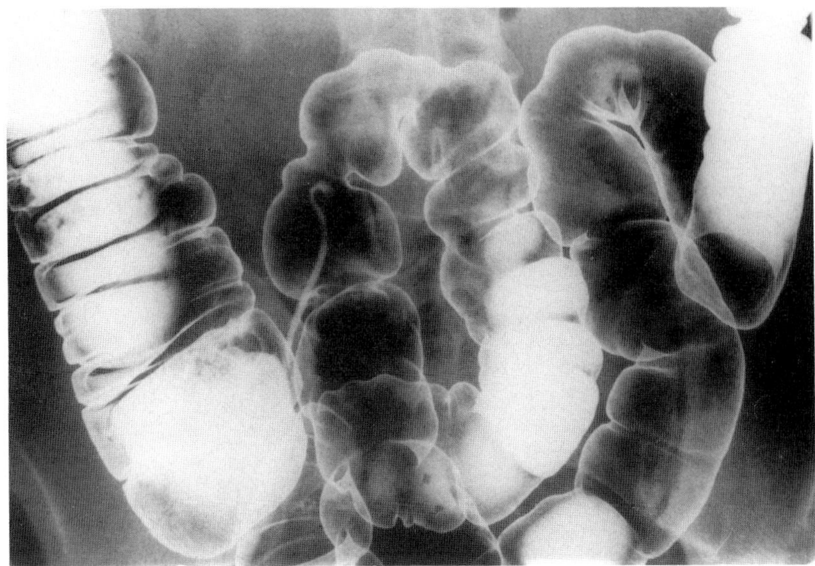

FIGURE 12.73. Elongated, cranially directed appendix. The most unfavorable position in case of perforation in appendicitis.

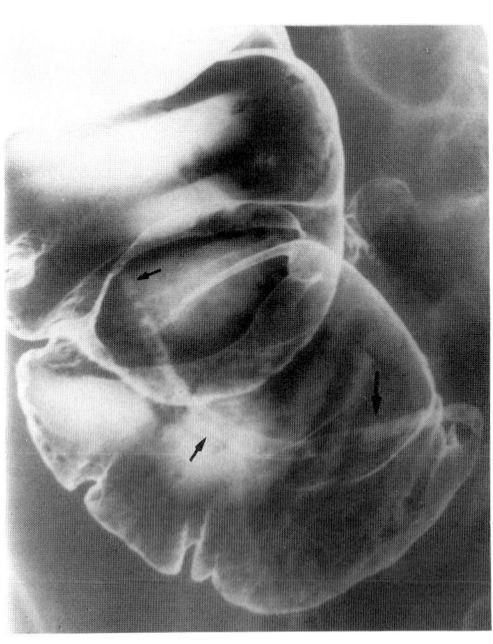

FIGURE 12.74. Retrocecal, laterally directed appendix (arrows).

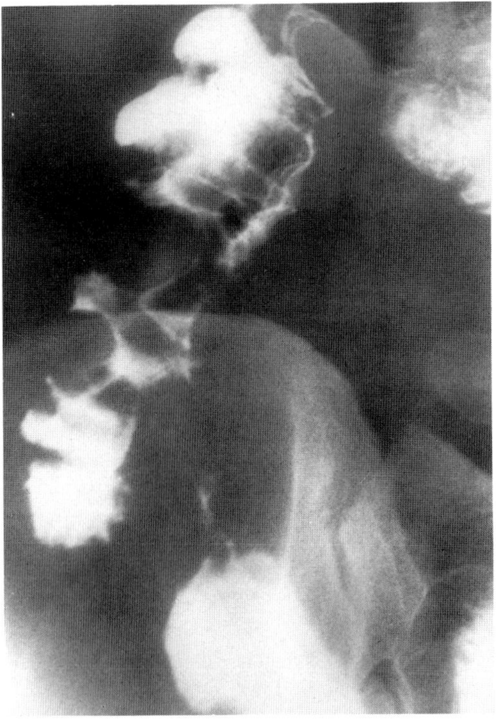

FIGURE 12.75. Tuberculosis of the ileocecal area resembling a neoplasm.

CHRONIC GRANULOMATOUS DISEASES OF THE ILEOCECAL AREA

Chronic Amebiasis

Acute amebiasis is not usually an indication for barium enema examination. Chronic amebiasis most frequently affects the ileocecal area and, in order of decreasing frequency, the ascending colon, rectum, and sigmoid colon. Mucosal infiltrations may transform into shallow ulcers, and then into deep ulcerations, penetrating up to the serosa with resultant fibrosis and scarring. Adhesions with adjacent intestinal loops follow fistulization. *Ameboma*, an amebic granuloma, is often cylindrical. Differentiation from Crohn's disease, tuberculosis, actinomycosis, and neoplasm may be difficult. Since they are responsive to medical treatment, amebomas are not surgically removed. The radiologic pattern of diffuse involvement of the large intestine resembles ulcerative colitis.

Tuberculosis

Enlargement of both solitary and aggregated lymphoid follicles is an early sign of tuberculosis, particularly when the terminal ileum is involved. An ulcerative form is characterized by deep longitudinal and transverse ulcerations. Polypoid growths mimicking a neoplasm are seen in a hyperplastic, pseudotumorous form (Fig. 12.75).

Actinomycosis

Actinomycosis of the colon is very rare. The ileocecal area is affected in almost all instances. Clinical and radiologic findings are similar to alimentary tract tuberculosis.

DIVERTICULA OF THE APPENDIX

The prevalence of appendiceal diverticulosis is 1.4% (Fig. 12.76). As a rule, these are acquired diverticula which rarely cause complications. Congenital appendiceal diverticula are solitary, and one hundred times less frequent than acquired. Complications of diverticula include diverticulitis, perforation, and bleeding. *Pseudomyxoma peritonei* can occur if an appendix is obstructed and perforates.

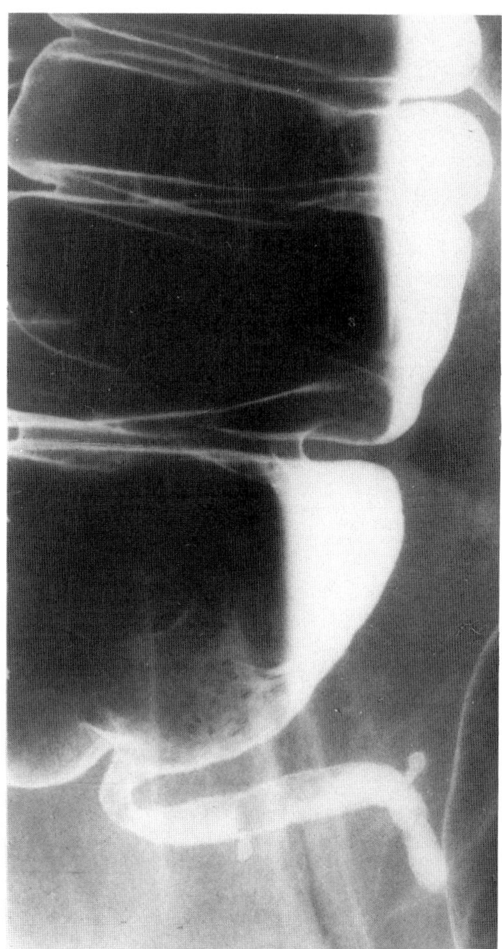

Figure 12.76. Diverticula of the appendix.

APPENDICITIS

Appendicitis may result from obstruction of the appendiceal lumen, secondary to edema, hyperplasia of lymphoid tissue, appendicoliths (Fig. 12.77), or an ingested foreign body. However, in a majority of cases, the etiology remains obscure. Radiologic symptoms may be helpful in establishing a diagnosis. On plain films, a gas-fluid level in the terminal ileum without significant bowel dilatation may result from local paresis. Gas-fluid levels in the cecum and terminal ileum, observed in only 15% of normal patients, can be demonstrated in 50% of patients with acute appendicitis. Under normal circumstances, gas may fill an appendix

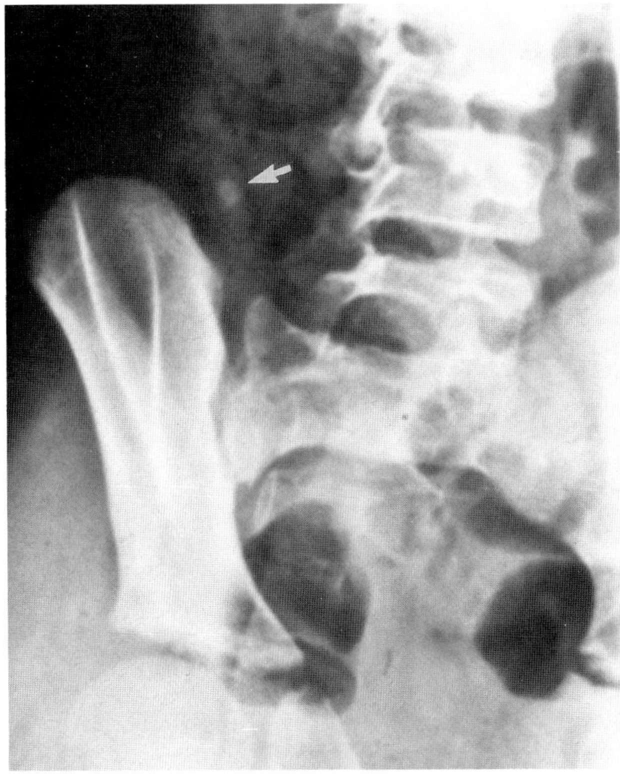

Figure 12.77. Appendicolith at the ostium of an appendix with an elevated cecum (arrow).

only transiently. A subhepatically positioned appendix may be filled with gas without underlying pathology. However, a gangrenous unperforated appendix can be distended by gas and may contain an air-fluid level in the lumen.

Opinions differ in regard to the radiologic diagnosis of chronic appendicitis. Failure of the appendix to fill with barium, immobility of the appendix on palpation, with segmentation of the contrast column, or prolonged retention of barium, might imply chronic appendicitis. However, none of these signs is very specific.

The position of an appendix corresponds to the position of the cecum during embryonic development. In 70% of cases the appendix is intraperitoneal and directed toward the pouch of Douglas. When the cecum has descended incompletely, the appendix is retroperitoneal, in front of the right kidney (Figs. 4.61 and 12.74). In such cases appendicitis can spread to the kidney region. A retrocecal appendix directed cephalad may be intraperitoneal. More than half of retrocecal appendices are not freely movable on palpation.

Graded compression US demonstrates a distended, noncompressible appendix whose diameter is larger than 7 mm in acute appendicitis (Fig. 12.78). Computed tomography fails to visualize a narrowed appendix, unless surrounded by abundant adipose tissue. In complicated appendicitis, such as with abscess or phlegmon, CT findings are characterized by a thickening of the appendiceal wall and of the mesentery together with possible displacement of the cecum. The most common cause for any intraperitoneal abscess is complicated appendicitis. Appendiceal abscesses are commonly located pericecally (Fig. 12.79). Computed tomography can locate extraserosal inflammatory masses in the alimentary canal and in the mesentery. Phlegmonae and abscesses in unexpected locations such as in the retroperitoneal space and in the mesentery may also result from complicated appendicitis.

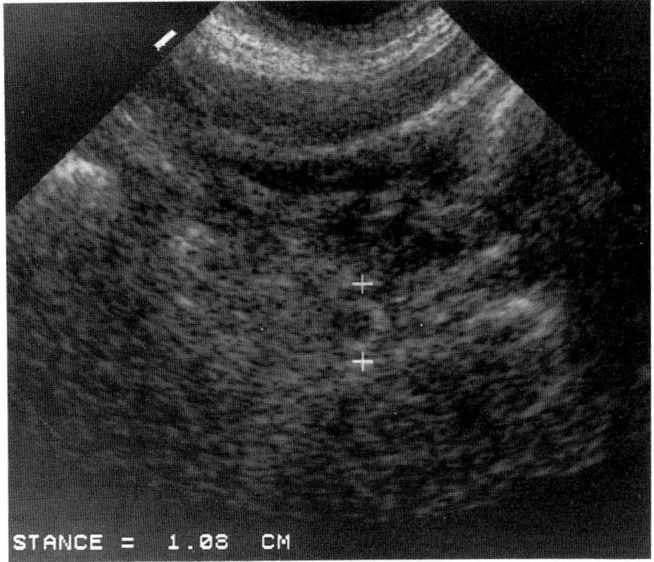

Figure 12.78. Typical "bulls-eye" ultrasound appearance of acute appendicitis (cursors). (Courtesy of W.L. Wells, MD, Louisiana State University, New Orleans.)

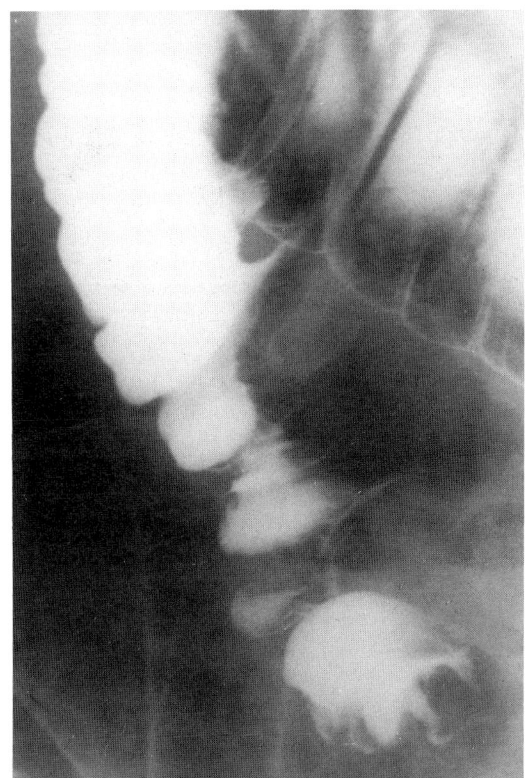

Figure 12.79. Large pericolonic appendiceal abscess compresses the cecum and the ascending colon.

MUCOCELE OF THE APPENDIX

The appendiceal lumen can be extremely distended and filled with sterile mucus. Fibrosis pervades the appendiceal wall, and, when encrusted with calcium salts, the appendix may be visible as a ring shadow on plain films. Prevalence of such an appendiceal mucocele was merely 0.15% in approximately 30,000 autopsies. Mucoceles most probably result from appendiceal obstruction, associated with excessive mucus secretion or an appendiceal cystadenoma. The appendix fails to fill with barium and may create an impression on the floor of the cecum. Differential diagnosis includes intussusception of the appendix, abscess, and neoplasm.

Pseudomyxoma peritonei can result from a mucinous ovarian carcinoma or from perforation of an appendiceal mucocele. Epithelial cells implant on the peritoneal surface and secrete gelatinous ascites. Dense gelatinous collections can cover the entire peritoneal surface and may fill the peritoneal cavity.

INTUSSUSCEPTION OF THE APPENDIX

A coiled-spring sign is characteristic of barium extending between the intussusceptum and the intussuscipiens. However, similar findings may also be observed with inversion of an appendiceal stump, mucocele and carcinoma of the appendix, endometriosis, and acute appendicitis. The majority of appendiceal invaginations into the cecum are asymptomatic and transient (Fig. 12.80).

NEOPLASMS

The most common polypoid lesions in the terminal ileum are inflammations, whereas in the cecum these are neoplasms. However, dysgammaglobulinemia or agammaglobulinemia

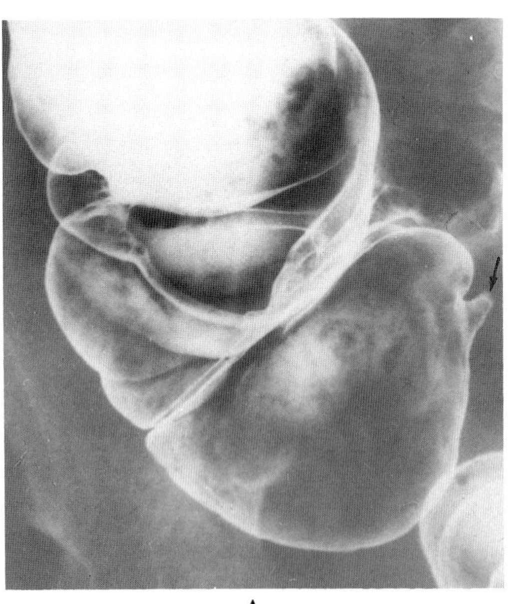

A

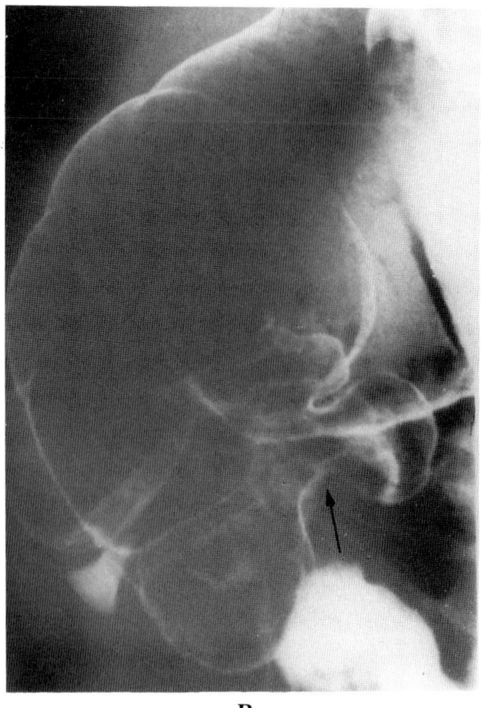

B

Figure 12.80. (A) Appendiceal stump. (B) Invagination of the appendix (arrow) resembles a tumor at the tip of the cecum.

may present as follicular lymphoid hyperplasia of the terminal ileum. Polypoid growths are more difficult to diagnose in the cecum than in other sections of the large bowel, since protrusion or enlargement of the ileocecal valve caused by various etiologies may mimic a neoplasm (Table 12.5). Retrograde prolapse of the ileocecal valve is not pathologic, but may also radiographically resemble a neoplasm. Carcinoma of the ileocecal valve is not common (Fig. 12.69). Cecal carcinoma commonly extends through the bowel wall and spreads into regional lymph nodes. A polypoid neoplasm of the cecal floor can appear as an iceberg emerging from an accumulation of barium on a double-contrast study with the patient in the upright position (Fig. 12.81). Intestinal lymphoma is more common in the terminal ileum than in the cecum; in the latter it is usually polypoid. A polypoid growth of the cecal floor can be an appendiceal stump or mucocele, a neoplasm, tuberculosis, or endometriosis (Table 12.5). However, obliteration of the cecal lumen results, in the majority of cases, from a malignant tumor. Alimentary canal carcinoids most frequently grow in the appendix and are not likely to metastasize.

Metastases to the ileocecal area, such as those of melanoma, may occur (Fig. 12.82).

TABLE 12.5. TUMOROUS GROWTHS OF THE ILEOCECAL REGION

Benign
Retrograde prolapse of the ileocecal valve
Appendiceal stump
Inverted appendiceal stump
Ileocecal intussusception
Appendiceal mucocele
Amebiasis and actinomycosis
Periappendiceal and pericecal abscesses
Benign neoplasm
Malignant
Carcinoma
Carcinoid
Lymphoma
Villous adenoma
Metastatic disease

OBSTRUCTIONS OF THE ILEOCECAL AREA

Ileocecal intussusception is the most common cause of obstruction in the ileocecal area of children. It may result from enlarged lymph-

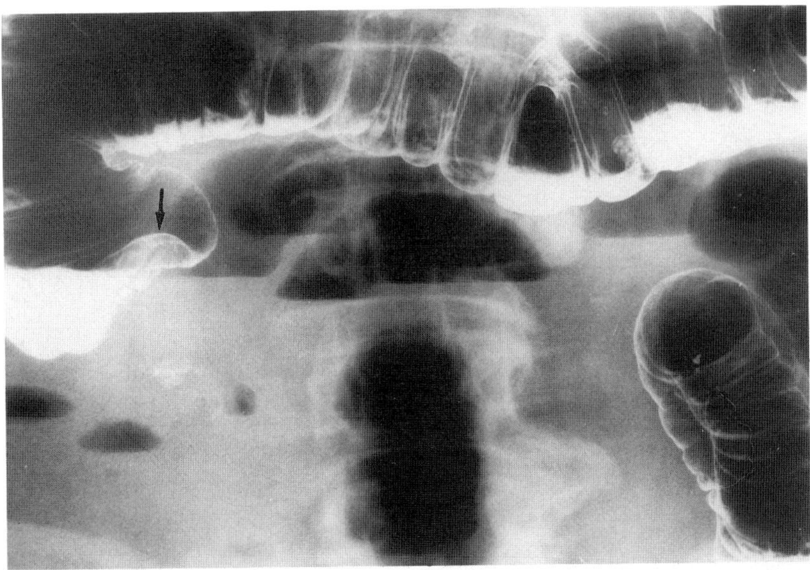

FIGURE 12.81. Carcinoma of the floor of the cecum (arrow) results in proximal mechanical obstruction.

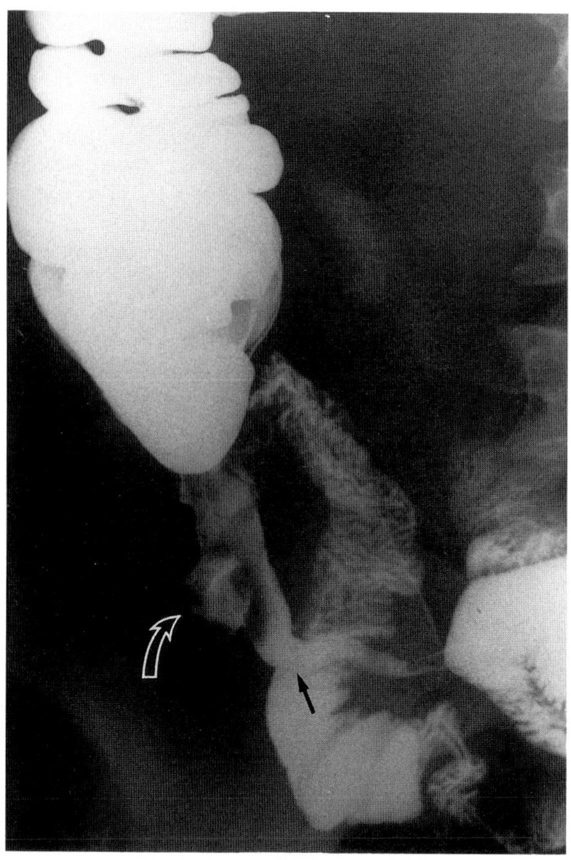

A

Figure 12.82. Malignant melanoma metastatic to the cecum. (A) Barium studies demonstrate narrowing of the cecum with a large ulceration (open arrow). Tip of the cecum (black arrow). (B) CT examination. (Used by permission, Plavsic B, Robinson AE. Variations in gastrointestinal melanoma metastases. Acta Radiol. Diagn. 1990;31: 493.)

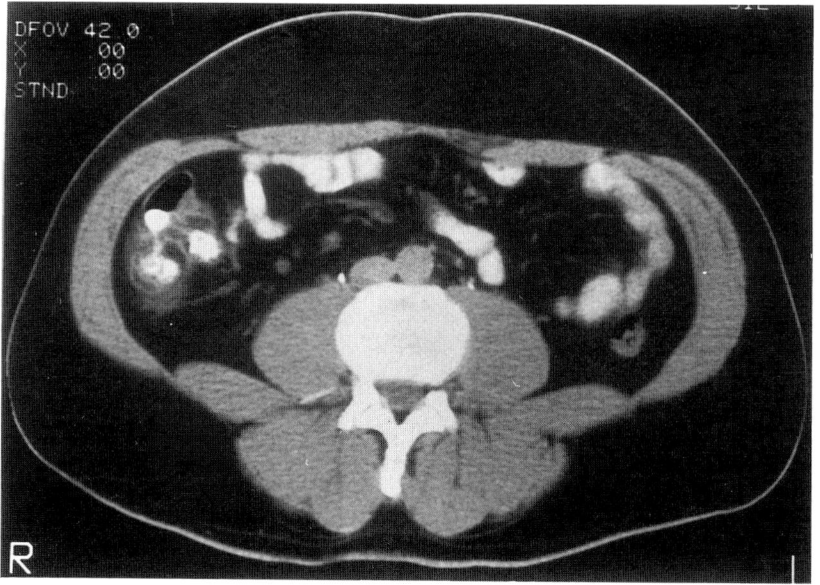

B

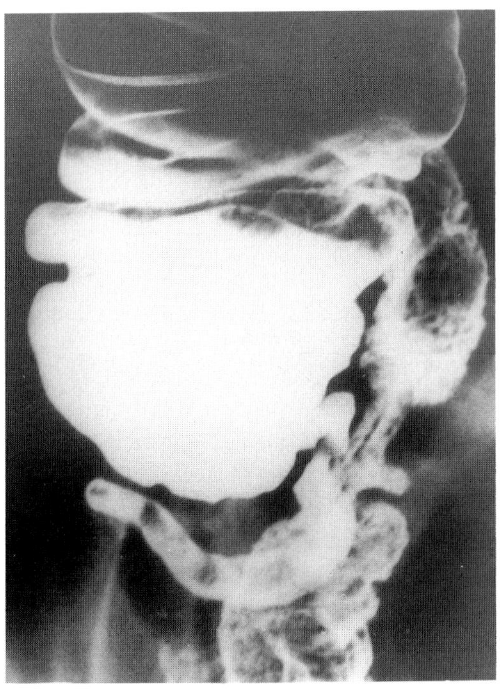

A

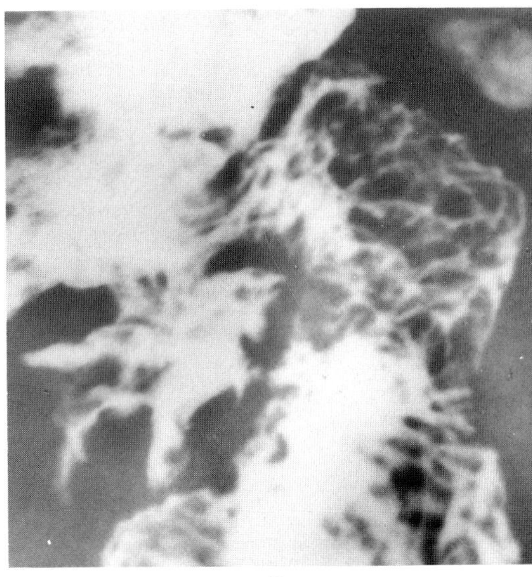

B

FIGURE 12.83. Enlarged lymphoid follicles in the terminal ileum. (A) Crohn's disease. Air bubbles in the appendix. (B) Immunoproliferative disorder.

oid tissue (Fig. 12.83). However, in adults, obstruction is most frequently the result of a neoplasm, mainly carcinoma and lymphoma. Obstructions may also be due to stricture from inflammatory diseases such as Crohn's disease.

VOLVULUS OF THE RIGHT COLON

Torsion of the cecum and/or proximal colon up to the hepatic flexure is due to volvulus of the right colon. Radiologic confirmation is important, since unrecognized right colon volvulus has been proved to be fatal. In contrast to sigmoid colon volvulus, which can be usually reduced by flexible endoscopy or contrast enema, right colon volvulus commonly requires surgical relief.

Cecal volvulus accounts for less than 5% of alimentary canal obstructions. Approximately 10% of large intestine volvulus occurs in the right colon. Demonstration of a cecum distended by gas is important and this can readily be done from plain films of the abdomen. A right colon volvulus is most likely to occur in the third and fourth decade of life, and results from failed fixation of the right colon to the posterior abdominal wall. This anomaly has been verified in 15% of an unselected population. Cecal volvulus may also result from insufficient air aspiration during colonoscopy. There are three types of right colon volvulus (Diagram 12.5A,B and C).

Most commonly, the cecum is in the left hypochondriac region or epigastric region (Figs. 12.84 and 12.85). Gas or gas-fluid levels are seen in the cecum and terminal ileum. In the supine position, the distended right colon is in the left portion of the abdomen, with the loop appearing "open" medially. In sigmoid colon volvulus, the loop is, in contrast, located more centrally, and is "closed," resembling a coffee bean (Diagram 12.5D and E).

When the right colon is twisted medially and anteriorly, it may be dilated to a width of more than 10 cm (Fig. 12.86). This is called *cecal ileus* and is followed by a cecal perforation rate of 20%. The duration of distension is a more important factor in the development of

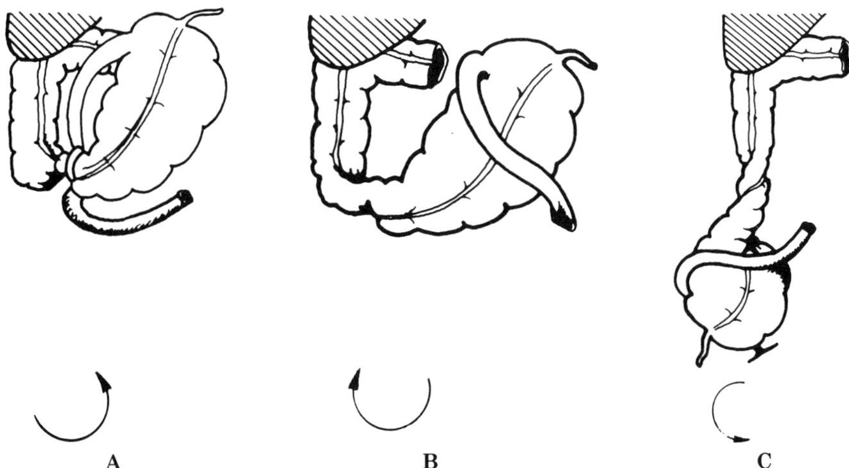

DIAGRAM 12.5. (A,B,C) Forms of right colon volvulus.

perforation than the extent. Cecal ileus is not merely a result of mechanical obstruction, but is a combination of paresis and mechanical obstruction of a mobile, partially twisted cecum.

Right colon volvulus often results in obstruction of the terminal ileum. Without coexisting peritonitis, signs of small bowel obstruction are usually not present in sigmoid colon volvulus. However, when an ileocecal valve is incompetent, or sigmoid volvulus is long-lasting, it can be accompanied by distension of the small intestine.

The diagnosis of volvulus in any section of the large intestine can be confirmed by a barium enema. The contrast column narrows and does not propagate into more proximal segments at the site of torsion. With incomplete volvulus, barium may penetrate into a twisted intestinal loop. Reduction of a cecal volvulus may occur following repeated barium enemas. Other obstructions of the left colon may result in cecal distension. In addition, barium enema readily separates right colon volvulus from a gas distended stomach.

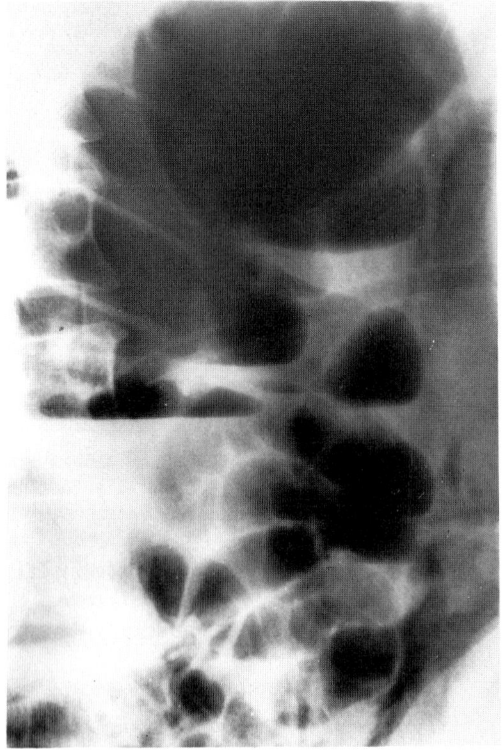

FIGURE 12.84. Volvulus of the right colon. Unfixed cecum and proximal ascending colon are in the left hypochondriac region. Gas distended loops of small bowel. (See Diagram 12.5A.)

RADIOLOGY OF THE RECTUM

For years, rectal and anal canal pathology was assessed by digitorectal, direct proctoscopic, and endoscopic examinations. However,

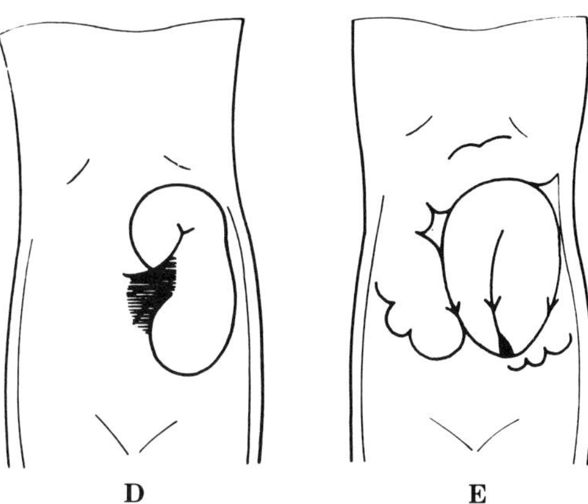

DIAGRAM 12.5 *continued.* Differentiating (D) right colon volvulus from (E) sigmoid volvulus. (Used by permission, Frimann-Dahl J. Volvulus of the right colon. Acta Radiol. 1954;41:141.)

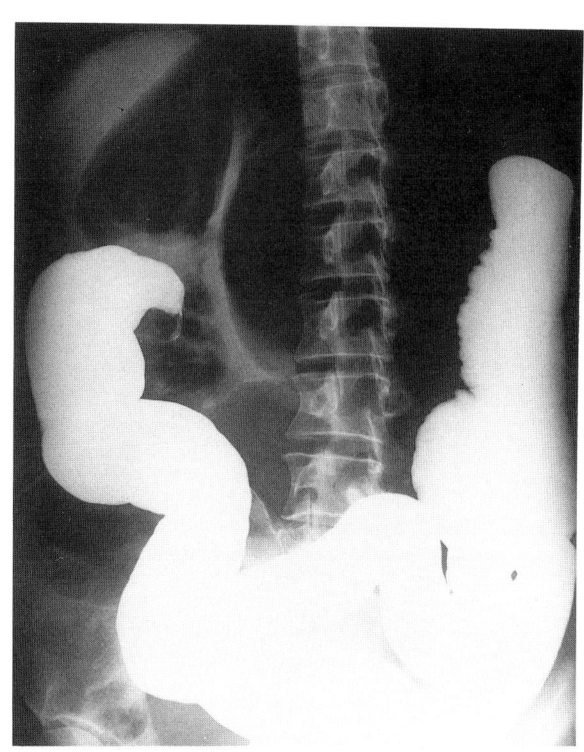

FIGURE 12.85. Barium enema of right colon volvulus. (See Diagram 12.5B.)

double-contrast studies allow excellent demonstration of the rectum. The results of a double-contrast study do not differ significantly from those of endoscopy. The large volume of the lumen makes single-contrast studies unsuitable for examination of the rectum, since most of the X-rays will be absorbed even if a diluted barium suspension is used (Fig. 12.87).

The presacral or retrorectal space, between the posterior wall of rectum and the anterior aspect of the sacrum, is normally 2–15 mm wide on films taken with an X-ray tube–film

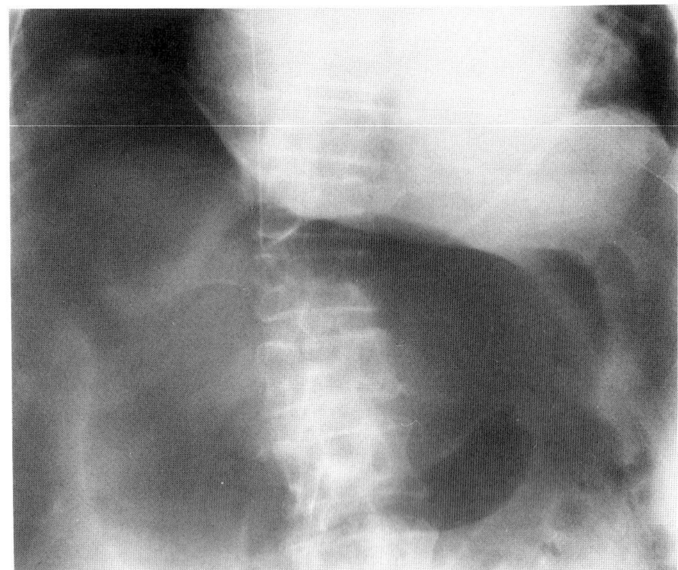

FIGURE 12.86. Volvulus of the right colon. Significant distension of the cecum. Supine plain abdominal film. (See Diagram 12.5C.)

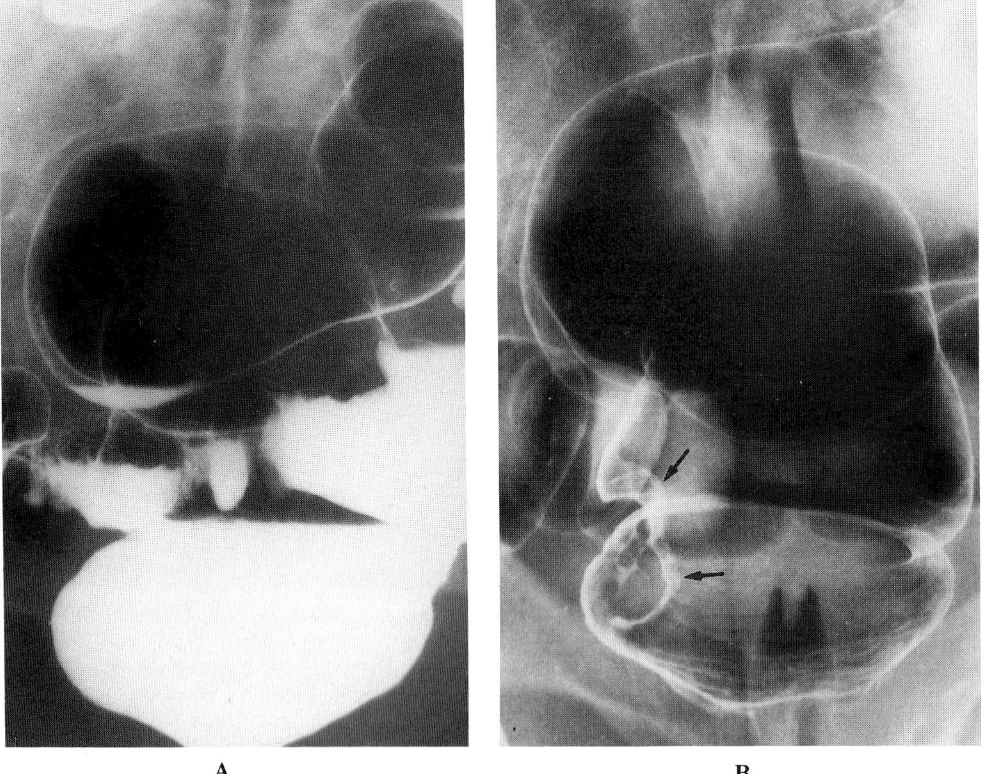

A B

FIGURE 12.87. (A) Rectum filled with barium appears normal. (B) Double-contrast examination reveals a large carcinoma (arrows).

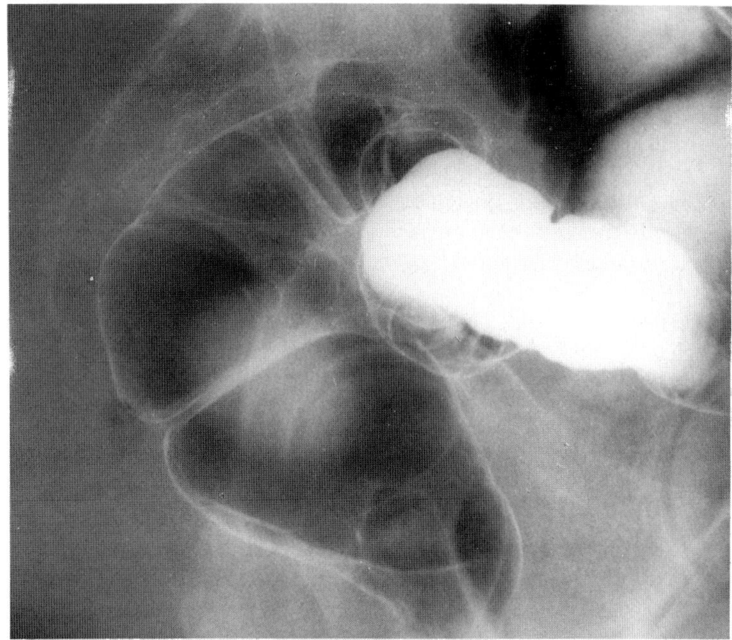

FIGURE 12.88. Normal retrorectal (presacral) space.

distance of 2 m (Fig. 12.88). A 15–20 mm width should arouse suspicion of a pathologic process, and values above 20 mm are considered absolutely abnormal. An abnormally large space is not a specific finding and may result from inflammatory edema of presacral adipose tissue, rectal carcinoma or other malignancies, enlarged lymph nodes, or thrombosis of the inferior vena cava.

The pathology of the rectum does not differ morphologically from that of other sections of the colon. However, a sturdy, complete, longitudinal muscular coating makes rectal diverticula (Fig. 12.89) an almost unknown entity. There is a predilection for certain pathologies, such as ulcerative colitis or carcinoma.

RECTAL HEMORRHOIDS

Hemorrhoids are dilated veins of the anal and perianal venous plexuses in the inferior mesenteric and the internal iliac veins. Dilated veins in the inferior hemorrhoidal plexuses are referred to as external hemorrhoids, whereas internal hemorrhoids are widenings in the superior hemorrhoidal plexus. Both can result from

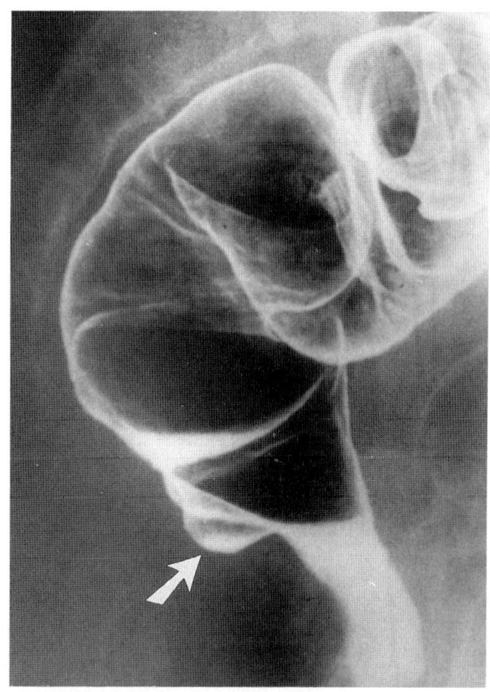

FIGURE 12.89. Diverticulum (arrow) on the posterior aspect of the rectal wall.

long-standing increased venous pressure as the result of obstipation, pregnancy, or portal hypertension. Anal columns of the anal canal and distal rectum consist primarily of hemorrhoidal veins. Internal hemorrhoids located in this region interrupt continuity of longitudinal folds in the anal canal but do not alter the mucosal relief in the manner that a neoplasm would.

Hemorrhoids significantly affect more than 3% of the adult population, the middle-aged and elderly being more involved. Internal hemorrhoids are diagnosed by digitorectal examination, endoscopy, or double-contrast enema. On double-contrast studies they present as solitary or multiple, spherical, oval, or, less often, serpiginous formations (Fig. 12.90). They change shape and size with changes in intra-abdominal pressure.

Hemorrhoids are often the cause of anal bleeding. Radiologic examination is utilized to exclude coincidental lesions such as colorectal carcinoma.

IDIOPATHIC ULCERATIVE PROCTITIS

Ulcerative proctitis closely resembles ulcerative colitis but is confined to the rectum and only occasionally affects the sigmoid colon in continuity. Clinical signs tend to be milder and progression is slower compared to ulcerative colitis. The lesions of colitis and proctitis are identical; hyperemia of the rectal mucosa, resulting in a granular appearance, is followed by ulcers of various dimensions, from small, rose-thorn ulcerations, to deep transmural ulcerations. However, ulcerations do not often penetrate deeper than the main muscular coat (Fig. 12.91). Transverse rectal folds frequently

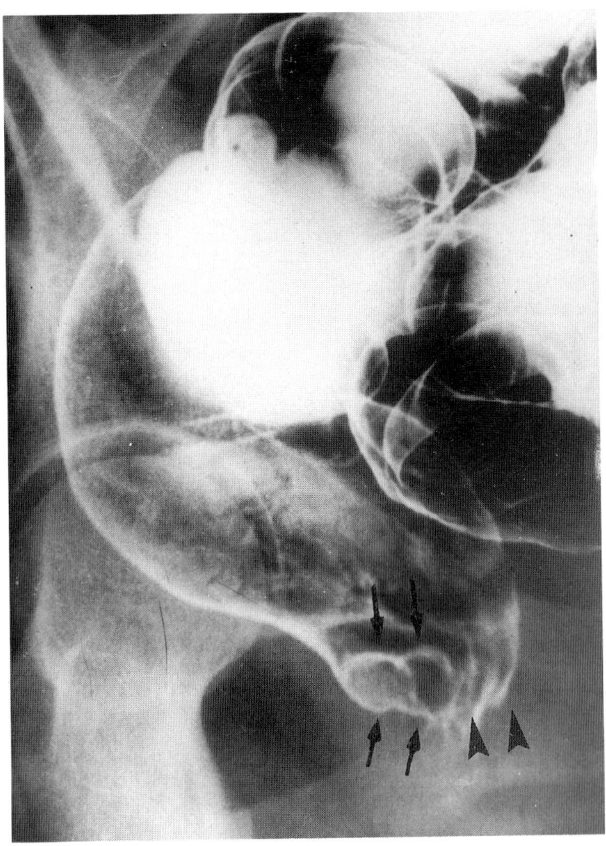

FIGURE 12.90. Internal hemorrhoids (arrows). Anal columns are also seen (arrowheads).

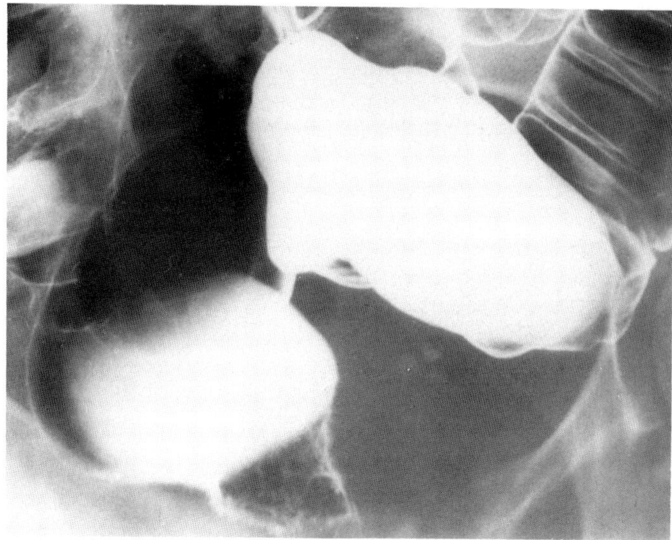

A

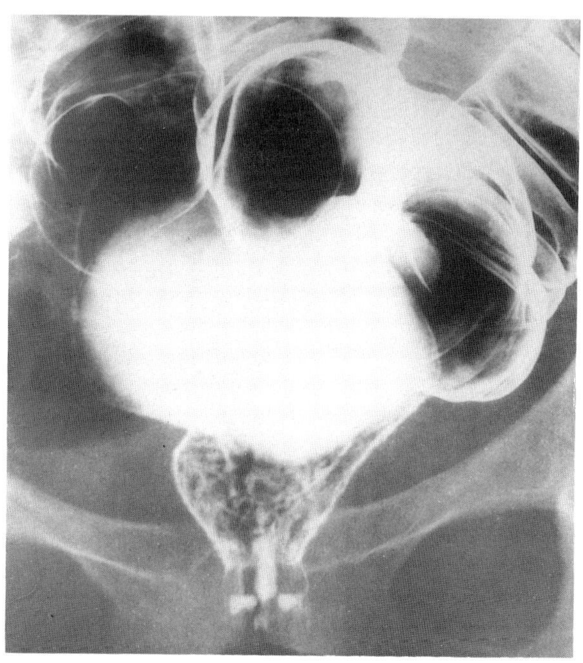

B

FIGURE 12.91. Ulcerative proctitis. (A) Faded transverse folds of the rectum. Irregular, nodular mucosal surface with small rose-thorn ulcers. (B) Granular mucosal surface of the rectum without ulcers.

vanish. Polypoid hyperplastic growth of the remaining mucosa may mimic polyps of other etiologies. Narrowing of the rectum occurs in the late stages. However, the natural history of ulcerative proctitis is unpredictable.

NEOPLASMS OF THE RECTUM

Barium enema is important for the diagnosis and localization of rectal neoplasms. They can appear 2–10 cm more proximal on double-contrast studies than on proctoscopy. Measurements of the anal canal length are also important for surgery. All of the macroscopic types of gastrointestinal polyps and carcinomas (annular, polypoid, and ulcerative) occur in the rectum as well (Figs. 12.92–12.95). In addition, cloacogenic carcinoma, a rare lesion, arises from the anal ductus, a transitional cloacogenic remnant (Fig. 12.96). These neoplasms are situated in the distal rectum and may represent

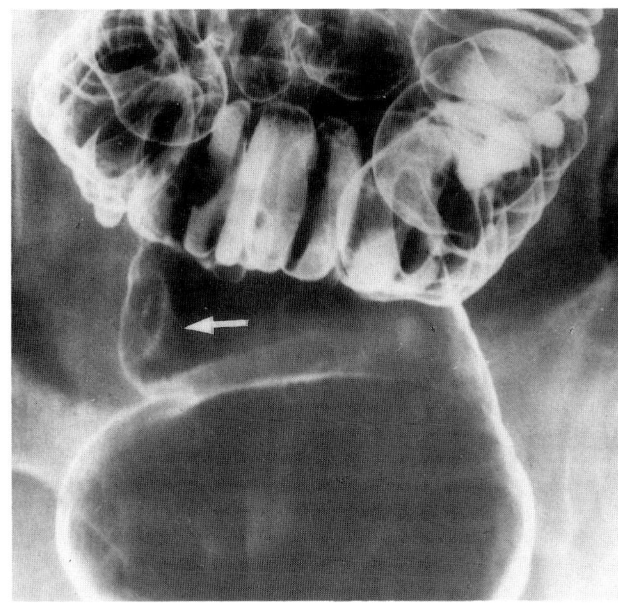

Figure 12.92. Sessile rectal polyp resembles a hat in the oblique projection (arrow).

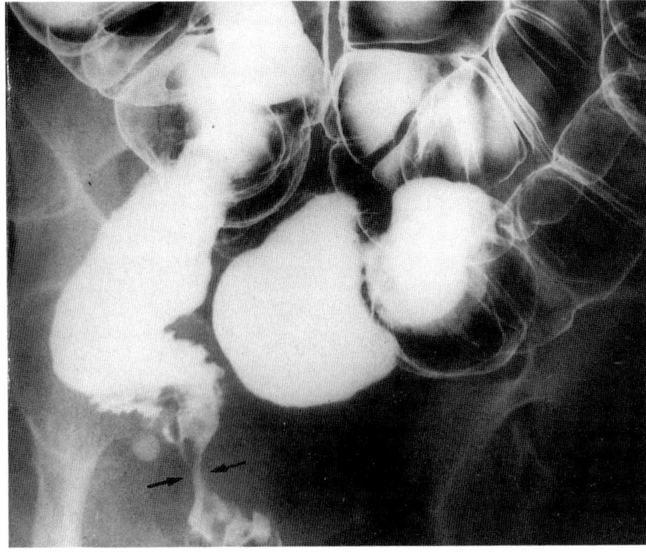

Figure 12.93. Annular carcinoma of the rectum. (A) Double-contrast barium enema (arrows).

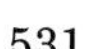

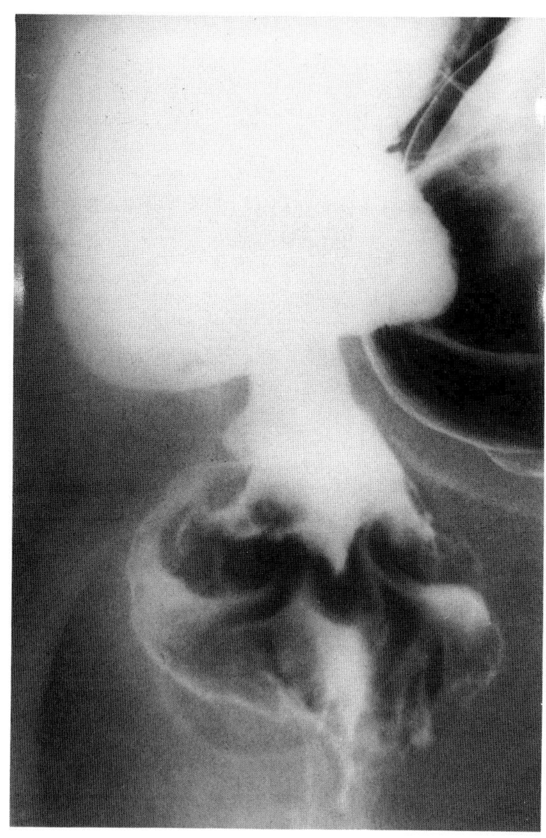

Figure 12.93 *continued.* Annular carcinoma of the rectum. (B) Typical appearance. Stenosis may result in inability to evacuate excess barium for a double-contrast study. (C) CT examination.

B

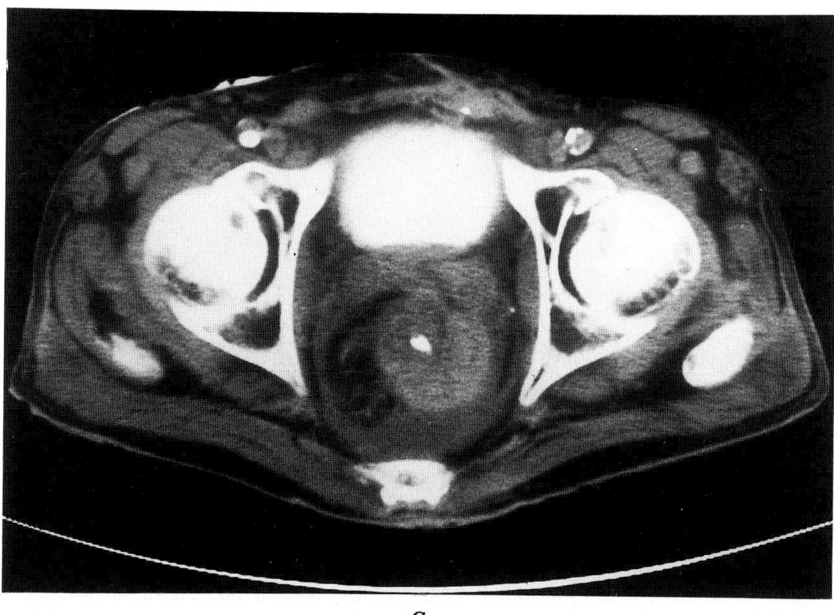

C

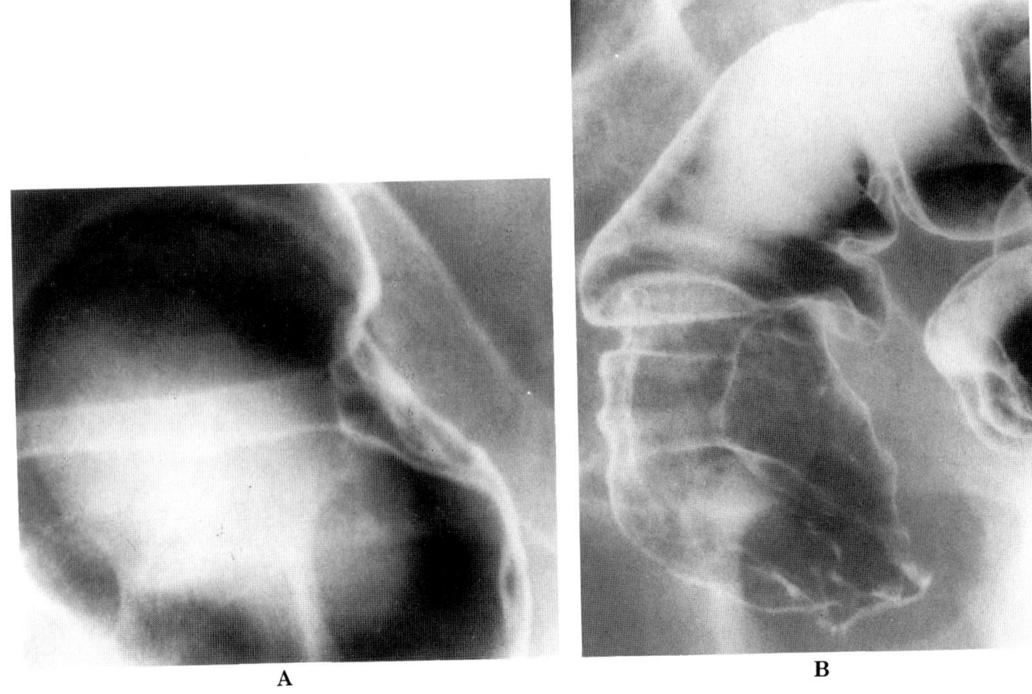

Figure 12.94. (A) and (B) Polypoid rectal carcinoma.

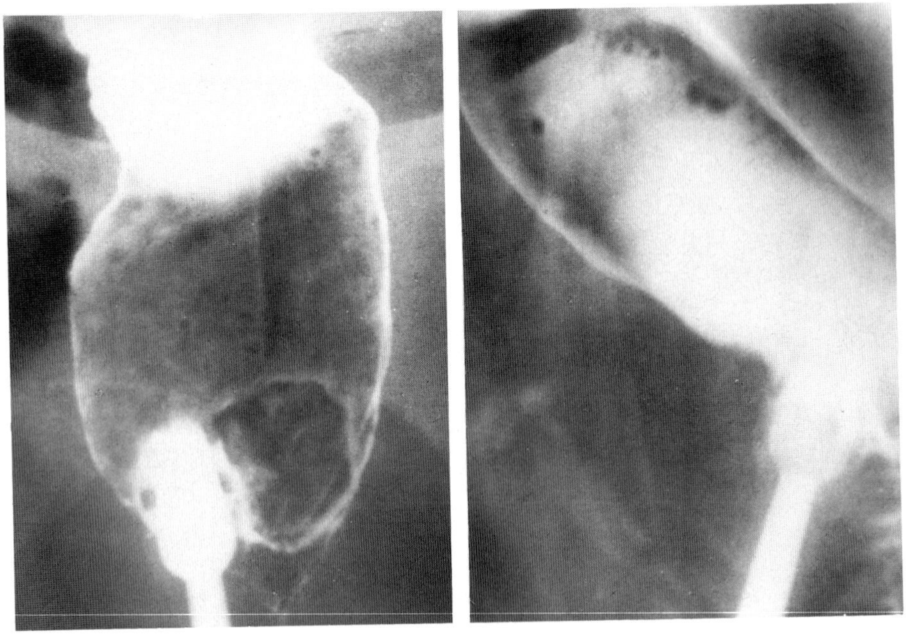

Figure 12.95. Carcinoma of the anterior aspect of the rectum demonstrated in P-A and profile projection.

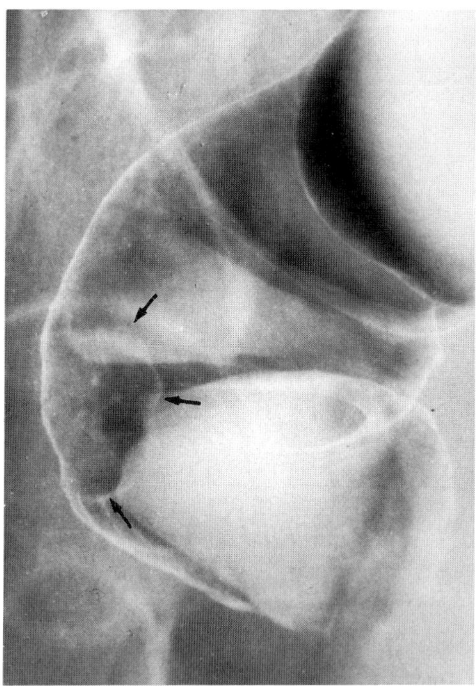

FIGURE 12.96. Cloacogenic carcinoma (arrows).

polypoid or plaque-like masses. Like adenocarcinoma and lymphoma, cloacogenic carcinoma may widen the presacral space.

The rectum and adjacent structures can be well demonstrated by CT studies after anal air insufflation, with or without oral administration of a positive contrast medium. Magnetic resonance imaging also yields good results in visualizing the rectum.

Rectal *carcinoids* are rounded neoplasms with a better prognosis than carcinoma (Fig. 12.97).

Neoplasms like lipoma and other benign mesenchymal tumors are very rare and can be readily demonstrated by CT (Fig. 12.98).

Lymphomas often occupy longer sections of the rectum and present as bulky masses infiltrating the rectal wall and protruding into the lumen (Fig. 12.99).

Metastatic neoplasms most frequently spread into the rectum by direct invasion from adjacent anatomic structures (Fig. 12.100). Conversely, primary rectal neoplasms may infiltrate adjacent organs.

Anal papillae, resulting from inflammation, are smooth, polypoid masses arising from the

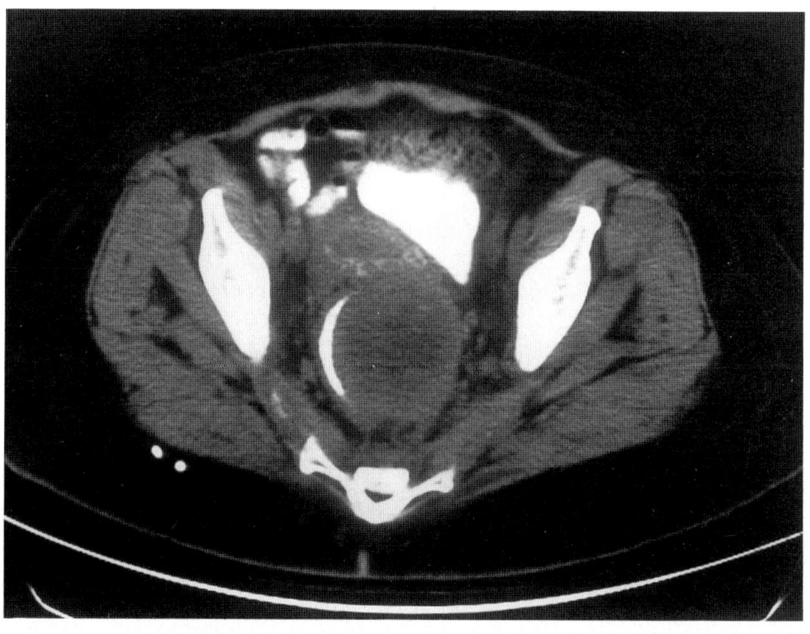

FIGURE 12.97. Carcinoid of the rectum. CT examination.

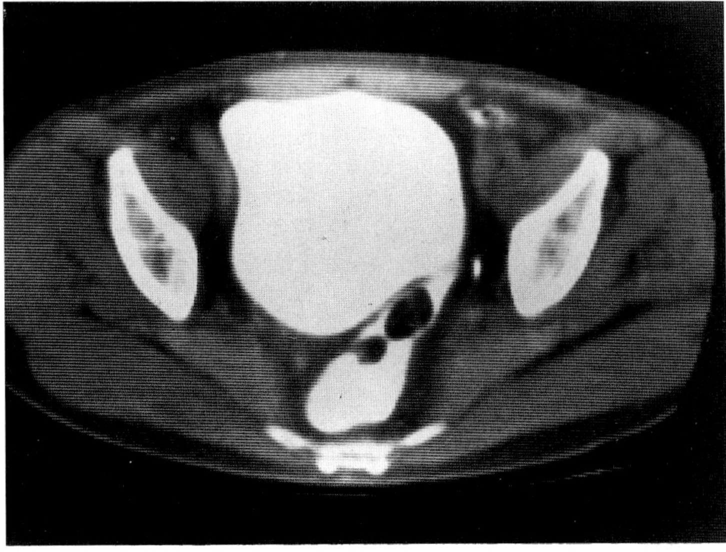

FIGURE 12.98. Lipomas of the sigmoid colon and rectum. CT examination.

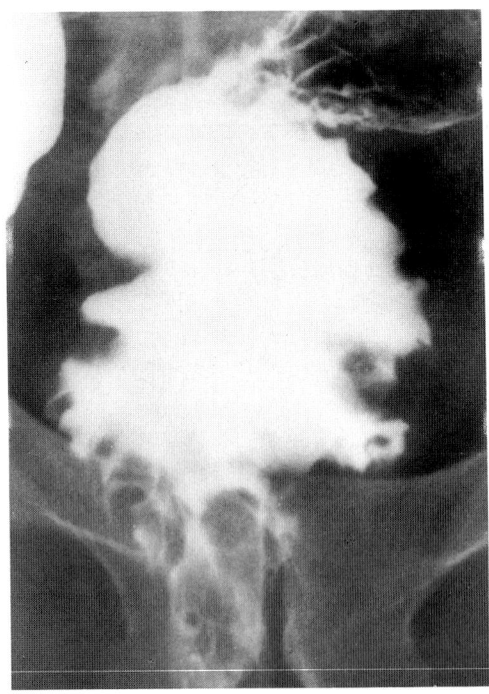

FIGURE 12.99. Lymphoma of the rectum. Rigidity of the wall interfered with evacuation of excess barium.

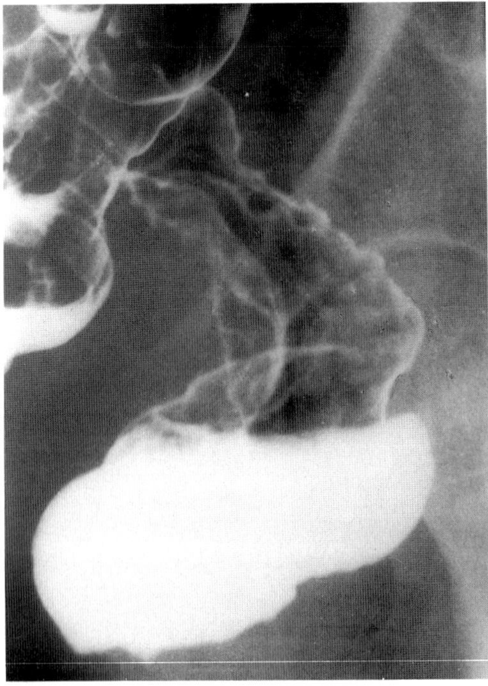

FIGURE 12.100. Ovarian carcinoma infiltrating the proximal rectum and the distal sigmoid colon.

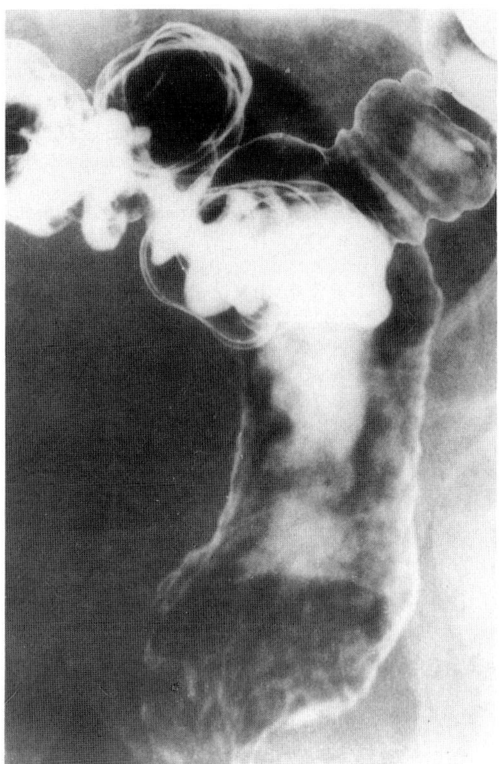

FIGURE 12.101. Chronic radiation injury to the rectum. Stenosis, loss of compliance of the wall, and mucosal irregularities.

base of the rectal columns, and may mimic polypoid carcinomas or hemorrhoids.

Since it is immobile, the rectum may be injured by external beam radiation of adjacent malignant neoplasms. Early changes are characterized by mucosal edema and small ulcerations. In a chronic phase, progressive narrowing of the lumen may occur due to fibrosis (Fig. 12.101).

Bibliography

Agha FP, Francis JR, Simms SM. Cystic lymphangioma of the colon. AJR. 1983;141:709.

Almy TP. Diverticular disease of the colon—the new look. Gastroenterology. 1965;49:109.

Bacon HE, Lowell EJ, Trimpi HD. Villous papillomas of the colon and rectum. Surgery. 1954;35:77.

Baker SR, Alterman DD. False-negative barium enema in patients with sigmoid cancer and coexistent diverticula. Gastrointest Radiol. 1985;10:171.

Balikian JR, Uthman SM, Khorui NF. Intestinal amebiasis. AJR. 1974;122:245.

Balthazar EJ. Congenital positional anomalies of the colon: radiographic diagnosis and clinical implications; abnormalities of fixation. Gastrointest Radiol. 1977;2:49.

Balthazar EJ. Carcinoid tumors of the alimentary tract, I: radiologic diagnosis. Gastrointest Radiol. 1978;3:1978.

Balthazar EJ, Megibow A, Schinella RA, Gordon R. Laminations of the CT diagnosis of acute diverticulitis: comparison of CT, contrast enema and pathologic findings in 16 patients. AJR. 1990;154: 281.

Bartone NF, Grieco RV, Vasilas A. A review of roentgen signs in lesions affecting the cecum. Radiology. 1960;84:285.

Beggs I, Thomas BM. Diagnosis of carcinoma of the colon by barium enema. Clin Radiol. 1983;34:423.

Berenbaum SL, Subbaro J. The hypertrophied ileocecal valve. Am J Dig Dis. 1955;22:307.

Bernstein MA, Feczko PJ, Halpert RD, Simms SM, Ackerman LV. Distribution of colonic polyps: increased incidence of proximal lesions in older patients. Radiology. 1985;155:35.

Boles RS, Hodes PJ. Endometriosis of the small and large intestine. Gastroenterology. 1958;34:367.

Bolin S, Franzen L, Nilsson E, Sjodahl R. Carcinoma of the colon and rectum. Tumors missed by radiological examination in 61 patients. Cancer. 1988; 61:1999.

Bresnihan ER, Simpkins KC. Villous adenoma of the large bowel, benign and malignant. Br J Radiol. 1975;48:801.

Buffo GC, Clair MR, Bonheim P. Diverticulosis of the vermiform appendix. Gastrointest Radiol. 1986; 11:108.

Butch RJ, Wittenberg J, Mueller PR, Simeone JF, Meyer JE, Ferrucci JT Jr. Presacral masses after abdominoperineal resection for colorectal carcinoma: the need for needle biopsy. AJR. 1985;144: 309.

Cahill KM. Amebiasis. NY State J Med. 1963;63: 2247.

Carrera CF, Young S, Lewicki AM. Intestinal tuberculosis. Gastrointest Radiol. 1976;1:147.

Case JT. The roentgen study of colonic diverticula. AJR. 1929;21:207.

Chrispin AR, Fry JK. The presacral space shown by barium enema. Br J Radiol. 1963;36:319.

Collins DC. A study of 50,000 specimens of the human vermiform appendix. Surg Gynecol Obst. 1955;101:437.

Connor R, Jones B, Fischman EK, Siegelman SS. Pneumatosis intestinalis—role of computed to-

mography in diagnosis and management. J Comput Assist Tomogr. 1984;8:269.
Coscina WF, Arger PH, Herlinger H, Levine MS, Coleman BG, Mintz MC. CT diagnosis of villous adenoma. J Comput Assist Tomogr. 1986;10:764.
Crooks DJM, Brown WR. The distribution of intestinal nodular lymphoid hyperplasia in immunoglobulin deficiency. Clin Radiol. 1980;31:701.
Dassel PM. Innocuous filling of the intestinal glands of the colon during barium enema (spiculation) simulating organic disease. Radiology. 1962;84: 877.
Dawson IMP, Cornes JS, Morson BC. Primary malignant lymphoid tumors of the intestinal tract. Br J Surg. 1961;48:80.
Demos TC, Fleisah ME. Coiled-spring sign of the cecum in acute appendicitis. AJR. 1986;146:45.
Dreyfuss JR, Benacerraf B. Saddle cancers of the colon and their progression to annular carcinomas. Radiology. 1978;129:289.
DuBrow PA, Frank PH. Barium evaluation of anal canal in patients with inflammatory bowel disease. AJR. 1983;140:1151.
Dukes CE. The classification of cancer of the rectum. J Path Bact. 1932;35:323.
Ekberg O. Ileocecal abnormalities in appendiceal abscess. Acta Radiol Diagn. 1978;19:343.
Ellerbroeck C, Smith WL. Neonatal small left colon in infant with cystic fibrosis. Ped Radiol. 1986;16: 162.
Feczko PJ, Berenstein MA, Halpert RD, Ackerman LV. Small colonic polyps. A reappraisal of their significance. Radiology. 1984;152:301.
Fedyshin P, Kelvin FM, Rice RP. Nonspecificity of barium enema findings in acute appendicitis. AJR. 1984;99:102.
Feldberg MAM, Hendricks MJ, van Waes PFGM. Role of CT in diagnosis and management of complications of diverticular disease. Gastrointest Radiol. 1985;10:370.
Fiegel LS, Fiegel SJ. Sigmoid volvulus: variations in the roentgen pattern. AJR. 1959;81:683.
Fischer MS. A roentgen sign of gangrenous appendicitis. AJR. 1959;81:639.
Fisk JD, Shulman HM, Greening RR, McDonald GB, Sale GE, Thoma ED. Gastrointestinal radiographic features of human graft-vs-host disease. AJR. 1981;136:329.
Fleischner FG, Bernstein CH. Roentgenanatomical studies of the normal ileocecal valve. Radiology. 1950;54:43.
Fleischner FG, Ming SC, Hanken EM. Revised concepts on diverticular disease of the colon, I: Diverticulosis; emphasis on tissue derangement and its relation to the irritable colon syndrome. Radiology. 1964;83:859.
Forssel G. Studies of the mechanism of movement of the mucous membrane of the digestive tract. AJR. 1923;10:87.
Frank PH, Riddel RH, Fecako PP, Levin B. Radiologic detection of colonic dysplasia (pre-carcinoma) in chronic ulcerative colitis. Gastrointest Radiol. 1978;3:209.
Fraser RD, Pierce CB. The differentiation of diverticulitis and carcinoma of the large bowel. A roentgenologic problem. J Can Assoc Radiol. 1950;1:39.
Frimann-Dahl J. Volvulus of the right colon. Acta Radiol. 1954;41:141.
Gardiner GA, Bird CR. Nonspecific ulcers of the colon resembling annular carcinoma. Radiology. 1980;137:331.
Gedgaudas KR, Maglinte DDT. Aphthous lesions in nodular lymphoma of the colon. South Med J. 1986;79:907.
Gelfand DW. Complications of gastrointestinal radiologic procedures, I: Complications of routine fluoroscopic studies. Gastrointest Radiol. 1980;5: 293.
Gelfand DW, Chen YM, Ott DJ. Detection of colonic polyps on single-contrast barium enema study: emphasis on the elderly. Radiology. 1987;164: 333.
Gianturco C. High-voltage technique in the diagnosis of polypoid growths of the colon. Radiology. 1950;55:27.
Gilbertson VA, Nelms JM. The prevention of invasive cancer of the rectum. Cancer. 1974;34:336.
Gilsanz V. Displacement of the appendix in intussusception. AJR. 1984;142:407.
Ginai AZ. Experimental evaluation of various available contrast agents for use in gastrointestinal tract in case of suspected leakage. Effect on pleura. Br J Radiol. 1986;59:887.
Gomberg JS, Friedman AC, Radecki PD. MRI differentiation of recurrent colo-rectal carcinoma from postoperative fibrosis. Gastrointest Radiol. 1986; 11:361.
Gordon BS, Clayman D. Barium granuloma of the rectum. Gastroenterology. 1957;32:943.
Grayson CE. Enlargement of the ileocecal valve. AJR. 1958;78:823.
Hall PA, Murfitt J, Pollock DJ. Caecal lipomas mimicking colonic angiodysplasia. Br J Radiol. 1985; 58:1213.
Heiken JP, Zuckerman GR, Balfe DM. The hypertrophied anal papilla: recognition on air-contrast barium enema examinations. Radiology. 1984;151: 315.
Heilburn N, Bernstein CB. Difficulties in the roentgen diagnosis of cecal tumors. AJR. 1962;87:693.
Hennild V, Kjaergard, Hensen LK. Radiologic evaluation of the continent (S-pouch) ileal reservoir

with anal anastomosis. Acta Radiol Diagn. 1986; 27:301.

Hillaed AE, Mann FA, Becker JM, Nelson JA. The ileoanal J pouch: radiographic evaluation. Radiology. 1985;155:591.

Himal HS, Wise JD, Cardella C. Localized colonic perforation following renal transplantation. Dis Colon Rectum. 1983;26:461.

Htoo AM. The radiological diagnosis of polyps in the presence of diverticular disease. Br J Radiol. 1979;52:263.

Hughes LE. Complications of diverticular disease: inflammation, obstruction and bleeding. Clin Gastroenterol. 1975;4:147.

Husband JE, Hodson NJ, Parson CA. The use of computed tomography in recurrent rectal tumors. Radiology. 1980;134:677.

Jeffrey RB, Federle MP, Stein SM, Crass RA. Intramural hematoma of the cecum following blunt trauma. J Comput Assist Tomogr. 1982;6:404.

Johnson CD, Carlson HC, Taylor WF, Weiland LP. Barium enemas of carcinoma of the colon: sensitivity of double- and single-contrast studies. AJR. 1983;140:1143.

Johnson CD, Rice RP, Kelvin FM, Foster WL, Williford ME. The radiologic evaluation of gross cecal distention: emphasis on cecal ileus. AJR. 1985;145:1211.

Jones B, Fishman EK, Siegelman SS: Computed tomography and appendiceal abscess: special applicability in the elderly. J Comput Assist Tomogr. 1983;7:434.

Keller CE, Halpert RD, Feczko PJ, Simms SM. Radiologic recognition of colonic diverticula simulating polyps. AJR. 1984;143:93.

Kelvin FM, Maglinte DDT. Colorectal carcinoma: a radiologic and clinical review. Radiology. 1987; 164:1.

Kelvin FM, Max RJ, Norton GA, Oddson TA, Rice RF, Thompson WM, Garbutt JT. Lymphoid follicular pattern of the colon in adults. AJR. 1979; 133:821.

Kenney PJ, Koehler RE, Shackelford GD. The clinical significance of large lymphoid follicles of the colon. Radiology. 1982;142:41.

Kirsh D, Drosd RE. Roentgen change in disease of the appendices epiploicae. AJR. 1959;81:640.

Kyaw MM, Gallagher T, Haines JO. Cloacogenic carcinoma of anorectal junction: a roentgenographic diagnosis. AJR. 1972. 1972;115:384.

Lane N, Fenoglio CM. I Observations on the adenoma as precursor to ordinary large bowel carcinoma. Gastrointest Radiol. 1976;1:111.

Laufer I. The double-contrast enema: myths and misconceptions. Gastrointest Radiol. 1977;1:19.

Laufer I, Smith NW, Mullens JE. The radiological demonstration of colorectal polyps undetected by endoscopy. Gastroenterology. 1976;70:167.

Levine MS, Trenkner SW, Herlinger H, Mishkin JD, Reynolds JC. Coiled-spring sign of appendiceal intussusception. Radiology. 1985;155:41.

Lieberman JM, Haaga JR. Computed tomography of diverticulitis. J Comput Assist Tomogr. 1983;7: 431.

Lynn TE, Dockerty MB, Wangh JMA. A clinicopathologic study of epiploic appendages. Surg Gynecol Obstet. 1956;103:423.

Macrae FA, Tan GK, Williams CB. Towards colonoscopy: a report on the complications of 5000 diagnostic or therapeutic colonoscopies. Gut. 1983; 24:376.

Maglinte DDT, Bush MI, Arnta EV, Bullington GE. Retained barium in the appendix; diagnostic and clinical significance. AJR. 1981;137:529.

Maglinte DDT, Keller KJ, Miller RE, Chernish SM. Colon and rectal carcinoma: spatial distribution and detection. Radiology. 1983;147:669.

Mahboubi S, Schnaufer L. The barium enema examination and rectal manometry in Hirschprung's disease. Radiology. 1979;130:643.

Margulis AR, Jovanovich A. The roentgen diagnosis of submucous lipomas of the colon. AJR. 1960;84: 1114.

Matsuura K, Nakata H, Takeda N, Nakata S, Shimoda Y. Innominate lines of the colon. Radiology. 1977;123:581.

Max RJ, Kelvin FM. Nonspecificity of discrete colonic ulceration on double-contrast barium enema study. AJR. 1980;134:1265.

Megibow AJ, Streiter ML, Balthazar EJ, Bosniak MA. Pseudomembranous colitis—diagnosis by computed tomography. J Comput Assist Tomogr. 1984;8:281.

Meszaros WT. Leiomyosarcoma of the colon. AJR. 1963;89:766.

Meyers MA, Whalen JP. Roentgen significance of the duodenocolic relationships: an anatomic approach. AJR. 1973;117:263.

Miller RE. Detection of colon carcinoma and the barium enema. JAMA. 1974;230:1195.

Miller RE, Lehman G. Polypoid colonic lesions undetected by endoscopy. Radiology. 1978;129:295.

Mindelzun RE, Hicks SM. Adult Hirschprung disease: radiographic findings. Radiology. 1986;160: 623.

Mintz MC, Selzer SE. Oral administration of contrast medium for rectal opacification in pelvic computed tomography. J Comp Tomogr. 1984;8:73.

Moffat RE, Gourley WK. Ileal lymphatic metastases from cecal carcinoma. Radiology. 1980;135:55.

Morgenstern L, Lee ES. Spatial distribution of colonic carcinoma. Arch Surg. 1978;113:1142.

Morson BC. The polyp-cancer sequence in the large bowel. Proc Soc Med. 1974;67:451.

Nagasaki A, Ikeda K, Hayashida Y. Radiologic diagnosis of Hirschprung's disease utilizing rectosphincteric reflex. Ped Radiol. 1984;14:384.

Nielsen VT, Vetner M, Harslov E. Collagenous colitis. Histopathology. 1980;4:83.

Nivatvougs S, Fry DS. How far does the proctosigmoidoscope reach. A prospective study of 1000 patients. N Engl J Med. 1980;303:380.

Norman DA, Morrison EB, Meyers WB. Massive gastrointestinal hemorrhage from diverticulum of the appendix. Dig Dis Sci. 1980;25:145.

O'Connell DJ, Thompson AJ. Lymphoma of the colon: the spectrum of radiologic changes. Gastrointest Radiol. 1978;2:377.

Olson RM, Perenchevich NP, Malcolm AW, Chaffey JT, Wilson RE. Patterns of recurrence following curative resection of adenocarcinoma of the colon and rectum. Cancer. 1980;45:2969.

Ott DJ, Albin DS, Gelfand DW, Meshan I. Predictive value of a diagnosis of colonic polyp on the double-contrast barium enema. Gastrointest Radiol. 1983; 8:75.

Ott DJ, Chen YM, Gelfand DW, Wu WC, Munitz HA. Single-contrast barium enema in the detection of colonic polyps. AJR. 1986;146:993.

Ott DJ, Gelfand DW, Chen YM, Munitz HA. Colonoscopy and the barium enema: a radiologic viewpoint. South Med J. 1985;78:1033.

Ott DJ, Gelfand DW, Wu WC, Munitz HA, Chen YM. How important is radiographic detection of diminutive polyps of the colon? AJR. 1986;146: 875.

Poppel MH, Adler H, Jacobson HG, Stein J, Lawrence LR. Mucous colon. Radiology. 1955;65:50.

Preston DJ, Lennard-Jones JE, Thomas GM. Towards a radiologic definition of idiopathic megacolon. Gastrointest Radiol. 1985;10:167.

Puglisi BS, Kauffman HM, Stewart ET, Dodds WJ, Adams MB, Komorowski RA. Colonic perforation in renal transplant patients. AJR. 1985;145: 555.

Radin RD, Halls JM. Cecal volvulus: a complication of colonoscopy. Gastrointest Radiol. 1986;11:110.

Rao AR, Kagan AR, Chan PM, Gilbert HA, Nussbaum H, Hintz BL. Patterns of recurrence following curative resection done for adenocarcinoma of the rectum and sigmoid colon. Cancer. 1981;48: 1492.

Rex DK, Lehman GA, Lappas JC, Miller RE. Sensitivity of double-contrast barium study for left colon polyps. Radiology. 1986;158:69.

Ribchester JM, Ward A. Solitary diverticulum of transverse colon masquerading as polyp. Br Med J. 1978;2:665.

Rosenberg SA, Diamond HD, Jaslowitz B, Craver LF. Lymphosarcoma: Review of 1269 cases. Medicine (Baltimore). 1961;40:31.

Rosenfield NS, Ablow RC, Markowitz RJ, Di Pietro M, Seashore JH, Toulonkian RJ, Cicchetti DV. Hirschprung disease – accuracy of the barium enema examination. Radiology. 1984;150:393.

Rubin AL, Carroll BA, Snow HD. The harmful effects of aqueous contrast agents on the gastrointestinal tract. Study of mechanisms and means of counteraction. Invest Radiol. 1981;16:50.

Rubin S, Dann DS, Ezekial CH, Vincent J. Retrograde prolapse of the ileocecal valve. AJR. 1962; 87:706.

Sachar DB, Greenstein AJ. Cancer in ulcerative colitis. Good news and bad news. Ann Intern Med. 1981;95:642.

Sasson L. Entrance of barium into intestinal glands during barium enema. JAMA. 1960;173:343.

Sato T, Sakai Y, Sonoyama A, Kawamoto S, Motoomi O, Kajita A, Tanaka H, Nakanishi K, Fujino Y, Fujita M. Radiologic spectrum of rectal carcinoid tumors. Gastrointest Radiol. 1984;9:23.

Schatzki R. The roentgenologic differential diagnosis between cancer and diverticulitis of the colon. Radiology. 1940;34:657.

Schwab FJ, Glick SN, Teplich SK. Reduction of cecal volvulus by multiple barium enemas. Gastrointest Radiol. 1985;10:185.

Siroospour D, Berardi RS. Volvulus of the sigmoid colon: a ten-year study. Dis Colon Rectum. 1976;19: 535.

Sisking BN, Burrell MI, Richter JO, Radin DR. CT appearance of giant sigmoid diverticulum. J Comput Assist Tomogr. 1986;10:534.

Smith THR, Tyler JM. CT demonstration of a giant colonic diverticulum. Gastrointest Radiol. 1987; 12:73.

Stevenson GW, Goodacre R, Jackson R, Ragbeer M, Rowland R. Dysplasia to carcinoma transformation in ulcerative colitis. AJR. 1984;143:108.

Sty JR, Chushid MJ, Babitt DP, Werlin SL: Involvement of the colon in chronic granulomatous disease in childhood. Radiology. 1979;132:618.

Swinton NW, Counts RL. Cancer of the colon and rectum; statistical study with end-results. JAMA. 1956;161:1142.

Taefey SA, Carlson HC. The fluoroscopic barium enema in colonic polyp detection. AJR. 1983;141: 1279.

Taglbjaerg PS, Thaysen EH. Collagenous colitis: an ultrastructural study of a case. Gastroenterology. 1982;82:561.

Templeton AW. Colon sphincters simulating organic disease. Radiology. 1960;75:237.

Thoeni RF, Vencrux AC. The anal canal: distinction

of internal hemorrhoids from small cancers by double-contrast enema examination. Radiology. 1982;145:17.

Thoeni RF, Fell SC, Engelstad B, Sherlock TR. Ileoanal pouches: comparison of CT, scintigraphy and contrast enemas for diagnosing postsurgical complications. AJR. 1990;154:73.

Trollope ML, Lindenauer SM. Diverticulosis of the vermiform appendix. A collective review. Dis Colon Rectum. 1974;17:200.

Wagonfeld JB, Baker AL, Reed JS, Platz CE, Kirsher JB. Acute dilatation of the colon in malignant lymphoma. Gastroenterology. 1976;70:264.

Waneck R, Lachner G, Jantsch H, Kovats E, Schiessel R. Lateral distant view for improved accuracy in locating rectal tumors. AJR. 1984;142:519.

Weber HM. The diagnosis of early intestinal cancer. AJR. 1950;64:929.

Wegener M, Borsch G, Schmidt G. Colorectal adnomas: distribution, incidence of malignant transformation, and rate of recurrence. Dis Colon Rectum. 1986;29:383.

Williams CB, Hunt RH, Loose H, Riddell RH, Sakai Y, Swarbrick ET. Colonoscopy in the management of colon polyps. Br J Surg. 1974;61:673.

Williams I. Innominate grooves in the surface of the mucosa. Radiology. 1965;84:877.

Williams SM, Berk RN, Harned RK. Radiologic features of multinodular lymphoma of the colon. AJR. 1984;143:87.

Wolf BS, Marshak RH. Roentgen features of diffuse lymphosarcoma of the colon. Radiology. 1969;75: 733.

Yousefzadeh DK, Teplich G. Urticaria of the colon. Radiology. 1979;132:315.

Zboralske FF, Bessolo RJ. Metastatic carcinoma of the mesentery and gut. Radiology. 1967;88:302.

Zinkin LD. A critical review of the classifications and staging of colorectal cancer. Dis Colon Rectum. 1983;26:37.

Index